Diet and Immune Function

Diet and Immune Function

Special Issue Editors

Elizabeth A Miles
Philip Calder
Caroline E Childs

MDPI • Basel • Beijing • Wuhan • Barcelona • Belgrade

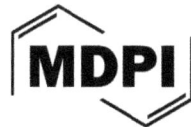

Special Issue Editors
Elizabeth A Miles
University of Southampton
UK

Philip Calder
University of Southampton
UK

Caroline E Childs
University of Southampton
UK

Editorial Office
MDPI
St. Alban-Anlage 66
4052 Basel, Switzerland

This is a reprint of articles from the Special Issue published online in the open access journal *Nutrients* (ISSN 2072-6643) from 2018 to 2019 (available at: https://www.mdpi.com/journal/nutrients/special_issues/diet-immune)

For citation purposes, cite each article independently as indicated on the article page online and as indicated below:

LastName, A.A.; LastName, B.B.; LastName, C.C. Article Title. *Journal Name* **Year**, *Article Number*, Page Range.

ISBN 978-3-03921-612-3 (Pbk)
ISBN 978-3-03921-613-0 (PDF)

© 2020 by the authors. Articles in this book are Open Access and distributed under the Creative Commons Attribution (CC BY) license, which allows users to download, copy and build upon published articles, as long as the author and publisher are properly credited, which ensures maximum dissemination and a wider impact of our publications.

The book as a whole is distributed by MDPI under the terms and conditions of the Creative Commons license CC BY-NC-ND.

Contents

About the Special Issue Editors vii

Diet and Immune Function
Reprinted from: *Nutrients* **2019**, *11*, 1933, doi:10.3390/nu11081933 1

Bethan Dalton, Iain C. Campbell, Raymond Chung, Gerome Breen, Ulrike Schmidt and Hubertus Himmerich
Inflammatory Markers in Anorexia Nervosa: An Exploratory Study
Reprinted from: *Nutrients* **2018**, *10*, 1573, doi:10.3390/nu10111573 10

Paulina Torres-Castro, Mar Abril-Gil, María J. Rodríguez-Lagunas, Margarida Castell, Francisco J. Pérez-Cano and Àngels Franch
TGF-β2, EGF, and FGF21 Growth Factors Present in Breast Milk Promote Mesenteric Lymph Node Lymphocytes Maturation in Suckling Rats
Reprinted from: *Nutrients* **2018**, *10*, 1171, doi:10.3390/nu10091171 26

Lourdes Santiago-López, Adrián Hernández-Mendoza, Verónica Mata-Haro, Belinda Vallejo-Córdoba, Abraham Wall-Medrano, Humberto Astiazarán-García, María del Carmen Estrada-Montoya and Aarón F. González-Córdova
Effect of Milk Fermented with *Lactobacillus fermentum* on the Inflammatory Response in Mice
Reprinted from: *Nutrients* **2018**, *10*, 1039, doi:10.3390/nu10081039 42

Starin McKeen, Wayne Young, Jane Mullaney, Karl Fraser, Warren C. McNabb and Nicole C. Roy
Infant Complementary Feeding of Prebiotics for the Microbiome and Immunity
Reprinted from: *Nutrients* **2019**, *11*, 364, doi:10.3390/nu11020364 55

Francesca Sassi, Cristina Tamone and Patrizia D'Amelio
Vitamin D: Nutrient, Hormone, and Immunomodulator
Reprinted from: *Nutrients* **2018**, *10*, 1656, doi:10.3390/nu10111656 78

Nour Yahfoufi, Nawal Alsadi, Majed Jambi and Chantal Matar
The Immunomodulatory and Anti-Inflammatory Role of Polyphenols
Reprinted from: *Nutrients* **2018**, *10*, 1618, doi:10.3390/nu10111618 92

Ga Young Lee and Sung Nim Han
The Role of Vitamin E in Immunity
Reprinted from: *Nutrients* **2018**, *10*, 1614, doi:10.3390/nu10111614 115

Nina Wærling Hansen and Anette Sams
The Microbiotic Highway to Health— New Perspective on Food Structure, Gut Microbiota, and Host Inflammation
Reprinted from: *Nutrients* **2018**, *10*, 1590, doi:10.3390/nu10111590 133

Vinicius Cruzat, Marcelo Macedo Rogero, Kevin Noel Keane, Rui Curi and Philip Newsholme
Glutamine: Metabolism and Immune Function, Supplementation and Clinical Translation
Reprinted from: *Nutrients* **2018**, *10*, 1564, doi:10.3390/nu10111564 151

Silvia Maggini, Adeline Pierre and Philip C. Calder
Immune Function and Micronutrient Requirements Change over the Life Course
Reprinted from: *Nutrients* **2018**, *10*, 1531, doi:10.3390/nu10101531 . . . . **182**

Joseph C. Avery and Peter R. Hoffmann
Selenium, Selenoproteins, and Immunity
Reprinted from: *Nutrients* **2018**, *10*, 1203, doi:10.3390/nu10091203 . . . . **209**

Julio Plaza-Díaz, Luis Fontana and Angel Gil
Human Milk Oligosaccharides and Immune System Development
Reprinted from: *Nutrients* **2018**, *10*, 1038, doi:10.3390/nu10081038 . . . . **229**

Wiebke Alker and Hajo Haase
Zinc and Sepsis
Reprinted from: *Nutrients* **2018**, *10*, 976, doi:10.3390/nu10080976 . . . . **246**

Mensiena B. G. Kiewiet, Marijke M. Faas and Paul de Vos
Immunomodulatory Protein Hydrolysates and Their Application
Reprinted from: *Nutrients* **2018**, *10*, 904, doi:10.3390/nu10070904 . . . . **263**

Marcelo Macedo Rogero and Philip C. Calder
Obesity, Inflammation, Toll-Like Receptor 4 and Fatty Acids
Reprinted from: *Nutrients* **2018**, *10*, 432, doi:10.3390/nu10040432 . . . . **285**

About the Special Issue Editors

Elizabeth A Miles is Lecturer in Nutritional Immunology at the University of Southampton. She has researched the influences of early nutrition and the maternal diet in pregnancy on offspring health and development. Her early research demonstrated that the neonatal immune responses of babies who subsequently developed allergic symptoms were different from babies who did not. Dr. Miles' research has also showed that the supplementation of healthy humans with omega-3 polyunsaturated fatty acids results in a dose-dependent increase in omega-3 fatty acids in plasma and immune cells and decreases ex vivo immune and inflammatory mediator production. Furthermore, increasing the intake of omega-3 fatty acids in pregnancy in families with an increased risk of allergic disease results in a decrease in ex vivo production of mediators involved in the allergic response. Dr Miles has published over 76 peer-reviewed research papers, 4 book chapters and 17 reviews based on her research interests.

Philip Calder is Professor of Nutritional Immunology at the University of Southampton, UK. He is an internationally recognized researcher on the metabolism and functionality of fatty acids with an emphasis on the roles of omega-3 fatty acids and on the influence of diet and nutrients on the immune and inflammatory responses. His research addresses both life course and translational considerations. He has received many awards and prizes for his work including the prestigious Danone International Prize for Nutrition (2016). Professor Calder was President of the International Society for the Study of Fatty Acids and Lipids (2009–2012), Chair of the Scientific Committee of the European Society for Clinical Nutrition and Metabolism (2012–2016) and President of the Nutrition Society (2016–2019). He will be President of the Federation of European Nutrition Societies (2019–2023). He was previously Editor-in-Chief of the *British Journal of Nutrition* and is currently an Associate Editor of several journals, including *Journal of Nutrition and Clinical Science*.

Caroline E Childs is Lecturer in Nutritional Sciences at the University of Southampton. Her research to date has focused on nutrients such as dietary fatty acids, probiotics and prebiotics and has assessed the effect of nutrient interventions on outcomes such as tissue composition, immune function, inflammatory status, immunosenescence and the gut microbiota. In 2010, she was named as one of the top three young investigators in the category "Lipids and Nutrition" at the International Society for the Study of Fatty Acids and Lipids conference. Dr Childs is Co-Chair of ILSI Europe's Nutrition, Immunity and Inflammation Task Force and a member of the ILSI Europe Expert Group on Determinants of Immune Competence. Dr Childs is a Nutrition Society Ambassador for the University of Southampton and Regional Representative for the Association for Nutrition. She is an editorial board member of *The Journal of Nutrition* and sits on the *Editorial Advisory Board of Nutrition Bulletin*.

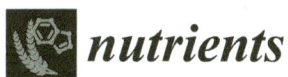

Editorial

Diet and Immune Function

Caroline E. Childs [1], Philip C. Calder [1,2] and Elizabeth A. Miles [1,*]

[1] Human Development and Health, Faculty of Medicine, University of Southampton, Southampton SO16 6YD, UK
[2] NIHR Southampton Biomedical Research Centre, University Hospital Southampton NHS Foundation Trust and University of Southampton, Southampton SO16 6YD, UK
* Correspondence: e.a.miles@soton.ac.uk; Tel.: +44(0)23-8120-6925

Received: 9 August 2019; Accepted: 15 August 2019; Published: 16 August 2019

Abstract: A well-functioning immune system is critical for survival. The immune system must be constantly alert, monitoring for signs of invasion or danger. Cells of the immune system must be able to distinguish self from non-self and furthermore discriminate between non-self molecules which are harmful (e.g., those from pathogens) and innocuous non-self molecules (e.g., from food). This Special Issue of Nutrients explores the relationship between diet and nutrients and immune function. In this preface, we outline the key functions of the immune system, and how it interacts with nutrients across the life course, highlighting the work included within this Special Issue. This includes the role of macronutrients, micronutrients, and the gut microbiome in mediating immunological effects. Nutritional modulation of the immune system has applications within the clinical setting, but can also have a role in healthy populations, acting to reduce or delay the onset of immune-mediated chronic diseases. Ongoing research in this field will ultimately lead to a better understanding of the role of diet and nutrients in immune function and will facilitate the use of bespoke nutrition to improve human health.

Keywords: nutrition; immunity; macronutrients; micronutrients; microbiome; life course; probiotic; prebiotic; inflammation

---

1. Overview of the Immune System

Broadly, cells of the immune system may be divided into those of the innate and those of the adaptive immune response. The innate response is the first response to an invading pathogen. Cells of the innate immune response include phagocytes (e.g., macrophages and monocytes), neutrophils, dendritic cells, mast cells, eosinophils, and others. The innate response is rapid, but not specialised and is generally less effective than the adaptive immune response.

The adaptive immune response has the ability to specifically recognise a pathogen and 'remember' it if exposed to it again. T cells are critical in antigen recognition and the co-ordination of the immune response. T cells are present in an array of subtypes that coordinate different types of immune responses. Broadly, they are divided into the cytotoxic T cells (bearing the CD8 receptor), which are involved in direct killing of infected damaged cells and tumour cells, and the T helper cells. T helper (Th) cells bear the CD4 receptor and are important in coordinating the responses of other immune cells. There are a number of subtypes of Th cells, defined by the cytokines they produce. Initial studies identified two subsets, the Th1 cells, which produced interferon gamma (IFN-γ) and interleukin (IL)-2 and were important in antiviral and cellular immune responses, and the Th2 subset producing IL-4, IL-5, and IL-13 and involved in humoral (antibody) and anti-parasitic responses (but also in allergic responses) [1]. It is now apparent that there are a number of other Th subtypes, which do not fall into these categories. This includes Th17 cells, which produce IL-17A, IL-17F, and IL-22 and are important in fighting extracellular pathogens (bacteria and fungi) [2]. There are also T regulatory cells

(Treg), which are CD4-bearing T cells vital in maintaining immune tolerance to allow the immune system to ignore non-harmful non-self (such as food, pollen, and environmental antigens such as latex). Thus, the role of T cells is coordinating an appropriate immune response following immune stimulation or challenge.

The other lymphocytes of the adaptive immune system are the B cells, which are responsible for antibody or immunoglobulin (Ig) production. Like T cells, B cells respond specifically to an antigen. They can differentiate into short-lived plasma cells, which produce Igs in the short term, or can become long-lived plasma cells. Igs are pathogen-specific molecules, which help the immune system to recognise and destroy pathogens. The B cells can differentiate into plasma cells, which produce one of five classes of Ig (IgM, IgD, IgG, IgA, and IgE). Each class of Ig has a specialised role [3]. IgM is the first Ig expressed during development, is often found as a multimeric molecule (e.g., pentameric), and can bind an antigen to identify it for destruction by immune cells. IgD is found in low concentrations in the plasma and the specialist role of IgD is not yet clear. IgG is the predominant Ig class and can persist for long periods. It has important roles in antigen labelling, resulting in more effective removal. IgA can be found in the serum (mostly as a monomer) and at mucosal surfaces (normally as a dimer). At the mucosal surface, IgA protects against bacteria and or viruses, preventing infection. IgA also has an important role in neutralising food antigens and helping to maintain immune tolerance to food antigens (preventing the development of food allergy) [4]. IgE has a role in clearance of extracellular parasites (e.g., helminths) but when produced inappropriately to innocuous environmental and food antigens, has an important role in IgE-mediated allergy. B cells go through a process called class switching to set the class of Ig that the plasma cells derived from them will produce. B cell class switching is controlled by the cytokines present, particularly IL-4, IL-6, and IFN-γ secreted from Th cells [5].

T and B cells can specialise to become memory cells, which persist permanently or for very long periods and are able to recognise the antigen if encountered again and elicit a rapid, pathogen-specific immune response.

The effective deployment of the immune system against pathogens or harmful signals and the swift resolution of the immune response is required for survival. The fighting of infection is only one piece of the puzzle. A fulminating immune response is costly in terms of energy expended and results in damage to the host tissues; thus, rapid and complete resolution of an immune response is also key. Cytokines play a role in resolution of immune responses. IL-10, which is produced by a range of immune cells including Tregs, has anti-inflammatory actions including suppressing inflammatory cytokine production [6].

The instigation of an immune response and the activities of the immune cells results in inflammation (seen as redness, swelling, and the feeling of heat and pain), which are signs of the damage to the tissue going on whilst the immune system does its work. This is an expected outcome of an effective immune response. Increasingly there is concern that modern lifestyle changes have resulted in the promotion of ongoing, low-grade, whole-body (systemic) inflammation caused by immune and other cells (e.g., adipocytes, the cells that store lipids in fat tissue) [7]. Such exposures may include diet quality and quantity [8].

2. The Role of Nutrition in Immune Function

Adequate and appropriate nutrition is required for all cells to function optimally and this includes the cells in the immune system. An "activated" immune system further increases the demand for energy during periods of infection, with greater basal energy expenditure during fever for example. Thus, optimal nutrition for the best immunological outcomes would be nutrition, which supports the functions of immune cells allowing them to initiate effective responses against pathogens but also to resolve the response rapidly when necessary and to avoid any underlying chronic inflammation. The immune system's demands for energy and nutrients can be met from exogenous sources i.e., the diet, or if dietary sources are inadequate, from endogenous sources such as body stores. Some micronutrients and dietary components have very specific roles in the development and maintenance of an effective immune system throughout the life course or in reducing chronic inflammation. For example, the amino acid arginine is essential for the generation of nitric oxide by macrophages, and the micronutrients vitamin A and zinc regulate cell division and so are essential for a successful proliferative response within the immune system.

Undernutrition is well understood to impair immune function, whether as a result of food shortages or famines in developing countries, or as a result of malnutrition arising from periods of hospitalisation in developed countries. The extent of impairment that results will depend upon the severity of the deficiency, whether there are nutrient interactions to consider, the presence of infection, and the age of the subject [9]. A single nutrient can also exert multiple diverse immunological effects, such as in the case of vitamin E, where it has a role as both antioxidant, inhibitor of protein kinase C activity, and potentially interacting with enzymes and transport proteins [10]. For some micronutrients, excessive intake can also be associated with impaired immune responses. For example, supplementation with iron can increase morbidity and mortality of those in malaria endemic regions. As well as nutrition having the potential to effectively treat immune deficiencies related to poor intake, there is a great deal of research interest in whether specific nutrient interventions can further enhance immune function in sub-clinical situations, and so prevent the onset of infections or chronic inflammatory diseases.

3. Gut-Associated Lymphoid Tissue

The majority of immune cells within the human body are found within the gut-associated lymphoid tissue (GALT), reflecting the importance of this immune tissue in maintaining host health. In ingesting food, we expose ourselves to near constant and massive antigenic stimulation, and our immune system must be able to provide strong and protective immunity against invasive pathogens, while tolerating food proteins and commensal bacteria. In order to achieve this, the GALT contains a variety of sensing and effector immune functions. Dendritic cells and M cells sample the gut content, while plasma B cells within the lamina propria produce IgA, providing protection against pathogenic organisms. Specialised immune regions known as Peyer's patches, rich in immune cells, allow for communication between immune cells resident within the GALT, propagation of signals to the wider systemic immune system, and the recruitment or efflux of immune cells [11].

Within the gut lumen itself, the human gut microbiome will provide antigens and signals with the potential to interact with resident and systemic immune cells. The composition of the gut microbiome changes over the life course, in response to dietary components, and to environmental factors such as antibiotic exposure. Dietary interventions targeted at the gut microbiome include probiotics and prebiotics. Probiotics are defined as "live microorganisms, which, when consumed in adequate amounts, confer a health benefit of the host" [12] while prebiotics, "a substrate that is selectively utilized by host microorganisms conferring a health benefit" [13], tend to be non-digestible oligosaccharides such as fructo-oligosaccharides and galacto-oligosaccharides. Provision of plant-based diets may enhance the diversity of nutrients that reach the gut microbiome, with the indigestibility of plant cell walls enabling peptides and lipids, which may otherwise have been absorbed in the upper digestive tract to reach the microbiome [14]. There may be circumstances in which immune cells of the GALT come into direct contact with nutrients or gut microbiota, such as in the case of reduced epithelial integrity, or 'leaky gut' observed in both acute and chronic gut inflammation [15]. Such changes in gut permeability may be influenced by micronutrient status such as that of vitamin D [16].

A number of nutrients and dietary interventions have demonstrated the capacity to improve measures of gut health or to reduce gut inflammation. Protein hydrolysates have been demonstrated to enhance barrier function and IgA production in animal models, and as a result may have applications for incorporation within hypo-allergenic infant formula and clinical nutrition for those with conditions such as inflammatory bowel disease [17]. Animal models of gut inflammation have identified that providing probiotic bacteria can reduce inflammation, with reductions in proinflammatory Th1 and Th17 cytokines such as IL-17 and IFN-γ, and enhanced production of inflammation resolving cytokine

IL-10 [18]. Prebiotics can also enhance barrier function, in addition to their role as substrates for bacterial metabolism [19]. Santiago-Lopez et al. have investigated the effect of fermented milk on a murine model of inflammatory bowel disease [18] and demonstrated a reduction in serum IL-17 and IFN-γ following fermented milk consumption when compared with the control group.

4. Immune Function Over the Life course

The developing foetus and neonates have an immature immune system, with poor antibody production and a low proliferative response to challenge. *In utero*, the foetus can gain passive protection from its mother via antibodies, which cross the placenta. This is the basis by which infants in the UK are provided with early protection against whooping cough, with mothers offered vaccination in their third trimester, in order to provide passive immunity to their infants until they reach the age of infant vaccinations. While immature, the foetal immune system can produce antibodies, and allergens can reach the developing foetus, and allergen-specific IgE can be detected in cord blood samples [20]. Another signature of the immaturity of the immune system in early life is the susceptibility of neonates to infections, and the associated higher burden of morbidity and mortality.

The development of the immune system in early life will be influenced by both feeding practices and environmental exposures. Breastfeeding provides further passive immunity to the infant, for example via transfer of antibodies and cytokines. Breast milk components can also stimulate maturation of the gut-associated lymphoid tissue, with breast milk known to be rich in bifidogenic oligosaccharides and to contain its own unique microbiota. Human milk oligosaccharides (HMOs) are synthesised from lactose in the mammary gland, and the specific HMO profile will vary between individuals and across contexts and changes over the time course of lactation [21]. These HMOs have been found to confer health benefits to infants by inhibiting the adhesion of microorganisms to the intestinal mucosa, enhancing the production of short-chain fatty acids by bacteria within the microbiome, and inhibiting inflammation [22]. Other immune active components of breast milk are also likely to be involved in immune system maturation, with studies identifying that the growth factors epidermal growth factor, fibroblast growth factor 21, and transforming growth factor-β2 can change lymphocyte phenotypes in new-born rats when provided as supplements by oral gavage [23].

In infancy, diverse environmental factors will impact upon immune system development; identified factors include pet ownership, antibiotic use, and the timing of introduction of foods [24]. The opportunity for introduction of prebiotic oligosaccharides during the introduction of foods has been explored, with the suggestion that this could provide a unique opportunity to influence the developing microbiome and thereby interact with the developing immune system [19]. These early years of life are a critical period in the development of the immune system, particularly for T cell function, with the thymus maturing and reaching its maximum size relative to body weight in infancy [25].

As we move through the life course towards later life, a decline in immune function is observed among older adults. As was the case in infancy, older adults are more susceptible to infections, and have more serious complications as a result than younger people. This declining immune function is known as immunosenescence and reflects deterioration of both the acquired and innate immune systems [26]. Declining T cell function with age arises from thymic involution and decreased thymic output, resulting in fewer naive T cells and more memory cells in the circulation [27]. Ageing is also associated with increased inflammation in the absence of infection and has been found to predict hospitalisation and death [28]. A number of micronutrient deficiencies have been identified as contributors to such declining immunity, and so may provide opportunities for targeted interventions to restore immune function [29].

5. Chronic Systemic Inflammation

Chronic systemic inflammation is a key underlying feature for a range of chronic non-communicable disease conditions such as cardiovascular disease, stroke, and autoimmune disorders such as rheumatoid arthritis. This chronic inflammation is positively correlated with aging and other co-morbidities (e.g., obesity, cardiovascular disease, insulin resistance). Interestingly, in a study in healthy adults, increasing age was found to be a risk factor for chronic systemic inflammation, independent of other risk factors such as body mass index, blood pressure, and blood lipid profiles [30].

The rising worldwide prevalence of obesity in children and adults is of grave concern. Obesity and over nutrition are strongly associated with chronic inflammation, metabolic perturbation, and higher risk for a number of chronic diseases including cardiovascular disease, stroke, type 2 diabetes mellitus, and chronic liver disease. This metabolism-induced inflammation associated with obesity is termed metaflammation, and the Western diet is a known risk factor [31,32]. The Western diet is characterised by a diet high in sugar, trans and saturated fats, but low in complex carbohydrates, fibre, micronutrients, and other bioactive molecules such as polyphenols and omega 3 polyunsaturated fatty acids. The mechanisms by which the Western diet predispose individuals to metaflammation are still under investigation. However, one mechanism which has been reported is the increased uptake of lipopolysaccharide (LPS, a constituent of gram-negative bacterial cells walls), from microbes in the gut because of increased gut leakiness. This LPS is sensed by cells of the innate immune system through toll-like receptor 4 (TLR4). Activation of TLR4 by LPS will induce an inflammatory response by the immune cells. Certain nutrients, notably long-chain omega 3 polyunsaturated fatty acids, can interfere with TLR4 activation and, thus, can ameliorate this inflammatory signal. Rogero et al. describe the relationship between obesity and inflammation and explores the immune pathway for this mechanism and the anti-inflammatory roles of omega 3 fatty acids in this process [33].

Interestingly, in juxtaposition with the review by Rogero et al. on inflammation in obesity, Dalton and colleagues report a study into systemic inflammation in individuals with the serious psychological eating disorder, anorexia nervosa [34]. They show that in a severely undernourished state, there are indications of systemic inflammation with an increased serum concentration of IL-6 when compared with healthy control participants. IL-6 is a classically inflammatory cytokine produced by immune and other cells. Whether this inflammation is the result of the impact of undernutrition or whether the clinical condition is the result of pre-existing inflammation is a matter that remains to be determined. It has been shown that patients with clinical depression have increased systemic inflammation suggesting that inflammation may have a bearing on mental health and wellbeing [35].

In contrast with the Western diet, the Mediterranean diet is rich in vegetables, fruit, nuts, legumes, fish, and 'healthy' dietary fats. The Mediterranean diet is associated with a reduced risk of chronic disease such as cardiovascular disease, cancer, and more recently Alzheimer's disease [36]. A range of bioactive compounds found in fruits and vegetables have been reported to offer one explanation for the protective effect of diets rich in fruits and vegetables (e.g., Mediterranean diet) on the reduction of risk for developing non-communicable diseases attributed to chronic inflammation (e.g., cardiovascular disease). One family of molecules, which are known to have a role in regulation of inflammation are the dietary polyphenols [37]. Yahfoufi et al. explain the mechanisms by which polyphenols can be immunomodulatory and anti-inflammatory and explore the evidence for the role of dietary polyphenols in reducing the risk of cardiovascular disease, some neurological diseases, and cancer [38].

6. Nutrition in the Clinical Setting

In clinical settings, acute inflammation may be a sudden, severe, and overwhelming process. If not controlled, this severe systemic inflammation results in sepsis, culminating in multiple organ failure and death. Sepsis is a major global cause of death killing approximately 6 million people per year and is estimated to be the cause of 30% of neonatal deaths [39]. In this Special Issue of Nutrients, the role of zinc in sepsis is discussed [40]. Zinc is known to be an important micronutrient for the immune system. It has a role as a cofactor with both catalytic and structural roles in many proteins [41]. Even a mild deficiency in zinc has been associated with widespread defects in both the adaptive and innate immune response [42]. During sepsis, zinc homeostasis is profoundly altered with zinc moving from the serum into the liver. Alker and Haase consider this phenomenon and the implications for therapeutic options to improve outcomes in patients presenting with sepsis [40].

Selenium is a trace element that, like zinc, has critical functional, structural, and enzymatic roles, in a range of proteins. Poor selenium status is associated with a higher risk for range of chronic diseases including cancer and cardiovascular disease [43]. In addition to critical roles in many non-immune tissues within the body, selenium is important for optimal immune function. Avery and Hoffman explain the role of selenium in immunobiology and the mechanisms by which selenoproteins regulate immunity. The evidence for the significance of selenium status in infectious diseases including human immunodeficiency virus infection is reviewed [44].

Glutamine is a nonessential amino acid that provides an important energy source for many cell types including those involved in immune responses. It also serves as a precursor for nucleotide synthesis, particularly relevant for rapidly dividing cells such as the immune cells during an immune response. During infection, the rate of glutamine consumption by immune cells is equivalent or greater than that for glucose. Glutamine has roles in the functions of a number of immune cells including neutrophils, macrophages, and lymphocytes [45]. In catabolic conditions (e.g., infection, inflammation, trauma), glutamine is released into the circulation, an essential process controlled by metabolic organs such as the liver, gut, and skeletal muscles. Despite this adaptation, a significant depletion of glutamine is seen in the plasma and tissues in critical illness, which has provided a rationale for the use of in clinical nutrition supplementation of critically ill patients. How glutamine homeostasis is maintained and when and how to utilise glutamine in the clinical setting is explored in a review by Cruzat et al. [45].

The vitamin D receptor (VDR) is a nuclear receptor that can directly affect gene expression [46]. The presence of VDR in the majority of immune cells immediately suggests an important role for this micronutrient in immune cell activities [47]. Furthermore, vitamin D-activating enzyme 1-α-hydroxylase (CYP27B1), which results in the active metabolite 1 α,25-dihydroxyvitamin D_3 (1,25$(OH)_2D_3$), is expressed in many types of immune cells. Ligation of VDR by 1,25$(OH)_2D_3$ can elicit the production of antimicrobial proteins and influence cytokine production by immune cells [47,48]. Sassi, Tamone, and d'Amelio have reviewed the evidence for the role of the nutrient vitamin D in the innate and adaptive immune systems [16].

7. Conclusions

In this Special Issue of Nutrients, the collected works provide a breadth of reviews and research indicating the key influence of nutrients and nutrition on immune responses in health and disease and across the life course. Nutrients may impact directly or indirectly upon immune cells causing changes in their function or may exert effects via changes in the gut microbiome. A better understanding of the role of nutrients in immune function will facilitate the use of bespoke nutrition to improve human health.

Author Contributions: Conceptualization, E.A.M.; writing—original draft preparation, E.A.M. and C.E.C.; writing—review and editing, E.A.M., P.C.C., and C.E.C.

Funding: This article received no external funding.

Acknowledgments: This article received no specific grant from any funding agency, commercial or not-for-profit sectors.

Conflicts of Interest: C.E.C. is member of the ILSI Europe Expert Group on Determinants of Immune Competence and Co-Chair of ILSI Europe's Nutrition, Immunity and Inflammation Task Force. C.E.C. receives research funding from HOST Therabiomics and honoraria to speak at an event organised by Yakult. P.C.C. has research funding from Bayer, has received research study products from Christian Hansen, and acts as a consultant/adviser to BASF, DSM, Cargill, Smartfish and Pfizer. E.A.M. has no conflicts of interest to declare.

References

1. Romagnani, S. T-cell subsets (Th1 versus Th2). *Ann. Allergy Asthma Immunol.* **2000**, *85*, 9–18. [CrossRef]
2. Zhu, J.; Yamane, H.; Paul, W.E. Differentiation of effector CD4 T cell populations. *Annu. Rev. Immunol.* **2010**, *28*, 445–489. [CrossRef] [PubMed]

3. Schroeder, H.W., Jr.; Cavacini, L. Structure and function of immunoglobulins. *J. Allergy Clin. Immunol.* **2010**, *125*, 41–52. [CrossRef]
4. Berin, M.C. Mucosal antibodies in the regulation of tolerance and allergy to foods. *Semin. Immunopathol.* **2012**, *34*, 633–642. [CrossRef] [PubMed]
5. Vazquez, M.I.; Catalan-Dibene, J.; Zlotnik, A. B cells responses and cytokine production are regulated by their immune microenvironment. *Cytokine* **2015**, *74*, 318–326. [CrossRef]
6. Saraiva, M.; O'Garra, A. The regulation of IL-10 production by immune cells. *Nat. Rev. Immunol.* **2010**, *10*, 170–181. [CrossRef] [PubMed]
7. Calder, P.C.; Ahluwalia, N.; Brouns, F.; Buetler, T.; Clement, K.; Cunningham, K.; Esposito, K.; Jonsson, L.S.; Kolb, H.; Lansink, M.; et al. Dietary factors and low-grade inflammation in relation to overweight and obesity. *Br. J. Nutr.* **2011**, *106*, 5–78. [CrossRef]
8. Calder, P.C.; Bosco, N.; Bourdet-Sicard, R.; Capuron, L.; Delzenne, N.; Dore, J.; Franceschi, C.; Lehtinen, M.J.; Recker, T.; Salvioli, S.; et al. Health relevance of the modification of low grade inflammation in ageing (inflammageing) and the role of nutrition. *Ageing Res. Rev.* **2017**, *40*, 95–119. [CrossRef]
9. Calder, P.C.; Jackson, A.A. Undernutrition, infection and immune function. *Nutr. Res. Rev.* **2000**, *13*, 3–29. [CrossRef]
10. Lee, G.Y.; Han, S.N. The Role of Vitamin E in Immunity. *Nutrients* **2018**, *10*, 1614. [CrossRef]
11. Macdonald, T.T.; Monteleone, G. Immunity, inflammation, and allergy in the gut. *Science* **2005**, *307*, 1920–1925. [CrossRef] [PubMed]
12. Hill, C.; Guarner, F.; Reid, G.; Gibson, G.R.; Merenstein, D.J.; Pot, B.; Morelli, L.; Canani, R.B.; Flint, H.J.; Salminen, S.; et al. Expert consensus document. The International Scientific Association for Probiotics and Prebiotics consensus statement on the scope and appropriate use of the term probiotic. *Nat. Rev. Gastroenterol. Hepatol.* **2014**, *11*, 506–514. [CrossRef] [PubMed]
13. Gibson, G.R.; Hutkins, R.; Sanders, M.E.; Prescott, S.L.; Reimer, R.A.; Salminen, S.J.; Scott, K.; Stanton, C.; Swanson, K.S.; Cani, P.D.; et al. Expert consensus document: The International Scientific Association for Probiotics and Prebiotics (ISAPP) consensus statement on the definition and scope of prebiotics. *Nat. Rev. Gastroenterol. Hepatol.* **2017**, *14*, 491–502. [CrossRef] [PubMed]
14. Hansen, N.W.; Sams, A. The Microbiotic Highway to Health-New Perspective on Food Structure, Gut Microbiota, and Host Inflammation. *Nutrients* **2018**, *10*, 1590. [CrossRef] [PubMed]
15. Bischoff, S.C.; Barbara, G.; Buurman, W.; Ockhuizen, T.; Schulzke, J.D.; Serino, M.; Tilg, H.; Watson, A.; Wells, J.M. Intestinal permeability—A new target for disease prevention and therapy. *BMC Gastroenterol.* **2014**, *14*, 189. [CrossRef] [PubMed]
16. Sassi, F.; Tamone, C.; D'Amelio, P. Vitamin D: Nutrient, Hormone, and Immunomodulator. *Nutrients* **2018**, *10*, 1656. [CrossRef] [PubMed]
17. Kiewiet, M.B.G.; Faas, M.M.; de Vos, P. Immunomodulatory Protein Hydrolysates and Their Application. *Nutrients* **2018**, *10*, 904. [CrossRef]
18. Santiago-Lopez, L.; Hernandez-Mendoza, A.; Mata-Haro, V.; Vallejo-Cordoba, B.; Wall-Medrano, A.; Astiazaran-Garcia, H.; Estrada-Montoya, M.D.C.; Gonzalez-Cordova, A.F. Effect of Milk Fermented with Lactobacillus fermentum on the Inflammatory Response in Mice. *Nutrients* **2018**, *10*, 1039. [CrossRef]
19. McKeen, S.; Young, W.; Mullaney, J.; Fraser, K.; McNabb, W.C.; Roy, N.C. Infant Complementary Feeding of Prebiotics for the Microbiome and Immunity. *Nutrients* **2019**, *11*, 364. [CrossRef]
20. Kamemura, N.; Tada, H.; Shimojo, N.; Morita, Y.; Kohno, Y.; Ichioka, T.; Suzuki, K.; Kubota, K.; Hiyoshi, M.; Kido, H. Intrauterine sensitization of allergen-specific IgE analyzed by a highly sensitive new allergen microarray. *J. Allergy Clin. Immunol.* **2012**, *130*, 113–121. [CrossRef]
21. Donovan, S.M.; Comstock, S.S. Human Milk Oligosaccharides Influence Neonatal Mucosal and Systemic Immunity. *Ann. Nutr. Metab.* **2016**, *69*, 42–51. [CrossRef] [PubMed]
22. Plaza-Diaz, J.; Fontana, L.; Gil, A. Human Milk Oligosaccharides and Immune System Development. *Nutrients* **2018**, *10*, 1038. [CrossRef] [PubMed]
23. Torres-Castro, P.; Abril-Gil, M.; Rodriguez-Lagunas, M.J.; Castell, M.; Perez-Cano, F.J.; Franch, A. TGF-beta2, EGF, and FGF21 Growth Factors Present in Breast Milk Promote Mesenteric Lymph Node Lymphocytes Maturation in Suckling Rats. *Nutrients* **2018**, *10*, 1171. [CrossRef] [PubMed]

24. Kim, H.; Sitarik, A.R.; Woodcroft, K.; Johnson, C.C.; Zoratti, E. Birth Mode, Breastfeeding, Pet Exposure, and Antibiotic Use: Associations With the Gut Microbiome and Sensitization in Children. *Curr. Allergy Asthma Rep.* **2019**, *19*, 22. [CrossRef] [PubMed]
25. Kuper, C.F.; van Bilsen, J.; Cnossen, H.; Houben, G.; Garthoff, J.; Wolterbeek, A. Development of immune organs and functioning in humans and test animals: Implications for immune intervention studies. *Reprod. Toxicol.* **2016**, *64*, 180–190. [CrossRef] [PubMed]
26. Crooke, S.N.; Ovsyannikova, I.G.; Poland, G.A.; Kennedy, R.B. Immunosenescence: A systems-level overview of immune cell biology and strategies for improving vaccine responses. *Exp. Gerontol.* **2019**, *124*, 110632. [CrossRef] [PubMed]
27. Berzins, S.P.; Uldrich, A.P.; Sutherland, J.S.; Gill, J.; Miller, J.F.; Godfrey, D.I.; Boyd, R.L. Thymic regeneration: Teaching an old immune system new tricks. *Trends Mol. Med.* **2002**, *8*, 469–476. [CrossRef]
28. Salanitro, A.H.; Ritchie, C.S.; Hovater, M.; Roth, D.L.; Sawyer, P.; Locher, J.L.; Bodner, E.; Brown, C.J.; Allman, R.M. Inflammatory biomarkers as predictors of hospitalization and death in community-dwelling older adults. *Arch. Gerontol. Geriatr.* **2012**, *54*, 387–391. [CrossRef]
29. Maggini, S.; Pierre, A.; Calder, P.C. Immune Function and Micronutrient Requirements Change over the Life Course. *Nutrients* **2018**, *10*, 1531. [CrossRef]
30. Miles, E.A.; Rees, D.; Banerjee, T.; Cazzola, R.; Lewis, S.; Wood, R.; Oates, R.; Tallant, A.; Cestaro, B.; Yaqoob, P.; et al. Age-related increases in circulating inflammatory markers in men are independent of BMI, blood pressure and blood lipid concentrations. *Atherosclerosis* **2008**, *196*, 298–305. [CrossRef]
31. Hotamisligil, G.S. Inflammation, metaflammation and immunometabolic disorders. *Nature* **2017**, *542*, 177–185. [CrossRef] [PubMed]
32. Christ, A.; Latz, E. The Western lifestyle has lasting effects on metaflammation. *Nat. Rev. Immunol.* **2019**, *19*, 267–268. [CrossRef] [PubMed]
33. Rogero, M.M.; Calder, P.C. Obesity, Inflammation, Toll-Like Receptor 4 and Fatty Acids. *Nutrients* **2018**, *10*, 432. [CrossRef] [PubMed]
34. Dalton, B.; Campbell, I.C.; Chung, R.; Breen, G.; Schmidt, U.; Himmerich, H. Inflammatory Markers in Anorexia Nervosa: An Exploratory Study. *Nutrients* **2018**, *10*, 1573. [CrossRef] [PubMed]
35. Dantzer, R.; O'Connor, J.C.; Freund, G.G.; Johnson, R.W.; Kelley, K.W. From inflammation to sickness and depression: When the immune system subjugates the brain. *Nat. Rev. Neurosci.* **2008**, *9*, 46–56. [CrossRef] [PubMed]
36. Dinu, M.; Pagliai, G.; Casini, A.; Sofi, F. Mediterranean diet and multiple health outcomes: An umbrella review of meta-analyses of observational studies and randomised trials. *Eur. J. Clin. Nutr.* **2018**, *72*, 30–43. [CrossRef] [PubMed]
37. Rahman, I.; Biswas, S.K.; Kirkham, P.A. Regulation of inflammation and redox signaling by dietary polyphenols. *Biochem. Pharmacol.* **2006**, *72*, 1439–1452. [CrossRef]
38. Yahfoufi, N.; Alsadi, N.; Jambi, M.; Matar, C. The Immunomodulatory and Anti-Inflammatory Role of Polyphenols. *Nutrients* **2018**, *10*, 1618. [CrossRef]
39. World Health Organization Sepsis. Available online: https://www.who.int/news-room/fact-sheets/detail/sepsis (accessed on 26 July 2019).
40. Alker, W.; Haase, H. Zinc and Sepsis. *Nutrients* **2018**, *10*, 976. [CrossRef]
41. Andreini, C.; Banci, L.; Bertini, I.; Rosato, A. Counting the zinc-proteins encoded in the human genome. *J. Proteome Res.* **2006**, *5*, 196–201. [CrossRef]
42. Ibs, K.H.; Rink, L. Zinc-altered immune function. *J. Nutr.* **2003**, *133*, 1452–1456. [CrossRef] [PubMed]
43. Rayman, M.P. Selenium and human health. *Lancet* **2012**, *379*, 1256–1268. [CrossRef]
44. Avery, J.C.; Hoffmann, P.R. Selenium, Selenoproteins, and Immunity. *Nutrients* **2018**, *10*, 1203. [CrossRef] [PubMed]
45. Cruzat, V.; Macedo Rogero, M.; Noel Keane, K.; Curi, R.; Newsholme, P. Glutamine: Metabolism and Immune Function, Supplementation and Clinical Translation. *Nutrients* **2018**, *10*, 1654. [CrossRef] [PubMed]
46. Haussler, M.R.; Whitfield, G.K.; Haussler, C.A.; Hsieh, J.C.; Thompson, P.D.; Selznick, S.H.; Dominguez, C.E.; Jurutka, P.W. The nuclear vitamin D receptor: Biological and molecular regulatory properties revealed. *J. Bone Miner. Res. Off. J. Am. Soc. Bone Miner. Res.* **1998**, *13*, 325–349. [CrossRef] [PubMed]

47. Baeke, F.; Takiishi, T.; Korf, H.; Gysemans, C.; Mathieu, C. Vitamin D: Modulator of the immune system. *Curr. Opin. Pharmacol.* **2010**, *10*, 482–496. [CrossRef] [PubMed]
48. Wang, T.T.; Nestel, F.P.; Bourdeau, V.; Nagai, Y.; Wang, Q.; Liao, J.; Tavera-Mendoza, L.; Lin, R.; Hanrahan, J.W.; Mader, S.; et al. Cutting edge: 1,25-dihydroxyvitamin D3 is a direct inducer of antimicrobial peptide gene expression. *J. Immunol.* **2004**, *173*, 2909–2912. [CrossRef] [PubMed]

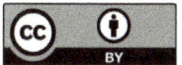

© 2019 by the authors. Licensee MDPI, Basel, Switzerland. This article is an open access article distributed under the terms and conditions of the Creative Commons Attribution (CC BY) license (http://creativecommons.org/licenses/by/4.0/).

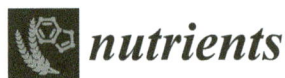

Article

Inflammatory Markers in Anorexia Nervosa: An Exploratory Study

Bethan Dalton [1,*], Iain C. Campbell [1], Raymond Chung [2,3], Gerome Breen [2,3], Ulrike Schmidt [1,4] and Hubertus Himmerich [1,4]

1. Section of Eating Disorders, Department of Psychological Medicine, Institute of Psychiatry, Psychology & Neuroscience, King's College London, London SE5 8AF, UK; iain.campbell@kcl.ac.uk (I.C.C.); ulrike.schmidt@kcl.ac.uk (U.S.); hubertus.himmerich@kcl.ac.uk (H.H.)
2. MRC Social, Genetic, and Developmental Psychiatry Centre, Institute of Psychiatry, Psychology & Neuroscience, King's College London, London SE5 8AF, UK; raymond.chung@kcl.ac.uk (R.C.); gerome.breen@kcl.ac.uk (G.B.)
3. National Institute for Health Research Biomedical Research Centre for Mental Health, Institute of Psychiatry, Psychology & Neuroscience at the Maudsley Hospital and King's College London, London SE5 8AF, UK
4. South London and Maudsley NHS Foundation Trust, Bethlem Royal Hospital, Monks Orchard Road, Beckenham, Kent BR3 3BX, UK
* Correspondence: bethan.l.dalton@kcl.ac.uk; Tel.: +44-0207-848-0183

Received: 28 September 2018; Accepted: 23 October 2018; Published: 24 October 2018

Abstract: Inflammation has been suggested to play a pathophysiological role in anorexia nervosa (AN). In this exploratory cross-sectional study, we measured serum concentrations of 40 inflammatory markers (including cytokines, chemokines, and adhesion molecules) and brain-derived neurotrophic factor (BDNF) in people with AN (n = 27) and healthy controls (HCs) (n = 13). Many of these inflammatory markers had not been previously quantified in people with AN. Eating disorder (ED) and general psychopathology symptoms were assessed. Body mass index (BMI) and body composition data were obtained. Interleukin (IL)-6, IL-15, and vascular cell adhesion molecule (VCAM)-1 concentrations were significantly elevated and concentrations of BDNF, tumor necrosis factor (TNF)-β, and vascular endothelial growth factor (VEGF)-A were significantly lower in AN participants compared to HCs. Age, BMI, and percentage body fat mass were identified as potential confounding variables for several of these inflammatory markers. Of particular interest is that most of the quantified markers were unchanged in people with AN, despite them being severely underweight with evident body fat loss, and having clinically significant ED symptoms and severe depression and anxiety symptoms. Future research should examine the replicability of our findings and consider the effect of additional potential confounding variables, such as smoking and physical activity, on the relationship between AN and inflammation.

Keywords: anorexia nervosa; inflammatory markers; inflammation; cytokines; chemokines; adhesion molecules

1. Introduction

Anorexia nervosa (AN) is a serious psychiatric disorder characterised by low body weight due to food restriction and weight-control behaviours, such as excessive exercise and self-induced vomiting, together with an intense fear of weight gain and disturbed body perception [1]. Altered concentrations of inflammatory markers, in particular cytokines, have been reported in people with AN [2,3]. Cytokines are cell signalling molecules produced by a range of cells (e.g., microglia, astrocytes) in the brain and the periphery (e.g., by macrophages and T-lymphocytes) and are essential in coordinating responses to infection [4]. In addition, changes in the circulating concentrations and production of cytokines have been associated with a range of disease states, including obesity [5] and diabetes [6], as well as depression [7], schizophrenia [8], and eating disorders (EDs) [2,3].

Research in AN has primarily focused on pro-inflammatory cytokines, which promote and up-regulate inflammatory reactions [4]. Recent meta-analyses have concluded that the pro-inflammatory cytokines tumor necrosis factor (TNF)-α and interleukin (IL)-6, are elevated in people with AN, compared to healthy individuals (for reviews see: [2,3]). However, few studies have quantified the concentrations of cytokines in other categories, such as T-helper (T_H)-1, T_H2, and anti-inflammatory cytokines (e.g., IL-10), the latter of which play an immunomodulatory role by reducing inflammation [9]. An example of one such cytokine yet to be measured in people with AN is TNF-β, which is produced by T_H1 cells. TNF-β performs a variety of important roles in immune regulation [10,11], but has also been implicated in the regulation of the commensal gut microbiota [12–14], which appears to be involved in the pathology of AN [15–17]. Additionally, a number of cytokines implicated in other disorders, such as depression and obesity, are yet to be measured in AN. One example is IL-17, a T_H17 cytokine that has been reported to predict treatment response in people with depression [18], and seems to be involved in the pathophysiology of schizophrenia [19] and the molecular and cellular effects of antipsychotics [20].

Chemokines are a subcategory of smaller cytokines known to induce chemotaxis, with some also having a homeostatic function in relation to haematopoiesis, immune surveillance, and adaptive immune system responses [21,22]. The chemokines RANTES, monocyte chemoattractant protein (MCP)-1, and fractalkine have been measured in two studies in people with AN [23,24]. Similarly, adhesion molecules, which mediate the binding of cells in the immune system [25], have been measured in one study in a sample of people with AN [26]. Circulating concentrations of vascular cell adhesion molecule (VCAM)-1 have been reported to be elevated in people with AN compared to healthy participants, but intercellular adhesion molecule (ICAM)-1 did not differ between the groups.

Cytokines and chemokines impact several biological domains implicated in the pathophysiology of AN, including the modulation of neurotransmitter systems, neuroendocrine functioning, and neural plasticity [27–31]. For example, in the depression literature, it has been hypothesised that elevated pro-inflammatory cytokine levels may lead to symptoms of depression, partly via their disruption of growth factor production, e.g., brain-derived neurotropic factor (BDNF) [32] and vascular endothelial growth factor (VEGF)-A [33], which has a subsequent effect on adult neurogenesis [28,34]. Disruption to these biological processes can then lead to alterations in mental state, including affect, learning and memory, and behaviour (e.g., depressive-like behaviours) [28,35].

A number of factors, including body mass index (BMI), age, medication, and smoking status, have been reported to influence cytokine concentrations [36]. These may be potential confounding factors in studies of the role of cytokines in AN, particularly given the low weight seen in AN, the tendency for research in EDs to focus on adolescents and young adults [2], and research indicating that people with EDs report higher rates of smoking than healthy controls [37]. Previous studies have not assessed the potential impact of depression symptoms on cytokine concentrations in AN. A pro-inflammatory profile has been identified in people with depression [38] and the comorbidity between AN and unipolar depression is of significant clinical relevance, as approximately 40% of people receiving treatment for AN also suffer from depression [39]. Therefore, it is unclear as to whether the alterations observed in cytokine concentrations are due to the AN or symptoms of comorbid disorders, such as depression.

Few studies have considered a broad range of cytokines and other markers involved in inflammatory processes and their potential role in the biological profile of AN. Therefore, in this exploratory cross-sectional study, we measured a variety of inflammatory markers in a sample of AN participants and healthy controls (HCs) to determine whether these markers are altered in AN. Several of these inflammatory markers have not been previously quantified in people with AN. A secondary objective was to test for the effects of potential confounders on concentrations of the inflammatory markers, including age and BMI, and explore the effect of current symptom severity on markers of inflammation in people with AN.

2. Materials and Methods

2.1. Participants and Study Design

Between 2010 and 2013, 55 participants with AN (outpatients $n = 27$; day-patients $n = 10$; inpatients $n = 18$) and 30 HCs were recruited as part of the "Relationship between Overactivity, Stress and Anxiety in Anorexia Nervosa" (ROSANA) study [40,41]. Female adults with a primary diagnosis of AN (restricting or binge-eating/purging type) and a BMI < 17.5 kg/m^2 were recruited within the first four weeks of treatment for AN via Specialist Eating Disorder Services in and around London. HCs ($n = 30$) were recruited via an e-mail circular to students and staff at King's College London. Exclusion criteria for HCs were a history of or current mental health disorder, including EDs, and the presence of physical illness, which were assessed in the initial research session using a specially designed record form and the research version of the Structured Clinical Interview for Diagnostic and Statistical Manual of Mental Disorders (DSM)-IV Axis I Disorders [42], described below. All participants provided informed consent before study participation. The study was conducted in accordance with the Declaration of Helsinki and the study received ethical approval from the South East London Research Ethics Committee (REC ref: 09/H0807/4).

2.2. Measures

2.2.1. Demographic Characteristics and Screening

A specially designed record form was used to collect demographic data and additional information relating to the inclusion and exclusion criteria described above, e.g., the presence of medical conditions. To determine smoking status, participants were asked if they smoked and if so, to report the number of cigarettes smoked per day. For AN participants, illness duration (in this case, time since diagnosis) was also recorded. All participants completed the research version of the Structured Clinical Interview for DSM-IV Axis I Disorders [42], a validated structured interview, to confirm diagnosis in the AN participants and identify a history of and/or current mental health problems in the HCs.

2.2.2. Anthropometry

Height and body weight were measured, and from these measurements, BMI (kg/m^2) was calculated. Body composition was also measured using a portable and non-invasive Inbody S10 machine (Inbody Co., Ltd., Seoul, Korea) which uses the Bioelectrical Impedance Analysis (BIA) measurement method. Following the input of height and weight details, this machine provides data on muscle and fat, bone mineral content, intracellular and extracellular water, protein, and minerals. The calculations used to do this are based on the assumption that the body is a cylindrical-shaped conductor. Resistance is low in lean tissue (as it contains the majority of intracellular and extracellular fluid and is thus a good conductor of electrical current), and fat mass is high in resistance as it is does not contain any water (and thus does not conduct electrical current). Based on the assumption that impedance (resistance) is proportional to total body water, predictive equations then determine total body water, total body fat, and lean tissue mass. Given that adipose tissue has been implicated in the genesis of cytokines and produces certain pro-inflammatory cytokines (e.g., IL-6), we focused on the association between inflammatory markers and body fat percentage and did not include other body composition parameters in our analyses.

2.2.3. Eating Disorder Behaviours and General Psychopathology

ED symptoms were assessed using the Eating Disorder Examination-Questionnaire (EDE-Q) [43]. This questionnaire has 36-items assessing ED symptoms and behaviours over the previous 28 days.

A global score can be calculated, and items can also be categorised and scored into the following four subscales: restraint, eating concern, weight concern, and shape concern. Related psychopathology was assessed using the Depression Anxiety Stress Scale 21-Version (DASS-21) [44]. This is a 21-item questionnaire measuring symptoms of general psychopathology over the previous seven days. As well as a total score, a score for the three subscales—depression, anxiety, and stress—can be calculated.

Additional measures related to physical activity were also collected and findings are reported elsewhere [40,41].

2.2.4. Inflammatory Markers

Blood samples were collected, and serum was stored at $-80\ ^{\circ}$C prior to use. Serum was thawed at room temperature and the concentrations of 42 inflammatory markers were quantified simultaneously using multiplex ELISA-based technology provided by the Meso Scale Discovery V-PLEX Human Biomarker 40-Plex Kit and a customised human duplex kit assaying BDNF and interferon (IFN)-α, following the manufacturer's instructions (Meso Scale Diagnostics, LLC., Rockville, MD, USA). Cases and controls were randomised across batches, and plates were scanned on the Mesoscale Scale Discovery MESO Quickplex SQ 120 reader at the MRC SGDP Centre, Institute of Psychiatry, Psychology & Neuroscience, King's College London. The inflammatory markers measured in the 40-plex array were: basic fibroblast growth factor (bFGF), C-reactive protein (CRP), Eotaxin, Eotaxin-3, Fms-like tyrosine kinase (Flt)-1, granulocyte-macrophage colony-stimulating factor (GM-CSF), ICAM-1, IFN-γ, IL-1α, IL-1β, IL-2, IL-4, IL-5, IL-6, IL-7, IL-8, IL-10, IL-12/IL-23p40, IL-12p70, IL-13, IL-15, IL-16, IL-17A, interferon γ-induced protein (IP)-10, MCP-1, MCP-4, macrophage inflammatory protein (MIP)-1α, MIP-1β, placental growth factor (PlGF), serum amyloid A (SAA), thymus and activation-regulated chemokine (TARC), tyrosine kinase (Tie)-2, TNF-α, TNF-β, VCAM-1, VEGF-A, VEGF-C, and VEGF-D. The assay for macrophage-derived chemokine (MDC) was not included in the current panel due to quality control issues.

2.3. Statistical Analysis

Thirty-two AN and 14 HC participants had available blood samples. One HC participant was excluded from the analyses due to having a BMI below 18.5 kg/m^2, i.e., in the underweight range. Five AN participants were excluded from analyses due to reported autoimmune and/or inflammatory diseases. Therefore, the current cross-sectional analyses are based on a sample consisting of 27 participants with a diagnosis of AN and 13 HCs.

Standard curves were used to determine absolute quantities (pg/mL) of each inflammatory marker. All statistical analyses were performed in Stata 15 [45].

2.3.1. Cross-Sectional Comparisons

For demographics and clinical characteristics, group comparisons were assessed using t-tests or Mann-Whitney U-tests depending on the distribution of the data. Log-transformation of inflammatory marker values was conducted due to the presence of outliers and non-normal distributions; however, data remained non-normal for most of the measured molecules. Therefore, Mann-Whitney U-tests were employed to compare concentrations of inflammatory markers between the AN and HC groups. IFN-α was only detected in three samples (two HC and one AN); the results are therefore not presented.

2.3.2. Exploratory Regression Analyses

Absolute quantities of the inflammatory markers (pg/mL) were log-transformed to allow for regression analyses. To identify marker-specific confounders, linear regressions were performed for each log-transformed inflammatory marker (as the dependent variable) with each potential confounding variable (age, BMI, percentage fat mass) separately in the whole sample. To test the effect of illness severity on inflammatory marker concentrations, we performed linear regressions in the AN participants, with the log-transformed inflammatory marker as the dependent variable and illness duration or ED symptoms, as measured by the EDE-Q, as the independent variable. To test the effect of general psychopathology on inflammatory marker concentrations, linear regressions in the AN participants, with the log-transformed inflammatory marker as the dependent variable and the total DASS-21 score as the independent variable, were conducted. For both sets of analyses, studentized residuals greater than ±3 standard deviations were deemed to be outliers and were removed, and assumptions were tested and met.

The level of significance was set at $p < 0.05$, and as this was an exploratory study, levels of significance were not adjusted for multiple testing.

3. Results

Demographic, anthropometric, and clinical characteristics of the AN participants and HCs are presented in Table 1. All participants were female. Mean age did not significantly differ between the AN and HC groups ($U = 144$, $z = -1.36$, $p = 0.1735$). Seven participants with AN reported being a current smoker, with an average of 9.14 ± 5.90 cigarettes smoked per day. As expected, AN participants had lower BMI ($t(38) = 7.88$, $p < 0.001$) and percentage body fat ($U = -22$, $z = 3.63$, $p = 0.0003$) scores, and higher EDE-Q scores (global score: $U = 85.5$, $z = -4.87$, $p < 0.001$) than HCs. The EDE-Q global score for the AN participants was greater than the commonly used clinical cut-off score of 4 e.g., [46,47]. AN participants also reported greater depression, anxiety, and stress than HCs on the DASS-21 (total score: $U = 92.5$, $z = -4.67$, $p < 0.001$). Proposed cut-off scores [44] suggest that the level of severity that AN participants reported was severe for depression, anxiety, and stress.

Table 1. Demographic, anthropometric, and clinical characteristics for AN participants and HCs.

Demographic, Anthropometric, and Clinical Characteristics	Healthy Controls ($n = 13$)	Anorexia Nervosa ($n = 27$)	p Value
Demographics			
Age (years) (mean ± SD)	25.54 ± 4.52	31.48 ± 11.40	0.1735
Current smoker (n)	0 [a]	7	
Anthropometrics			
BMI (kg/m^2) (mean ± SD)	20.88 ± 1.68	15.33 ± 2.25	<0.0010
Body fat (%) (mean ± SD)	17.08 ± 6.05 [b]	7.76 ± 6.07	0.0003
Clinical characteristics			
Duration of diagnosis, years (mean ± SD)		11.64 ± 11.54 [c]	
AN-R/AN-BP (n)		12/15	
Current outpatient/inpatient (n)		16/11	
EDE-Q Global (mean ± SD)	0.66 ± 0.70	4.20 ± 1.27	<0.0010
EDE-Q Restraint (mean ± SD)	0.62 ± 0.88	4.04 ± 1.77	<0.0010
EDE-Q Eating Concern (mean ± SD)	0.26 ± 0.48	3.82 ± 1.28	<0.0010
EDE-Q Weight Concern (mean ± SD)	0.74 ± 0.83	4.13 ± 1.59	<0.0010
EDE-Q Shape Concern (mean ± SD)	1.02 ± 0.85	4.82 ± 1.24	<0.0010
DASS-21 Total (mean ± SD)	13.85 ± 13.89	72.30 ± 33.32	<0.0010
DASS-21 Depression (mean ± SD)	3.54 ± 5.43	24.59 ± 13.73	<0.0010
DASS-21 Anxiety (mean ± SD)	3.08 ± 4.94	19.48 ± 11.84	0.0001
DASS-21 Stress (mean ± SD)	7.23 ± 5.20	28.22 ± 10.69	<0.0010

[a] $n = 6$ missing; [b] $n = 1$ missing; [c] $n = 3$ missing. Abbreviations: HCs—healthy controls; AN—anorexia nervosa; SD—standard deviation; BMI—body mass index; AN-R—anorexia nervosa restricting type; AN-BP—anorexia nervosa binge-eating/purging type; EDE-Q—Eating Disorder Examination—Questionnaire; DASS-21—Depression Anxiety and Stress Scales-21 Version.

3.1. Inflammatory Markers

3.1.1. Cross-Sectional Comparison

The median concentrations (pg/mL) of the quantified inflammatory markers, along with the interquartile range, and minimum and maximum values, for HCs and AN participants are shown in Table 2. Median serum levels of TNF-β ($U = 76$, $z = 2.87$, $p = 0.004$) and VEGF-A ($U = 102$, $z = 2.12$, $p = 0.030$) were lower in AN participants than in HCs. Median concentrations of IL-6 ($U = 92$, $z = -2.41$, $p = 0.016$), IL-15 ($U = 85$, $z = -2.61$, $p = 0.009$), and VCAM-1 ($U = 106$, $z = -2.01$, $p = 0.032$) were found to be higher in AN participants compared to HCs. No other inflammatory parameters were found to differ between groups.

Table 2. Median serum concentrations (pg/mL), with interquartile range (IQR), minimum and maximum values, of inflammatory markers for HCs and AN participants.

Inflammatory Marker	Healthy Controls					Anorexia Nervosa					p Value
	N	Median	IQR	Min	Max	N	Median	IQR	Min	Max	
a. Concentrations significantly lower in AN compared to HCs											
BDNF	13	17,375.24	7862.72	10,526.40	21,884.09	27	12,799.75	5947.87	7792.55	23,003.72	0.0315
TNF-β	13	0.86	0.32	0.43	53.22	27	0.60	0.19	0.16	1.22	0.0041
VEGF-A	13	471.96	220.76	205.98	749.41	27	288.82	155.41	133.70	973.73	0.0338
b. Concentrations significantly higher in AN compared to HCs											
IL-6	13	0.38	0.29	0.10	1.11	27	0.49	0.90	0.20	3.35	0.0159
IL-15	13	2.54	0.39	1.91	3.18	27	2.90	0.81	1.57	5.24	0.0090
VCAM-1	13	612,378.30	92,337.87	402,297.20	739,682.80	27	709,059.60	220,832.10	434,057.50	1,069,997.00	0.0448
c. Concentrations not significantly different between groups											
bFGF	13	11.01	10.73	2.17	21.13	27	12.13	13.39	1.15	65.25	0.3334
CRP	13	332,422.10	1,497,240.00	38,821.00	4,878,443.00	27	342,975.80	5,408,764.00	39,716.48	37,500,000.00	0.9424
Eotaxin	13	208.55	61.81	136.51	285.80	27	175.47	123.38	101.36	511.08	0.8511
Eotaxin-3	13	20.55	6.48	9.95	112.91	27	15.15	14.22	5.14	60.87	0.1058
Flt-1	13	61.83	11.64	27.93	86.21	27	68.69	28.37	11.99	117.06	0.1224
GM-CSF	13	0.15	0.21	0.02	0.88	22	0.19	0.17	0.01	0.35	0.8779
ICAM-1	13	658,988.00	183,427.10	517,283.10	861,717.20	27	701,224.80	244,044.70	415,274.60	977,044.00	0.1224
IFN-γ	13	3.94	1.64	2.11	6.84	27	4.64	5.72	2.11	64.28	0.1448
IL-1α	13	1.13	1.32	0.41	3.51	27	1.01	0.64	0.44	6.00	0.4105
IL-1β	9	0.20	0.33	0.04	1.86	21	0.19	0.19	0.01	4.07	0.7343
IL-2	6	0.12	0.24	0.03	0.43	13	0.15	0.16	0.01	0.85	0.9301
IL-4	13	0.08	0.07	0.01	0.20	25	0.05	0.05	0.00	5.24	0.1481
IL-5	12	1.09	0.87	0.43	3.45	24	1.29	1.01	0.07	4.39	0.7626
IL-7	13	13.66	6.11	8.76	20.13	27	12.58	6.80	5.82	26.20	0.8966
IL-8	13	33.51	62.10	8.44	503.23	27	23.09	92.94	5.80	388.41	0.4271
IL-10	13	0.18	0.10	0.06	0.41	27	0.28	0.26	0.04	4.40	0.3120
IL-12/IL-23p40	13	117.69	49.83	72.15	250.50	27	92.00	50.59	38.72	220.89	0.0806
IL-12p70	11	0.18	0.09	0.01	0.53	25	0.19	0.25	0.01	1.06	0.7572
IL-13	9	2.95	3.25	1.53	10.34	17	2.44	3.13	0.76	6.35	0.2692
IL-16	13	160.52	58.89	99.73	291.95	27	183.59	194.22	127.93	463.24	0.1702

Table 2. Cont.

Inflammatory Marker	Healthy Controls					Anorexia Nervosa					p Value
					c. Concentrations not significantly different between groups						
IL-17A	13	1.78	1.94	0.36	3.85	27	1.91	1.51	0.63	43.83	0.9539
IP-10	13	110.93	57.70	75.89	175.65	27	115.99	108.88	72.71	596.43	0.3191
MCP-1	13	208.55	126.78	140.94	406.88	27	191.53	77.31	121.51	345.28	0.3480
MCP-4	13	142.79	80.25	54.04	212.93	27	120.65	83.26	53.61	290.55	0.6133
MIP-1α	13	25.01	7.73	16.36	56.15	27	23.02	15.10	15.68	66.68	0.8624
MIP-1β	13	102.15	62.83	34.70	280.41	27	81.06	44.32	41.10	271.72	0.3334
PlGF	13	3.38	1.57	1.91	6.06	27	3.85	1.81	1.71	6.21	0.6754
SAA	13	2,683,488.00	1,218,569.00	318,141.50	13,200,000.00	27	2,681,116.00	9,488,702.00	525,220.00	164,000,000.00	0.8061
TARC	13	365.16	319.52	168.47	690.47	27	370.33	378.45	68.69	7680.34	0.7617
Tie-2	13	5847.41	2784.74	4065.41	8455.58	27	6212.88	3028.74	2440.01	10,077.48	0.7617
TNF-α	13	1.59	0.50	0.91	2.70	27	1.64	1.08	0.61	2.95	0.8966
VEGF-C	13	574.92	119.71	242.97	739.49	27	449.26	243.10	277.52	852.72	0.2919
VEGF-D	13	790.06	358.08	383.69	1126.91	27	757.22	413.20	458.68	1906.49	0.8061

Abbreviations: IQR—interquartile range; min—minimum; max—maximum; AN—anorexia nervosa; HC—healthy controls; BDNF—brain-derived neurotrophic factor; TNF—tumor necrosis factor; VEGF—vascular endothelial growth factor; IL—interleukin; VCAM-1—vascular cell adhesion molecule-1; bFGF—basic fibroblast growth factor; CRP—C-reactive protein; Flt-1—Fms-like tyrosine kinase-1; GM-CSF—granulocyte-macrophage colony-stimulating factor; ICAM-1—intercellular adhesion molecule-1; IFN-γ—interferon- γ; IP-10—interferon γ-induced protein-10; MCP—monocyte chemoattractant protein; MIP—macrophage inflammatory protein; PlGF—placental growth factor; SAA—serum amyloid A; TARC—thymus and activation-regulated chemokine; Tie-2—tyrosine kinase-2.

3.1.2. Identification of Marker-Specific Confounding Variables

The full findings of the regressions assessing age, BMI, and percentage fat mass as potential confounders of the serum concentrations of inflammatory markers across all participants are shown in Table S1. Age significantly influenced the serum concentrations of Eotaxin-3 ($F(1, 37) = 5.68$, $p = 0.0224$), IFN-γ ($F(1, 33) = 7.91$, $p = 0.0082$), MCP-1 ($F(1, 38) = 8.87$, $p = 0.0050$), MIP1-α ($F(1, 38) = 4.48$, $p = 0.0408$), SAA ($F(1, 38) = 6.99$, $p = 0.0119$), and TNF-α ($F(1, 38) = 5.07$, $p = 0.0302$). BMI significantly predicted concentrations of IL-4 ($F(1, 34) = 4.73$, $p = 0.0367$), IL-6 ($F(1, 38) = 9.48$, $p = 0.0039$), IL-10 ($F(1, 37) = 6.67$, $p = 0.0139$), IL-12/IL-23p40 ($F(1, 38) = 10.97$, $p = 0.0020$), IL-15 ($F(1, 38) = 9.54$, $p = 0.0037$), TNF-β ($F(1, 35) = 7.45$, $p = 0.0098$), and VEGF-C ($F(1, 37) = 6.17$, $p = 0.0177$). Percentage fat mass significantly influenced IL-6 ($F(1, 38) = 8.83$, $p = 0.0052$), IL-12/IL-23p40 ($F(1, 37) = 10.05$, $p = 0.0031$), TNF-β ($F(1, 35) = 4.93$, $p = 0.0331$), and VEGF-C ($F(1, 38) = 5.00$, $p = 0.0315$). Age, BMI, and percentage fat mass were not found to be associated with concentrations of any of the remaining inflammatory markers.

3.1.3. Effect of Illness Severity

Full results from the regressions determining the effect of illness severity, in relation to illness duration, ED symptoms, and general psychopathology, on serum concentrations of the inflammatory markers in AN participants only are shown in Table S2. Illness duration of AN participants significantly predicted serum concentrations of IL-4 ($F(1, 18) = 15.82$, $p = 0.0009$), IL-12/IL-23p40 ($F(1, 21) = 6.70$, $p = 0.0172$), MCP-1 ($F(1, 21) = 6.40$, $p = 0.0194$), and VEGF-A ($F(1, 22) = 5.55$, $p = 0.0278$). Severity of ED symptoms in AN participants, as measured by the EDE-Q, predicted serum concentrations of IP-10 ($F(1, 23) = 12.60$, $p = 0.0017$) and PlGF ($F(1, 25) = 4.44$, $p = 0.0454$). Level of general psychopathology (symptoms of depression, anxiety, and stress, as measured by the DASS-21) significantly predicted Eotaxin ($F(1, 25) = 4.64$, $p = 0.0410$), IL-7 ($F(1, 25) = 4.60$, $p = 0.0419$), IL-8 ($F(1, 25) = 10.08$, $p = 0.0040$), IP-10 ($F(1, 25) = 6.06$, $p = 0.0211$), MCP-1 ($F(1, 25) = 5.43$, $p = 0.0282$), and TARC ($F(1, 22) = 9.18$, $p = 0.0062$) concentrations. No other inflammatory markers were significantly associated with illness duration or severity of ED and general psychopathology symptoms.

3.2. Brain-Derived Neurotrophic Factor

Median serum levels of BDNF were reduced in AN participants compared to HCs ($U = 101$, $z = 2.15$, $p = 0.0320$). Concentrations of BDNF were significantly influenced by BMI ($F(1, 38) = 13.86$, $p = 0.0007$) and percentage body fat mass ($F(1, 38) = 7.08$, $p = 0.0114$), but not by age, as shown in Table S1. Illness duration, ED symptom severity, and general psychopathology symptoms were not associated with serum concentrations of BDNF (see Table S2).

4. Discussion

4.1. Summary of Findings

We measured a range of markers involved in inflammatory processes, including cytokines, chemokines, acute-phase reactants, and cell adhesion molecules, in people with AN and HCs. Median concentrations of BDNF, IL-6, IL-15, TNF-β, VCAM-1, and VEGF-A were found to differ between AN and HCs, with IL-6, IL-15, and VCAM-1 being elevated in AN, and BDNF, TNF-β, and VEGF-A being reduced, compared to HCs. No other inflammatory markers differed between AN participants and HCs. Our exploratory analyses also identified potential confounding variables of these markers, including age, BMI, and percentage fat mass, which should be considered in future studies. Illness severity, both with respect to ED and general psychopathology symptoms, predicted concentrations of certain inflammatory markers that were not found to differ between AN participants and HCs. Of the markers with significant cross-sectional differences, illness duration predicted serum concentrations of VEGF-A.

4.1.1. Inflammatory Markers

Given that the AN patients in this sample are seriously unwell, as evidenced by their low BMI, the loss of fat mass, and the presence of clinically significant ED and severe depression and anxiety symptoms, the finding that most inflammatory markers ($n = 33$) were unchanged may seem somewhat surprising. However, it has been proposed that the functioning of the immune system is relatively preserved in AN, despite malnutrition [48]. For example, extensive evidence suggests that patients with AN tend to be free from infectious diseases, and rarely have colds and/or flu (at least until very advanced stages of the disease) [48,49], which is in contrast to the heightened risk of infection observed in those with typical malnutrition. A recent in vitro study of immune parameters in people with AN reported that despite reductions in some immune cell populations, AN is also associated with enhanced antioxidant potential and anti-inflammatory status, in comparison to HCs [50]. This may contribute to the preservation of immune system functioning reported in AN. However, it needs to be considered that data derived from in vitro methods may not reflect how cells would respond in vivo. An additional contributing factor could be a relatively sustained/unaffected gut barrier function in AN [51], in spite of the distinct alterations of the gut microbiome and low gut microbiome diversity reported in AN patients [15]. A 'leaky gut' is associated with low-grade inflammation (i.e., leaking of bacteria and/or their components from the gut into circulation is thought to elicit an inflammatory response) [52,53]; therefore, sustained gut permeability will reduce the likelihood of an inflammatory response.

To the best of our knowledge, this is the first time serum concentrations of IL-15, TNF-β, and VEGF-A have been measured and were found to be altered in AN patients. Therefore, we have discussed the potential significance of these findings in more detail.

IL-15, a T cell growth factor, has been suggested to be involved in the modulation of serotonergic transmission [54,55], which may underlie the depressive symptoms and sleep disturbances that are often present in people with AN, and fits with existing evidence of serotonergic alterations in AN [56,57]. Elevations of IL-15 levels have also been reported in patients with schizophrenia [58], which is interesting in light of the possible genetic overlaps between AN and schizophrenia that have been identified in genome-wide association study (GWAS) data [59]. IL-15 has also been implicated in cross-talk between fat and muscle and reported to have an anabolic role, i.e., decreasing fat and increasing muscle mass [60]. It is unclear, therefore, why it is increased in the anorectic group given that they show a severe loss of body fat. It may, for example, be raised as a way of trying to maintain muscle mass in the ill state.

TNF-β (also known as lymphotoxin-α) has several roles in immune regulation [10] and is involved in the regulation of cell survival, proliferation, differentiation, and apoptosis [11]. A TNF-β polymorphism (+252G/A) has been proposed to increase the risk of developing schizophrenia [61]. TNF-β also has a role in maintaining lipid homeostasis, which is potentially important in AN. However, what is perhaps of most interest is that it is involved in regulating intestinal microbiota [12–14], especially as the gut microbiome has been implicated in the pathophysiology of AN e.g., [15].

VEGF-A induces angiogenesis, vasculogenesis, and endothelial cell growth, and also influences vascular permeability, similar to VCAM-1 [62]. Altered levels of VEGF-A have also been found in patients with depression [63] and schizophrenia [64]. Lastly, VEGF-A has been suggested to enhance adult neurogenesis and hippocampus-dependent learning and memory [33], which may be important in both responsivity to illness and in relation to therapy.

Taken together, changes in IL-15, TNF-β, and VEGF-A could potentially contribute to the development of AN symptoms, such as low mood and disturbed sleep, as well as its clinical consequences, such as impaired learning and memory. Furthermore, they provide a link between the biological pathophysiology of AN with depression and schizophrenia, which are clinically- and genetically-related psychiatric disorders. This association may be suggestive of inflammatory markers being indicators of transdiagnostic symptoms, such as low mood, rather than specific psychiatric diagnoses. Also, such a biological association between these disorders could have clinical and therapeutic relevance. For example, we could consider the question as to whether antipsychotics, such as olanzapine, which is approved for the treatment of schizophrenia and alters cytokine production [65], might help patients with AN [31,66]. This may also be of particular interest in AN as olanzapine has been shown to alter the gut microbiome, which could additionally contribute to weight gain [67–70].

The findings of increased IL-6 and VCAM-1 serum concentrations in our sample of people with AN compared to HCs are of less novelty, but indicate the reliability of our findings, as these results have also been reported previously.

As described, there are already a number of studies that have consistently identified an association between AN and the pro-inflammatory cytokine IL-6 [2]. IL-6 is an inducer of the acute-phase response, which has been shown to have suppressive effects on food intake [71] and inhibit adipogenesis [72]. Our results replicated the findings of increased concentrations of IL-6 in people with AN, as compared to HCs.

Víctor et al. [26] previously reported increased VCAM-1 serum levels in patients with AN. VCAM-1 is a cell adhesion molecule with a key role in leukocyte recruitment from blood into tissue and is thus important for cellular immune response [73]. Because of its wide distribution in human tissues and organs, VCAM-1 has been implicated in the development of a variety of pathophysiological states in the brain and in the body periphery, including autoimmune diseases, cardiovascular disease, and infections [74].

It is unclear why these particular inflammatory markers are altered in people with AN compared to HCs. However, there are a number of potential factors which may contribute to these alterations, including stress and neuroendocrine functioning, genetics, the gut microbiota, early life stress, and negative health behaviours (e.g., disturbed sleep, altered diet, smoking) [75].

4.1.2. Brain-Derived Neurotrophic Factor

The reduced serum concentrations of BDNF in AN participants compared to HCs is consistent with previous findings [76]. BDNF is a neurotrophin implicated in both central and peripheral nervous system development. It is well-established that BDNF and cytokines cross-regulate each other. Certain pro-inflammatory cytokines can suppress the expression of BDNF [34] and BDNF-dependent synaptic plasticity [32]. It is thought that the detrimental effect of pro-inflammatory cytokines on neuroplasticity may be mediated by BDNF [34]. Taking together the evidence in AN of elevated pro-inflammatory cytokines [2,3], reduced concentrations of BDNF and VEGF-A [76], and reduced hippocampal volumes [77,78], a key area for adult neurogenesis, it could be hypothesised that this mechanism may be at play in AN, as proposed in the depression literature [34,79]. This hypothesis would be consistent with the high prevalence (approximately 40%) of depression in patients with AN [39].

4.1.3. Marker-Specific Confounding Variables

Our exploratory regression analyses found that BMI significantly predicted BDNF, IL-4, IL-6, IL-10, IL-12/IL-23p40, IL-15, TNF-β, and VEGF-C concentrations. BDNF, IL-6, IL-12/IL-23p40, TNF-β, and VEGF-C were also significantly predicted by percentage fat mass. Previous studies assessing IL-6 in AN have failed to control for BMI in cross-sectional analyses. Therefore, we cannot be certain that the alterations we identified in concentrations of BDNF, IL-6, IL-15, and TNF-β are attributable to AN, rather than simply BMI or percentage fat mass. We also identified age as a significant confounder of Eotaxin-3, IFN-γ, MCP-1, MIP1-α, SAA, and TNF-α. Therefore, studies in larger samples with adequate power should ensure that BMI, and other confounding variables, such as age and percentage fat mass, are incorporated into analyses as covariates to further explore this relationship. Research is also needed to consider the effect of additional potential confounding variables on the relationship between AN and inflammation. Physical activity, for example, may be particularly pertinent in AN patients, given that excessive exercise is often a key feature of the disorder.

4.2. Strengths and Limitations

This study is the first to measure several inflammatory markers in patients with AN, including IL-15 and TNF-β, identifying several alterations in inflammatory markers in AN that warrant future research in larger samples. We also assessed illness severity, in terms of illness duration; ED symptoms, including psychological and anthropometric measures; and associated psychopathology (e.g., depression and anxiety), in our participants. Few previous studies have included such variables [2], which in the current study have allowed us to explore the relationship between illness severity and inflammatory markers. In addition, for the HCs, the median values of a number of the assessed markers are similar to those observed in previous studies, suggesting that our HC group is a valid comparison group.

Several limitations should be noted. The sample is small, which limits the power in this study and due to the exploratory nature, we did not correct for multiple testing, thus increasing the likelihood of receiving a significant result. Additionally, while the AN and HC groups did not differ in mean age, it must be mentioned that the AN group had a larger age range (18–67 years) than the HCs (20–36 years). The AN sample included both inpatients and outpatients; differences between these treatment settings in the opportunity to engage in ED behaviours, such as calorie restriction, self-induced vomiting, and excessive exercise, may effect cytokine concentrations e.g., [80,81]. As BIA measurements of body composition are influenced by fluid and electrolyte status (for which there are known imbalances in AN and these parameters are reported to be particularly affected in early refeeding), the accuracy of BIA measurements of body composition may be limited, particularly in the AN group [82,83]. For practical reasons, it was not possible to ensure blood samples were drawn at a specific time of day and as cytokine production and release is reported to occur in a circadian manner, it is possible that some natural variations may have occurred [84]. As previously described, the inflammatory markers measured in the current study can be affected by a number of pre-analytical factors [36], including age, BMI, smoking, and medication. We did not have data on medication for all participants; however, research has shown that antidepressant and antipsychotic medication can influence cytokine concentrations and production [20,85]. As these medications are prescribed to AN patients to target comorbid features of AN, such as depression and/or to induce weight gain [31], it would be important to identify medication status and incorporate this into analyses as a potential covariate. However, the limited power in this study precludes more complex analyses, such as incorporating several confounding variables or considering the effect of nominal confounders, such as smoking status, on inflammatory markers. Overall, future investigations of inflammatory markers in AN need to ensure that such confounders are assessed and reported, and if possible, accounted for in statistical analyses.

5. Conclusions

This exploratory study measured a broad range of inflammatory markers, many of which had not been previously assessed in AN. IL-15, VEGF-A, and TNF-β, for the first time, were shown to be altered in people with AN in comparison to HCs. Previous findings regarding an elevation of IL-6 and VCAM-1 and a reduction in BDNF in AN participants were replicated. We also considered age, BMI, and percentage fat mass as potential confounding variables of concentrations of the inflammatory markers. Our findings suggest that future research should include covariates in analyses of this relationship to explore whether this may account for some of the group differences in inflammatory markers observed in the current study. Finally, given that these inflammatory markers function as part of a complex network, future studies in larger samples should consider developing a composite score of cytokine concentrations.

Supplementary Materials: The following are available online at http://www.mdpi.com/2072-6643/10/11/1573/s1: Table S1: Findings from the linear regressions of potential confounders—age, BMI, percentage fat mass (independent variable)—on log-transformed values of inflammatory markers (dependent variable) in the whole sample; Table S2: Findings from the linear regressions of illness severity (independent variable) on log-transformed values of inflammatory markers (dependent variable) in AN patients only.

Author Contributions: Conceptualization, G.B., U.S., and H.H.; Data curation, B.D.; Formal analysis, B.D.; Funding acquisition, I.C.C., G.B., U.S., and H.H.; Investigation, B.D., I.C.C., R.C., and U.S.; Methodology, I.C.C., R.C., and U.S.; Project administration, U.S.; Supervision, I.C.C., G.B., U.S., and H.H.; Writing–original draft, B.D.; Writing—review & editing, B.B., I.C.C., R.C., G.B., U.S., and H.H.

Funding: The ROSANA study was supported by an National Institute for Health Research (NIHR) Programme Grant for Applied Research (RP-PG-0606-1043). The current study was funded by a studentship awarded to Bethan Dalton by the Department of Psychological Medicine, King's College London (KCL) and the Institute of Psychiatry, Psychology and Neuroscience (IoPPN), KCL. Iain Campbell, Raymond Chung, Gerome Breen, and Ulrike Schmidt receive salary support from the NIHR Mental Health Biomedical Research Centre at South London and Maudsley NHS Foundation Trust and KCL. Ulrike Schmidt is supported by an NIHR Senior Investigator Award. The views expressed are those of the author(s) and not necessarily those of the NHS, the NIHR, or the Department of Health and Social Care. The APC was funded locally by monies supplied by Hubertus Himmerich.

Acknowledgments: We thank the participants of the ROSANA study and the research team who collected the data between 2009 and 2013.

Conflicts of Interest: The authors declare no conflict of interest.

References

1. American Psychiatric Association. *Diagnostic and Statistical Manual of Mental Disorders*, 5th ed.; American Psychiatric Publishing: Arlington, VA, USA, 2013.
2. Dalton, B.; Bartholdy, S.; Robinson, L.; Solmi, M.; Ibrahim, M.A.A.; Breen, G.; Schmidt, U.; Himmerich, H. A meta-analysis of cytokine concentrations in eating disorders. *J. Psychiatr. Res.* **2018**, *103*, 252–264. [CrossRef] [PubMed]
3. Solmi, M.; Veronese, N.; Favaro, A.; Santonastaso, P.; Manzato, E.; Sergi, G.; Correll, C.U. Inflammatory cytokines and anorexia nervosa: A meta-analysis of cross-sectional and longitudinal studies. *Psychoneuroendocrinology* **2015**, *51*, 237–252. [CrossRef] [PubMed]
4. Dinarello, C.A. Proinflammatory cytokines. *Chest* **2000**, *118*, 503–508. [CrossRef] [PubMed]
5. Schmidt, F.M.; Weschenfelder, J.; Sander, C.; Minkwitz, J.; Thormann, J.; Chittka, T.; Mergl, R.; Kirkby, K.C.; Fasshauer, M.; Stumvoll, M.; et al. Inflammatory cytokines in general and central obesity and modulating effects of physical activity. *PLoS ONE* **2015**, *10*, e0121971. [CrossRef] [PubMed]
6. Xiao, J.; Li, J.; Cai, L.; Chakrabarti, S.; Li, X. Cytokines and diabetes research. *J. Diabetes Res.* **2014**, *2014*, 920613. [CrossRef] [PubMed]
7. Lichtblau, N.; Schmidt, F.M.; Schumann, R.; Kirkby, K.C.; Himmerich, H. Cytokines as biomarkers in depressive disorder: Current standing and prospects. *Int. Rev. Psychiatry* **2013**, *25*, 592–603. [CrossRef] [PubMed]
8. Müller, N.; Weidinger, E.; Leitner, B.; Schwarz, M.J. The role of inflammation in schizophrenia. *Front. Neurosci.* **2015**, *9*, 372. [CrossRef] [PubMed]
9. Opal, S.M.; DePalo, V.A. Anti-inflammatory cytokines. *Chest* **2000**, *117*, 1162–1172. [CrossRef] [PubMed]
10. Ruddle, N.H. Lymphotoxin and TNF: How it all began-a tribute to the travelers. *Cytokine Growth Factor Rev.* **2014**, *25*, 83–89. [CrossRef] [PubMed]
11. Bauer, J.; Namineni, S.; Reisinger, F.; Zoller, J.; Yuan, D.; Heikenwalder, M. Lymphotoxin, NF-κB, and cancer: The dark side of cytokines. *Dig. Dis.* **2012**, *30*, 453–468. [CrossRef] [PubMed]
12. McCarthy, D.D.; Summers-Deluca, L.; Vu, F.; Chiu, S.; Gao, Y.; Gommerman, J.L. The lymphotoxin pathway: Beyond lymph node development. *Immunol. Res.* **2006**, *35*, 41–54. [CrossRef]
13. Upadhyay, V.; Fu, Y.X. Lymphotoxin signalling in immune homeostasis and the control of microorganisms. *Nat. Rev. Immunol.* **2013**, *13*, 270–279. [CrossRef] [PubMed]
14. Kruglov, A.A.; Grivennikov, S.I.; Kuprash, D.V.; Winsauer, C.; Prepens, S.; Seleznik, G.M.; Eberl, G.; Littman, D.R.; Heikenwalder, M.; Tumanov, A.V. Nonredundant function of soluble $LT\alpha_3$ produced by innate lymphoid cells in intestinal homeostasis. *Science* **2013**, *342*, 1243–1246. [CrossRef] [PubMed]
15. Borgo, F.; Riva, A.; Benetti, A.; Casiraghi, M.C.; Bertelli, S.; Garbossa, S.; Anselmetti, S.; Scarone, S.; Pontiroli, A.E.; Morace, G.; et al. Microbiota in anorexia nervosa: The triangle between bacterial species, metabolites and psychological tests. *PLoS ONE* **2017**, *12*, e0179739. [CrossRef] [PubMed]
16. Herpertz-Dahlmann, B.; Seitz, J.; Baines, J. Food matters: How the microbiome and gut-brain interaction might impact the development and course of anorexia nervosa. *Eur. Child Adolesc. Psychiatry* **2017**, *26*, 1031–1041. [CrossRef] [PubMed]

17. Lam, Y.Y.; Maguire, S.; Palacios, T.; Caterson, I.D. Are the gut bacteria telling us to eat or not to eat? Reviewing the role of gut microbiota in the etiology, disease progression and treatment of eating disorders. *Nutrients* **2017**, *9*, E602. [CrossRef] [PubMed]
18. Jha, M.K.; Minhajuddin, A.; Gadad, B.S.; Greer, T.L.; Mayes, T.L.; Trivedi, M.H. Interleukin 17 selectively predicts better outcomes with bupropion-SSRI combination: Novel T cell biomarker for antidepressant medication selection. *Brain Behav. Immun.* **2017**, *66*, 103–110. [CrossRef] [PubMed]
19. Borovcanin, M.; Jovanovic, I.; Radosavljevic, G.; Djukic Dejanovic, S.; Bankovic, D.; Arsenijevic, N.; Lukic, M.L. Elevated serum level of type-2 cytokine and low IL-17 in first episode psychosis and schizophrenia in relapse. *J. Psychiatr. Res.* **2012**, *46*, 1421–1426. [CrossRef] [PubMed]
20. Himmerich, H.; Schonherr, J.; Fulda, S.; Sheldrick, A.J.; Bauer, K.; Sack, U. Impact of antipsychotics on cytokine production in-vitro. *J. Psychiatr. Res.* **2011**, *45*, 1358–1365. [CrossRef] [PubMed]
21. Turner, M.D.; Nedjai, B.; Hurst, T.; Pennington, D.J. Cytokines and chemokines: At the crossroads of cell signalling and inflammatory disease. *Biochim. Biophys. Acta* **2014**, *1843*, 2563–2582. [CrossRef] [PubMed]
22. Borish, L.C.; Steinke, J.W. 2. Cytokines and chemokines. *J. Allergy Clin. Immunol.* **2003**, *111*, S4604–S4675. [CrossRef]
23. Pisetsky, D.S.; Trace, S.E.; Brownley, K.A.; Hamer, R.M.; Zucker, N.L.; Roux-Lombard, P.; Dayer, J.M.; Bulik, C.M. The expression of cytokines and chemokines in the blood of patients with severe weight loss from anorexia nervosa: An exploratory study. *Cytokine* **2014**, *69*, 110–115. [CrossRef] [PubMed]
24. Zhang, S.; Tang, H.; Gong, C.; Liu, J.; Chen, J. Assessment of serum CX3CL1/fractalkine level in Han Chinese girls with anorexia nervosa and its correlation with nutritional status: A preliminary cross-sectional study. *J. Investig. Med.* **2017**, *65*, 333–337. [CrossRef] [PubMed]
25. Murphy, K.; Travers, P.; Walport, M. *Janeway's Immunobiology*, 7th ed.; Garland Science, Taylor & Francis Group: Abingdon, UK, 2009.
26. Víctor, V.M.; Rovira-Llopis, S.; Saiz-Alarcon, V.; Sanguesa, M.C.; Rojo-Bofill, L.; Banuls, C.; de Pablo, C.; Alvarez, A.; Rojo, L.; Rocha, M.; et al. Involvement of leucocyte/endothelial cell interactions in anorexia nervosa. *Eur. J. Clin. Investig.* **2015**, *45*, 670–678. [CrossRef] [PubMed]
27. Jeon, S.W.; Kim, Y.K. Neuroinflammation and cytokine abnormality in major depression: Cause or consequence in that illness? *World J. Psychiatry* **2016**, *6*, 283–293. [CrossRef] [PubMed]
28. Capuron, L.; Miller, A.H. Immune system to brain signaling: Neuropsychopharmacological implications. *Pharmacol. Ther.* **2011**, *130*, 226–238. [CrossRef] [PubMed]
29. Stuart, M.J.; Singhal, G.; Baune, B.T. Systematic review of the neurobiological relevance of chemokines to psychiatric disorders. *Front. Cell. Neurosci.* **2015**, *9*, 357. [CrossRef] [PubMed]
30. Kowalska, I.; Karczewska-Kupczewska, M.; Straczkowski, M. Adipocytokines, gut hormones and growth factors in anorexia nervosa. *Clin. Chim. Acta* **2011**, *412*, 1702–1711. [CrossRef] [PubMed]
31. Himmerich, H.; Treasure, J. Psychopharmacological advances in eating disorders. *Expert Rev. Clin. Pharmacol.* **2018**, *11*, 95–108. [CrossRef] [PubMed]
32. Tong, L.; Prieto, G.A.; Kramár, E.A.; Smith, E.D.; Cribbs, D.H.; Lynch, G.; Cotman, C.W. BDNF-dependent synaptic plasticity is suppressed by IL-1β via p38 MAPK. *J. Neurosci.* **2012**, *32*, 17714–17724. [CrossRef] [PubMed]
33. Licht, T.; Keshet, E. Delineating multiple functions of VEGF-A. in the adult brain. *Cell. Mol. Life Sci.* **2013**, *70*, 1727–1737. [CrossRef] [PubMed]
34. Calabrese, F.; Rossetti, A.C.; Racagni, G.; Gass, P.; Riva, M.A.; Molteni, R. Brain-derived neurotrophic factor: A bridge between inflammation and neuroplasticity. *Front. Cell. Neurosci.* **2014**, *8*, 430. [CrossRef] [PubMed]
35. Donzis, E.J.; Tronson, N.C. Modulation of learning and memory by cytokines: Signaling mechanisms and long term consequences. *Neurobiol. Learn. Mem.* **2014**, *115*, 68–77. [CrossRef] [PubMed]
36. Dugué, B.; Leppanen, E.; Grasbeck, R. Preanalytical factors and the measurement of cytokines in human subjects. *Int. J. Clin. Lab. Res.* **1996**, *26*, 99–105. [CrossRef] [PubMed]
37. Anzengruber, D.; Klump, K.L.; Thornton, L.; Brandt, H.; Crawford, S.; Fichter, M.M.; Halmi, K.A.; Johnson, C.; Kaplan, A.S.; LaVia, M.; et al. Smoking in eating disorders. *Eat. Behav.* **2006**, *7*, 291–299. [CrossRef] [PubMed]
38. Dowlati, Y.; Herrmann, N.; Swardfager, W.; Liu, H.; Sham, L.; Reim, E.K.; Lanctot, K.L. A meta-analysis of cytokines in major depression. *Biol. Psychiatry* **2010**, *67*, 446–457. [CrossRef] [PubMed]

39. Ulfvebrand, S.; Birgegard, A.; Norring, C.; Hogdahl, L.; von Hausswolff-Juhlin, Y. Psychiatric comorbidity in women and men with eating disorders results from a large clinical database. *Psychiatry Res.* **2015**, *230*, 294–299. [CrossRef] [PubMed]
40. Keyes, A.; Woerwag-Mehta, S.; Bartholdy, S.; Koskina, A.; Middleton, B.; Connan, F.; Webster, P.; Schmidt, U.; Campbell, I.C. Physical activity and the drive to exercise in anorexia nervosa. *Int. J. Eat. Disord.* **2015**, *48*, 46–54. [CrossRef] [PubMed]
41. Schmidt, U.; Sharpe, H.; Bartholdy, S.; Bonin, E.M.; Davies, H.; Easter, A.; Goddard, E.; Hibbs, R.; House, J.; Keyes, A.; et al. Treatment of anorexia nervosa: A multimethod investigation translating experimental neuroscience into clinical practice. In *Programme Grants for Applied Research*; NIHR Journals Library: Southampton, UK, 2017.
42. First, M.B.; Gibbon, M.; Spitzer, R.L.; Williams, J.B.W. *User's Guide for the Structured Clinical Interview for DSM-IV Axis I Disorders—Research Version*; Biometrics Research Department, New York State Psychiatric Institute: New York, NY, USA, 1996.
43. Fairburn, C. *Appendix: Eating Disorder Examination Questionnaire (EDE-Q. Version 6.0) In Cognitive Behaviour Therapy and Eating Disorders*; Guilford Press: New York, NY, USA, 2008.
44. Lovibond, S.; Lovibond, P. *Manual for the Depression Anxiety Stress Scales*, 2nd ed.; Psychology Foundation: Sydney, Australia, 1995.
45. StataCorp. *Stata Statistical Software: Release 15*; StataCorp LLC: College Station, TX, USA, 2017.
46. Luce, K.H.; Crowther, J.H.; Pole, M. Eating Disorder Examination Questionnaire (EDE-Q): Norms for undergraduate women. *Int. J. Eat. Disord.* **2008**, *41*, 273–276. [CrossRef] [PubMed]
47. Mond, J.M.; Hay, P.J.; Rodgers, B.; Owen, C. Eating Disorder Examination Questionnaire (EDE-Q): Norms for young adult women. *Behav. Res. Ther.* **2006**, *44*, 53–62. [CrossRef] [PubMed]
48. Marcos, A. The immune system in eating disorders: An overview. *Nutrition* **1997**, *13*, 853–862. [CrossRef]
49. Slotwinska, S.M.; Slotwinski, R. Immune disorders in anorexia. *Cent. Eur. J. Immunol.* **2017**, *42*, 294–300. [CrossRef] [PubMed]
50. Omodei, D.; Pucino, V.; Labruna, G.; Procaccini, C.; Galgani, M.; Perna, F.; Pirozzi, D.; De Caprio, C.; Marone, G.; Fontana, L.; et al. Immune-metabolic profiling of anorexic patients reveals an anti-oxidant and anti-inflammatory phenotype. *Metabolism* **2015**, *64*, 396–405. [CrossRef] [PubMed]
51. Mörkl, S.; Lackner, S.; Meinitzer, A.; Mangge, H.; Lehofer, M.; Halwachs, B.; Gorkiewicz, G.; Kashofer, K.; Painold, A.; Holl, A.K.; et al. Gut microbiota, dietary intakes and intestinal permeability reflected by serum zonulin in women. *Eur. J. Nutr.* **2018**. [CrossRef] [PubMed]
52. Alam, R.; Abdolmaleky, H.M.; Zhou, J.R. Microbiome, inflammation, epigenetic alterations, and mental diseases. *Am. J. Med. Genet. B Neuropsychiatr. Genet.* **2017**, *174*, 651–660. [CrossRef] [PubMed]
53. Żak-Gołąb, A.; Kocelak, P.; Aptekorz, M.; Zientara, M.; Juszczyk, L.; Martirosian, G.; Chudek, J.; Olszanecka-Glinianowicz, M. Gut microbiota, microinflammation, metabolic profile, and zonulin concentration in obese and normal weight subjects. *Int. J. Endocrinol.* **2013**, *2013*, 674106. [CrossRef] [PubMed]
54. Pan, W.; Wu, X.; He, Y.; Hsuchou, H.; Huang, E.Y.; Mishra, P.K.; Kastin, A.J. Brain interleukin-15 in neuroinflammation and behavior. *Neurosci. Biobehav. Rev.* **2013**, *37*, 184–192. [CrossRef] [PubMed]
55. Wu, X.; Hsuchou, H.; Kastin, A.J.; He, Y.; Khan, R.S.; Stone, K.P.; Cash, M.S.; Pan, W. Interleukin-15 affects serotonin system and exerts antidepressive effects through IL15Rα receptor. *Psychoneuroendocrinology* **2011**, *36*, 266–278. [CrossRef] [PubMed]
56. Gauthier, C.; Hassler, C.; Mattar, L.; Launay, J.M.; Callebert, J.; Steiger, H.; Melchior, J.C.; Falissard, B.; Berthoz, S.; Mourier-Soleillant, V.; et al. Symptoms of depression and anxiety in anorexia nervosa: Links with plasma tryptophan and serotonin metabolism. *Psychoneuroendocrinology* **2014**, *39*, 170–178. [CrossRef] [PubMed]
57. Kaye, W.H.; Frank, G.K.; Bailer, U.F.; Henry, S.E.; Meltzer, C.C.; Price, J.C.; Mathis, C.A.; Wagner, A. Serotonin alterations in anorexia and bulimia nervosa: New insights from imaging studies. *Physiol. Behav.* **2005**, *85*, 73–81. [CrossRef] [PubMed]
58. de Witte, L.; Tomasik, J.; Schwarz, E.; Guest, P.C.; Rahmoune, H.; Kahn, R.S.; Bahn, S. Cytokine alterations in first-episode schizophrenia patients before and after antipsychotic treatment. *Schizophr. Res.* **2014**, *154*, 23–29. [CrossRef] [PubMed]

59. Bulik-Sullivan, B.; Finucane, H.K.; Anttila, V.; Gusev, A.; Day, F.R.; Loh, P.R.; Duncan, L.; Perry, J.R.; Patterson, N.; Robinson, E.B.; et al. An atlas of genetic correlations across human diseases and traits. *Nat. Genet.* **2015**, *47*, 1236–1241. [CrossRef] [PubMed]
60. Pedersen, B.K. Muscles and their myokines. *J. Exp. Biol.* **2011**, *214*, 337–346. [CrossRef] [PubMed]
61. Kadasah, S.; Arfin, M.; Rizvi, S.; Al-Asmari, M.; Al-Asmari, A. Tumor necrosis factor-α and -β genetic polymorphisms as a risk factor in Saudi patients with schizophrenia. *Neuropsychiatr. Dis. Treat.* **2017**, *13*, 1081–1088. [CrossRef] [PubMed]
62. Ferrara, N. Vascular endothelial growth factor: Basic science and clinical progress. *Endocr. Rev.* **2004**, *25*, 581–611. [CrossRef] [PubMed]
63. Sharma, A.N.; da Costa e Silva, B.F.; Soares, J.C.; Carvalho, A.F.; Quevedo, J. Role of trophic factors GDNF, IGF-1 and VEGF in major depressive disorder: A comprehensive review of human studies. *J. Affect. Disord.* **2016**, *197*, 9–20. [CrossRef] [PubMed]
64. Frydecka, D.; Krzystek-Korpacka, M.; Lubeiro, A.; Stramecki, F.; Stanczykiewicz, B.; Beszlej, J.A.; Piotrowski, P.; Kotowicz, K.; Szewczuk-Boguslawska, M.; Pawlak-Adamska, E.; et al. Profiling inflammatory signatures of schizophrenia: A cross-sectional and meta-analysis study. *Brain Behav. Immun.* **2018**, *71*, 28–36. [CrossRef] [PubMed]
65. Kluge, M.; Schuld, A.; Schacht, A.; Himmerich, H.; Dalal, M.A.; Wehmeier, P.M.; Hinze-Selch, D.; Kraus, T.; Dittmann, R.W.; Pollmacher, T. Effects of clozapine and olanzapine on cytokine systems are closely linked to weight gain and drug-induced fever. *Psychoneuroendocrinology* **2009**, *34*, 118–128. [CrossRef] [PubMed]
66. Himmerich, H.; Au, K.; Dornik, J.; Bentley, J.; Schmidt, U.; Treasure, J. Olanzapine treatment for patients with anorexia nervosa. *Can. J. Psychiatry* **2017**, *62*, 506–507. [CrossRef] [PubMed]
67. Davey, K.J.; Cotter, P.D.; O'Sullivan, O.; Crispie, F.; Dinan, T.G.; Cryan, J.F.; O'Mahony, S.M. Antipsychotics and the gut microbiome: Olanzapine-induced metabolic dysfunction is attenuated by antibiotic administration in the rat. *Transl. Psychiatry* **2013**, *3*, e309. [CrossRef] [PubMed]
68. Davey, K.J.; O'Mahony, S.M.; Schellekens, H.; O'Sullivan, O.; Bienenstock, J.; Cotter, P.D.; Dinan, T.G.; Cryan, J.F. Gender-dependent consequences of chronic olanzapine in the rat: Effects on body weight, inflammatory, metabolic and microbiota parameters. *Psychopharmacology* **2012**, *221*, 155–169. [CrossRef] [PubMed]
69. Flowers, S.A.; Evans, S.J.; Ward, K.M.; McInnis, M.G.; Ellingrod, V.L. Interaction between atypical antipsychotics and the gut microbiome in a bipolar disease cohort. *Pharmacotherapy* **2017**, *37*, 261–267. [CrossRef] [PubMed]
70. Morgan, A.P.; Crowley, J.J.; Nonneman, R.J.; Quackenbush, C.R.; Miller, C.N.; Ryan, A.K.; Bogue, M.A.; Paredes, S.H.; Yourstone, S.; Carroll, I.M.; et al. The antipsychotic Olanzapine interacts with the gut microbiome to cause weight gain in mouse. *PLoS ONE* **2014**, *9*, e115225. [CrossRef] [PubMed]
71. Wong, S.; Pinkney, J. Role of cytokines in regulating feeding behaviour. *Curr. Drug Targets* **2004**, *5*, 251–263. [CrossRef] [PubMed]
72. Ohsumi, J.; Sakakibara, S.; Yamaguchi, J.; Miyadai, K.; Yoshioka, S.; Fujiwara, T.; Horikoshi, H.; Serizawa, N. Troglitazone prevents the inhibitory effects of inflammatory cytokines on insulin-induced adipocyte differentiation in 3T3-L1 cells. *Endocrinology* **1994**, *135*, 2279–2282. [CrossRef] [PubMed]
73. Wittchen, E.S. Endothelial signaling in paracellular and transcellular leukocyte transmigration. *Front. Biosci.* **2009**, *14*, 2522–2545. [CrossRef]
74. Allavena, R.; Noy, S.; Andrews, M.; Pullen, N. CNS elevation of vascular and not mucosal addressin cell adhesion molecules in patients with multiple sclerosis. *Am. J. Pathol.* **2010**, *176*, 556–562. [CrossRef] [PubMed]
75. Bauer, M.E.; Teixeira, A.L. Inflammation in psychiatric disorders: What comes first? *Ann. N. Y. Acad. Sci.* **2018**. [CrossRef] [PubMed]
76. Brandys, M.K.; Kas, M.J.H.; van Elburg, A.A.; Campbell, I.C.; Adan, R.A.H. A meta-analysis of circulating BDNF concentrations in anorexia nervosa. *World J. Biol. Psychiatry* **2011**, *12*, 444–454. [CrossRef] [PubMed]
77. Burkert, N.T.; Koschutnig, K.; Ebner, F.; Freidl, W. Structural hippocampal alterations, perceived stress, and coping deficiencies in patients with anorexia nervosa. *Int. J. Eat. Disord.* **2015**, *48*, 670–676. [CrossRef] [PubMed]

78. Connan, F.; Murphy, F.; Connor, S.E.; Rich, P.; Murphy, T.; Bara-Carill, N.; Landau, S.; Krljes, S.; Ng, V.; Williams, S.; et al. Hippocampal volume and cognitive function in anorexia nervosa. *Psychiatry Res.* **2006**, *146*, 117–125. [CrossRef] [PubMed]
79. Audet, M.-C.; Anisman, H. Interplay between pro-inflammatory cytokines and growth factors in depressive illnesses. *Front. Cell. Neurosci.* **2013**, *7*, 68. [CrossRef] [PubMed]
80. Canavan, B.; Salem, R.O.; Schurgin, S.; Koutkia, P.; Lipinska, I.; Laposata, M.; Grinspoon, S. Effects of physiological leptin administration on markers of inflammation, platelet activation, and platelet aggregation during caloric deprivation. *J. Clin. Endocrinol. Metab.* **2005**, *90*, 5779–5785. [CrossRef] [PubMed]
81. Raschke, S.; Eckel, J. Adipo-myokines: Two sides of the same coin–mediators of inflammation and mediators of exercise. *Mediat. Inflamm.* **2013**, *2013*, 320724. [CrossRef] [PubMed]
82. Kyle, U.G.; Bosaeus, I.; De Lorenzo, A.D.; Deurenberg, P.; Elia, M.; Manuel Gomez, J.; Lilienthal Heitmann, B.; Kent-Smith, L.; Melchior, J.C.; Pirlich, M.; et al. Bioelectrical impedance analysis-part II: Utilization in clinical practice. *Clin. Nutr.* **2004**, *23*, 1430–1453. [CrossRef] [PubMed]
83. Ackland, T.R.; Lohman, T.G.; Sundgot-Borgen, J.; Maughan, R.J.; Meyer, N.L.; Stewart, A.D.; Muller, W. Current status of body composition assessment in sport: Review and position statement on behalf of the ad hoc research working group on body composition health and performance, under the auspices of the I.O.C. Medical Commission. *Sports Med.* **2012**, *42*, 227–249. [CrossRef] [PubMed]
84. Labrecque, N.; Cermakian, N. Circadian clocks in the immune system. *J. Biol. Rhythms* **2015**, *30*, 277–290. [CrossRef] [PubMed]
85. Munzer, A.; Sack, U.; Mergl, R.; Schonherr, J.; Petersein, C.; Bartsch, S.; Kirkby, K.C.; Bauer, K.; Himmerich, H. Impact of antidepressants on cytokine production of depressed patients in vitro. *Toxins* **2013**, *5*, 2227–2240. [CrossRef] [PubMed]

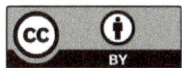

© 2018 by the authors. Licensee MDPI, Basel, Switzerland. This article is an open access article distributed under the terms and conditions of the Creative Commons Attribution (CC BY) license (http://creativecommons.org/licenses/by/4.0/).

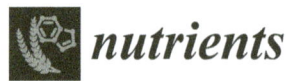

Article

TGF-β2, EGF, and FGF21 Growth Factors Present in Breast Milk Promote Mesenteric Lymph Node Lymphocytes Maturation in Suckling Rats

Paulina Torres-Castro [1,2], Mar Abril-Gil [1,2], María J. Rodríguez-Lagunas [1,2], Margarida Castell [1,2], Francisco J. Pérez-Cano [1,2,*] and Àngels Franch [1,2]

1. Physiology Section, Department of Biochemistry and Physiology, Faculty of Pharmacy and Food Science, University of Barcelona, 08028 Barcelona, Spain; mtorreca29@alumnes.ub.edu (P.T.-C.); mariadelmar.abril@ub.edu (M.A.-G.); mjrodriguez@ub.edu (M.J.R.-L.); margaridacastell@ub.edu (M.C.); angelsfranch@ub.edu (À.F.)
2. Nutrition and Food Safety Research Institute (INSA·UB), 08921 Santa Coloma de Gramenet, Spain
* Correspondence: franciscoperez@ub.edu; Tel.: +34-934-024-505

Received: 6 August 2018; Accepted: 24 August 2018; Published: 27 August 2018

Abstract: Breast milk, due to its large number of nutrients and bioactive factors, contributes to optimal development and immune maturation in early life. In this study, we aimed to assess the influence of some growth factors present in breast milk, such as transforming growth factor-β2 (TGF-β2), epidermal growth factor (EGF), and fibroblast growth factor 21 (FGF21), on the immune response development. Newborn Wistar rats were supplemented daily with TGF-β2, EGF, or FGF21, throughout the suckling period. At day 14 and 21 of life, lymphocytes from mesenteric lymph nodes (MLNs) were isolated, immunophenotyped, and cultured to evaluate their ability to proliferate and release cytokines. The main results demonstrated that supplementation with TGF-β2, EGF, or FGF21 modified the lymphocyte composition in MLNs. At day 14, all supplementations were able to induce a lower percentage of natural killer (NK) cells with the immature phenotype (CD8$^+$), and they reduced the CD8αα/CD8αβ ratio at day 21. Moreover, the cytokine pattern was modified by the three treatments, with a down regulation of interleukin (IL)-13 secretion. These results showed the contribution of these growth factors in the lymphocytes MLNs immune maturation during the neonatal period.

Keywords: growth factors; breast milk; immunonutrition; cytokines; lymphocytes

1. Introduction

At time of birth, the intestine is immature, not only anatomically, but also metabolically and immunologically [1–3]. Intestinal development is a key process in early life because it includes important functions related to growth and survival. It is important to develop mechanisms to digest and absorb nutrients in an efficient way [4]. Moreover, the intestine begins hosting the gut microbiota and establishing appropriate host immune responses against pathogens [2]. The intestinal maturation process can be conditioned through synergy of several factors, such as genetics, microbial colonization, and nutrition [1–3].

Breast milk is the gold standard to feed the newborn because it includes a rich number of components, which are essential for optimal growth and development [5]. It also contains a high number of bioactive factors, which participate in the immune maturation process of infants [2,6]. Among these components, immunoglobulins (Igs), cytokines, and growth factors (GFs) have an important role [7–9]. In this sense, the effects of several GFs present in maternal milk that promote intestinal maturation have been described, although their impact on immune development is still unclear [9].

On the one hand, the transforming growth factor-β (TGF-β) family members have multifunctional actions involved in maintaining intestinal homeostasis, regulating inflammation, and allergy development [10–12]. TGF-βs act on different types of leukocytes, to control the initiation and resolution of immune responses through the recruitment, activation, and survival of cells [12,13]. TGF-β2 is the predominant isoform present in human and rat breast milk; it reaches the neonatal intestine where, at birth, endogenous production is low and increases towards weaning [3,10,12]. In infants, breast milk TGF-βs play an important role in developing immune response and promoting oral tolerance development [12].

On the other hand, one of the most abundant GFs in breast milk is the epidermal growth factor (EGF), the concentration of which is 500 times more than other GFs present in breast milk [14]. Its concentration is very high in colostrum and it decreases significantly during suckling, both in human and rodent milk, suggesting that EGF plays a role in the promotion of early neonatal intestinal growth [2,15]. In fact, EGF is a key intestinal regulator in protecting intestinal barrier integrity, essential for the absorption of nutrients and the exclusion of pathogens, in both humans and animals [14,16,17]. EGF is a polyfacetic molecule, which acts by regulating different processes, such as cell growth, survival, migration, apoptosis, proliferation, and differentiation. In early life, milk EGF seems to be one of the crucial components involved in the prevention of necrotizing enterocolitis (NEC) [1,14].

EGF and TGF-β together with the immunosuppressive interleukin (IL)-10, also present in breast milk, are involved in the functional development of the gastrointestinal mucosa, tolerance acquisition, and inflammation downregulation in damaged intestinal cells [6,7].

In recent years, new components present in breast milk have been discovered. This is the case of the fibroblast growth factor 21 (FGF21), which belongs to the hormone-like subgroup within the FGF superfamily, and has been found in rodent and human milk [16]. The FGF21 present in milk, seems to be involved in local actions in the neonatal intestine. It is a highly active pleiotropic factor, involved in multiple aspects of metabolism through a variety of mechanisms, where it regulates both the expression and activity of digestive enzymes, and the synthesis and release of several intestinal hormone factors [16,18]. All these effects make FGF21 a good candidate to be studied, due to its possible contribution to neonatal intestinal function.

Overall, because TGF-β2, EGF, and FGF21 are biologically active factors found in breast milk and are suggested to be involved in neonatal intestine maturation; our hypothesis is that they could also have an important role in the immune development process in early life. Therefore, the main objective of the current study was to ascertain whether the effect of a daily supplementation with these compounds could promote immune response development, during the suckling period in rats. The effects of the supplementations on mesenteric lymph nodes (MLNs), an inductor site of the gut associated lymphoid tissue (GALT), were studied specifically during and at the end of the suckling period, in terms of lymphocyte phenotypic composition and on the immune functionality, such as their lymphoproliferative and cytokine production abilities.

2. Materials and Methods

2.1. Animals

Pregnant Wistar rats (G15) were obtained from Janvier Labs (Le Genest-Saint-Isle, France), and were individually housed in cages under controlled conditions of temperature and humidity in a 12:12 h light:dark cycle with access to food and water *ad libitum*. The pregnant rats were monitored daily and allowed to deliver naturally. The day after birth was reported as day 1. The studies were performed in accordance with institutional guidelines, for the care and use of laboratory animals, and were approved by the Ethical Committee for Animal Experimentation (CEEA) at the University of Barcelona (UB) and Catalonia Government (CEEA-UB Ref. 220/15, UB/DAAM 8521).

2.2. Dietary Supplementation

The suckling pups were unified in litters of nine pups per mother and were randomized into four groups, formed by three litters each (n = 27 pups/group). This sample size was required for each group, as previous studies have demonstrated the remarkable role of variability among litters [19]. The Appraising Project Office's program, from the Universidad Miguel Hernández de Elche (Alicante) was used for such estimation, to detect statistically significant differences among groups, assuming there was no dropout rate and a type I error of 0.05 (two-sided).

Besides the reference group (REF group), three supplemented groups based on nutritional intervention were created: the transforming growth factor-β2 (TGF-β2), epidermal growth factor (EGF), and the fibroblast growth factor 21 (FGF21). All animals were identified daily, weighed, and supplemented by oral gavage with a volume of 10 mL/kg/day during the suckling period, from day 1 to day 21 of age. The suckling pups were separated from their mothers 30 min before oral administration, to allow gastric emptying. All daily handling was done at the same period of the day, to avoid modifications in biological rhythms. All actions were performed as described in previous studies in the group, References [19,20].

TGF-β2, EGF, and FGF21 groups were supplemented with recombinant human TGF-β2, recombinant rat EGF, and recombinant human FGF21 (all from Peprotech®, Rocky Hill, NJ, USA). The products were reconstituted according to the manufacturer's recommendations.

The dose of TGF-β2 was 35 µg/kg/day, which was based on the amount of TGF-β2 found in the last lactation rat milk (62 ng/mL), and the milk intake by pups within 4–14 days of age [3]. The dose of EGF was 100 µg/kg/day, which had been demonstrated to be effective as a treatment in a rat model of NEC [21]. Finally, the dose of FGF21 was 5 µg/kg/day, an amount that was established in relation to TGF-β2, which has been found in a 1:10 ratio FGF21:TGF-β2 [10,16]. The REF group received a matched volume of the vehicle used for the GFs administration (1% bovine serum albumin (BSA) in phosphate buffer saline (PBS)).

2.3. Measurement of Growth and Development

Body weight was registered daily throughout the study. Two end points were established, at day 14 and at the end of the suckling period at day 21. At these times, prior to sacrifice, the pups were anesthetized with intramuscular ketamine (90 mg/kg; Imalgene®, Merial, Barcelona, Spain) and xylazine hydrochloride (10 mg/kg, Rompun®, Bayer, Barcelona, Spain); and body length (nose-anal) was measured. These data allowed the calculation of morphologic variables, such as the body mass index (BMI, g/cm^2) and Lee index, for assessing obesity in rats (($g^{1/3}$/cm) × 1000).

2.4. Sample Collection and Processing

Once anesthetized, MLNs and small intestine (SI) were obtained through a ventral laparotomy. The SI was weighed, measured, and divided into three equal length portions. Gut washes (GWs) were obtained from the distal SI. Briefly, the intestine was flushed with cold PBS and cut into 5 mm pieces. The tissue was incubated with PBS (10 min, 37 °C, shaking), centrifuged (538 g, 10 min, 4 °C), and later, supernatant was collected and stored at −20 °C until Igs quantification.

2.5. Quantification of Intestinal IgA and IgM by ELISA

The IgA and IgM content were quantified in GWs from day 21 of study, by ELISA Quantitation Set (Bethyl Laboratories, Inc., Montgomery, MD, USA), as previously described in Reference [19]. GWs were diluted at 1:20 (IgA) and 1:10 (IgM). Data were expressed as µg/g of tissue.

2.6. Lymphocyte Isolation from Mesenteric Lymph Nodes

The MLNs were placed in complete culture medium, containing Roswell Park Memorial Institute (RPMI 1640, Sigma-Aldrich, St. Louis, MO, USA) 10% fetal bovine serum (FBS, Sigma-Aldrich, St. Louis,

MO, USA), 1% L-glutamine (Sigma-Aldrich, St. Louis, MO, USA), 1% penicillin streptomicin (PenStrep; Sigma-Aldrich, St. Louis, MO, USA), and 0.05 mM 2-β-mercaptoethanol (Merck, Darmstadt, Germany). MLNs lymphocytes were obtained in sterile conditions by passing the tissue through a cell strainer (40 µm, BD Biosciences, San Diego, CA, USA). The cell suspensions were centrifuged (538 g, 10 min, 4 °C), and the pellet was resuspended with complete RPMI medium. The cell counts and viabilities were determined using an automated cell counter, after staining the cells with trypan blue (Countess™, Invitrogen, Madrid, Spain), following usual laboratory procedures, as described in Reference [22]. The lymphocytes were immediately used to characterize their phenotype, and to determine their ability to proliferate and secrete cytokines.

2.7. Mesenteric Lymph Node Cells Stimulation and Proliferation Assay

MLNs cell activation was performed in sterile conditions, using 96-well tissue culture plates (TPP®, Trasadingen, Switzerland), which were pre-incubated with 200 µL/well of monoclonal antibodies (mAbs) anti-CD3 (10 µg/mL, BD Biosciences, San Diego, CA, USA) and anti-CD28 (2 µg/mL, BD Biosciences, San Diego, CA, USA) (2 h, 37 °C, 5% CO_2). Then, MLNs lymphocyte suspensions (5 × 10^4 cells/mL) were added to each well. A total of eight wells were used for each sample: four pre-incubated with the mitogenic mAbs (stimulated cells, SC) and four without pre-incubation (non-stimulated cells, NSC). The plates were incubated for 48 h, at 37 °C and 5% CO_2. Four hours before the end time of the incubation, 5-bromo-2′-deoxyuridine (BrdU, 20 µL/well, Merck, Darmstadt, Germany) was added to measure its incorporation as an indicator of DNA synthesis in a colorimetric immunoassay.

The plates were centrifuged (210 g, 5 min) and supernatants were collected and stored at −80 °C, until cytokine analysis. After fixation, the anti-BrdU mAbs and peroxidase conjugated anti-BrdU mAbs and 3,3′,5,5′-tetramethylbenzidine (TMB) were added, following the manufacturer's recommendations of the BrdU Cell Proliferation Assay Kit (Merck, Darmstadt, Germany). The absorbance (Abs) was measured at 450 nm (Multiskan MS, Labsystems, Helsinki, Finland). Data were expressed as a proliferation rate as follows: Proliferation rate = (A/B), where, A = ((Abs-SC − Abs-NSC)/Abs-NSC) $_{supplemented\ group}$, and B = ((Abs-SC − Abs-NSC)/Abs-NSC) $_{reference\ group}$.

2.8. Quantification of Cytokine Secretion by Mesenteric Lymph Node Lymphocytes

Supernatants collected after the cell stimulation process described above, were used for the quantification of IL-2, IL-4, IL-10, IL-13, IL-17A, interferon (IFN)-γ, and tumor necrosis factor (TNF)-α concentration using a ProcartaPlex® Multiplex Immunoassay, according to the manufacturer's instructions (eBioscience, San Diego, CA, USA) and as previously described in Reference [19]. Each analyte's concentration was detected using the MAGPIX instrument (Luminex Corp., Austin, TX, USA), in the facilities of the Scientific and Technological Centers of the University of Barcelona (CCiT-UB), and the results were analyzed using xPONENT® 4.2 software (Luminex Corp., Austin, TX, USA). The limits of detection were as follows: 2.10–8600 pg/mL for IL-2; 0.85–3500 pg/mL for IL-4; 14–55,700 pg/mL for IL-10; 3.17–13,000 pg/mL for IL-13; 2.61–2675 pg/mL for IL-17A; 4.35–17,800 pg/mL for IFN-γ; and 3.08–12,600 pg/mL for TNF-α.

2.9. Immunofluorescence Staining and Flow Cytometry Analysis

Lymphocytes from MLNs (5 × 10^4 cells) were immunophenotyped by multiple immunofluorescence staining technique. Mouse anti-rat mAbs conjugated to fluorescein isothiocyanate (FITC), phycoerythrin (PE), peridinin-chlorophyll-a protein (PerCP), allophycocyanin (APC) or APC-cyanine(Cy)7 were used, as in previous studies [19]. For cell subset differentiation, five different mAbs panels were used; Panel 1: TCRαβ/NKR-P1A/CD8α; Panel 2: CD8α/CD8β/TCRγδ; Panel 3: αE integrin/CD62L/CD8α/CD4; Panel 4: CD45RA/TLR4/CD8α/CD4/CD25; and Panel 5: CD25/CD4/Foxp3. With the first panel, NK cells (NKR-P1A$^+$ TCRαβ$^-$), natural killer T (NKT) cells (NKR-P1A$^+$ TCRαβ$^+$), and TCRαβ$^+$ cells (TCRαβ$^+$ NKR-P1A$^-$) could be differentiated, which in combination with the TCRγδ+ cells (obtained from Panel 2) constituted the total of T cells. B cells (CD45RA+) were identified with Panel 4. The mAbs used in this study are detailed in the Supplementary Materials (Table S1).

Briefly, cells were incubated with a mixture of 10 µL of saturating concentrations of each mouse anti-rat mAbs in PBS pH 7.2, containing 2% FBS and 0.1% sodium azide (Merck, Darmstadt, Germany), at 4 °C in darkness for 20 min. For T reg evaluation, an intracellular staining was performed. For that, cells previously labeled with anti-CD4-PE and anti-CD25-FITC mAbs, were fixed/permeabilized using a specific buffer kit (eBioscience, San Diego, CA, USA). Then, intracellular staining with anti-Foxp3-APC mAb was carried out, under the same conditions as extracellular staining. After washing, all stained cells were fixed with 0.5% paraformaldehyde (Panreac, Barcelona, Spain) and stored at 4 °C in darkness, until analysis by flow cytometry. For each sample, a positive control staining using each isotype matched mAbs and a negative control without staining were included. Analyses were performed in a Gallios™ Cytometer (Beckman Coulter, Miami, FL, USA) in the CCiT-UB. Data were assessed by FlowJo® version 10 software (Tree Star Inc., Ashland, Covington, KY, USA). Results were expressed as percentages of positive cells in the lymphocyte population, selected according to their forward- and side-scatter characteristics (FSC/SSC) using previous studies protocols [19], or in a selected population. The gating strategy was specific for each panel used, but overall, markers (e.g., CD8α in Panel 1, αE integrin, and CD62L in Panel 3) were evaluated in specific gate subsets (e.g., NK, NKT, or T cells in Panel 1, and CD8 or CD4 cells in Panel 3).

2.10. Statistical Analysis

Statistical analyses were performed using the IBM Social Sciences Software Program (SPSS, version 22.0, Chicago, IL, USA). Levene's and Shapiro–Wilk tests were applied to assess variance equality and normal distribution, respectively. When the results demonstrated equality of variance and normal distribution, a one-way analysis of variance (ANOVA) test was performed. Nonparametric tests were carried out when normal distribution and equality of variance did not exist. Specifically, Kruskal–Wallis and Mann–Whitney U tests were used to assess significance for independent samples. Significant differences were established at $p < 0.05$. Data in the text, tables, and figures are expressed as the mean ± standard error of the mean (S.E.M).

3. Results

3.1. Animal Growth

Body growth was assessed in the three groups receiving supplementation (TGF-β2, EGF, and FGF21), and compared with those receiving the vehicle (REF). Body weight increased during suckling period in the REF group ($p < 0.05$) and the supplementations did not affect this growth pattern (Supplementary Materials, Figure S1). With respect to morphometric variables and SI growth, there were no differences among the studied groups at any age considered (Table 1).

Table 1. Morphometric variables and small intestinal growth.

		BMI	Lee Index	SI Relative Weight	SI Relative Length
		(g/cm^2)	(($\sqrt[3]{}$g/cm) × 1000)	(%)	(%)
Day 14	REF	0.365 ± 0.009	332.9 ± 3.473	3.51 ± 0.05	118.29 ± 5.49
	TGF-β2	0.373 ± 0.010	336.9 ± 3.844	3.59 ± 0.14	114.34 ± 4.28
	EGF	0.340 ± 0.007	327.0 ± 2.845	3.48 ± 0.06	122.64 ± 2.91
	FGF21	0.371 ± 0.009	337.4 ± 4.044	3.18 ± 0.06	105.59 ± 5.31
Day 21	REF	0.404 ± 0.010 ᵠ	319.5 ± 2.551 ᵠ	4.15 ± 0.24 ᵠ	89.57 ± 3.12 ᵠ
	TGF-β2	0.404 ± 0.009 ᵠ	320.8 ± 3.225 ᵠ	4.25 ± 0.09 ᵠ	85.65 ± 2.20 ᵠ
	EGF	0.404 ± 0.007 ᵠ	322.9 ± 2.574	4.38 ± 0.07 ᵠ	88.34 ± 2.20 ᵠ
	FGF21	0.420 ± 0.011 ᵠ	329.0 ± 4.053	4.78 ± 0.17 ᵠ	89.97 ± 4.01 ᵠ

BMI: body mass index. SI: small intestine. TGF-β2: transforming growth factor-β2. EGF: epidermal growth factor. FGF21: fibroblast growth factor 21. Results are expressed as mean ± standard error of the mean (S.E.M) ($n = 9$).
ᵠ $p < 0.05$ vs. day 14 at same group.

All groups increased BMI, SI relative weight, and SI relative length with age ($p < 0.05$, day 21 vs. day 14). Regarding the Lee index, only the animals from the REF group and those supplemented with TGF-β2, showed significant differences associated with age ($p < 0.05$), but the supplementation with EGF and FGF21 did not display such a significant age difference.

3.2. IgA and IgM Concentration in Gut Wash

Intestinal secretory IgA and IgM were determined at day 21 of life. At that age, the pups' intestinal levels were not entirely influenced by maternal breast milk, as happens earlier in life when breast milk (very rich in IgA) is the only source of food. Nevertheless, none of the interventions (TGF-β2, EGF, and FGF21 supplemented groups) showed significant differences regarding IgA or IgM, compared to the REF group (Supplementary Materials, Figure S2).

3.3. Mesenteric Lymph Node Lymphocytes Composition

The proportion of the main lymphocyte subsets in MLN was established during (day 14) and at the end of (day 21) suckling period. On both days, most of the MLN cells (~75%) were T cells, the majority of them being TCRαβ$^+$ cells and only ~3% TCRγδ$^+$ cells; B cells counted for about 15–18%, NK and NKT cells represented subpopulations with less than 3% of total lymphocytes, and Treg cells were ~4% (Table 2).

Table 2. Main lymphocyte subsets in mesenteric lymph nodes.

		Reference	TGF-β2	EGF	FGF21
Day 14	T cells (%)	75.90 ± 1.80	77.90 ± 1.39	74.36 ± 1.88	79.60 ± 1.50
	T TCRαβ$^+$ (%)	72.90 ± 1.98	75.24 ± 1.29	71.22 ± 1.94	75.90 ± 1.20
	T TCRγδ$^+$ (%)	3.00 ± 0.20	2.66 ± 0.20	3.14 ± 0.23	3.70 ± 0.40
	NK (%)	1.63 ± 0.30	1.22 ± 0.08	1.35 ± 0.12	1.42 ± 0.17
	NKT (%)	1.15 ± 0.14	1.18 ± 0.20	0.94 ± 0.05	0.98 ± 0.06
	B cells (%)	17.65 ± 1.65	16.19 ± 1.40	19.62 ± 1.23	15.86 ± 1.07
Day 21	T cells (%)	74.60 ± 1.36	75.86 ± 1.10	75.29 ± 1.20	76.41 ± 0.69
	T TCRαβ$^+$ (%)	71.57 ± 1.44	73.28 ± 1.14	72.93 ± 1.26	73.10 ± 0.77
	T TCRγδ$^+$ (%)	3.07 ± 0.15	2.58 ± 0.15	2.36 ± 0.13 *,Ψ	3.31 ± 0.13
	NK (%)	0.95 ± 0.07 Ψ	0.79 ± 0.06 Ψ	0.77 ± 0.08 Ψ	1.05 ± 0.07
	NKT (%)	1.57 ± 0.07 Ψ	1.55 ± 0.11	1.39 ± 0.21	1.63 ± 0.18 Ψ
	B cells (%)	14.67 ± 0.71	14.30 ± 0.64	12.95 ± 1.19 Ψ	13.23 ± 0.62

Results are expressed as mean ± S.E.M ($n = 9$). * $p < 0.05$ vs. reference (REF) group at same age; Ψ $p < 0.05$ vs. day 14 at same group.

Although at 14 days there were no differences among the supplemented groups, some differences could be seen at 21 days (Table 2). At the end of the suckling period, only the EGF supplementation showed a significant decrease in the percentage of TCRγδ$^+$ cells, compared to the REF group ($p < 0.05$). Moreover, the REF and groups supplemented with TGF-β2 and EGF decreased the NK cell proportion, in comparison to the same group at 14 days ($p < 0.05$). The animals from the REF and FGF21 groups increased the percentage of NKT cells with age, and only those from the EGF group were able to decrease the proportion of TCRγδ$^+$ and B cell percentages at day 21 ($p < 0.05$ vs. day 14).

The percentage of CD8$^+$ cells and the CD8αα/CD8αβ ratio from MLNs lymphocytes, were determined as indicators of immune maturation (Figure 1). The proportion of CD8$^+$ cells did not show significant differences, either associated with age (day 14 vs. day 21) or to any of the supplementations, compared to the REF group (Figure 1a). However, regarding the results from CD8αα/CD8αβ ratio, the EGF supplementation induced a significant increase at 14 days ($p < 0.05$ vs. REF, Figure 1b). At day 21, in all supplemented groups, the CD8αα/CD8αβ ratio had decreased when they were compared to their respective group at day 14, but no differences among the interventions and the REF groups were found (Figure 1b).

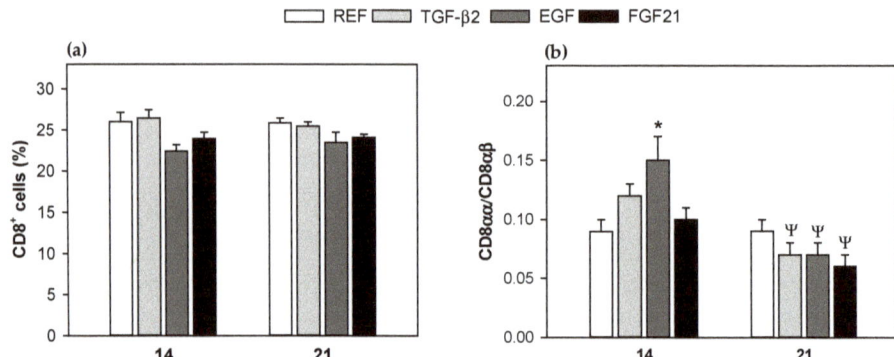

Figure 1. Proportion of CD8$^+$ cells and ratio CD8αα/CD8αβ in mesenteric lymph nodes at 14 and 21 days of life. (**a**) % CD8$^+$ cells; (**b**) The ratio CD8αα/CD8αβ was calculated as the quotient of the percentages of CD8αα cells and CD8αβ cells in CD8$^+$ cells (%). Results are expressed as mean ± standard error of the mean (S.E.M) (n = 9). Statistical differences: * $p < 0.05$ vs. reference group (REF group) at same age; $^\Psi$ $p < 0.05$ vs. same group at day 14. TGF-β2: transforming growth factor-β2. EGF: epidermal growth factor. FGF21: fibroblast growth factor 21.

Further analysis of CD8$^+$ and CD8$^-$ subsets revealed some changes associated with the supplementations (Figure 2).

Regarding the TCRαβ$^+$ subsets (CD8$^+$ and CD8$^-$, respectively, Figure 2a,b), no changes due to supplementation were found either at 14 or at 21 days, with respect to the REF group. Only, the supplementation with FGF21 decreased the proportion of TCRαβ$^+$ CD8$^-$ (~8%), when values from day 21 were compared to day 14 (Figure 2a, $p < 0.05$). The TCRγδ$^+$ CD8$^-$ cell percentage (Figure 2c), increased due to supplementation with EGF and FGF21 at 14 days, with only the latter achieving statistical significance, but these changes were not observed at the end of the suckling period (day 21). However, both interventions showed a 50% decrease in the TCRγδ$^+$ CD8$^-$ cell proportion associated with age ($p < 0.05$, day 21 vs. day 14). Moreover, the TCRγδ$^+$ CD8$^+$ cell proportion in the EGF group (Figure 2d), was lower than the REF group at day 21 ($p < 0.05$). In relation to the NKT population (CD8$^-$ and CD8$^+$ subsets), only the NKT CD8$^-$ subset showed changes associated with age for all groups (Figure 2e), but not due to the supplementations.

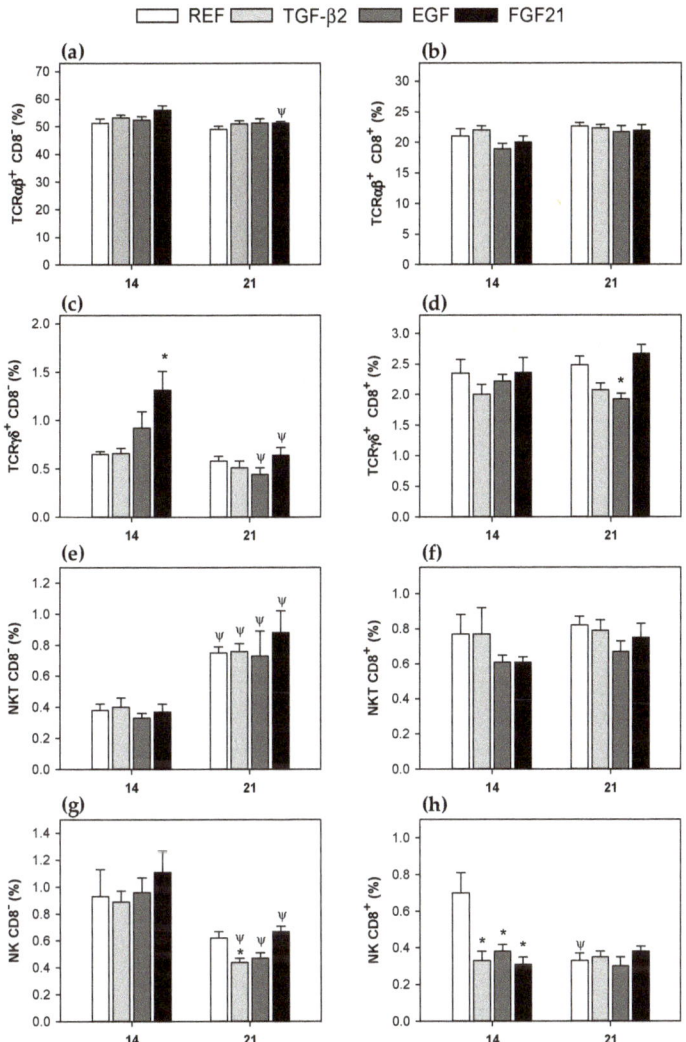

Figure 2. Percentages of CD8$^+$ and CD8$^-$ lymphocyte subsets in mesenteric lymph nodes at 14 and 21 days of life. (**a**) TCRαβ$^+$ CD8$^-$; (**b**) TCRαβ$^+$ CD8$^+$; (**c**) TCRγδ$^+$ CD8$^-$; (**d**) TCRγδ$^+$ CD8$^+$; (**e**) NKT CD8$^-$; (**f**) NKT CD8$^+$; (**g**) NK CD8$^-$; and (**h**) NK CD8$^+$. Results are expressed as mean ± S.E.M ($n = 9$). Statistical difference: * $p < 0.05$ vs. REF group at same age; $^\Psi$ $p < 0.05$ vs. same group at day 14.

However, NKT CD8$^+$ cell proportions were not affected (Figure 2f). Results from the NK cell population showed that in supplemented groups, there was a decrease in NK CD8$^-$ cell proportions related to age (Figure 2g, $p < 0.05$, day 21 vs. day 14), and that only supplementation with TGF-β2 induced a significant decrease compared with the REF group at 21 days (Figure 2g, $p < 0.05$ vs. REF). The phenotype of the intestinal NK cells based on CD8 expression, could be considered as immature (NK CD8$^+$) or more mature (NK CD8$^-$). The three supplementations were able to decrease the proportion of NK cells expressing CD8 at 14 days (Figure 2h), which reached similar values to those from reference 21-day-old rats. Thus, only the REF group decreased its percentage of NK CD8$^+$ cells at 21 days, with respect to day 14 (Figure 2h).

The lymphocytes' commitment to the mucosal compartment were studied by means of the proportion of cells expressing two adhesion molecules of importance in the intestinal homing; thus, the total percentage of cells bearing the selectin CD62L and the αE integrin were determined (Figure 3).

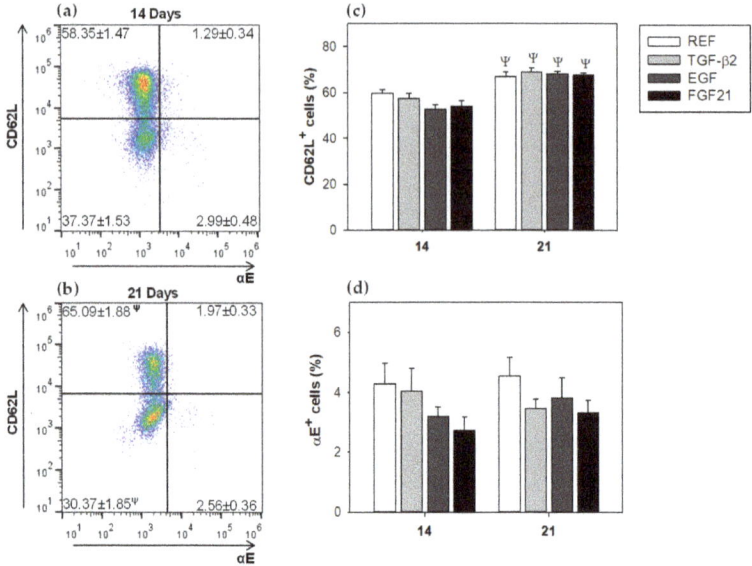

Figure 3. Surface expression of αE integrin and CD62L selectin, in mesenteric lymph nodes at 14 and 21 days of life. (**a**) CD62L/αE integrin surface expression at 14 days, (**b**) CD62L/αE integrin surface expression at 21 days, (**c**) CD62L$^+$ cells (%) and (**d**) αE$^+$ cells (%). Results are expressed as mean ± S.E.M (n = 9). Statistical difference: $^\Psi$ p > 0.05 vs. same group at day 14.

Figure 3a,b show the molecular pattern of αE/CD62L on day 14 and 21. The CD62L molecule was expressed on both days in high proportion of cells (~60%). Although the percentage of CD62L$^+$ cells increased significantly with age in all studied groups (Figure 3a–c, p < 0.05), none of the supplemented groups induced significant differences, when they were compared to the REF group at the same age. The αE$^+$ cells were present in a proportion lower than 5% at both studied times (Figure 3b–d) and were not modified by any GFs administration (Figure 3d).

The percentages of integrin αE$^+$ cells and selectin CD62L$^+$ cells in CD8$^+$, CD4$^+$, and B cells were further studied (Table 3). None of the supplemented groups showed significant differences, compared to the REF group at the same age. All studied groups increased CD62L$^+$ CD8$^+$ and CD62L$^+$ CD4$^+$ percentages with age (p < 0.05, day 21 vs. day 14). The REF group increased (~15%) αE$^+$ B cells subset proportion, with respect to the same group at 14 days, whereas all supplemented groups decreased (~20%) this subset with age (p < 0.05). In addition, the supplementation with EGF and FGF21, decreased the percentage of αE expression in CD4$^+$ cells with age. Although there was a tendency to increase with age, the proportion of CD62L$^+$ in B cells in all groups, it was only significant in the TGF-β2 group (p < 0.05).

At the end of the suckling period, activated CD4 cells (Foxp3$^-$ CD25$^+$ CD4$^+$ cells) and Treg cells (Foxp3$^+$ CD25$^+$ CD4$^+$ cells) were also studied, and no changes were found due to diets (day 21), with all groups together having a mean percentage of 1.22 ± 0.12 and 3.81 ± 0.11, respectively.

Table 3. Surface expression of the αE integrin and the CD62L selectin in CD4+, CD8+, and B cells in mesenteric lymph nodes.

		14 Days			
		Reference	TGF-β2	EGF	FGF21
%αE	CD8+	2.75 ± 0.72	2.92 ± 0.49	2.94 ± 0.52	2.88 ± 0.44
	CD4+	2.81 ± 0.39	3.07 ± 0.45	4.46 ± 0.34	3.80 ± 0.26
	B cells	15.98 ± 1.61	18.33 ± 1.39	18.92 ± 2.50	20.32 ± 3.12
%CD62L	CD8+	65.27 ± 1.56	62.38 ± 3.47	59.25 ± 2.52	59.21 ± 3.55
	CD4+	59.55 ± 1.76	55.41 ± 2.36	53.61 ± 1.37	53.65 ± 2.40
	B cells	48.43 ± 2.77	46.6 ± 2.05	38.77 ± 2.08	37.29 ± 4.78
		21 Days			
		Reference	TGF-β2	EGF	FGF21
%αE	CD8+	3.84 ± 0.48	2.98 ± 1.04	3.70 ± 0.48	3.97 ± 0.66
	CD4+	2.83 ± 0.75	2.61 ± 0.52	1.94 ± 0.18 $^\Psi$	2.52 ± 0.30 $^\Psi$
	B cells	18.43 ± 1.83 $^\Psi$	13.03 ± 1.55 $^\Psi$	14.95 ± 1.69 $^\Psi$	15.75 ± 1.16 $^\Psi$
%CD62L	CD8+	71.49 ± 1.38 $^\Psi$	72.10 ± 1.93 $^\Psi$	70.78 ± 2.19 $^\Psi$	72.88 ± 2.37 $^\Psi$
	CD4+	66.02 ± 1.74 $^\Psi$	68.24 ± 1.64 $^\Psi$	66.66 ± 0.42 $^\Psi$	66.80 ± 1.22 $^\Psi$
	B cells	56.79 ± 2.25	60.92 ± 2.17 $^\Psi$	60.82 ± 3.92	57.61 ± 2.37

Results are expressed as mean ± S.E.M (n = 9). $^\Psi$ $p < 0.05$ vs. day 14 at same group.

3.4. Proliferation and Cytokine Production by Mesenteric Lymph Nodes Cells

To determine the functional capacity of MLN lymphocytes, we studied their proliferative response and their ability to secrete cytokines on days 14 and 21. With regard to the proliferation of MLNs cells on days 14 and 21, GFs supplementations were not able to significantly modify such lymphocyte function induced by anti-CD3 and anti-CD28 mAbs (Supplementary Materials, Figure S3). However, cytokine production was influenced by GFs supplementation (Table 4).

The pattern of cytokines released from MLNs cells at day 14, showed a high secretion of IFN-γ, followed by IL-10. In the conditions tested, the secretion of IL-2, IL-4, IL-13, IL-17A, and TNF-α was lower than 90 pg/mL. IL-10/TNF-α (anti-inflammatory/pro-inflammatory cytokines) and IFN-γ/IL-4 (Th1/Th2) ratios were also calculated. No changes in the cytokine pattern at day 14 were detected by GFs supplementation. However, at day 21, some changes appeared due to supplementations and due to age. IL-2 production was 5–10 times higher due to age in the REF, TGF-β2, and EGF groups ($p < 0.05$ day 21 vs. day 14). IL-4 levels were ~50% lower in the EGF group at day 21, than those at day 14 ($p < 0.05$). The groups that received EGF and FGF21 for 21 days, decreased the IL-10 content ~1.5 times with respect to their values at day 14 ($p < 0.05$). IL-13 secretion was lower at day 21 with respect to day 14, in the EGF and FGF21 groups ($p < 0.05$), and the three GFs groups showed lower values than those present in the REF group ($p < 0.05$). The lower levels of IFN-γ production at day 21 compared to day 14 were only significant in the REF group, which accounted for a 50% reduction ($p < 0.05$). Moreover, TNF-α release decreased (~30%) with age in the REF, TGF-β2, and FGF21 groups, whereas supplementation with EGF increased TNF-α production ($p < 0.05$ vs. REF group).

The IL-10/TNF-α ratio decreased according to age in the EGF and FGF21 groups, and in the EGF group, values were significantly lower than the REF group ($p < 0.05$).

Table 4. Cytokine production by mesenteric lymph node cells after in vitro stimulation.

(pg/mL)	14 Days			
	Reference	TGF-β2	EGF	FGF21
IL-2	42.71 ± 5.96	39.24 ± 5.66	50.45 ± 6.66	56.72 ± 11.04
IL-4	89.82 ± 13.00	57.14 ± 7.81	82.65 ± 12.47	74.97 ± 12.18
IL-10	879.82 ± 239.40	688.01 ± 145.14	1450.87 ± 296.29	1326.99 ± 217.06
IL-13	25.38 ± 5.64	17.53 ± 3.03	31.91 ± 4.28	26.18 ± 4.03
IL-17A	71.98 ± 26.92	70.22 ± 20.16	60.12 ± 13.61	50.82 ± 9.53
IFN-γ	10323.26 ± 2391.46	8302.75 ± 1964.09	9329.17 ± 1662.87	7882.51 ± 2810.34
TNF-α	8.76 ± 0.98	9.48 ± 0.68	9.19 ± 1.16	7.40 ± 0.25
IL-10/TNF-α	115.00 ± 33.11	79.71 ± 21.80	170.87 ± 43.10	178.05 ± 29.25
IFN-γ/IL-4	110.35 ± 20.65	195.32 ± 61.39	124.85 ± 37.55	103.80 ± 26.93
(pg/mL)	21 Days			
	Reference	TGF-β2	EGF	FGF21
IL-2	390.57 ± 141.49 ^{Ψ}	383.80 ± 89.21 ^{Ψ}	244.79 ± 80.37 ^{Ψ}	270.16 ± 114.54
IL-4	70.52 ± 10.51	52.21 ± 7.69	48.52 ± 1.91 ^{Ψ}	66.60 ± 8.80
IL-10	705.45 ± 63.95	514.70 ± 55.30	508.26 ± 61.43 ^{Ψ}	542.36 ± 78.82 ^{Ψ}
IL-13	19.51 ± 2.44	12.92 ± 0.74 *	9.91 ± 1.24 *,^{Ψ}	9.83 ± 1.65 *,^{Ψ}
IL-17A	59.97 ± 7.14	46.91 ± 4.03	52.30 ± 10.7022	41.24 ± 11.77
IFN-γ	4231.26 ± 365.41 ^{Ψ}	4488.50 ± 416.14	6900.74 ± 1129.78	4595.11 ± 1058.87
TNF-α	6.63 ± 0.11 ^{Ψ}	6.55 ± 0.20 ^{Ψ}	10.02 ± 0.40 *	5.91 ± 0.38 ^{Ψ}
IL-10/TNF-α	106.47 ± 9.73	80.13 ± 9.55	50.48 ± 5.72 *,^{Ψ}	95.64 ± 17.03 ^{Ψ}
IFN-γ/IL-4	64.25 ± 9.61	111.99 ± 25.23	147.25 ± 27.9166	81.50 ± 25.37

Results are expressed as mean ± S.E.M (n = 9). * $p < 0.05$ vs. REF group at same age; ^{Ψ} $p < 0.05$ vs. day 14 at same group.

4. Discussion

At birth, the immune system is immature, as evidenced by a poor antibody production and low proliferative response of immune cells. In addition, there are mucosal immune impairments, such as low intestinal IgA content, reduced number of B lymphocytes in the intestinal mucosa, and few intestinal T cells [23]. Immune development is driven, among other factors, by components of breast milk. It is known that growth factors, such as TGF-β2 and EGF, regulate the immune response in early life and confer protective effects against gut mucosal inflammation by enhancing oral tolerance [1,2,7]. FGF21, which is also present in maternal milk, is a less-studied component and could be involved in such effects as well [16]. The current study aimed to evaluate whether supplementation with TGF-β2, EGF, or FGF21 had a role in immune maturation in early life. A rat pup model was used to evaluate the effect of a daily supplementation with TGF-β2, EGF, or FGF21 during suckling on the GALT, particularly in the MLNs, which is an inductor site of intestinal immune response. We assessed the immune maturation by functions, such as lymphoproliferation, cytokine production ability, and establishing lymphocyte MLNs composition.

Regarding growth, the body weight of pups was not modified due to supplementation with any of the GFs studied. These results were in line with other investigations, in which rats receiving either TGF-β2 [10] or EGF [24,25] during the first two weeks of life did not change their body weight. Likewise, although a study showed that the body weight of FGF21-knockout mice compared to wild-type 3-month-old mice was not different [26], its physiological role as a weight regulating factor was discussed [18]. Overall, it seems that the tested GFs, under the conditions we used, did not have a key role in the growth of neonates.

Intestinal length and weight are useful tools for evaluating the primary impact of a nutrient on the maturation of the rat small intestine [27]. The GFs supplementation in the current study did not affect these variables. However, it has been reported that suckling rats receiving intraperitoneal administration of EGF (100 µg/kg) for only two days, increased stomach and intestinal weights [24]; and that rat pups receiving oral administration of EGF through formula at concentrations exceeding the reported concentrations of EGF in rodent milk, enhanced intestinal growth (weight and length) [15]. Thus, in agreement with our results, only high doses of these compounds seem to be able to modify intestinal growth.

Although no impact on the body and intestinal growth due to any of these GFs was observed, some effects of TGF-β2, EGF, or FGF21 on immune variables have been shown to be specific; and therefore, the influence of each GF tested on MLN lymphocyte maturation will be discussed separately.

Transforming growth factor-β (TGF-β) has a wide range of biological activities and among them, it has an important role in cell proliferation and differentiation. TGF-β acts as a cytokine having predominantly suppressive effects on the growth of T and B lymphocytes. In this study, the supplementation of suckling rats with TGF-β2 did not have a significant influence on unspecific MLNs proliferative cell response. This result contrasted with a report showing that suckling rats receiving a whey-enriched TGF-β formula, down-regulated the MLNs lymphocyte proliferative response to specific antigen after being sensitized [28]. On the other hand, we observed that MLNs cells after TGF-β2 supplementation did not modify the changes in IL-2 and TNF-α secretion associated with age, but attenuated IL-13 production at day 21 with respect to reference animals. The attenuation on IL-13 production, a Th2 cytokine linked to allergic processes [29–31], agrees with results showing that Brown Norway rat pups receiving a formula with TGF-β2 between 4 and 18 days of life shifted the immune response from a Th2 type towards a Th1 profile [13]. Likewise, it is known that low levels of IL-13 in colostrum and mature milk are associated with less eczema in early life [32]. Thus, our results suggested that early TGF-β2 intake could play an important role in the prevention of Th2 mediated alterations, such as allergy.

In the current study, the TGF-β2 supplementation was already able to modulate MLN lymphocyte composition in suckling rats. It decreases the proportion of the immature phenotype of the intestinal NK cells (NK CD8$^+$) on day 14 at levels observed later (day 21); which indicated a positive action on the intestinal immune maturation. This developmental pattern, decreasing CD8 expression in the NK cell surface with age, has previously described in rat neonatal intraepithelial lymphocytes (IEL) and MLN cells [19,27]. In line with this, we found that, although no changes in total CD8$^+$ cells were observed due to TGF-β2 supplementation, a lower CD8αα/CD8αβ ratio at day 21, compared to day 14 appeared. This ratio has been described to be reduced according to age in healthy MLNs cells from suckling rats [19], thus our results may suggested a promotion of the intestinal immune system maturation. This contrasts with results in BALB/c mice pups, showing higher CD8$^+$ T cell proportions when their lactating mothers were treated with mAbs, against TGF-β twice a week from delivery until weaning [33]. On the other hand, we did not find changes in the MLNs Treg (CD4$^+$ CD25$^+$ Foxp3$^+$) cell proportion. However, some authors have suggested that oral tolerance induced by breastfeeding could depend on TGF-β signaling from breast milk, which would be able to up-regulate Foxp3$^+$ cells [33].

Regarding the intestinal humoral immune response, it is known that IgA is poorly produced by the neonate mucosal immune system [1,28], and that TGF-β1 and TGF-β2 from mammalian milk are able to stimulate the synthesis of mucosal IgA [28,33]. Thus, TGF-β acting in synergy with IL-10, can promote IgA production and oral tolerance induction [28]. However, our results did not show significant changes in the intestinal IgA and IgM content of the suckling rats. This lack of effect could be due to the fact that breast milk contains IgA and IgM, which are transferred to the pups, and then these milk antibodies in the intestine would mask the pups' own levels. For this reason, intestinal IgA and IgM assessment cannot be a good marker of nutritional supplementation at this level.

Epidermal growth factor (EGF) is a peptide that modulates a variety of biological responses, such as cell proliferation and differentiation [14]. It is known that it has a clear effect on epithelium, where it accelerates maturation and stimulates cell proliferation [34–36]. However, in the current study, we have not detected any effect of the EGF supplementation on the proliferative response of MLNs cells in the suckling pups. There is evidence that EGF prevents and reduces the incidence and severity of NEC by modulating important transcription factors for cytokine regulation [37], and it is known that the balance of pro-inflammatory and anti-inflammatory cytokines may play a key role in the development of NEC [17]. This effect may be attributable to a down-regulation of pro-inflammatory IL-18 and to an increase of anti-inflammatory IL-10 at the site of injury [17,37]. Here we found that, 21-day EGF supplementation increased TNF-α and decreased IL-13 production by MLNs cells. The changes in these two cytokines, contained in maternal milk [32,38], could be associated with positive effects. Indeed, decreased IL-13 can be useful in the prevention of allergy, as stated for TGF-β2 [29–31]. Moreover, EGF supplementation kept the levels of TNF-α on day 21 at the same level as that on day 14, which could play in favor of its own effects because it is known that EGF receptor (EGF-R) is up-regulated by TNF-α [39]. Regarding MLNs cell composition, EGF supplementation shares some maturate effects with TGF-β2, such as the induction of lower levels of NK CD8$^+$ cells and CD8αα/CD8αβ ratio.

Finally, focusing on fibroblast growth factor 21 (FGF21), recent studies showed that its function is not limited to the regulation of metabolism, but that it is also involved in the protection of multiple physiological processes, such as oxidation, inflammation, atherosclerosis, and aging processes [40]. A recent study demonstrated that, in the spleen of mice with collagen-induced arthritis (CIA), FGF21 reduces the expression of inflammatory cytokines, such as IL-17, TNF-α, IL-1β, IL-6, IL-8, and MMP3, whereas IL-10 levels were increased, compared to PBS treated CIA mice [41]. In line with this, we have not found any significant difference with respect to non-supplemented animals on MLNs inflammatory cytokines, but the FGF21 supplementation decreased IL-13 at 21 days, as we also found with the other GFs, suggesting, therefore, its role in preventing allergic events.

It is known that FGF21 is present in breast milk and does not contribute to systemic levels in mouse neonates, but appears to act locally on the mouse neonatal intestine [16]; and it is unknown whether this factor plays an important role in the maturation of the immune system. We found that suckling rats receiving FGF21 promoted maturation of the early life intestinal immune system by accelerating the decrease in the proportion of NK CD8$^+$ cells and the decrease in the CD8αα/CD8αβ cell ratio in MLNs, as well as TGF-β2 and EGF. This is the first time that the immunomodulatory effect of FGF21 has been demonstrated in early life.

5. Conclusions

In conclusion, our study demonstrated that supplementation with TGF-β2, EGF, or FGF21 during the suckling period had an immunoregulatory effect. Although some specific effects appeared, the three growth factors were able to modulate similar aspects of MLN cells, such as promoting lymphocyte maturation, as observed by increasing NK cells with a more mature phenotype (CD8$^-$) and reducing IL-13 production, which could be useful in avoiding allergic processes. Further studies should be carried out to establish the effect of the supplementation of TGF-β2, EGF, or FGF21 on the response of suckling pups in other parts of the intestinal immune system, such as in the intestinal epithelium or even at the systemic level.

Supplementary Materials: The following are available online at http://www.mdpi.com/2072-6643/10/9/1171/s1, Figure S1: Growth curve of all studied groups during the suckling period (from 1 to 21 days of life), Figure S2: IgA and IgM concentration in gut wash from 21-day-old animals after the different nutritional interventions, Figure S3: Proliferation of mesenteric lymph nodes lymphocytes at 14 and 21 days of life, Table S1: List of monoclonal antibodies (mAbs) used for immunophenotyping the mesenteric lymph nodes (MLN) cells.

Author Contributions: M.J.R.-L., M.C., F.J.P.-C., and À.F. conceived and designed the experiments; P.T.-C. and M.A.-G. performed the experiments; P.T.-C., F.J.P.-C., and À.F. analyzed the data and wrote the manuscript. F.J.P.-C. and À.F. have primary responsibility for the final content. All the authors reviewed and approved the final version of the manuscript.

Funding: This study was supported by a grant from the Spanish Ministry of Economy, Industry and Competitiveness (AGL2013-48459-P). Paulina Torres-Castro holds a fellowship from the National Secretary of Higher Education, Science, Technology and Innovation of Ecuador (SENESCYT-DMPF-2015-1666-CO).

Acknowledgments: The authors thank Lidia Marín-Morote for their help with the laboratory work. The authors also thank J. Comas and his laboratory technicians from the Scientific and Technological Centres of the University of Barcelona (CCiT-UB) for their assistance in the cytometry service.

Conflicts of Interest: The authors declare no conflict of interest.

References

1. Turfkruyer, M.; Verhasselt, V. Breast milk and its impact on maturation of the neonatal immune system. *Curr. Opin. Infect. Dis.* **2015**, *28*, 199–206. [CrossRef] [PubMed]
2. García, C.; Duan, R.D.; Brévaut-Malaty, V.; Gire, C.; Millet, V.; Simeoni, U.; Bernard, M.; Armand, M. Bioactive compounds in human milk and intestinal health and maturity in preterm newborn: An overview. *Cell. Mol. Biol.* **2013**, *59*, 108–131. [CrossRef] [PubMed]
3. Penttila, I.A.; van Spriel, A.B.; Zhang, M.F.; Xian, C.J.; Steeb, C.B.; Cummins, A.G.; Zola, H.; Read, L.C. Transforming growth factor-β levels in maternal milk and expression in postnatal rat duodenum and ileum. *Pediatr. Res.* **1998**, *44*, 524–531. [CrossRef] [PubMed]
4. Buddington, R.K.; Sangild, P.T. Companion animals symposium: Development of the mammalian gastrointestinal tract, the resident microbiota, and the role of diet in early life. *J. Anim. Sci.* **2011**, *89*, 1506–1519. [CrossRef] [PubMed]
5. Jacobi, S.K.; Odle, J. Nutritional factors influencing intestinal health of the neonate. *Adv. Nutr.* **2012**, *3*, 687–696. [CrossRef] [PubMed]
6. Castellote, C.; Casillas, R.; Ramírez-Santana, C.; Pérez-Cano, F.J.; Castell, M.; Moretones, M.G.; López-Sabater, M.C.; Franch, À. Premature delivery influences the immunological composition of colostrum and transitional and mature human milk. *J. Nutr.* **2011**, *141*, 1181–1187. [CrossRef] [PubMed]
7. Field, C.J. The immunological components of human milk and their effect on immune development in infants. *J. Nutr.* **2005**, *135*, 1–4. [CrossRef] [PubMed]
8. Andreas, N.J.; Kampmann, B.; Mehring Le-Doare, K. Human breast milk: A review on its composition and bioactivity. *Early Hum. Dev.* **2015**, *91*, 629–635. [CrossRef] [PubMed]
9. Ballard, O.; Morrow, A.L. Human milk composition: Nutrients and bioactive factors. *Pediatr. Clin. N. Am.* **2013**, *60*, 49–74. [CrossRef] [PubMed]
10. Penttila, I.A.; Flesch, I.E.; McCue, A.L.; Powell, B.C.; Zhou, F.H.; Read, L.C.; Zola, H. Maternal milk regulation of cell infiltration and interleukin 18 in the intestine of suckling rat pups. *Gut* **2003**, *52*, 1579–1586. [CrossRef] [PubMed]
11. Sanjabi, S.; Oh, S.A.; Li, M.O. Regulation of the immune response by TGF-β: From conception to autoimmunity and infection. *Cold Spring Harb. Perspect. Biol.* **2017**, *9*, a022236. [CrossRef] [PubMed]
12. Penttila, I.A. Milk-derived transforming growth factor-beta and the infant immune response. *J. Pediatr.* **2010**, *156*, S21–S25. [CrossRef] [PubMed]
13. Penttila, I. Effects of transforming growth factor-beta and formula feeding on systemic immune responses to dietary β-lactoglobulin in allergy-prone rats. *Pediatr. Res.* **2006**, *59*, 650–655. [CrossRef] [PubMed]
14. Tang, X.; Liu, H.; Yang, S.; Li, Z.; Zhong, J.; Fang, R. Epidermal growth factor and intestinal barrier function. *Mediat. Inflamm.* **2016**, *2016*, 1927348. [CrossRef] [PubMed]
15. Berseth, C.L. Enhancement of intestinal growth in neonatal rats by epidermal growth factor in milk. *Am. J. Physiol.* **1987**, *253*, G662–G665. [CrossRef] [PubMed]
16. Gavaldà-Navarro, A.; Hondares, E.; Giralt, M.; Mampel, T.; Iglesias, R.; Villarroya, F. Fibroblast growth factor 21 in breast milk controls neonatal intestine function. *Sci. Rep.* **2015**, *5*, 13717. [CrossRef] [PubMed]
17. Coursodon, C.F.; Dvorak, B. Epidermal growth factor and necrotizing enterocolitis. *Curr. Opin. Pediatr.* **2012**, *24*, 160–164. [CrossRef] [PubMed]
18. Kharitonenkov, A.; DiMarchi, R. Fibroblast growth factor 21 night watch: Advances and uncertainties in the field. *J. Intern. Med.* **2017**, *281*, 233–246. [CrossRef] [PubMed]
19. Grases-Pintó, B.; Abril-Gil, M.; Rodríguez-Lagunas, M.J.; Castell, M.; Pérez-Cano, F.J.; Franch, À. Leptin and adiponectin supplementation modifies mesenteric lymph node lymphocyte composition and functionality in suckling rats. *Br. J. Nutr.* **2018**, *119*, 486–495. [CrossRef] [PubMed]
20. Rigo-Adrover, M.D.M.; Van Limpt, K.; Knipping, K.; Garssen, J.; Knol, J.; Costabile, A.; Franch, À.; Castell, M.; Pérez-Cano, F.J. Preventive effect of a synbiotic combination of galacto- and fructooligosaccharides mixture with *Bifidobacterium breve* M-16V in a model of multiple rotavirus infections. *Front. Immunol.* **2018**, *9*, 1318. [CrossRef] [PubMed]

21. Maynard, A.A.; Dvorak, K.; Khailova, L.; Dobrenen, H.; Arganbright, K.M.; Halpern, M.D.; Kurundkar, A.R.; Maheshwari, A.; Dvorak, B. Epidermal growth factor reduces autophagy in intestinal epithelium and in the rat model of necrotizing enterocolitis. *Am. J. Physiol. Liver Physiol.* **2010**, *299*, G614–G622. [CrossRef] [PubMed]
22. Camps-Bossacoma, M.; Pérez-Cano, F.J.; Franch, À.; Untersmayr, E.; Castell, M. Effect of a cocoa diet on the small intestine and gut-associated lymphoid tissue composition in an oral sensitization model in rats. *J. Nutr. Biochem.* **2017**, *42*, 182–193. [CrossRef] [PubMed]
23. Basha, S.; Surendran, N.; Pichichero, M. Immune responses in neonates. *Expert Rev. Clin. Immunol.* **2014**, *10*, 1171–1184. [CrossRef] [PubMed]
24. Hormi, K.; Lehy, T. Transforming growth factor-alpha in vivo stimulates epithelial cell proliferation in digestive tissues of suckling rats. *Gut* **1996**, *39*, 532–538. [CrossRef] [PubMed]
25. Pollack, P.F.; Goda, T.; Colony, P.C.; Edmond, J.; Thornburg, W.; Korc, M.; Koldovský, O. Effects of enterally fed epidermal growth factor on the small and large intestine of the suckling rat. *Regul. Pept.* **1987**, *17*, 121–132. [CrossRef]
26. Camporez, J.P.; Asrih, M.; Zhang, D.; Kahn, M.; Samuel, V.T.; Jurczak, M.J.; Jornayvaz, F.R. Hepatic insulin resistance and increased hepatic glucose production in mice lacking FGF21. *J. Endocrinol.* **2015**, *226*, 207–217. [CrossRef] [PubMed]
27. Pérez-Cano, F.J.; Franch, À.; Castellote, C.; Castell, M. The suckling rat as a model for immunonutrition studies in early life. *Clin. Dev. Immunol.* **2012**, *2012*, 537310. [CrossRef] [PubMed]
28. Zhang, M.F. The Role of Milk Transforming Growth Factor-β (TGF-β) in the Development of the Infant Gut and Gut Mucosal Immune System. Ph.D. Thesis, University of Adelaide, Adelaide, Australia, 2000.
29. Wills-Karp, M.; Luyimbazi, J.; Xu, X.; Schofield, B.; Neben, T.Y.; Karp, C.L.; Donaldson, D.D. Interleukin-13: Central mediator of allergic asthma. *Science* **1998**, *282*, 2258–2261. [CrossRef] [PubMed]
30. Kubo, T.; Morita, H.; Sugita, K.; Akdis, C.A. Introduction to mechanisms of allergic diseases. In *Middleton's Allergy Essentials*; Holgate, S., Sheikh, A., Eds.; Elsevier: New York, NY, USA, 2017; pp. 1–27. ISBN 978-0-323-37579-5.
31. Bao, K.; Reinhardt, R.L. The differential expression of IL-4 and IL-13 and its impact on type-2 immunity. *Cytokine* **2015**, *75*, 25–37. [CrossRef] [PubMed]
32. Munblit, D.; Treneva, M.; Peroni, D.G.; Colicino, S.; Chow, L.Y.; Dissanayeke, S.; Pampura, A.; Boner, A.L.; Geddes, D.T.; Boyle, R.J.; et al. Immune components in human milk are associated with early infant immunological health outcomes: A prospective three-country analysis. *Nutrients* **2017**, *9*, 532. [CrossRef] [PubMed]
33. Sakaguchi, K.; Koyanagi, A.; Kamachi, F.; Harauma, A.; Chiba, A.; Hisata, K.; Moriguchi, T.; Shimizu, T.; Miyake, S. Breast-feeding regulates immune system development via transforming growth factor-β in mice pups. *Pediatr. Int.* **2018**, *60*, 224–231. [CrossRef] [PubMed]
34. Dvorak, B.; Halpern, M.D.; Holubec, H.; Williams, C.S.; McWilliam, D.L.; Dominguez, J.A.; Stepankova, R.; Payne, C.M.; McCuskey, R.S. Epidermal growth factor reduces the development of necrotizing enterocolitis in a neonatal rat model. *Am. J. Physiol. Gastrointest. Liver Physiol.* **2002**, *282*, G156–G164. [CrossRef] [PubMed]
35. Weaver, L.T.; Walker, W.A. Epidermal growth factor and the developing human gut. *Gastroenterology* **1988**, *94*, 845–847. [CrossRef]
36. Wong, W.M.; Wright, N.A. Epidermal growth factor, epidermal growth factor receptors, intestinal growth, and adaptation. *JPEN J. Parenter. Enteral Nutr.* **1999**, *23*, S83–S88. [CrossRef] [PubMed]
37. Halpern, M.D.; Dominguez, J.A.; Dvorakova, K.; Holubec, H.; Williams, C.S.; Meza, Y.G.; Ruth, M.C.; Dvorak, B. Ileal cytokine dysregulation in experimental necrotizing enterocolitis is reduced by epidermal growth factor. *J. Pediatr. Gastroenterol. Nutr.* **2003**, *36*, 126–133. [CrossRef] [PubMed]
38. Hanson, L.Å.; Korotkova, M. The role of breastfeeding in prevention of neonatal infection. *Semin. Neonatol.* **2002**, *7*, 275–281. [CrossRef] [PubMed]
39. Takeyama, K.; Dabbagh, K.; Lee, H.M.; Agustí, C.; Lausier, J.A.; Ueki, I.F.; Grattan, K.M.; Nadel, J.A. Epidermal growth factor system regulates mucin production in airways. *Proc. Natl. Acad. Sci. USA* **1999**, *96*, 3081–3086. [CrossRef] [PubMed]

40. Yan, J.; Wang, J.; Huang, H.; Huang, Y.; Mi, T.; Zhang, C.; Zhang, L. Fibroblast growth factor 21 delayed endothelial replicative senescence and protected cells from H_2O_2-induced premature senescence through SIRT1. *Am. J. Transl. Res.* **2017**, *9*, 4492–4501. [PubMed]
41. Li, S.M.; Yu, Y.H.; Li, L.; Wang, W.F.; Li, D.S. Treatment of CIA mice with FGF21 down-regulates TH17-IL-17 axis. *Inflammation* **2016**, *39*, 309–319. [CrossRef] [PubMed]

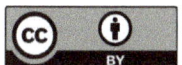

© 2018 by the authors. Licensee MDPI, Basel, Switzerland. This article is an open access article distributed under the terms and conditions of the Creative Commons Attribution (CC BY) license (http://creativecommons.org/licenses/by/4.0/).

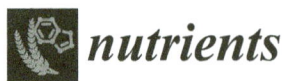

Article

Effect of Milk Fermented with *Lactobacillus fermentum* on the Inflammatory Response in Mice

Lourdes Santiago-López [1], Adrián Hernández-Mendoza [1], Verónica Mata-Haro [2], Belinda Vallejo-Córdoba [1], Abraham Wall-Medrano [3], Humberto Astiazarán-García [4], María del Carmen Estrada-Montoya [1] and Aarón F. González-Córdova [1,*]

[1] Laboratorio de Química y Biotecnología de Productos Lácteos, Centro de Investigación en Alimentación y Desarrollo A. C. (CIAD), Carretera a La Victoria Km. 0.6, Hermosillo, Sonora 83304, Mexico; lulu140288@gmail.com (L.S.-L.); ahernandez@ciad.mx (A.H.-M.); vallejo@ciad.mx (B.V.-C.); carmenes@ciad.mx (M.d.C.E.-M.)

[2] Laboratorio de Microbiología e Inmunología, Centro de Investigación en Alimentación y Desarrollo A. C. (CIAD), Carretera a La Victoria Km. 0.6, Hermosillo, Sonora 83304, Mexico; vmata@ciad.mx

[3] Departamento de Ciencias Químico-Biológicas, Instituto de Ciencias Biomédicas, Universidad Autónoma de Ciudad Juárez, Anillo Envolvente del PRONAF y Estocolmo s/n, Ciudad Juárez 32310, Chihuahua, Mexico; awall@uacj.mx

[4] Laboratorio de Patología Experimental, Centro de Investigación en Alimentación y Desarrollo A. C. (CIAD), Carretera a la Victoria Km. 0.6, Hermosillo, Sonora 83304, Mexico; hastiazaran@ciad.mx

* Correspondence: aaronglz@ciad.mx; Tel./Fax: +52-662-289-2400

Received: 12 July 2018; Accepted: 6 August 2018; Published: 8 August 2018

Abstract: Currently, the effect of fermented milk on the T-helper 17 response in inflammatory bowel diseases (IBDs) is unknown. The aim of the present study was to evaluate the effect of milks fermented with *Lactobacillus fermentum* on the Th1/Th17 response in a murine model of mild IBD. Exopolysaccharide (EPS), lactic acid (LA), and total protein (TP) contents and bacterial concentration were determined. Male C57Bl/6 mice intragastrically received either raw (FM) or pasteurized (PFM) fermented milk before and during a dextran sulfate infusion protocol. Blood, spleen, and colon samples were collected at Weeks 6 and 10. IL-6, IL-10, and TNFα were determined in serum, and IL-17, IL-23, and IFNγ were determined in intestinal mucosa and serum. The FM groups did not differ in cell concentration, LA, or TP content ($p > 0.05$); FM-J28 had the highest EPS content. Spleen weight and colon length did not differ among the FM groups ($p > 0.05$). In the FM-J20 and PFM-J20 groups, IL-17 and IFNγ decreased, and the IL-10 concentration was enhanced ($p < 0.05$) at Week 6. IL-6, TNFα, IL-23, and IFNγ did not differ in serum and mucosa ($p > 0.05$), and IL-17 was lowest in FM-J28 and FM-J20. Therefore, FM appears to potentially play a role in decreasing the Th17 response. However, further studies are needed to elucidate the FM-mediated anti-inflammatory mechanisms in IBD.

Keywords: fermented milk; Th1/Th17 response; inflammatory process

1. Introduction

Inflammatory bowel diseases (IBDs) are characterized by chronic and uncontrolled inflammation in the intestinal mucosa. Different factors have been evidenced to affect the immune system at the mucosal level [1]. For example, inflammatory mediators such as cytokines play an important role in the adaptive immune response at the intestinal mucosal level. The modulation of biological cellular functions may initiate downstream signaling pathways and mediate cellular proliferation and differentiation [2]. In particular, Th1 and Th17 cells have been implicated in the development of IBD. Th1 is characterized by the presence of interferon-γ (IFNγ) and Th17 by the presence of interleukin

(IL)-17, IL-21, and IL-22 [3]. Cytokines such as IL-6, TGF-β, and IL-23 promote the development of Th17 cells in IBD [4]. One study related Th1 and Th17 responses to the pathogenesis of IBD and suggested that Th1 cells may enhance the production of Th17 cells. In this previous study, a higher concentration of Th17 vs. Th1 cells was reported in a colitis model with CBirl TCR transgenic mice, which are immunodominant susceptible to flagellin microbiota [5]. In contrast, another study examining the cytokine profiles of Th1 and Th17 in a colitis model found that IL-4 and IL-10 levels were enhanced while IL-17 levels were reduced [6].

In another study, the pathogenic action of IL-23 was demonstrated. In IL-23R-deficient mice, reduced Reg3b protein expression in intestinal mucosa was shown to directly affect antimicrobial activity. In addition, IL-23-dependent Reg3b triggers an influx of IL-22, regulating the number of neutrophils in the lamina propia and restoring IL-22 secretion. This finding is important given the role of IL-23 in neutralizing the Th17 response in IBD [7].

Moreover, the administration of probiotics was shown to possibly modulate the inflammatory process through the Th1-Th2-Th17 response. Zheng et al. [8] reported that *Bifidobacterium breve* and *Lactobacillus rhamnosus* reduce Th17 and increase the Th2 cell subset in human peripheral blood mononuclear cells. In addition, the active components of probiotics were shown to be responsible for enhancing the numbers of CD4 + FoxP3 + regulatory T cells in mesenteric lymph nodes and for decreasing the cytokines tumor necrosis factor-α (TNFα), IFNγ, and IL-10 in Peyer's patches and the large intestine. In another study, probiotics were shown to play an important role in the down-regulation of the nuclear factor kappa B (NFkB) pathway in RAW 264.7 cells to prevent TNFα expression in a lipopolysaccharide-induced model [9].

Several additional studies have documented the regulation of the immune response in IBDs by administering probiotics [10–14]. However, few studies have documented the effects of fermented milk on the Th17 response, which regulates various inflammatory processes at the intestinal level. In one case, Dahi-fermented milk containing a probiotic reduced myeloperoxidase (MPO) activity and TNFα, IL-6, and IFNγ levels [14]. Meanwhile, milk with fermented *Lactobacillus rhamnosus* GG reduced colonic inflammation and injury and stimulated the activation of epidermal growth factor receptor (EGFR) and protein kinase B (Akt), which may be attributed to the release of p40 and p75 proteins during fermentation [15].

These latter studies demonstrated the potential role of milk fermented with probiotics on the inflammatory process. However, the effect of fermented milk on the Th1/Th17 response has not been reported. The aim of the present study was to evaluate the effect of milk fermented with *Lactobacillus fermentum* (J20 and J28) on the Th1/Th17 response in a murine model of inflammation.

2. Materials and Methods

2.1. Preparation of Fermented Milk

The *Lactobacillus fermentum* strains J20 and J28 were cultured in MRS broth (De Man, Rogosa and Sharpe, Difco) for 12 h at 37 °C. Posteriorly, to elaborate the fermented milk, the strains were sub-cultured twice in commercial milk (1% v/v) and incubated for 24 h and 12 h at 37 °C. Then, commercial skimmed milk was inoculated (3% v/v) with the 12-h cultures and incubated for 48 h at 37 °C. Finally, the fermented milks (FMs) were placed in a cold water bath or submitted to heat treatment (75 °C, 15 min) to obtain pasteurized fermented milk (PFM), which was subsequently submersed in a cold water bath to inactivate bacteria. The samples were stored at 4 °C. A control pH treatment was prepared with acidified milk (AM) by adding 800 μL of lactic acid (~90%, Sigma-Aldrich, Mexico City, Mexico) to skimmed milk to obtain a similar lactic acid concentration as FM.

2.2. Characterization of Fermented Milk

Bacterial cell concentration, lactic acid (LA) content, and total protein (TP) content were determined in the FMs and PFMs. The cell concentrations were determined at 48 h of fermentation by counts on plates of MRS agar. The LA and TP contents were determined by AOAC techniques 2000. The titratable acidity was expressed as percent LA titrated in 10 mL of fermented milk, using NaOH (0.1 N) and phenolphtalein as the indicator. TP was quantified by the Kjeldahl method using a nitrogen-to-protein conversion factor of 6.25.

2.3. Determination of Exopolysaccharide

The exopolysaccharides (EPS) were precipitated from the supernatant of FM at 48 h of fermentation. Samples were centrifuged ($3600\times g$, 60 min, 10 °C), and the supernatants were recovered. Afterwards, trichloroacetic acid solution (20% v/v, Sigma-Aldrich) was added to the supernatants, which were incubated for 2 h at 4 °C. Precipitated proteins were removed by centrifugation ($3600\times g$, 60 min, and 10 °C). Next, the supernatants were treated with two volumes of cold ethanol, followed by 12 h of incubation at 4 °C. The EPS were recovered by centrifugation and posteriorly suspended in 1 mL of milli-Q water. The total EPS content was estimated for each sample by the phenol-sulfuric method using glucose as the standard [16].

2.4. Animal Study

Seventy mice C57Bl/6 (weight 30 g, six weeks old) were obtained from BIOINVERT (Mexico City, Mexico). The mice were randomly allocated into seven groups ($n = 10$/group) using a simple randomization procedure (computerized random numbers) based on their initial weight to obtain statistically equal groups (ANOVA, $p > 0.05$). Intestinal chronic inflammation was induced by the administration of dextran sulfate sodium (DSS). The mice were divided into the following treatment groups: (1) negative control (water); (2) DSS group; (3) AM + DSS (AM); (4) FM-J20 + DSS (FM-J20); (5) PFM-J20 + DSS (PFM-J20); (6) FM-J28 + DSS (FM-J28); and (7) PFM-J28 + DSS (PFM-J28). Half of the animals from each group were tested in a model of mild inflammation (six weeks) to evaluate the course of inflammation. The other mice were tested up to the end of the experimental period to evaluate chronic/systemic inflammation. Mice were housed in a controlled environment (22 °C, 12 h/12 h light/dark cycle) and fed a conventional diet and water *ad libitum*. This study, including the corresponding animal experiment, was approved by the Bioethics Committee of the Research Center for Food and Development (CIAD for its Spanish acronym), Hermosillo, Sonora, Mexico (CE/002/2015).

Mice were intragastrically fed 800 µL/day/mouse of either FM or water (control groups) for 10 weeks. To induce chronic inflammation, mice were intragastrically fed with 3% (w/v) DSS (40 kDa; Sigma-Aldrich) dissolved in sterile water. Mice were treated with four cycles of DSS. For each cycle, mice were fed with 200 µL/day/mouse for seven days; subsequently, between each cycle, mice drank water normally for seven days [6] (Figure 1). Body weight and water and food consumption were recorded daily. Half of the animals per group were euthanized at Week 6, while the rest of the mice underwent two additional rounds of DSS administration and milk feeding and were euthanized at Week 10.

The body weight initial ranged from 27.2 ± 4.9 g to 30.0 ± 3.1 g. The body weight gain was 4.2 ± 9.2 g and was highest for water group and lowest for the LFJ28 group.

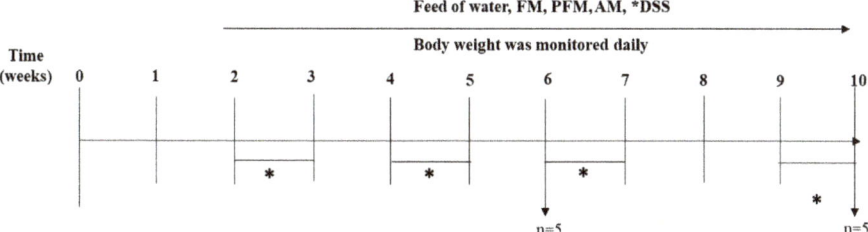

Figure 1. Experimental design. FM + DSS, PFM + DSS, and AM experimental groups of mice received daily treatments from Week 1 to Week 10. Mice received DSS in Week 2, 4, 6, and 9. *DSS administration period

2.4.1. Serum, Organ, and Mucosa Collection

After mice were euthanized ($n = 5$), the spleen and colon were removed. Spleens were weighed, and the colon lengths were measured. Blood samples were collected by cardiac puncture. The blood samples were allowed to clot at room temperature for 30 min before centrifugation (3500 rpm, 5 min, 4 °C), and the serum was collected and stored at −80 °C until further analysis.

For the mucosal collection, segments of the distal colon were removed from mice, cut open longitudinally, and mixed with 1 mL of fresh RPMI 1640 medium (Sigma-Aldrich) supplemented with penicillin–streptomycin (1%). Then, the samples were incubated at 37 °C for 24 h. The culture supernatants were harvested by centrifugation ($3600 \times g$, 10 min, 10 °C), and stored at −20 °C until being assayed [17].

2.4.2. Quantification of Cytokines

Murine IFNγ minimum detectable dose (MDD 1.8 pg/mL), IL-17 (MDD, 5 pg/mL), IL-22, and IL-23 (MDD 2.28 pg/mL) were evaluated in samples of serum and mucosal tissues by ELISA (R&D System). Serum samples were also used for quantification of IL-6 (MDD 1.4 pg/mL), IL-10 (MDD 6.8 pg/mL), TNFα (MDD 0.9 pg/mL), IFNγ (MDD 0.5 pg/mL), and IL-17 (0.8 pg/mL) (CBA kits, R & D Systems, San Jose, CA, USA) by flow cytometry (BD FACSCantoTM II, San Jose, CA, USA).

2.4.3. Histological Analysis

A histological examination of distal colon samples was performed by triplicate observations of three samples from the distal colon of each animal. Specifically, 0.5 cm of each sample were fixed in 10% buffered formalin, dehydrated in ethanol, paraffin embedded, and continuously sliced. Then, samples were deparaffinized, rehydrated, and stained with hematoxylin and eosin staining. The samples were evaluated under a $10\times$ light-fluorescent microscope (LEICA DM2000, Leica Mycrosystems Inc., Chicago, IL, USA) to observe morphological changes to colonic tissue and the imagens were processed in the LEICA V2 program.

2.5. Statistical Analysis

EPS, LA, TP, cell concentration, spleen weight, and colon length were analyzed by one-way ANOVAs. Differences among means per group were analyzed using Tukey–Kramer tests and were considered significant when $p < 0.05$. The cytokine values were analyzed using the non-parametric Kruskal–Wallis test; the data were presented as medians and considered significant when $p < 0.05$. The cytokine concentrations were determined by ELISA using ELISAanalysis.com software; the concentrations from CBA kits were analyzed using the BD FACSArrayTM bioanalyzer (Becton Dickinson, San Jose, CA, USA) Statistical differences were analyzed in the Minitab V.16.1.1. package.

3. Results and Discussion

Several studies have reported that an anti-inflammatory response may be attributed to the presence of LA bacteria and their cell components [18]. Additionally, other components, such as EPS released during the fermentation process [19] and LA present in the matrix of FM [20], may generate an anti-inflammatory response. Therefore, cell concentration, LA, EPS, and TP content from both FMs were analyzed and are described in Table 1. Notably, several bacteria are known to synthesize EPS; the EPS are associated with the cell surface or are present as slime. Some studies have reported on the role of EPS in protecting against desiccation and toxic compounds. In addition, an important characteristic of probiotics is the presence of EPS, which allows adhesion to solid surfaces and biofilm formation [16].

Under fermentation conditions, it was previously suggested that EPS production was associated with bacterial growth. In the present study, EPS production was determined at 48 h of fermentation, which corresponded with the highest cell concentration (9 log CFU/mL) for both FMs. FM-J28 showed the highest EPS concentration ($p < 0.05$). Some studies have described other conditions that may influence EPS production, such as type of bacteria, carbon source, and temperature of incubation [21]. Moreover, it has since been suggested that EPS may enhance the anti-inflammatory effect [19]. We determined that *Lactobacillus fermentum* was able to produce EPS under these fermentation conditions even though cell concentration, LA, and TP did not show significant differences ($p > 0.05$) among the milks fermented with different strains or the milks fermented with different strains that underwent pasteurization.

Table 1. Cell concentrations, total protein in fermented milk and metabolites derived from the fermentation process.

Fermented Milk	Cell Concentration (Log CFU/mL)	Lactic Acid (%)	Exopolysaccharides (mg/mL)	Total Protein (%)
FM-J20	9.0 ± 0.01 [a]	0.72 ± 0.01 [a]	50.99 ± 0.10 [a]	2.80 ± 0.04 [a]
PFM-J20	ND	0.75 ± 0.03 [a]	61.00 ± 0.15 [a]	2.71 ± 0.09 [a]
FM-J28	9.04 ± 0.01 [a]	0.90 ± 0.01 [a]	79.59 ± 0.05 [b]	3.01 ± 0.05 [a]
PFM-J28	ND	0.87 ± 0.01 [a]	77.30 ± 0.01 [b]	2.88 ± 0.07 [a]

ND = Not detected. The values are the means $\pm$ SD ($n = 3$). Different letters for a same parameter indicate statistical differences ($p < 0.05$) among dietary groups. Statistical differences were established by one-way ANOVAs and Tukey–Kramer Post Hoc tests. Raw (FM) and pasteurized (PFM) milks were fermented with *Lactobacillus fermentum* strains J20 and J28.

3.1. Anti-Inflammatory Response

Previous studies have demonstrated that, after four or five cycles of DSS administration, inflammation at the intestinal level may occur, affecting physiological parameters such as weight loss, intestine length, and the weight of other organs [22]. In the present study, the spleen of the DSS group had a significantly lower weight ($p < 0.05$) with respect to the water group at Week 6; however, it was not different ($p > 0.05$) compared to the groups administered with either FM. Conversely, in the end assay, the spleen weight did not significantly differ among groups ($p > 0.05$) (Figure 2). Furthermore, spleen weight at Weeks 6 and 10 for each group presented statistical differences ($p < 0.05$); the highest weight was found at Week 10 for the groups administered with DSS or FM + DSS.

The importance of the spleen as a secondary organ in the immune response may be highlighted. It is one of the sites where the immune response may be regulated and also stores immunological cells such as B and T cells, dendritic cells, and macrophages, which exert discrete functions [23]. Studies have demonstrated that, during inflammatory processes, spleen weight may increase because of immune activation or infection, leading to the hyperactivity of the spleen [12]. In the present study, the spleen weight increased in all treatments at Week 10, with exception of the water group; however, these differences were not significant ($p > 0.05$), indicating that the effect of DSS and FM treatments may be limited.

Colon length did not differ significantly among all groups ($p > 0.05$) nor between Weeks 6 and 10, which may indicate a low response to the inflammatory process during the study period.

The administration of DSS is known to reproducibly induce mild intestinal inflammation and the development of ulcers in mice, increasing neutrophil counts in the intestine [24]. In this regard, the capacity of Th17 cells to secrete IL-17 but not IFNγ or IL-4 has been described; these prior cells play an important role in the mediation of the inflammation process and tissue destruction [25,26]. Therefore, it is important to know their functions and develop strategies that block their response at local level, principally in IBDs [27].

The serum cytokine profiles at Week 6 showed a significant increase in IL-17 in the groups subjected to DSS-induced inflammation with respect to the water group ($p < 0.05$) (Figure 3A). Meanwhile, the concentration of IFNγ in the DSS group was enhanced compared to the water group at Week 6, yet decreased by Week 10 ($p < 0.05$) (Figure 3B). The concentration of IFN-γ in serum samples was enhanced at Week 6 for the DSS groups FM-J20 and PFM-J28. These values corresponded with an enhancement in the Th1 response, as various reports have documented. The inflammation process, as based on IL-17, was sufficient at Week 6; hence, by Week 10, the organisms were possibly able to regulate the inflammation process. In our study, for example, the FM-J28 group at Week 6 showed enhanced IL-17 but not IFN. This is a possible response mechanism to a low concentration of IFNγ. Finally, IL-22 and IL-23 were not detected.

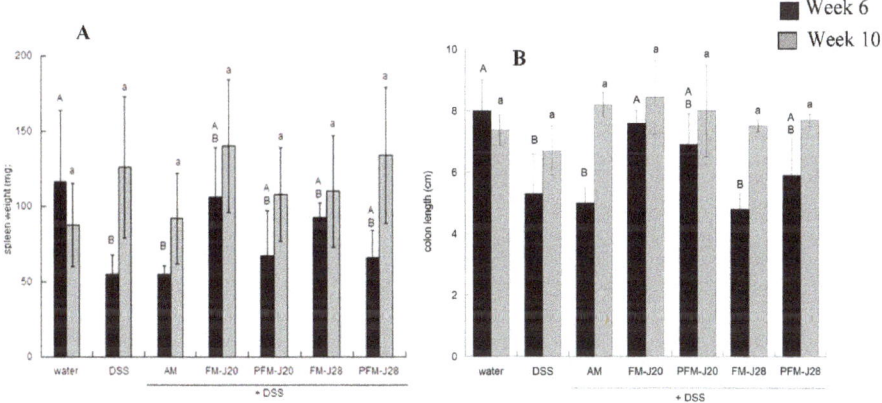

Figure 2. Effect of dextran sulfate sodium and fermented milk administration on spleen weight (**A**) and colon length (**B**) at Weeks 6 (black) and 10 (grey). Bars with an uppercase letter indicate statistical differences at Week 6 among treatments, and bars with a lowercase letter indicate statistical differences at Week 10 according to the Tukey–Kramer test ($p < 0.05$). The values are the means ± SD ($n = 5$).

The groups administered with FM-J20 and PFM-J20 showed the lowest concentration of IL-17 ($p < 0.05$) at Weeks 6 and 10. FM-J20 and PFM-J20 differed in the presence of viable bacterial cells, yet both FMs were able to decrease the concentration of IL-17, suggesting that different components from FM are involved in this effect. However, no statistical difference was encountered at Week 10 with respect to the DSS group ($p > 0.05$). Furthermore, IL-6 and TNFα did not show statistical differences among treatments and the control (DSS and water) at Weeks 6 and 10 ($p > 0.05$) (Figure 3C,D). However, the concentration of IL-10 cytokine did significantly differ ($p < 0.05$) (Figure 3E); the groups administered with PFM-J20 and FM J28 presented the highest concentration at Weeks 6 and 10, respectively.

It was previously reported that the expression of the genes that encode for IL-6, IL-1β, IL-23A, TGFβ, and STAT3 are involved in the differentiation of Th17 cells in a DSS-induced inflammation model [28]. Furthermore, studies have demonstrated that Th17 cells require specific cytokines such as

IL-23, which mediates the expansion of IL-17. On the other hand, low levels of IFNγ and IFNα may enhance the gene expression of IL-17 and IL-17-producing cells generated by IL-23 stimulation [29].

The findings reported in the present work are in agreement with those of other studies. For example, the administration of VSL#3 probiotics decreased TNFα and IL-6 and increased IL-10 serum levels in a DSS-induced colitis model of inflammation [10]. However, the concentration of inflammatory cytokines in our study is minor compared with other studies, which may indicate that the response following FM intake is lower in our inflammation model. Different compounds derived from FM are responsible for the anti-inflammatory effect [30,31]. For instance, milk fermented with *Lactobacillus rhamnosus* GG (LGG) was found to reduce colonic inflammation and injury and to also stimulate the activation of EGFR and Akt pathways while suppressing cytokine-induced apoptosis. This effect was attributed to the soluble proteins p40 and p75 present in milk fermented with LGG [15]. Furthermore, the immunoprotective effect of probiotic Dahi containing *Lactobacillus acidophilus* LaVK2 and *Bifidobacterium bifidum* BbVK3 on DSS-induced ulcerative colitis in mice was demonstrated to significantly reduce TNFα, IL-6, and IFNγ cytokines in colonic tissue [14].

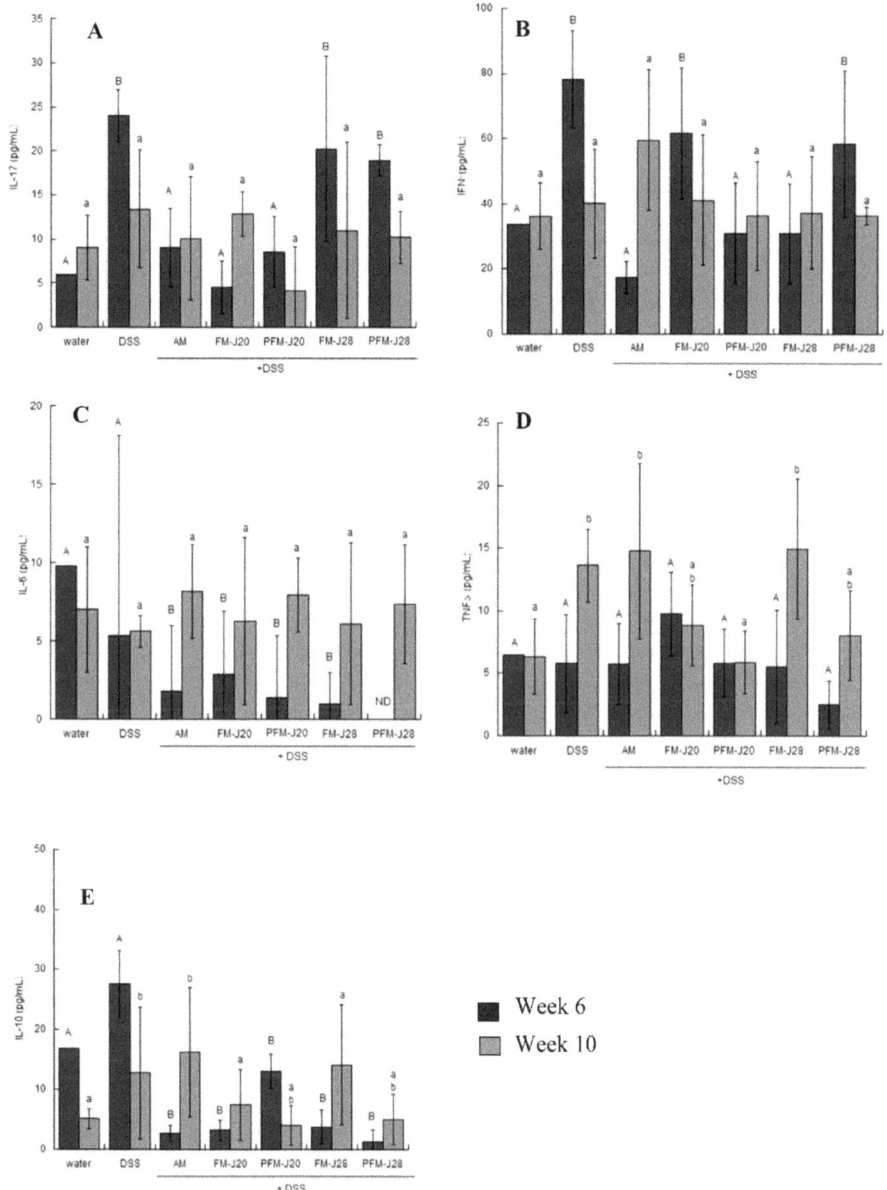

Figure 3. Effects of DSS and fermented milk administration on: IL-17 (**A**); and IFNγ (**B**) in serum samples, determined by ELISA; and on: IL-6 (**C**); TNFα (**D**); and IL-10 (**E**), determined by flow cytometry at Weeks 6 and 10. Bars with an uppercase letter indicate statistical differences at Week 6 among treatments, and bars with a lowercase letter indicate statistical differences at Week 10 ($p < 0.05$) according to the Kruskal–Wallis test. The values correspond to medians ± interquartile ranges for $n = 5$.

Several reports have shown the different mechanisms of action involved in the anti-inflammatory effect of probiotics, but few studies have demonstrated possible pathways at the cellular level.

One possible mechanism of action may be related with cell viability or cell wall components, which can be internalized into M cells, interact with dendritic cells, and then down-regulate the production of the pro-inflammatory cytokines IL-1β, IL-6, IL-17, TNFα, and IFNγ [32,33]. Furthermore, bioactive peptides have shown anti-inflammatory activity by down-regulating LPS-induced cytokine production in monocytes cells via the NF-kB pathway [34].

Moreover, LA may induce different inflammatory responses in LPS-stimulated RAW 264.7 cells. Some studies have reported its association with metabolic acidosis, which frequently complicates sepsis and septic shock and may be deleterious for cellular function. In this study, the AM group showed no statistical difference ($p > 0.05$) with respect to the control group and FM groups; however, it is important to carry out further studies on LA and its role in inflammatory processes.

In the determination of cytokines in samples of intestinal mucosal (Figure 4), FM-J20, FM-J28, and PFM-J28 showed statistical differences ($p < 0.05$) among treatments with respect to the controls (DSS and water). However, IFNγ levels were not statistically different ($p > 0.05$), and IL-23 was not detected at the mucosal level. These results correspond with those reported in other studies wherein the presence of IFNγ inhibited IL-17 [5]. IL-23 is important for the expansion, stabilization, and conditioning of the Th17 response; hence, the IL-23/17 axis may be considered as a hallmark and an attractive probiotic therapeutic target in IBD [32]. The study by Jadhav et al. [14] showed the lowest concentrations of TNFα, IL-6, and IFNγ in samples of colonic tissue from mice administered with Dahi (fermented dairy) + DSS as well as a group administered probiotic + DSS.

This effect has also been observed in mice following the administration of milk fermented with *Bifidobacterium* strains. In particular, these mice showed a lower concentration of TNFα in culture supernatants, while IL-10 increased in the FM group and also reduced the histological score compared to treatments with saline and unfermented milk [35]. A possible mechanism for the anti-inflammatory effect may be related to the inhibition or modulation of the expression of several genes such as NF-kB, RELB, and TNFα, which have been reported as active during inflammation processes [36].

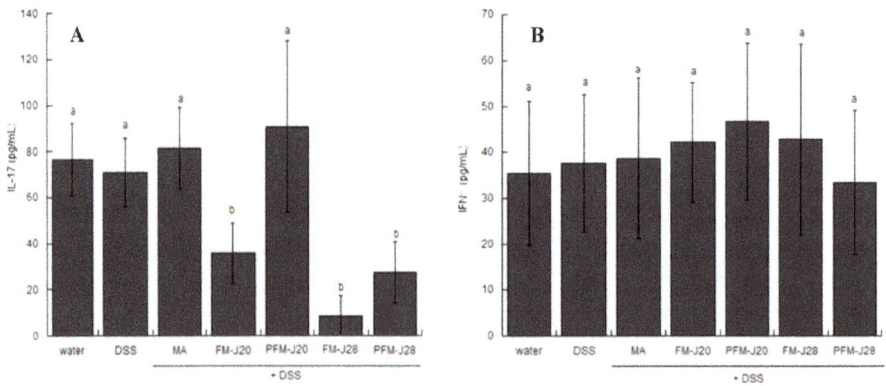

Figure 4. The effect of DSS and fermented milk administration on IL-17 (**A**) and IFNγ (**B**) determined by ELISA of colonic mucosa at Week 10. Different letters show statistical differences ($p < 0.05$) among treatments according to the Kruskal–Wallis test. The values are medians ± interquartile ranges ($n = 5$).

The binding of IL-10 to its receptor triggers phosphorylation-dependent activation of the transcription factor STAT3, which upregulates the gene expression of members of the SOCS family and proinflammatory cytokines such as TNFα and macrophage inflammatory protein 2. However, this process is possibly inhibited by the presence of bacteria or other components, such as EPS [37].

Histological Analysis

The DSS inflammation process is characterized by histological findings such as edema, infiltration of inflammatory cells into both the mucosa and submucosa, and destruction of epithelial cells [28]. Our results indicated that neither the administration of DSS or fermented milk affected the structure of mucosa or submucosa (Figure 5). A low number of inflammatory cells infiltrated (Figure 5B) but did not result in mucosal injury. Therefore, the histological analysis of samples confirmed that the inflammation process was not extensive; this finding may suggest that the presence of pro-inflammatory cytokines did not cause extensive changes. On the other hand, some studies have suggested that invasion of inflammatory cells into the mucosa produces increased concentrations of inflammatory cytokines such as TNFα, which then induce the expression of genes associated with inflammation [10]. In addition, DSS may induce the expression of COX-2, an enzyme responsible for the formation of prostanoids [38] that has been shown to be specifically induced in epithelial cells under IBD conditions [39].

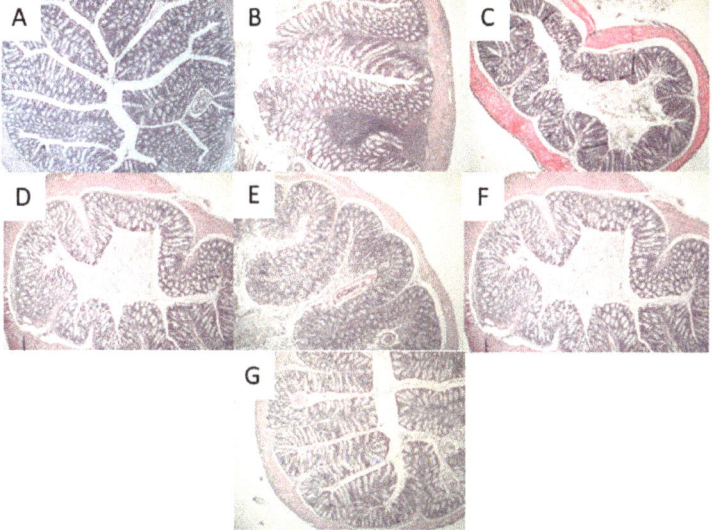

Figure 5. Histological analysis of cross sections of colon tissue samples stained with hematoxylin–eosin (10×): (**A**) water control group; (**B**) DSS group; (**C**) AM + DSS group; (**D**) FM-J20 + DSS group; (**E**) PFM-J20 + DSS group; (**F**) FM-J28 + DSS group; and (**G**) PFM-J28 + DSS group.

These findings show that FM administration may prevent intestinal inflammation by stabilizing mucosal immunity through different components or metabolites derived during the fermentation process [13]. In particular, the present results show that the administration of FM could mediate the Th1/Th17 response, but more studies are required to determine the possible metabolites involved and the activation pathways. The interaction of derivative compounds from fermentation, such as LA and EPS, as well as the presence of bacteria could result in an anti-inflammatory response that stimulates IL-10 production and inhibits TNFα despite the interaction of TLR2 and TLR4 and activation of NF-kB. For example, in one previous study, the presence of LA and *Lactobacillus casei* Shirota culture supernatants suppressed phosphorylation and degradation of I-kB-α [40].

4. Conclusions

In the present study, several strategies to reduce inflammation in an IBD model employing milk fermented with *Lactobacillus* strains were evaluated. The administration of milk fermented with *Lactobacillus fermentum* possibly decreased the inflammatory response at Week 6 because of the metabolites or cell components present in this product. However, further studies are needed to determine the modulation of Th1/Th17 by fermented milk. The findings in the present study show the potential regulatory effect of FM on the inflammatory process, although this effect was minor, possibly as a result of irregularity in the inflammatory process. Future studies are needed to establish an adequate model of inflammation that allows the Th17 response to be evaluated considering the other biomarkers involved in this response, including chemokines, transcription factors, and metabolites released during fermentation, as well as cell differentiation, which may all be responsible for promoting an anti-inflammatory response.

Author Contributions: A.F.G.-C., A.H.-M., V.M.-H., B.V.-C., A.W.-M., H.A.-G. and L.S.-L. designed the study. V.M.-H. and L.S.-L. contributed to the flow cytometer analysis of the samples. L.S.-L. wrote the manuscript. V.M.-H., A.H.-M. and A.F.G.-C. revised the manuscript. A.W.-M. contributed to the histological analysis. H.A.-G., B.V.-C. and M.d.C.E.-M. provided valuable scientific knowledge and advisory throughout the study.

Funding: This study was supported by the Mexican Council of Science and Technology (CONACyT; Mexico City) research project 240338 CONACyT.

Acknowledgments: The authors would like to thank Alejandro Santos-Espinosa, Alejandro Epigmenio-Chavez, Lilia María Beltrán-Barrientos, and Miguel Angel Rendón-Rosales for their technical assistance in this study. The authors would also like to thank the Mexican Council of Science and Technology (CONACyT) for the graduate scholarship provided to L. Santiago-López. Histological analyses were performed with equipment acquired with funding from the Comprehensive Institutional Strengthening Program (PIFI) 2007-2008, 2909 5001-004-09

Conflicts of Interest: The authors declare that they have no conflicts of interest regarding the publication of this paper.

References

1. Chami, B.; Yeung, A.W.S.; van Vreden, C.; King, N.J.C.; Bao, S. The role of CXCR3 in DSS-induced colitis. *PLoS ONE* **2014**, *9*, e101622. [CrossRef] [PubMed]
2. O'Shea, J.J.; Murray, P.J. Cytokine signaling modules in inflammatory responses. *Immunity* **2008**, *28*, 477–487. [CrossRef] [PubMed]
3. Ito, R.; Kita, M.; Shin-Ya, M.; Kishida, T.; Urano, A.; Takada, R.; Sakagami, J.; Imanishi, J.; Iwakura, Y.; Okanoue, T.; et al. Involvement of IL-17A in the pathogenesis of DSS-induced colitis in mice. *Biochem. Biophys. Res. Commun.* **2008**, *377*, 12–16. [CrossRef] [PubMed]
4. Weaver, C.T.; Elson, C.O.; Fouser, L.A.; Kolls, J.K. The Th17 Pathway and inflammatory diseases of the intestines, lungs, and skin. *Annu. Rev. Pathol. Mech. Dis.* **2013**, *8*, 477–512. [CrossRef] [PubMed]
5. Feng, T.; Qin, H.; Wang, L.; Benveniste, E.N.; Elson, C.O.; Cong, Y. Th17 cells induce colitis and promote Th1 cell responses through IL-17 induction of innate IL-12 and IL-23 production. *J. Immunol.* **2011**, *186*, 6313–6318. [CrossRef] [PubMed]
6. Alex, P.; Zachos, N.C.; Nguyen, T.; Gonzales, L.; Chen, T.E.; Conklin, L.S.; Centola, M.; Li, X. Distinct cytokines patterns identified from multiplex profiles of murine DSS and TNBS-Induced Colitis. *Inflamm. Bowel Dis.* **2009**, *15*, 341–352. [CrossRef] [PubMed]
7. Aden, K.; Rehman, A.; Falk-Paulsen, M.; Secher, T.; Kuiper, J.; Tran, F.; Pfeuffer, S.; Sheibani-Tezerji, R.; Breuer, A.; Luzius, A.; et al. Epithelial IL-23R signaling licenses protective IL-22 responses in intestinal inflammation. *Cell Rep.* **2016**, *16*, 2208–2218. [CrossRef] [PubMed]
8. Zheng, B.; van Bergenhegouwen, J.; Overbeek, S.; van de Kant, H.J.G.; Garssen, J.; Folkerts, G.; Vos, P.; Morgan, M.E.; Kraneveld, A.D. *Bifidobacterium breve* attenuates murine dextran sodium sulfate-induced colitis and increases regulatory T cell responses. *PLoS ONE* **2014**, *9*, e95441. [CrossRef] [PubMed]
9. Zakostelska, Z.; Kverka, M.; Klimesova, K.; Rossmann, P.; Mrazek, J.; Kopecny, J.; Hornova, M.; Srutkova, D.; Hudcovic, T.; Ridl, J.; et al. Lysate of probiotic *Lactobacillus casei* DN-114 001 ameliorates colitis by strengthening the gut barrier function and changing the gut microenvironment. *PLoS ONE* **2011**, *6*, e27961. [CrossRef] [PubMed]
10. Dai, C.; Zheng, C.Q.; Meng, F.J.; Zhou, Z.; Sang, L.X.; Jiang, M. VSL#3 probiotics exerts the anti-inflammatory activity via PI3k/Akt and NF-κB pathway in rat model of DSS-induced colitis. *Mol. Cell. Biochem.* **2013**, *374*, 1–11. [PubMed]

11. Chiba, Y.; Shida, K.; Nagata, S.; Wada, M.; Bian, L.; Wang, C.; Shimizu, T.; Yamashiro, Y.; Kiyoshima-Shibata, J.; Nanno, M.; et al. Well-controlled proinflammatory cytokine responses of Peyer's patch cells to probiotic *Lactobacillus casei*. *Immunology* **2010**, *130*, 352–362. [CrossRef] [PubMed]
12. Herías, M.V.; Koninkx, J.F.; Vos, J.G.; Huis in't Veld, J.H.; van Dijk, J.E. Probiotic effects of *Lactobacillus casei* on DSS-induced ulcerative colitis in mice. *Int. J. Food Microbiol.* **2005**, *103*, 143–155. [CrossRef] [PubMed]
13. Imaoka, A.; Umesaki, Y. Rationale for Using of *Bifidobacterium* probiotic strains-fermented milk against colitis based on animal experiments and clinical trials. *Probiotics Antimicrob. Proteins* **2008**, *1*, 8–14. [CrossRef] [PubMed]
14. Jadhav, S.R.; Shandilya, U.K.; Kansal, V.K. Immunoprotective effect of probiotic Dahi Containing *Lactobacillus acidophilus* and *Bifidobacterium bifidum* on dextran sodium sulfate-induced ulcerative colitis in mice. *Probiotics Antimicrob. Proteins* **2012**, *4*, 21–26. [CrossRef] [PubMed]
15. Yoda, K.; Miyazawa, K.; Hosoda, M.; Hiramatsu, M.; Yan, F.; He, F. *Lactobacillus* GG-fermented milk prevents DSS-induced colitis and regulates intestinal epithelial homeostasis through activation of epidermal growth factor receptor. *Eur. J. Nutr.* **2014**, *53*, 105–115. [CrossRef] [PubMed]
16. Tallon, R.; Bressollier, P.; Urdaci, M.C. Isolation and characterization of two exopolysaccharides produced by *Lactobacillus plantarum* EP56. *Res. Microbiol.* **2003**, *154*, 705–712. [CrossRef] [PubMed]
17. Nanda-Kumar, N.S.; Balamurugan, R.; Jayakanthan, K.; Pulimood, A.; Pugazhendhi, S.; Ramakrishna, B.S. Probiotic administration alters the gut flora and attenuates colitis in mice administered dextran sodium sulfate. *J. Gastroenterol. Hepatol.* **2008**, *23*, 1834–1839. [CrossRef] [PubMed]
18. Taverniti, V.; Guglielmetti, S. The immunomodulatory properties of probiotic microorganisms beyond their viability (ghost probiotics: Proposal of paraprobiotic concept). *Genes Nutr.* **2011**, *6*, 261–274. [CrossRef] [PubMed]
19. Hidalgo-Cantabrana, C.; Algieri, F.; Rodriguez-Nogales, A. Effect of a Ropy *Bifidobacterium animalis* subsp. *lactis* Strain orally administered on DSS-induced colitis mice Model. *Front. Microbiol.* **2016**, *7*, 868. [CrossRef] [PubMed]
20. Kellum, J.A.; Song, M.; Li, J. Lactic and hydrochloric acids induce different patterns of inflammatory response in LPS-stimulated RAW 264.7 cells. *Am. J. Physiol. Regul. Intregr. Comp. Physiol.* **2004**, *286*, 686–692. [CrossRef] [PubMed]
21. Degeest, B.; Janssens, B.; De Vuyst, L. Exopolysaccharide (EPS) biosynthesis by *Lactobacillus sakei* 0-1: Production kinetics, enzyme activities and EPS yields. *J. Appl. Microbiol.* **2001**, *91*, 470–477. [CrossRef] [PubMed]
22. Morgan, M.E.; Zheng, B.; Koolink, P.J.; van de Kant, H.J.G.; Haazen, L.C.; van Roest, M.; Garssen, J.; Folkerts, G.; Kraneveld, A.D. New Perspective on Dextran Sodium sulfate colitis: Antigen-specific T cell development during intestinal inflammation. *PLoS ONE* **2013**, *8*, e69936. [CrossRef] [PubMed]
23. Bronte, V.; Pittet, M. The spleen in local and systemic regulation of immunity. *Immunity* **2014**, *39*, 806–818. [CrossRef] [PubMed]
24. Ohtsuka, Y.; Sanderson, I. Dextran sulfate Sodium-Induced inflammation is enhanced by intestinal epithelial cell chemokine expression in mice. *Pediatr. Res.* **2003**, *53*, 143–147. [PubMed]
25. Fischer, A. Human immunodeficiency: Connecting STATA3, Th17 and human mucosal immunity. *Immunol. Cell Biol.* **2008**, *86*, 549–551. [CrossRef] [PubMed]
26. Tesmer, L.; Lundy, S.; Sarkar, S.; Fox, D. Th17 cells in human disease. *Immunol. Rev.* **2008**, *223*, 87–113. [CrossRef] [PubMed]
27. Crome, S.Q.; Wang, A.Y.; Levings, M.K. Translational mini-review series on Th17 cells: Function and regulation of human T helper 17 cells in health and disease. *Clin. Exp. Immunol.* **2010**, *159*, 109–119. [CrossRef] [PubMed]
28. Ogawa, A.; Andoh, A.; Araki, Y.; Bamba, T.; Fujiyama, Y. Neutralization of interleukin-17 aggravates dextran sulfate sodium-induced colitis in mice. *Clin. Immunol.* **2004**, *110*, 55–62. [CrossRef] [PubMed]
29. Liu, Z.J.; Yadav, P.K.; Su, J.L.; Wang, J.S.; Fei, K. Potential role of Th17 cells in the pathogenesis of inflammatory bowel disease. *World J. Gastroenterol.* **2009**, *15*, 5784–5788. [CrossRef] [PubMed]
30. Granier, A.; Goulet, O.; Hoarau, C. Fermentation products: Immunological effects on human and animal models. *Pediatr. Res.* **2013**, *74*, 238–244. [CrossRef] [PubMed]
31. Bordoni, A.; Danesi, F.; Dardevet, D.; Dupont, D.; Fernandez, A.S.; Gille, D.; Nunes, C.; Pinto, P.; Re, R.; Rémond, D.; et al. Dairy products and inflammation: A review of the clinical evidence. *Crit. Rev. Food Sci. Nutr.* **2017**, *57*, 2497–2525. [CrossRef] [PubMed]

32. Owaga, E.; Hsieh, R.-H.; Mugendi, B.; Masuku, S.; Shinh, C.-K.; Chang, J.-S. Th17 cells as potential probiotic therapeutic targets in inflammatory bowel diseases. *Int. J. Mol. Sci.* **2015**, *16*, 20841–20858. [CrossRef] [PubMed]
33. Lee, H.S.; Han, S.Y.; Bae, E.A.; Huh, C.H.S.; Ahn, Y.T.; Lee, J.H.K.; Kim, D.H. Lactic acid bacteria inhibit proinflammatory cytokine expression and bacterial glycosaminoglycan degradation activity in dextran sulfate sodium-induced colitic mice. *Int. Immunopharmacol.* **2008**, *8*, 574–580. [CrossRef] [PubMed]
34. Håversen, L.; Ohlsson, B.G.; Hahn-Zoric, M.; Hanson, L.Å.; Mattsby-Baltzer, I. Lactoferrin down-regulates the LPS-induced cytokine production in monocytic cells via NF-κB. *Cell. Immunol.* **2002**, *220*, 83–95. [CrossRef]
35. Matsumoto, S.; Watanabe, N.; Imaka, A.; Okabe, Y. Preventive effects of *Bifidobacterium* and *Lactobacillus*-fermented milk on the development of inflammatory bowel disease in senescence-accelerated mouse P1/Yit strain mice. *Digestion* **2001**, *64*, 92–99. [CrossRef] [PubMed]
36. Haileselassie, Y.; Navis, M.; Vu, N.; Qazi, K.R.; Rethi, B.; Sverremark-Ekström, E. Postbiotic modulation of retinoic acid imprinted mucosal-like dendritic cells by probiotic *Lactobacillus reuteri* 17938 in vitro. *Front. Immunol.* **2016**, *7*, 96. [CrossRef] [PubMed]
37. Mirpuri, J.; Sotnikov, I.; Denning, T.L.; Yarovinsky, F.; Parkos, C.A.; Denning, P.W.; Louis, N.A. *Lactobacillus rhamnosus* (LGG) regulates IL-10 signaling in the developing murine colon through upregulation of the IL-10R2 receptor subunit. *PLoS ONE* **2012**, *7*, e51955. [CrossRef] [PubMed]
38. Krieglstein, C.F.; Cerwinka, W.H.; Laroux, F.S.; Salter, J.W.; Russell, J.M.; Schuermann, G.; Grisham, M.B.; Ross, C.R.; Granger, D.N. Regulation of murine intestinal inflammation by reactive metabolites of oxygen and nitrogen: Divergent roles of superoxide and nitric oxide. *J. Exp. Med.* **2001**, *194*, 1207–1218. [CrossRef] [PubMed]
39. Menchen, L.; Colon, A.L.; Madrigal, J.L.; Beltran, L.; Botella, S.; Lizasoain, I.; Leza, J.C.; Moro, M.A.; Menchen, P.; Cos, E.; et al. Activity of inducible and neuronal nitric oxide synthases in colonic mucosa predicts progression of ulcerative colitis. *Am. J. Gastroenterol.* **2004**, *99*, 1756–1764. [CrossRef] [PubMed]
40. Watanabe, T.; Nishio, H.; Tanigawa, T.; Yamagami, H.; Okazaki, H.; Watanabe, K.; Tominaga, K.; Fujiwara, Y.; Oshitani, N.; Asahara, T.; et al. Probiotic *Lactobacillus casei* strain Shirota prevents indomethacin-induced small intestinal injury: Involvement of lactic acid. *Am. J. Physiol. Gastrointest. Liver Physiol.* **2009**, *297*, G506–G513. [CrossRef] [PubMed]

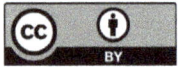

© 2018 by the authors. Licensee MDPI, Basel, Switzerland. This article is an open access article distributed under the terms and conditions of the Creative Commons Attribution (CC BY) license (http://creativecommons.org/licenses/by/4.0/).

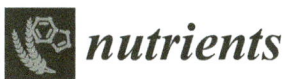

Review

Infant Complementary Feeding of Prebiotics for the Microbiome and Immunity

Starin McKeen [1,2,3], **Wayne Young** [1,2,3], **Jane Mullaney** [1,2,3], **Karl Fraser** [1,2,3], **Warren C. McNabb** [2,3] and **Nicole C. Roy** [1,2,3],*

1. AgResearch, Food Nutrition & Health, Grasslands Research Centre, Private Bag 11008, Palmerston north 4442, New Zealand; Starin.Mckeen@agresearch.co.nz (S.M.); Wayne.Young@agresearch.co.nz (W.Y.); Jane.Mullaney@agresearch.co.nz (J.M.); Karl.Fraser@agresearch.co.nz (K.F.)
2. Riddet Institute, Massey University, Private Bag 11222, Palmerston North 4442, New Zealand; W.McNabb@massey.ac.nz
3. High-Value Nutrition National Science Challenge, Auckland, New Zealand
* Correspondence: Nicole.Roy@agresearch.co.nz; Tel.: +64-6-3518-1101

Received: 7 January 2019; Accepted: 6 February 2019; Published: 9 February 2019

Abstract: Complementary feeding transitions infants from a milk-based diet to solid foods, providing essential nutrients to the infant and the developing gut microbiome while influencing immune development. Some of the earliest microbial colonisers readily ferment select oligosaccharides, influencing the ongoing establishment of the microbiome. Non-digestible oligosaccharides in prebiotic-supplemented formula and human milk oligosaccharides promote commensal immune-modulating bacteria such as *Bifidobacterium*, which decrease in abundance during weaning. Incorporating complex, bifidogenic, non-digestible carbohydrates during the transition to solid foods may present an opportunity to feed commensal bacteria and promote balanced concentrations of beneficial short chain fatty acid concentrations and vitamins that support gut barrier maturation and immunity throughout the complementary feeding window.

Keywords: weaning; oligosaccharides; non-digestible carbohydrates; metabolites; gut barrier; tolerance

1. Introduction

The strategic introduction of prebiotic compounds during weaning presents an opportunity to promote infant health and to support development via balanced co-maturation of the gut microbiome and host. Between 4 and 6 months of age, nutrient demands of growing infants surpass what is provided by breastmilk or formula alone [1–4]. Complementary foods accompany and gradually replace breastmilk and formula throughout the weaning period, providing essential nutrients to the developing digestive system and modulating microbial colonisation [1,5–8]. The young immune system is influenced by the gut microbiome and supported by metabolites produced during the microbial fermentation of prebiotic compounds, leading to a tolerance for commensal microbes and specific responses to pathogens [9–15]. Prebiotic compounds in breastmilk and supplemented formulas promote commensal immune-modulating bacteria, such as *Bifidobacterium*, and beneficial metabolites, such as short chain fatty acids (SCFAs) and vitamins [16–21]. Introducing non-digestible starches through complementary foods may present an opportunity to promote commensal bacteria and support microbial production of beneficial metabolites throughout the complementary feeding window, with lasting effects on health [22–24].

Prior to weaning, the healthy infant gut microbiome is shaped by maternal factors, such as mode of birth, environment, and first foods: breastmilk and infant formula [10,25–33]. The establishment of microbial species changes dramatically throughout the first 2–3 years of life before stabilising at an adult-like composition [7]. While individual variations in taxonomic composition persist, analogous genes consistently and predictably fill similar functional and metabolic niches as new foods are introduced and formula or breastfeeding ceases [7]. Commensal species that colonise the immature gut modulate gene expression of epithelial and immune cells and, in turn, are regulated by adaptive and innate immune responses in the mucosal immune system [14,26,31,34–42].

Breastmilk and some types of prebiotic-supplemented formulas provide non-digestible oligosaccharides (NDOs) to the gut microbiome, which exert a strong influence on the microbial composition and metabolism [43]. The introduction of starchy foods such as cereals, porridges, and pureed tubers is common practice due to the neutral tastes, smooth textures, and ease of swallowing as oral coordination develops [44]. The role of these starches in the community dynamics of the immature and unstable infant microbiome remains unknown.

Based on investigations into human milk oligosaccharides (HMOs) and NDOs, prebiotic whole foods may support immunity and immune development through a variety of direct and indirect mechanisms. While poorly characterised compared to oligosaccharides, starches may act as receptor analogues to pathogens, reducing the quantity of enteric pathogens that reach the gut epithelium and subsequent infection [45]. Starches also promote populations of bacteria of which some strains directly interact with immunomodulatory factors in the gut mucosa [46]. These and other commensal bacteria also ferment starches into metabolites such as SCFAs and vitamins, which have known benefits to gut barrier integrity, immune-regulation, and immune response [47].

This review summarises the current body of knowledge on the complementary feeding of prebiotic starches for the microbiome with a focus on the interactions of commensal species, microbial metabolites, and the development of the gut barrier and immune system.

2. The Need to Complementary Feed

Complementary feeding is the necessary inclusion of solid foods alongside the milk-based diet of infants during the transition to adult foods. The inclusion of solid foods is recommended to coincide with sufficient oral maturation and an imbalance between the nutrient requirements of infants and the nutritional provisions of breastmilk and formula, as demonstrated in Figure 1 [44]. Previously, it was thought that the inclusion of solid foods in the diet was driven by an increase in the demand for energy and protein between 4 and 6 months of age. However, Krebs and Hambidge (1986) found that infants' absorption of zinc from breastmilk is inadequate to meet factorial estimates of requirements based on healthy growth curves [3]. Similarly, iron requirements increase with erythrocyte mass and myoglobin in lean tissue from 4–12 months of age, surpassing the low concentrations (0.2–0.4 mg/L) of highly bioavailable (50%) iron in breastmilk at approximately 6 months of age [48].

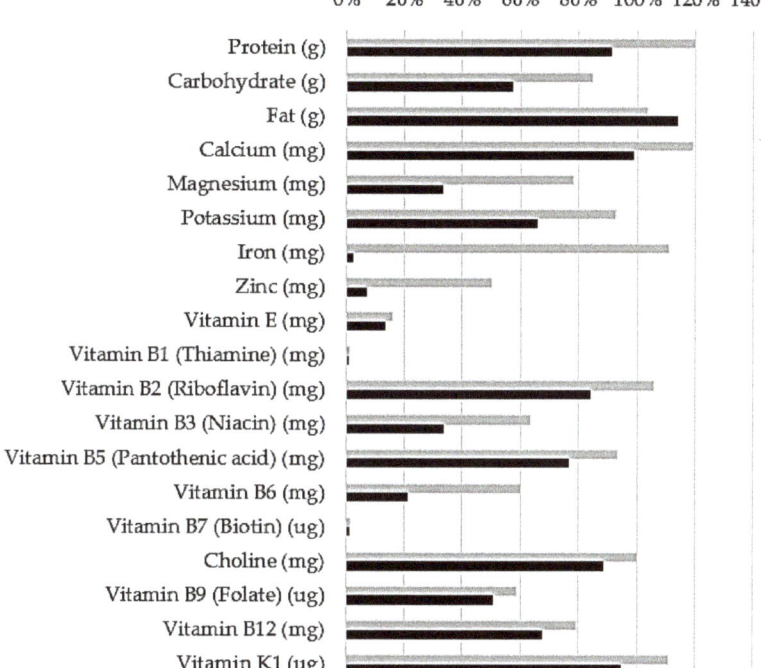

Figure 1. The percent of nutrient requirements based on the recommended daily intakes (RDIs) [49] that are met via average daily breastmilk consumption (750 mL from 0–6 months and 800 mL from 7–12 months) [50].

Timing of the introduction of solid foods has been investigated in both low- and high-income countries. Delaying solids until 6 months of age was previously thought to be associated with lower body mass index in high-income countries and with lower rates of allergy and decreased water-borne diarrheal disease in low- and middle-income countries [51,52]. However, recent studies in larger cohorts have challenged this assertion, proposing that individual oral maturation, nutrient requirements, and environmental disease burden should determine when to introduce solids [4]. Results from the PIAMA (Prevention and Incidence of Asthma and Mite Allergy) cohort in the Netherlands suggest that a short duration of breastfeeding (4 months or less) is associated with an increased risk for being overweight during childhood rather than the early introduction of solid foods, and the risk is not different between breastfed and formula-fed infants [53]. However, this study does not report on the types of solid foods that were introduced, the duration of the overlap of breastfeeding and solid feeding, or the potential mechanisms of metabolic programming.

In addition to nutritional provisions, breastmilk also provides non-nutritive and immune-modulatory factors that impart significant benefits, even in partial concentrations or shorter durations [12]. The health promoting properties of breastmilk include varying levels and types of carbohydrates, non-digestible HMOs, immunoglobulins (IgG, IgM, and isoforms of sIgA), amino acids, polyunsaturated fatty acids, monoglycerides, leuric acid, linoleic acid, cytokines, chemokines, soluble receptors, antibacterial proteins/peptides, and intact immune cells that are governed by maternal Lewis blood type, secretor status, and phase of lactation [54]. HMOs have received significant attention in infant nutrition for their ability to influence a variety of gut functions: epithelial integrity, mucosal integrity, susceptibility to pathogenic infection, microbial community structure, SCFA production, and vitamin synthesis. Over 2000 distinct HMO structures (Figure 2a) have been identified, with significant variation between individuals and phase of lactation, but a 9:1 ratio of galactooligosaccharides (GOS):fructoligosaccharides (FOS) is typical [55,56]. Infant formulas are continuing to develop based on an increasing understanding of the roles of each of these factors in microbiome maturation, brain development, and immunity. Synthetic and plant-derived GOS, FOS (Figure 2b), inulin, pectin, and β-glucans, either alone or in comparable ratios, are well characterised and have been primary targets of infant formula additive research and product development [56,57]. Staged and follow-on formulas that vary in composition according to the recommended daily allowances and the introduction of complementary foods are also increasingly recommended [2].

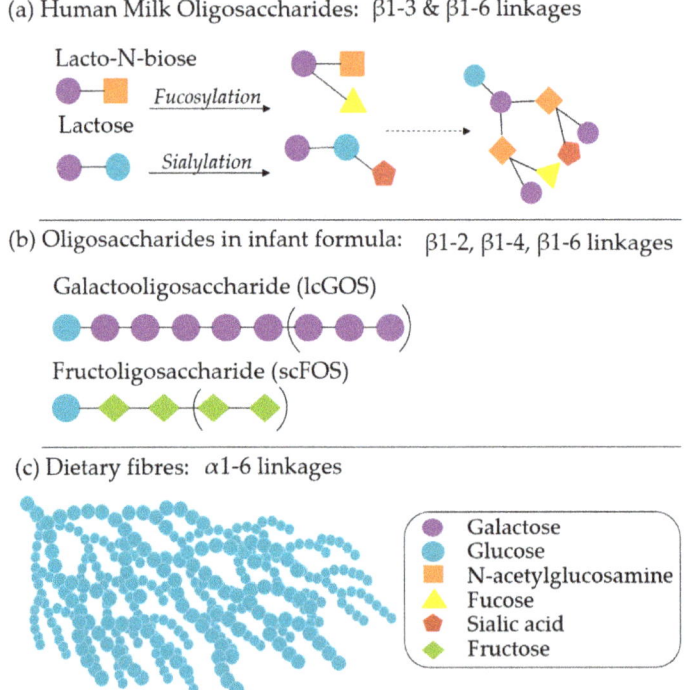

Figure 2. (a) The core structures of human milk oligosaccharides (HMOs), common modification pathways, and an example of a complex HMO, connected by β1-3 and β 1-6 linkages that are resistant to enzymatic cleavage by human-derived enzymes. (b) The structure of galactooligosaccharide (long chain) and fructoligosaccharide (short chain), which are common prebiotic molecules in supplemented infant formulas: β1-2, β1-4, and β1-6 linkages are resistant to enzymatic cleavage by human derived enzymes. (c) A model of dietary starch, characterized by glucose molecules connected by α1-6 linkages in a complex higher structure, which contributes to incomplete enzymatic cleavage by human enzymes.

Infant digestive systems are uniquely suited to digest macronutrients provided by breastmilk. The intestinal epithelium of neonates has narrow villi and small crypts (Figure 3), which duplicate and expand with age, a process which is influenced by components in breastmilk and host-microbe interactions [58]. The expansion of the epithelial surface during weaning is necessary to accommodate the increasing nutrient load, but dysregulation of this process can lead to hyperplastic crypts, blunted villi, inflammatory responses in the mucosa, and subsequent malabsorption of nutrients [59].

The enzymatic dynamics of infant digestion are poorly characterised due to wide variations between individuals over time and infrequent investigations with replicated results [60]. Lactose, fatty acids, and proteins are the most abundant macronutrients in milk, which are absorbed and utilised predominantly in the small intestine [20]. Lipase and trypsin (lipid and protein digestive enzymes) are present in concentrations comparable to adults and are sufficiently active at the less extreme pH (3.2) of the infant gut. However, amylase secretion and activity are distinct in infants. Compared to lipid and protein digestion, the ability to digest carbohydrates is limited to simple carbohydrates such as lactose and sucrose, rather than complex carbohydrates, until weaning. At weaning, salivary α-amylase and pancreatic α-amylase are present at reduced concentrations compared to that of adults [61]. However, glucoamylase (also referred to as amyloglucosidase), a brush border enzyme in the small intestine capable of cleaving α1,4-glycosidic bonds, is produced at 100–150% of adult concentrations at birth, which may compensate for the otherwise minimal starch hydrolysis [62,63]. Non-digestible structures such as HMOs and non-digestible carbohydrates (NDCs) resist complete enzymatic degradation and pass to the large intestine where they become available as a nutrient source for the enteric microbiota [64]. Breastfed infants also receive varying amounts of maternal amylase, as well as small concentrations of up to 50 other digestive enzymes, through breastmilk [65]. During weaning, infants that continue to consume breastmilk may have increased capacity to digest dietary starches compared to those receiving formulas, but this and the subsequent interactions with enteric microbes has yet to be investigated.

3. Gut Barrier Development

The epithelial barrier of the gut is formed by enterocytes, the primary absorptive cells with crypts and villi, connected by tight junctions (TJ). The absorption of nutrients occurs transepithelially (through) and paracellularly (between tight junction pores of ~4Å in healthy epithelia), requiring the specificity and structural functionality of TJ proteins [66]. Compromised barrier integrity is characteristic of inflammation and can lead to aberrant immune responses that have been implicated in the development of allergies [67]. Apart from the histomorphological analysis of tissue biopsies, epithelial integrity is measured in healthy infants by feeding non-digestible sugars, lactulose and mannitol, and then measuring their ratios in urine over a multi-hour collection to indicate paracellular sugar translocation into the bloodstream and subsequent excretion [68]. Faecal calprotectin has also been used as an indicator of barrier integrity; however, this is unreliable and highly variable among and within individuals and populations [68,69]. Faecal calprotectin levels are higher in infants than in adults, possibly indicative of the immature gut undergoing cellular division, replication, and differentiation, and are higher in breastfed infants than formula-fed infants [70]. Clinical investigations with reliable measurements of barrier integrity in infants are rare, particularly those that are sufficiently powered to understand the effects of foods and nutrients. To understand the mechanisms by which nutrients, probiotics, and microbial metabolites may affect epithelial integrity, in vitro experiments using single cell monolayers of Caco-2 cell lines are common and ex vivo tissue microscopy from porcine and murine models provide further insights but are limited in their ability to translate directly to humans.

HMOs and NDCs support barrier integrity by increasing TJs and promoting crypt and villus differentiation (Figure 3). The effects of prebiotics on structural integrity are best understood for GOS, which prevents loss of structure in Caco-2 monolayers when challenged by deoxynivanol (DON), a mycotoxin that inhibits protein synthesis and increases paracellular permeability [71]. Additionally, the stabilisation of claudin3, a TJ protein, and suppressed cytokine synthesis have been detected in GOS-treated media [72]. Formulations with higher ratios of short chain molecules provide the most protection to the epithelium, suggesting that complex resistant starch structures may not have direct, non-microbial mediated benefits on the epithelium [73].

Mucus Membrane

At the luminal surface of the enteric epithelium, the mucus layer provides a structural and functional barrier that provides lubrication and separates the microbiota from epithelial cells while allowing for the transport of nutrients and metabolites. Mucus is a complex heterogeneous suspension matrix with high concentrations of high molecular weight glycoproteins called mucins, which are secreted by goblet cells, and contains antimicrobial peptides, such as defensins [41]. Different types of mucins have different roles in the lumen: secreted mucins form the mucus layer over the epithelium, transmembrane mucins appear to be involved in signaling pathways, and some species of bacteria rely on mucins as an energy source [40].

Several bacterial products, including lipopolysaccharides and flagellin on gram-negative bacteria and lipoteichoic acids on gram positive bacteria, have been found to upregulate the mucin gene expression and to stimulate mucin secretion [74]. Some probiotics, such as specific strains of *Bifidobacterium* and *Lactobacillus*, successfully adhere to mucins and reach epithelial surfaces using non-flagellar appendages called tight adherence pili, which influence immune responses [75,76]. This contributes to differences between the discarded microbiome identified in faecal collections and the microbiome in the mucosa and at the epithelial surface [77,78]. Probiotic treatment, particularly with *Lactobacillus*, has been shown to increase mucin and defensin secretion in murine models and in vitro cell monolayers [79].

Prebiotics influence the composition of mucus by increasing the concentration of glycans [24], decreasing the luminal pH, and increasing mucin glycosylation and sulphation [80], which protects mucins from being degraded by host proteases and bacterial glycosidases (Figure 3) [81]. Mucus, specifically secreted MUC-2, has also demonstrated immune-regulatory signals by interfering with the expression of inflammatory cytokines but not tolerogenic cytokines by inhibiting gene transcription through nuclear factor NF-κB (the nuclear factor kappa-light-chain-enhancer of activated B cells) in dendritic cells (DCs) [82]. The mucus layer plays a significant role in microbial signaling, cross-feeding, microbe-host interactions, and enteric immunity but can only be partially simulated in in vitro experiments.

4. Establishment of the Microbiome and Immune System in the First Year of Life

Microbial community composition during the first year of life is dynamic, unstable, and susceptible to perturbations [6,83]. The gut is the largest immune organ in the human body, containing approximately 65% of immunologic tissues and up to 80% of the immunoglobulin-producing tissues of the body [84]. During gestation, the foetal immune system is downregulated, making neonates particularly susceptible to infection and aberrant immune responses. The epithelial barrier, mucosa, and environmental conditions, such as pH, provide the majority of protection against pathogens in the neonatal period (Figure 3) [85,86]. Healthy immune development in infants is characterised by a transition from innate type 1 immunity, dominated by non-specific macrophages and neutrophils, to adaptive type 2 immunity, characterised by specific T cells and B cells, which is fundamental to the establishment of tolerance: the ability to distinguish between beneficial commensal bacteria and harmful pathogens, leading to the appropriate scale and duration of responses to actual threats (Figure 3) [87]. Spatial and temporal interactions between the microbiome, microbial metabolites, and gut epithelial cells in the lumen, on the surface of epithelial cells, and in the interior components of the gut-associated lymphoid tissue (GALT), such as DCs, modulate balanced immune development, immune response, homeostasis, and disease (Figure 3) [88].

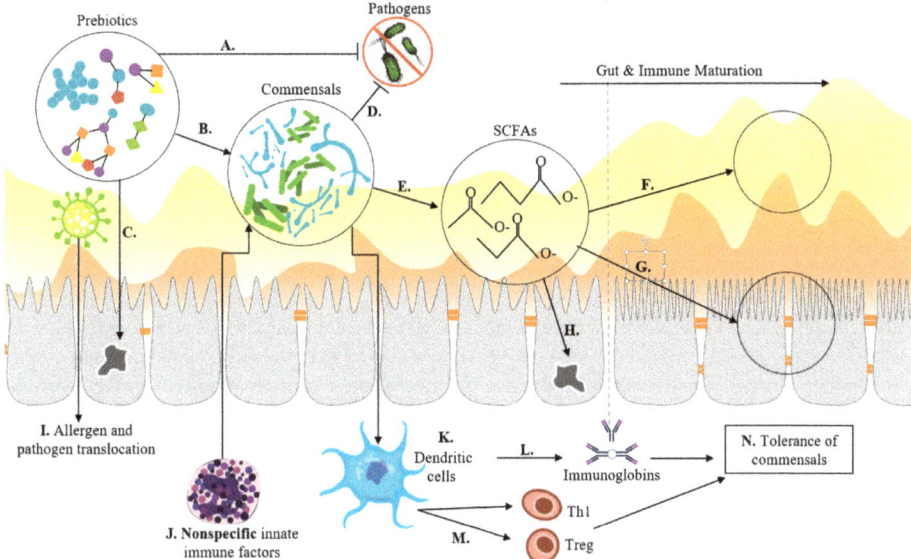

Figure 3. A schematic of multiple mechanisms by which prebiotics modulate immune and gut development. **A.** Prebiotics bind to pathogens as receptor analogues, preventing adhesion to the epithelial surface and subsequent infection. **B.** Prebiotics promote populations of commensal microbes, which outcompete pathogens for resources **D**, reducing infections. **C.** Prebiotics act directly upon the epithelium promoting the mRNA transcription of proteins involved in barrier integrity. **E.** Commensal microbes produce metabolites, such as short chain fatty acids (SCFAs), that decrease the lumen pH and increase mucus **F**, increase TJ proteins and crypt and villi development **G**, and serve as an energy source for enterocytes that form the epithelium **H**. In infants, the immature gut is susceptible to allergy and pathogen translocation **I** through leaky gut barrier. **J.** Non-specific immune factors, such as macrophages and neutrophils attack commensals and pathogens alike in poorly regulated inflammatory responses. During immune development, dendritic cells **K** sample commensal microbes, through Toll-Like Receptor (TLR) recognition, allowing for antigen specific immunoglobin production **L** and promoting the differentiation of T and B cells **M**, resulting in improved tolerance to commensals and targeted response to pathogens **N**.

4.1. Immune Ontogeny

Innate immunity favours Th2 responses and macrophage and neutrophil inflammatory activity, which use specific classes of Toll-Like Receptors (TLRs), such as TLR4, which are capable of recognising structurally conserved molecules on microbes [89]. As the immune system develops, additional mechanisms of microbe recognition with increased specificity and response cascades develop: C-type lectin receptors, pattern recognition receptors, TLR2, and TLR9 are expressed by immune cells, such as DCs, in the mucosa and epithelium [90]. These immune cells can be both upregulated and downregulated by exogenous factors, such as microbial metabolites of starch fermentation, and they demonstrate cross-regulatory activity amongst themselves by way of immune factors and regulatory cytokines [90].

Due to the poor specificity of the young immune system, commensal bacteria are rapidly killed by macrophages. However, DCs can retain small numbers of live commensals for several days, protecting them from innate immune responses while selectively inducing a protective IgA response that protects against mucosal penetration by commensals [91]. Mesenteric lymph nodes restrict these commensal-loaded DCs to the mucosal immune compartment, which allows for localised immune responses while preventing more damaging systemic responses [91]. DCs express TLRs, which have been implicated in gut homeostasis and inflammatory responses characteristic of food allergies, intestinal inflammation, and infections when poorly regulated [92]. Insufficient TLR exposure to commensals, as found through antibiotic-mediated dysbiosis in murine models, is also correlated with increased susceptibility to viral infections [93]. Infant TLR responses to commensal microbes differ from responses in adults, demonstrating the impaired production of inflammatory mediators and heightened production of inflammatory cytokines, such as IL-10 [85,87].

TLRs are susceptible to modulation by dietary starches in in vitro models. Different starch structures bind differentially to TLRs, activating NF-κB, and activator proteins (AP-1), but the strong immune-stimulating effects may also be attenuated by starch-exposed intestinal epithelial cells [94]. B2→1 fructans and High Maize 260 mainly stimulate TLR2, whereas Novelose 330 binds to TLR2 and TLR5 [95]. High Maize 260, which has a smaller average particle size of 12.8 μm, smooth surface, and high degree of molecular order was found to have a stronger regulatory effect on epithelial cells than Novelose 330, which has a larger average particle size of 46.6 μm and consists of destroyed and convoluted granules due to the retrogradation process. Despite the attenuating activity, TLRs continue to produce Th1 cytokines [94]. High-maize 260 is also more effective than inulin and sugar pectin in reducing chemokine release in response to *Sphingomonas paucimobilis* infections in vitro [96]. In vivo, the mucosal matrix is expected to drastically alter the exposure of epithelial cells to starch structures, limiting the applicability of these findings to in vivo mechanisms.

4.2. Microbiome Assembly

Pioneer species in the infant gut shape the early environment, which influences the dynamic succession of subsequent microbes and immune cascades. Nutrients, digestive processes, gases, and pH gradients throughout the gut modulate the microbial community, which in turn also influences the characteristics of some of these attributes. Microbiota resembling maternal oral microbiota may begin to colonise the infant gut in utero, for example low abundance commensal bacteria such as *Prevotella*, *Neisseria*, and *Escherichia Coli*, which have been found through the sequencing of amniotic fluids and placentas of preterm infants [97]. However, the mode of delivery is considered the first major event confirmed to seed the infant microbiome with lasting colonisers [7].

Vaginally delivered infants are predominantly colonised by *Bacteroides*, *Bifidobacterium*, *Parabacteroides*, and *Escherichia/Shigella*, several of which are obligate anaerobes. Infants delivered by caesarean section are enriched with *Enterobacter*, *Haemophilus*, *Staphylococcus*, *Streptococcus*, and *Veilonella*, which are associated with skin, oral, and environmental species [7], a larger proportion of which are aerobic. The differences in microbial community structure and gene content (i.e., the metagenome) between caesarean- and vaginally-delivered infants gradually decrease over the first year of life, but the differences in innate and adaptive immunity remain detectable for up to 2 years of age. Caesarean-delivered infants have lower levels of IgA-, IgG-, and IgM-secreting cells, indicating reduced adaptive immune responses, have lower levels of Th1 supporting chemokines, IFNγ and IL-8, and have decreased CD4+ T cell responses [12]. Caesarean-delivered infants, in particular those who were born by elective caesarean delivery instead of emergency delivery, are at higher risk for asthma, atopy, juvenile arthritis, and inflammatory bowel disease [98–100]. This effect is particularly pronounced for developing obesity where any caesarean delivery has been associated with a 15% increased risk for obesity, but there is a 30% increased risk in elective caesarean-delivered infants [101]. The risk for development of infectious diseases is not clear. Considering these differences, it is critical that microbiome studies in infants consider the mode of delivery, and this will be strengthened by accounting for differences between emergency and elective caesarean-delivered infants.

During the first several weeks of life, pioneer facultative anaerobic species, which have metabolic flexibility in the presence of oxygen, shift the environment to favour obligate anaerobic species by utilising oxygen to create a more anaerobic environment [102] and by reducing luminal substrates through redox (oxygen)-dependent genetic pathways that produce metabolites, such as acetate, which is often required or highly stimulatory for anaerobes [103]. The meconium of neonates is rich in facultative anaerobes such as *E. Coli*, but the faecal microbiota becomes more diverse with the appearance of obligate anaerobes such as *Bifidobacterium* and *Clostridium* within the first week [104]. In a cohort of 19 healthy breastfed full-term Japanese infants, the averaged percentage of obligate anaerobic bacteria in the gut progressed from 32% (1 day), 37% (7 days), 54% (1 month), 70% (3 months), 64% (6 months), to 99% at 3 years of age. Significant individual variations within this homogenous cohort diminished by 3 years of age [105,106]. This study did not specify the delivery modes of this cohort, and the consequent possibility of significant differences in the colonisation patterns of facultative and obligate anaerobes.

The effects of breastmilk and formula feeding on the infant microbiome and immunity are a popular topic of research. Breastfeeding has been associated with a decreased risk of necrotising enterocolitis, infections, and diarrhoea in early life and with a lower incidence of inflammatory bowel disease, type 2 diabetes, and obesity later in life compared to formula-fed infants [107]. Another meta-analysis found no association between breastmilk consumption and allergy, asthma, high blood pressure, or high cholesterol [108]. Considering the complexity of the immune-modulating factors of breastmilk, the identifying characteristics of the microbiome that contribute to these benefits is challenging. *Bifidobacterium* has consistently been found to exist in higher abundances in exclusively breastfed infants, whereas *Lactobacillus* has been reported to be higher in formula-fed infants in some studies [102,109], while at other times reported to be higher in breastfed infants [110]. Backhed et al. associated exclusive breastfeeding with lower phylogenetic diversity dominated by *Bifidobacterium* and *Lactobacillus* and lower relative abundances of *Clostridiales* and *Bacteroides* compared to mixed-fed infants [7]. Some of these differences may persist throughout the weaning phase as breastmilk and formula feeding continue with supplementation of solid foods.

In an effort to impart similar bifidogenic effects on formula-fed infants, the supplementation of infant formula with prebiotics, or prebiotics and probiotics, has become common. A 9:1 ratio of synthetic linear polymers of GOS:FOS is standard, but these prebiotics represent a simplistic uniform version of the HMO structures found in breastmilk [20]. Abrahamse-Berkeveld et al. (2016) found that a combination of short chain GOS (scGOS dp of 3–15), long chain FOS (lcFOS dp of 3–6), and *Bifidobacterium breve* increased the abundance of *Bifidobacterium* from 48% to 60% of the total bacterial species and reduced the percentage of *Clostridium lituseburense*/*C. histolyticum* from 2.6% to 2.0%. [46]. In an in vitro study, Leder et al. (1999) found that many different strains of *Bifidobacterium* are capable of utilizing scGOS, but of the species analysed, only *B. adolescentis* can utilise lcFOS, providing evidence of the selectivity between related commensal strains and prebiotic structures [111]. These investigations into the utilisation of HMOs and prebiotics in formula offer a starting point for exploring the effects of prebiotics provided by whole complementary foods.

Oligosaccharides also provide additional protection against pathogenic infection by acting as structural mimics of the pathogen binding sites that coat the surface of intestinal epithelial cells. Pathogenic bacteria such as *E. Coli* bind to oligosaccharides in the lumen, reducing the pathogen load available for adhesion to intestinal epithelial cells. In Caco-2 and human epithelial type 2 (Hep-2) cell lines, purified GOS reduced adhesion by 70% and 65% respectively. This effect was dose-dependent and reached a maximum at 16 mg/mL [45]. It is unclear if complex starches, such as resistant starch, have the same effect.

4.3. Functional Transitions during Complementary Feeding

Investigations into the functional differences between modes of feeding at the metagenomic and transcriptomic level are less common. Backhed et al. found differences in the relative abundance of functional genes in the faecal microbiome of breastfed and formula-fed infant that accounted for approximately 1.30% of the variation in KEGG Orthologs, which is substantial considering the expected constitutive expression of most genes [7]. This study did not specify the types of formulas used in this comparison, and the expression of genes during this dynamic age may be more facultative than constitutive due to the inherent instability of the immature infant microbiome.

The community structure and metabolic functions of the infant gut microbiota are strongly influenced by dietary prebiotics. The bifidogenic nature of breastmilk is well-established and has been attributed to HMOs [112]. HMO consumption has only been identified in select *Bacteroides* (*Bifidobacterium*) and *Lactobacillus* species, and different species and subspecies have been found to utilise different protein-substrate binding and enzymatic mechanisms to metabolise HMOs [113,114]. *B. longum* subsp. *infantis*, which is enriched in breastfed infants, express an overabundance of proteins that transport HMO substrates into the cell, where they are broken up into their constituent sugars before being metabolised. This limits the sugars that are available to other species within the microbiota [115]. *B. bifidum*, however, relies on a set of diverse membrane-associated extracellular glycosyl hydrolases, lacto-*N*-biosidase and endo-*N*-acetylgalactosaminidase [116], which have comparable enzymatic affinities for HMOs but may release monosaccharides such as lactose, fucose, and sialic acid into the lumen, which become available to other microbes [117].

Glycosylation patterns on HMOs influence the enzymatic activity that microbes employ. *B. breve* has been found to have a preference for sialylated HMOs over neutral HMOs, engaging enzymes that convert HMOs into multiple intracellular products, but it does not internalise the whole molecule [118]. *B. longum* has numerous genes for carbohydrate utilisation, including 30 glycosyl hydrolases that are likely involved in HMO degradation, though adult strains have indicated a preference for plant polysaccharides [119]. The transcriptomic analysis of *B. longum* SC596 when shifting from a neutral HMO substrate to a fucosylated HMO substrate found the gene expression was altered to resemble the intracellular import strategy of *B. infantis*, which may provide an example of the facultative gene expression of infant microbiota in response to dietary factors [20]. A meta-transcriptomic analysis of faecal samples from a single breastfed baby followed from birth to six months of age, during which formula, dairy, and solid foods were introduced, found that the carbohydrate fermentation activity of *Bifidobacterium*, based on β-galactosidase activity, decreases during weaning while that of the resident Firmicutes increases, which corresponds with changes in relative abundance of major and minor species [120].

At approximately 3 months of age, genes implicated in complex carbohydrate utilization are enriched compared to meconium samples, which favour lactose/galactose and sucrose uptake and utilisation based on a metagenomic analysis [6]. Just prior to introducing solid foods between 4 and 6 months of age, the gut microbiome derives energy through the degradation of simple sugars, lactose-specific transport, and carbohydrate uptake, as is expected for a milk-based diet. However, functional genes involved in plant-polysaccharide metabolism are present prior to the introduction of complementary weaning foods [6]. By 12 months of age, the infant microbiome is highly enriched with species and genes active in the degradation of complex sugars and starches [7]. For instance, *Bacteroides thetaiotaomicron*, an anaerobic glycan degrading enzyme producer of the Bacteroidetes phylum, can typically be detected at 12 months of age [6]. An additional study showed that the increased abundance of *Bifidobacterium* and decreased abundance of *Bacteroides* and *Clostridium* in breastfed infants compared to formula-fed and mixed-fed infants persists into the weaning phase [121].

Thompson et al. identified differences before and after the introduction of solid foods between the microbiomes of exclusively breastfed and non-exclusively breastfed infants [122]. *Veillonella*, *Roseburia*, and members of the *Lachnospiraceae* family appeared with the introduction of solids in breastfed infants, whereas *Streptococcus* and *Coprobacillus* were identified after the introduction of solids in non-exclusively breastfed infants [122]. Most notable of these findings was the increased relative abundance of *Bifidobacterium* after the inclusion of solids in non-exclusively breastfed infants, compared to a decreased relative abundance of *Bifidobacterium* after the inclusion of solids in exclusively breastfed infants, which may reflect differential effects of dietary oligosaccharides and starches during complementary feeding. Metabolic inferences using a PiCRUST analysis of this limited 16S dataset showed that only 24 gene clusters encoding enzymes were overrepresented in exclusively breastfed infants after the introduction of solid foods, including polysaccharide degradation, compared to 230 enzymatic gene clusters overrepresented in the non-exclusively breastfed microbiome, which were primarily involved in signal transduction regulatory systems [122]. This finding indicates differences in metabolic plasticity between exclusively breastfed and non-exclusively breastfed infants, though it is possible that the substantial immune factors in breastmilk have a stronger effect on which gene clusters are overrepresented in this small cohort.

Human faecal microbiota may develop the capacity to degrade a specific type of starch (Type III Resistant Starch) at weaning, as demonstrated in an in vitro fermentation study using faecal inoculum collected from breastfed and formula–fed infants before and during weaning [123]. However, species with the potential capacity to degrade starch have been found to be present at birth [6]. From a metagenome perspective, microbial networks of infants at 4 months are drastically different to those at 12 months, but polysaccharide degradation has been found to be more pronounced after the cessation of breastfeeding, rather than during the introduction of solid foods in breastfed infants [7]. It is possible that the cessation of HMO substrates decreases the need for the expression of HMO-degrading genes and reduces the competitive advantage of species selective for HMOs, allowing species with a preference for polysaccharide substrates to assume a greater ecological niche. However, neither the in vitro experiment nor the metagenomic analysis consider the nutrient availability and degradation that occurs in the proximal regions of the large intestine prior to analysis of the faecal microbiome.

Starch degradation in the large intestine is a cooperative process that includes enzymatic starch degradation into glucose, glycolysis leading to SCFAs and organic acids, and hydrogen production. Starch binding capacity and enzyme specificity underpin the ability of amylolytic microbes to metabolise starch structures [124]. The presence and function of cellulosomes, amylosomes, and starch utilisation system gene clusters have been investigated in keystone species belonging to the Firmicutes and Bacteroidetes families. Three broad classes of amylases have been identified in amylolytic bacteria that hydrolyse starch into D-glucose: α-amylase for α-1,4 linkages, type 1 pullanase for α-1,6 linkages, and amylopullalanases for α-1,4 and α-1,6 linkages [125]. Stable Isotope Probing (RNA-SIP), which allows for the tracking of ^{13}C-isotope labelled carbon utilisation through metabolite production, has identified complex trophic structures that implicate primary starch degraders, such as *Ruminococcus bromii*, in downstream carbon utilization by microbes found in the infant gut such as *Prevotella*, *Bifidobacterium*, and *Eubacterium rectale* [126]. The association of amylolytic enzymes with the cell wall and the ability to stabilize large molecules for cleavage may indicate the function of a given microbe within the trophic network [127,128]. For instance, extracellular protein complexes on *Bacteroides thetaiotamicron* imports starch molecules for internal degradation, limiting the extracellular release of mono and di-saccharides, compared to outer membrane protein complexes on *Clostridium butyricum* which degrade starches outside of the cell before importing the mono- and disaccharides for subsequent metabolism into SCFAs [47,129,130]. This variety of enzyme structures and systems points to the metabolic flexibility, which may be increased during dietary transitions such as weaning, that the microbiome utilises to maximise energy harvest.

Fermentation profiles vary by substrate structure, which changes throughout enzymatic degradation. Short oligosaccharide chains, such as scFOS, are more rapidly fermented than long oligosaccharide chains, such as inulin [131]. The rate of fermentation as measured by the SCFA production was highest during the first 4 hours in a faecal inoculum provided with scFOS substrate, whereas long chain inulin produced the most SCFA between 12–24 h [131]. Warren et al. (2018) expanded upon these findings by comparing digested to non-digested starches from a range of processed, un-processed, digested, and un-digested starch and resistant starch substrates. This study found that microbiota are able to ferment amorphous and crystalline starches equally well, perhaps attributable to the range of amylolytic enzymes found in the microbiome, and found no difference in the fermentation rates of the digested versus undigested substrates [132]. Both the 16S rRNA gene amplicon sequencing analysis of the inoculum and the SCFA analysis revealed differentiations according to time-points depending upon the classification of the starch substrate [132].

4.4. SCFAs

SCFAs are the primary class of microbial metabolites of starch degradation and are implicated in immune regulation. SCFAs function as an energy source for the host epithelium and other microbes, affect lipid metabolism, protect against infection, have anti-inflammatory properties, influence the gut-brain axis, facilitate immune cell metabolic reprogramming, and regulate immune cell transcription through epigenetic modifications [133]. SCFA production varies throughout the colon because of substrate availability, population dynamics, and microbial cross-feeding [134]. The fermentation of starch substrates by the gut microbial community is characterised by high acetate production, followed by propionate and relatively less butyrate, though ratios are highly variable [132,135]. RNA-SIP studies show that lactate is a precursor to both acetate and propionate and that acetate is precursor for butyrate via both the Co-A transferase pathway and the butyrate kinase pathway [136]. For example, *Bifidobacterium adolescentis* can degrade resistant starch leading to the byproducts lactate and acetate. Acetate is, in turn, used by *Eubacterium* spp., *Roseburia* spp., and *Coprococcus catus*, resulting in the production of butyrate. *Faecalibacterium prausnitzii*, an abundant butyrate producer in adults, has not been detected in infants younger than approximately 2 years of age [137]. Figure 4 demonstrates a simplified ecological network in which multiple species of bacteria commonly identified in infants perform parts of the metabolic pathways leading to biosynthesis of SCFAs.

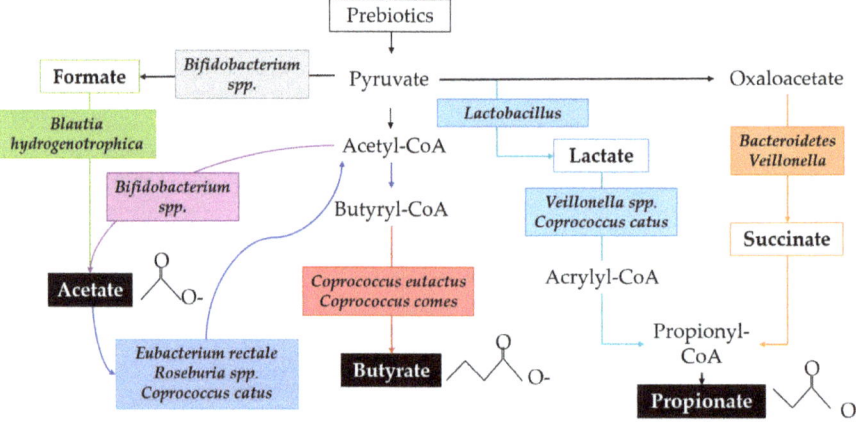

Figure 4. A simplified schematic of the biosynthesis of SCFAs by microbial species identified in human infants. Organic acid metabolites are outlined, and SCFAs are highlighted in black boxes. Species of bacteria found in the infant gut microbiome that are implicated in the corresponding pathway are italicised.

SCFAs begin shaping the enteric environment with the introduction of breastmilk and formula. Exclusive breastfeeding is associated with lower absolute concentrations of all SCFAs, except lactate [105]. Ratios of SCFAs within total concentrations have been found to be variable: exclusively breastfed infants are more likely to have higher proportions of acetate, while partially breastfed and formula-fed infants are more likely to have relatively higher proportions of propionate, and exclusively formula-fed infants are likely to have relatively higher proportions of butyrate [138]. However, measuring SCFAs in faecal samples only provides an indicator of the balance between SCFA production and absorption. Absorption is likely to vary with epithelial barrier integrity and maturity, which is known to be influenced by other factors in breastmilk [58,139].

SCFAs modulate immune factors through multiple mechanisms. They increase the expression of antimicrobial peptides excreted by epithelial cells; modulate the production of cytokines and chemokines; regulate the differentiation, recruitment, and activation of immune cells; and modulate the differentiation of T lymphocytes [21]. Commonly cited anti-inflammatory properties of SCFAs can be attributed to their ability to reduce the production and activity of pro-inflammatory cytokines such as TNF-α and IL-12, often by modulating activity of neutrophils, DCs, and macrophages [140]. Alternatively, SCFAs increase the production of other cytokines, such as IL-18, which has been implicated in the repair and maintenance of epithelial integrity [141].

Acetate is a minor energy source for gut epithelial cells, a major energy source for muscles and brain tissue, has anti-inflammatory properties, decreases the pH of the colon, and is used by cross-feeding species as a co-substrate to produce butyrate [139,142]. Numerous species of *Bifidobacterium* readily produce acetate from starchy substrates. Anti-inflammatory properties of acetate have been linked to the SCFA-dependent modulation of NF-κB in the COLO320DM adenocarcinoma cell lines, to decreased IL-6 protein release from organ culture, and to decreased LPS-stimulated TNFα from neutrophils. However, these dose-dependent effects are less pronounced for acetate than propionate and butyrate [143]. Acetate has also been identified as an important metabolite by which some subspecies of *Bifidobacterium* protect against infection, possibly by inhibiting the translocation of toxins from the gut lumen to the bloodstream [144]. Several in vitro studies suggest that the benefits of acetate are largely due to the enhanced epithelial integrity, which imparts protection from infection and inflammation. For instance, *B. longum infantis 157F*, which is found in breastfed infants and metabolises glucose to acetate, was found to protect against harmful protein translocation across a Caco-2 epithelial barrier in an in vitro cell-culture experiment [144].

Propionate has been associated with health benefits most particularly in adults [145]. Similar to acetate, propionate is a minor energy source for gut epithelial cells, decreases the pH of the colon, is anti-inflammatory, and has immune modulating properties that in vitro studies of TER in Caco-2 cell lines suggest are linked to beneficial effects on epithelial barrier integrity [146]. Additionally, propionate decreases liver lipogenesis, serum cholesterol levels, and colorectal carcinogenesis in other tissues. Insulin sensitivity improvements and increased satiety in adults has also been correlated with increased propionate levels [139,142,145]. These effects have not been investigated in weaning infants.

Butyrate is the preferred energy source for gut epithelial cells, meaning that little butyrate reaches systemic circulation. Butyrate also decreases the pH of the colon, promotes epithelial proliferation, prevents colorectal cancer cell proliferation, reduces oxidative stress, is anti inflammatory, and improves gut barrier function by stimulating the production of mucins, antimicrobial peptides, and TJ proteins [139,142]. Gantois et al. found that butyrate also downregulates the expression of virulence genes in *Salmonella enterica* and *typhimurium* [147]. Butyrate producing bacteria, such as *Eubacterium rectale*, *Roseburia spp*, and *Faecalibacterium prausnitzii* frequently utilise acetate as a substrate [148]. The effects of butyrate have been found to be paradoxical where low concentrations of butyrate (2 mM) promote gut barrier function, characterised by increased TER and decreased mannitol flux, but high doses (8 mM) may induce cell apoptosis and disrupt the intestinal barrier, as is characteristic of necrotising enteric colitis [149]. One study identified the benefits of butyrate to be characteristic of cellular differentiation because of the increased dome formation and alkaline phosphatase activity [146], whereas another identified cell migration, as is needed for epithelial repair, as a beneficial mechanism [149]. Both studies found that the effects were dependent on protein synthesis and gene transcription but not the beta-oxidation or activation of adenosine 3′, 5′-cyclic monophosphate [146,149].

Most investigations into SCFAs have focused on adult populations. In infants, SCFAs are considered beneficial, but faecal measurements are inappropriate to use as an indicator of a healthy microbiome due to its paradoxical effects at high concentrations and the importance of considering the balance of SCFA utilisation by epithelial cells and absorption into the blood stream.

4.5. Vitamins

Vitamins are an additional class of secondary metabolites produced by the microbiota with effects on immunity. Commensal bacteria have the capacity to synthesise essential vitamins, particularly from the B and K groups, the expression of which is distinct in infants compared to adults. The microbiota in neonates demonstrate the enrichment of genes involved in the production of Vitamin K2, retinol, folate, pyroxidal (B6), and biotin (B7), which are involved in bone, vision, tooth development, and glucose conversion are upregulated in the neonatal microbiome. Genes involved in the transport of B12, iron, hemin, and heme are also enriched in neonates but decline markedly with age, corresponding with increased nutritional demands for iron between 4 and 6 months of age. Throughout the weaning months, genes involved in the biosynthesis of thiamine (B1), pantothenate (B5), cobalamin (B12), and lysine increase [150]. Methionine degradation and leucine and tryptophan biosynthesis increase to reach levels comparable to mothers by 12 months of age [7].

It has been estimated that B vitamins are produced by 40–65% of human gut microbes, with some microbes having the capacity to produce all 8 B-vitamins and some demonstrating pathways that complemented those of other organisms [151]. These estimates were determined by aligning metagenomes from the human gut microbiome to an annotated genome on the PubSEED platform [151]. *Bifidobacteriales* contained the most conserved pattern of B1, B3, and B7 in approximately 35% of the genomes, whereas *Bacteroidetes* demonstrated biosynthetic pathways of all 8 vitamins present in 51% of the genomes [151]. *Prevotellaceae* produce B2, B5, and B7; *Lactobacillales* either contain no biosynthetic pathways, or were limited to B2; and *Clostridiales* produce only B12 [151]. The full folate biosynthesis (B9) pathway is present in 43% of genomes, which is distributed in nearly all *Bacteroidetes* genomes, in most Fusobacteria and *Proteobacteria*, and in partial pathways occuring in *Actinobacteria* and *Firmicutes* [151]. Vitamin K in one of two forms is reported to be produced by *Bacteroides*, *Enterobacter*, *Veillonella*, and *Eubacterium lentum*, though the bioavailability of bacterially-derived Vitamin K has not been established [152]. How these genes are differentially expressed in the infant microbiome and in response to specific types of complementary foods has yet to be explored.

The interactions between microbially-derived vitamins and immune cells are varied and poorly characterised. Of the known pathways, B6 has been found to serve as a cofactor in immunomodulatory pathways [153], B9 has been implicated in the maintenance of regulatory T cells [154], and B12 has been found to augment CD8+ T lymphocytes and NK cell activity in deficient patients [35,155]. Interestingly, the byproducts from vitamin synthesis pathways have also recently been implicated in immune cell recognition: mucosa-associated invariant T cells, which produce IL-17 and IFN-γ, are activated in response to microbe-derived products of the riboflavin biosynthetic pathway that are presented by a monomeric major histocompatibility complex class 1 (MHC-1)-like related molecule (MR1) [156]. These MHC and MHC-like molecules are imperative to discriminate self from non-self, enabling protective immunity [157].

5. Discussion and Conclusions

Complementary feeding merges neonatal nutrition with diverse childhood nutrition during a window of high variability and instability in the microbiome. Starchy foods are common complementary foods based on texture and palatability, but the health-promoting benefits of complex starches during this window are unknown. Currently, no harmful effects or negative outcomes of starch consumption during complementary feeding have been reported. However, certain common complementary foods that contain starch, such as rice and wheat, also contain nutrient-binding compounds such as phytic acid, which can be altered during processing [158]. Based on the evidence that prebiotic HMOs and NDCs alter the microbial community structure and microbial metabolism and promoted immunity and immune development, investigations into prebiotic complex starches are warranted. However, the utilisation and fermentation of starch structures occurs in a complex trophic network governed by keystone species, cross-feeding dynamics, host-microbe interactions, and biogeography of the gut lumen that are particularly dynamic during the rapid growth and colonisation phase of complementary feeding. Identifying the interactions and characteristics of a healthy infant gut that result in beneficial clinical outcomes remains challenging.

The mechanisms by which starch may contribute to immunity and immune development are varied. While some oligosaccharides are known to act as receptor analogues for pathogens, thus preventing adhesion to the epithelium and consequent infection, this effect has not been explored for complex starch structures from whole foods. Starch also promotes populations of commensal bacteria with direct immunomodulatory activity in the mucosa and at the intestinal epithelium. These commensal bacteria also produce metabolites, including SCFAs, vitamins, and small molecules that may beneficially alter the environment, support structural immunity at the epithelial barrier, and promote balanced and appropriate immune responses to commensals and pathogens. Building upon extensive research into HMOs and prebiotic-supplemented formulas by investigating transitions to more complex starch structures may offer functional insights into the mechanisms that underpin balanced microbiome-mediated immune development during the complementary feeding window and facilitate the development and application of functional complementary foods.

Author Contributions: Conceptualisation, S.M., W.Y., and N.C.R.; resources, N.C.R. and W.C.M.; writing—original draft preparation, S.M.; writing—review and editing, W.Y., K.F., J.M., N.C.R., and W.C.M.; supervision, W.Y., K.F., W.C.M., and N.C.R.; project administration, N.C.R. and W.C.M.; funding acquisition, N.C.R.

Funding: This research received no external funding.

Conflicts of Interest: The authors declare no conflict of interest.

References

1. Sen, P.; Mardinogulu, A.; Nielsen, J. Selection of complementary foods based on optimal nutritional values. *Sci. Rep.* **2017**, *7*, 5413. [CrossRef] [PubMed]
2. Lonnerdal, B.; Hernell, O. An opinion on "staging" of infant formula: A developmental perspective on infant feeding. *J. Pediatr. Gastroenterol. Nutr.* **2016**, *62*, 9–21. [CrossRef] [PubMed]
3. Krebs, N.F.; Hambidge, K.M. Zinc requirements and zinc intakes of breast-fed infants. *Am. J. Clin. Nutr.* **1986**, *43*, 288–292. [CrossRef] [PubMed]
4. Young, B.E.; Krebs, N.F. Complementary feeding: Critical considerations to optimize growth, nutrition, and feeding behavior. *Curr. Pediatr. Rep.* **2013**, *1*, 247–256. [CrossRef] [PubMed]
5. Cong, X.; Xu, W.; Janton, S.; Henderson, W.A.; Matson, A.; McGrath, J.M.; Maas, K.; Graf, J. Gut microbiome developmental patterns in early life of preterm infants: Impacts of feeding and gender. *PloS ONE* **2016**, *11*, e0152751. [CrossRef] [PubMed]
6. Koenig, J.E.; Spor, A.; Scalfone, N.; Fricker, A.D.; Stombaugh, J.; Knight, R.; Angenent, L.T.; Ley, R.E. Succession of microbial consortia in the developing infant gut microbiome. *Proc. Natl. Acad. Sci. USA* **2011**, *108* (Suppl. 1), 4578–4585. [CrossRef]
7. Backhed, F.; Roswall, J.; Peng, Y.; Feng, Q.; Jia, H.; Kovatcheva-Datchary, P.; Li, Y.; Xia, Y.; Xie, H.; Zhong, H.; et al. Dynamics and stabilization of the human gut microbiome during the first year of life. *Cell Host Microbe* **2015**, *17*, 852. [CrossRef]
8. Hill, C.J.; Lynch, D.B.; Murphy, K.; Ulaszewska, M.; Jeffery, I.B.; O'Shea, C.A.; Watkins, C.; Dempsey, E.; Mattivi, F.; Tuohy, K. Evolution of gut microbiota composition from birth to 24 weeks in the infantmet cohort. *Microbiome* **2017**, *5*, 4. [CrossRef]
9. Goulet, O. Potential role of the intestinal microbiota in programming health and disease. *Nutr. Rev.* **2015**, *73* (Suppl. 1), 32–40. [CrossRef]
10. Praveen, P.; Jordan, F.; Priami, C.; Morine, M.J. The role of breast-feeding in infant immune system: A systems perspective on the intestinal microbiome. *Microbiome* **2015**, *3*, 41. [CrossRef] [PubMed]
11. Walker, W.A. Initial intestinal colonization in the human infant and immune homeostasis. *Ann. Nutr. Metab.* **2013**, *63* (Suppl. 2), 8–15. [CrossRef]
12. Amenyogbe, N.; Kollmann, T.R.; Ben-Othman, R. Early-life host-microbiome interphase: The key frontier for immune development. *Front. Pediatr.* **2017**, *5*, 111. [CrossRef]

13. Clavel, T.; Gomes-Neto, J.C.; Lagkouvardos, I.; Ramer-Tait, A.E. Deciphering interactions between the gut microbiota and the immune system via microbial cultivation and minimal microbiomes. *Immunol. Rev.* **2017**, *279*, 8–22. [CrossRef] [PubMed]
14. Kaplan, J.L.; Shi, H.N.; Walker, W.A. The role of microbes in developmental immunologic programming. *Pediatr. Res.* **2011**, *69*, 465–472. [CrossRef]
15. Li, M.; Wang, M.; Donovan, S.M. Early development of the gut microbiome and immune-mediated childhood disorders. *Semin. Reprod. Med.* **2014**, *32*, 74–86. [CrossRef] [PubMed]
16. Bertelsen, R.J.; Jensen, E.T.; Ringel-Kulka, T. Use of probiotics and prebiotics in infant feeding. *Best Pract. Res. Clin. Gastroenterol.* **2016**, *30*, 39–48. [CrossRef]
17. Blacher, E.; Levy, M.; Tatirovsky, E.; Elinav, E. Microbiome-modulated metabolites at the interface of host immunity. *J. Immunol.* **2017**, *198*, 572–580. [CrossRef] [PubMed]
18. Kwak, M.J.; Kwon, S.K.; Yoon, J.K.; Song, J.Y.; Seo, J.G.; Chung, M.J.; Kim, J.F. Evolutionary architecture of the infant-adapted group of bifidobacterium species associated with the probiotic function. *Syst. Appl. Microbiol.* **2016**, *39*, 429–439. [CrossRef]
19. Sierra, C.; Bernal, M.J.; Blasco, J.; Martinez, R.; Dalmau, J.; Ortuno, I.; Espin, B.; Vasallo, M.I.; Gil, D.; Vidal, M.L.; et al. Prebiotic effect during the first year of life in healthy infants fed formula containing gos as the only prebiotic: A multicentre, randomised, double-blind and placebo-controlled trial. *Eur. J. Nutr.* **2015**, *54*, 89–99. [CrossRef]
20. Thomson, P.; Medina, D.A.; Garrido, D. Human milk oligosaccharides and infant gut bifidobacteria: Molecular strategies for their utilization. *Food Microbiol.* **2018**, *75*, 37–46. [CrossRef] [PubMed]
21. Corrêa-Oliveira, R.; Fachi, J.L.; Vieira, A.; Sato, F.T.; Vinolo, M.A.R. Regulation of immune cell function by short-chain fatty acids. *Clin. Transl. Immunol.* **2016**, *5*, e73. [CrossRef] [PubMed]
22. Maier, T.V.; Lucio, M.; Lee, L.H.; VerBerkmoes, N.C.; Brislawn, C.J.; Bernhardt, J.; Lamendella, R.; McDermott, J.E.; Bergeron, N.; Heinzmann, S.S.; et al. Impact of dietary resistant starch on the human gut microbiome, metaproteome, and metabolome. *mBio* **2017**, *8*. [CrossRef] [PubMed]
23. Tanaka, M.; Nakayama, J. Development of the gut microbiota in infancy and its impact on health in later life. *Allergol. Int.* **2017**, *66*, 515–522. [CrossRef] [PubMed]
24. Schroeder, B.O.; Birchenough, G.M.; Ståhlman, M.; Arike, L.; Johansson, M.E.; Hansson, G.C.; Bäckhed, F. Bifidobacteria or fiber protects against diet-induced microbiota-mediated colonic mucus deterioration. *Cell Host Microbe* **2018**, *23*, 27–40. [CrossRef] [PubMed]
25. Rogier, E.W.; Frantz, A.L.; Bruno, M.E.; Wedlund, L.; Cohen, D.A.; Stromberg, A.J.; Kaetzel, C.S. Lessons from mother: Long-term impact of antibodies in breast milk on the gut microbiota and intestinal immune system of breastfed offspring. *Gut Microbes* **2014**, *5*, 663–668. [CrossRef] [PubMed]
26. Rogier, E.W.; Frantz, A.L.; Bruno, M.E.; Wedlund, L.; Cohen, D.A.; Stromberg, A.J.; Kaetzel, C.S. Secretory antibodies in breast milk promote long-term intestinal homeostasis by regulating the gut microbiota and host gene expression. *Proc. Natl. Acad. Sci. USA* **2014**, *111*, 3074–3079. [CrossRef] [PubMed]
27. Cui, X.; Li, Y.; Yang, L.; You, L.; Wang, X.; Shi, C.; Ji, C.; Guo, X. Peptidome analysis of human milk from women delivering macrosomic fetuses reveals multiple means of protection for infants. *Oncotarget* **2016**, *7*, 63514–63525. [CrossRef]
28. Duranti, S.; Lugli, G.A.; Mancabelli, L.; Armanini, F.; Turroni, F.; James, K.; Ferretti, P.; Gorfer, V.; Ferrario, C.; Milani, C.; et al. Maternal inheritance of bifidobacterial communities and bifidophages in infants through vertical transmission. *Microbiome* **2017**, *5*, 66. [CrossRef]
29. Gonzalez-Perez, G.; Hicks, A.L.; Tekieli, T.M.; Radens, C.M.; Williams, B.L.; Lamouse-Smith, E.S. Maternal antibiotic treatment impacts development of the neonatal intestinal microbiome and antiviral immunity. *J. Immunol.* **2016**, *196*, 3768–3779. [CrossRef]
30. Hartwig, I.; Diemert, A.; Tolosa, E.; Hecher, K.; Arck, P. Babies galore; or recent findings and future perspectives of pregnancy cohorts with a focus on immunity. *J. Reprod. Immunol.* **2015**, *108*, 6–11. [CrossRef]
31. Romano-Keeler, J.; Weitkamp, J.H. Maternal influences on fetal microbial colonization and immune development. *Pediatri. Res.* **2015**, *77*, 189–195. [CrossRef] [PubMed]
32. Schlinzig, T.; Johansson, S.; Stephansson, O.; Hammarstrom, L.; Zetterstrom, R.H.; von Dobeln, U.; Cnattingius, S.; Norman, M. Surge of immune cell formation at birth differs by mode of delivery and infant characteristics-a population-based cohort study. *PloS ONE* **2017**, *12*, e0184748. [CrossRef]

33. Schwartz, C.; Chabanet, C.; Szleper, E.; Feyen, V.; Issanchou, S.; Nicklaus, S. Infant acceptance of primary tastes and fat emulsion: Developmental changes and links with maternal and infant characteristics. *Chem. Senses* **2017**, *42*, 593–603. [CrossRef] [PubMed]
34. Belkaid, Y.; Segre, J.A. Dialogue between skin microbiota and immunity. *Science* **2014**, *346*, 954–959. [CrossRef] [PubMed]
35. Brestoff, J.R.; Artis, D. Commensal bacteria at the interface of host metabolism and the immune system. *Nat. Immunol.* **2013**, *14*, 676–684. [CrossRef] [PubMed]
36. Kabat, A.M.; Srinivasan, N.; Maloy, K.J. Modulation of immune development and function by intestinal microbiota. *Trends Immunol.* **2014**, *35*, 507–517. [CrossRef]
37. Martin, R.; Nauta, A.J.; Ben Amor, K.; Knippels, L.M.; Knol, J.; Garssen, J. Early life: Gut microbiota and immune development in infancy. *Benef. Microbes* **2010**, *1*, 367–382. [CrossRef]
38. Paun, A.; Danska, J.S. Immuno-ecology: How the microbiome regulates tolerance and autoimmunity. *Curr. Opin. Immunol.* **2015**, *37*, 34–39. [CrossRef]
39. Ruff, W.E.; Kriegel, M.A. Autoimmune host-microbiota interactions at barrier sites and beyond. *Trends Mol. Med.* **2015**, *21*, 233–244. [CrossRef]
40. Shi, N.; Li, N.; Duan, X.; Niu, H. Interaction between the gut microbiome and mucosal immune system. *Mil. Med. Res.* **2017**, *4*, 14. [CrossRef]
41. Sjogren, Y.M.; Tomicic, S.; Lundberg, A.; Bottcher, M.F.; Bjorksten, B.; Sverremark-Ekstrom, E.; Jenmalm, M.C. Influence of early gut microbiota on the maturation of childhood mucosal and systemic immune responses. *Clin. Exp. Allergy* **2009**, *39*, 1842–1851. [CrossRef] [PubMed]
42. Turroni, F.; Milani, C.; Duranti, S.; Mancabelli, L.; Mangifesta, M.; Viappiani, A.; Lugli, G.A.; Ferrario, C.; Gioiosa, L.; Ferrarini, A.; et al. Deciphering bifidobacterial-mediated metabolic interactions and their impact on gut microbiota by a multi-omics approach. *ISME J.* **2016**, *10*, 1656–1668. [CrossRef] [PubMed]
43. Triantis, V.; Bode, L.; Van Neerven, R. Immunological effects of human milk oligosaccharides. *Front. Pediatr.* **2018**, *6*, 190. [CrossRef] [PubMed]
44. Prell, C.; Koletzko, B. Breastfeeding and complementary feeding: Recommendations on infant nutrition. *Deutsches Ärzteblatt Int.* **2016**, *113*, 435. [PubMed]
45. Shoaf, K.; Mulvey, G.L.; Armstrong, G.D.; Hutkins, R.W. Prebiotic galactooligosaccharides reduce adherence of enteropathogenic escherichia coli to tissue culture cells. *Infect. Immun.* **2006**, *74*, 6920–6928. [CrossRef] [PubMed]
46. Abrahamse-Berkeveld, M.; Alles, M.; Franke-Beckmann, E.; Helm, K.; Knecht, R.; Kollges, R.; Sandner, B.; Knol, J.; Ben Amor, K.; Bufe, A. Infant formula containing galacto-and fructo-oligosaccharides and bifidobacterium breve m-16v supports adequate growth and tolerance in healthy infants in a randomised, controlled, double-blind, prospective, multicentre study. *J. Nutr. Sci.* **2016**, *5*, e42. [CrossRef]
47. Swennen, K.; Courtin, C.M.; Delcour, J.A. Non-digestible oligosaccharides with prebiotic properties. *Crit. Rev. Food Sci. Nutr.* **2006**, *46*, 459–471. [CrossRef]
48. Dallman, P. Nutritional anemia of infancy: Iron, folic acid, and vitamin B12. *Nutri. Infancy Phila. Henley Belfus Inc* **1988**, 216–235.
49. Zealand, N. *Food and Nutrition Guidelines for Healthy Infants and Toddlers (Aged 0-2): Background Paper*; Ministry of Health: Wellington, New Zealand, 2008.
50. Allen, L.H. B vitamins in breast milk: Relative importance of maternal status and intake, and effects on infant status and function. *Adv. Nutr.* **2012**, *3*, 362–369. [CrossRef]
51. Schack-Nielsen, L.; Sorensen, T.; Mortensen, E.L.; Michaelsen, K.F. Late introduction of complementary feeding, rather than duration of breastfeeding, may protect against adult overweight. *Am. J. Clin. Nutr.* **2010**, *91*, 619–627. [CrossRef]
52. Ong, K.K.; Kennedy, K.; Castaneda-Gutierrez, E.; Forsyth, S.; Godfrey, K.M.; Koletzko, B.; Latulippe, M.E.; Ozanne, S.E.; Rueda, R.; Schoemaker, M.H.; et al. Postnatal growth in preterm infants and later health outcomes: A systematic review. *Acta Paediatr.* **2015**, *104*, 974–986. [CrossRef] [PubMed]
53. Pluymen, L.P.; Wijga, A.H.; Gehring, U.; Koppelman, G.H.; Smit, H.A.; van Rossem, L. Early introduction of complementary foods and childhood overweight in breastfed and formula-fed infants in the netherlands: The piama birth cohort study. *Eur. J. Nutr.* **2018**, 1–9. [CrossRef] [PubMed]
54. Georgi, G.; Bartke, N.; Wiens, F.; Stahl, B. Functional glycans and glycoconjugates in human milk. *Am. J. Clin. Nutr.* **2013**, *98*, 578S–585S. [CrossRef] [PubMed]

55. Engfer, M.B.; Stahl, B.; Finke, B.; Sawatzki, G.; Daniel, H. Human milk oligosaccharides are resistant to enzymatic hydrolysis in the upper gastrointestinal tract. *Am. J. Clin. Nutr.* **2000**, *71*, 1589–1596. [CrossRef] [PubMed]
56. Oozeer, R.; van Limpt, K.; Ludwig, T.; Ben Amor, K.; Martin, R.; Wind, R.D.; Boehm, G.; Knol, J. Intestinal microbiology in early life: Specific prebiotics can have similar functionalities as human-milk oligosaccharides. *Am. J. Clin. Nutr.* **2013**, *98*, 561S–571S. [CrossRef] [PubMed]
57. Boehm, G.; Moro, G. Structural and functional aspects of prebiotics used in infant nutrition. *J. Nutr.* **2008**, *138*, 1818S–1828S. [CrossRef] [PubMed]
58. Cummins, A.; Thompson, F. Effect of breast milk and weaning on epithelial growth of the small intestine in humans. *Gut* **2002**, *51*, 748–754. [CrossRef]
59. Keusch, G.T.; Denno, D.M.; Black, R.E.; Duggan, C.; Guerrant, R.L.; Lavery, J.V.; Nataro, J.P.; Rosenberg, I.H.; Ryan, E.T.; Tarr, P.I. Environmental enteric dysfunction: Pathogenesis, diagnosis, and clinical consequences. *Clin. Infect. Dis.* **2014**, *59*, S207–S212. [CrossRef]
60. Bourlieu, C.; Menard, O.; Bouzerzour, K.; Mandalari, G.; Macierzanka, A.; Mackie, A.R.; Dupont, D. Specificity of infant digestive conditions: Some clues for developing relevant in vitro models. *Crit. Rev. Food Sci. Nutr.* **2014**, *54*, 1427–1457. [CrossRef]
61. Sibley, E. Carbohydrate intolerance. *Curr. Opin. Gastroenterol.* **2004**, *20*, 162–167. [CrossRef]
62. Lebenthal, E.; Lee, P.C.; Heitlinger, L.A. Impact of development of the gastrointestinal tract on infant feeding. *J. Pediatr.* **1983**, *102*, 1–9. [CrossRef]
63. Lin, A.H.-M.; Nichols, B.L. The digestion of complementary feeding starches in the young child. *Starch* **2017**, *69*. [CrossRef]
64. Parracho, H.; McCartney, A.L.; Gibson, G.R. Probiotics and prebiotics in infant nutrition. *Proc. Nutr. Soc.* **2007**, *66*, 405–411. [CrossRef] [PubMed]
65. Dewit, O.; Dibba, B.; Prentice, A. Breast-milk amylase activity in english and gambian mothers: Effects of prolonged lactation, maternal parity, and individual variations. *Pediatr. Res.* **1990**, *28*, 502–506. [CrossRef] [PubMed]
66. Anderson, J.M.; Van Itallie, C.M. Physiology and function of the tight junction. *Cold Spring Harb. Perspect. Biol.* **2009**, *1*, a002584. [CrossRef] [PubMed]
67. Georas, S.N.; Rezaee, F. Epithelial barrier function: At the front line of asthma immunology and allergic airway inflammation. *J. Allergy Clin. Immunol.* **2014**, *134*, 509–520. [CrossRef] [PubMed]
68. Denno, D.M.; VanBuskirk, K.; Nelson, Z.C.; Musser, C.A.; Hay Burgess, D.C.; Tarr, P.I. Use of the lactulose to mannitol ratio to evaluate childhood environmental enteric dysfunction: A systematic review. *Clin. Infect. Dis.* **2014**, *59*, S213–S219. [CrossRef]
69. Rugtveit, J.; Fagerhol, M.K. Age-dependent variations in fecal calprotectin concentrations in children. *J. Pediatr. Gastroenterol. Nutr.* **2002**, *34*, 323. [CrossRef]
70. Dorosko, S.M.; MacKenzie, T.; Connor, R.I. Fecal calprotectin concentrations are higher in exclusively breastfed infants compared to those who are mixed-fed. *Breastfeed. Med.* **2008**, *3*, 117–119. [CrossRef]
71. De Walle, J.V.; Sergent, T.; Piront, N.; Toussaint, O.; Schneider, Y.-J.; Larondelle, Y. Deoxynivalenol affects in vitro intestinal epithelial cell barrier integrity through inhibition of protein synthesis. *Toxicol. Appl. Pharmacol.* **2010**, *245*, 291–298. [CrossRef]
72. Akbari, P.; Braber, S.; Alizadeh, A.; Verheijden, K.A.; Schoterman, M.H.; Kraneveld, A.D.; Garssen, J.; Fink-Gremmels, J. Galacto-oligosaccharides protect the intestinal barrier by maintaining the tight junction network and modulating the inflammatory responses after a challenge with the mycotoxin deoxynivalenol in human caco-2 cell monolayers and b6c3f1 mice. *J. Nutr.* **2015**, *145*, 1604–1613. [CrossRef] [PubMed]
73. Akbari, P.; Fink-Gremmels, J.; Willems, R.; Difilippo, E.; Schols, H.A.; Schoterman, M.H.C.; Garssen, J.; Braber, S. Characterizing microbiota-independent effects of oligosaccharides on intestinal epithelial cells: Insight into the role of structure and size: Structure-activity relationships of non-digestible oligosaccharides. *Eur. J. Nutr.* **2017**, *56*, 1919–1930. [CrossRef] [PubMed]
74. Cornick, S.; Tawiah, A.; Chadee, K. Roles and regulation of the mucus barrier in the gut. *Tissue Barriers* **2015**, *3*, e982426. [CrossRef] [PubMed]
75. Turroni, F.; Serafini, F.; Foroni, E.; Duranti, S.; Motherway, M.O.C.; Taverniti, V.; Mangifesta, M.; Milani, C.; Viappiani, A.; Roversi, T. Role of sortase-dependent pili of bifidobacterium bifidum prl2010 in modulating bacterium–host interactions. *Proc. Natl. Acad. Sci. USA* **2013**, *110*, 11151–11156. [CrossRef] [PubMed]

76. Walker, A. Probiotics stick it to the man. *Nat. Rev. Microbiol.* **2009**, *7*, 843. [CrossRef] [PubMed]
77. Haange, S.-B.; Oberbach, A.; Schlichting, N.; Hugenholtz, F.; Smidt, H.; von Bergen, M.; Till, H.; Seifert, J. Metaproteome analysis and molecular genetics of rat intestinal microbiota reveals section and localization resolved species distribution and enzymatic functionalities. *J. Proteome Res.* **2012**, *11*, 5406–5417. [CrossRef] [PubMed]
78. Zmora, N.; Zilberman-Schapira, G.; Suez, J.; Mor, U.; Dori-Bachash, M.; Bashiardes, S.; Kotler, E.; Zur, M.; Regev-Lehavi, D.; Brik, R.B.-Z. Personalized gut mucosal colonization resistance to empiric probiotics is associated with unique host and microbiome features. *Cell* **2018**, *174*, 1388–1405.e1321. [CrossRef] [PubMed]
79. Caballero-Franco, C.; Keller, K.; De Simone, C.; Chadee, K. The vsl#3 probiotic formula induces mucin gene expression and secretion in colonic epithelial cells. *Am. J. Physiol. Gastrointest. Liver Physiol.* **2007**, *292*, G315–G322.
80. Nofrarias, M.; Martinez-Puig, D.; Pujols, J.; Majo, N.; Perez, J.F. Long-term intake of resistant starch improves colonic mucosal integrity and reduces gut apoptosis and blood immune cells. *Nutrition* **2007**, *23*, 861–870. [CrossRef]
81. Brockhausen, I. Sulphotransferases acting on mucin-type oligosaccharides. *Biochem. Soc. Trans.* **2003**, *31*, 318–325. [CrossRef]
82. Shan, M.; Gentile, M.; Yeiser, J.R.; Walland, A.C.; Bornstein, V.U.; Chen, K.; He, B.; Cassis, L.; Bigas, A.; Cols, M. Mucus enhances gut homeostasis and oral tolerance by delivering immunoregulatory signals. *Science* **2013**, 1237910. [CrossRef]
83. Yassour, M.; Vatanen, T.; Siljander, H.; Hämäläinen, A.-M.; Härkönen, T.; Ryhänen, S.J.; Franzosa, E.A.; Vlamakis, H.; Huttenhower, C.; Gevers, D. Natural history of the infant gut microbiome and impact of antibiotic treatment on bacterial strain diversity and stability. *Sci. Transl. Med.* **2016**, *8*, 343ra381. [CrossRef] [PubMed]
84. Jeurink, P.V.; van Esch, B.C.; Rijnierse, A.; Garssen, J.; Knippels, L.M. Mechanisms underlying immune effects of dietary oligosaccharides. *Am. J. Clin. Nutr.* **2013**, *98*, 572S–577S. [CrossRef] [PubMed]
85. Kollmann, T.R.; Levy, O.; Montgomery, R.R.; Goriely, S. Innate immune function by toll-like receptors: Distinct responses in newborns and the elderly. *Immunity* **2012**, *37*, 771–783. [CrossRef] [PubMed]
86. Goenka, A.; Kollmann, T.R. Development of immunity in early life. *J. Infect.* **2015**, *71* (Suppl. 1), S112–S120. [CrossRef]
87. Duerkop, B.A.; Vaishnava, S.; Hooper, L.V. Immune responses to the microbiota at the intestinal mucosal surface. *Immunity* **2009**, *31*, 368–376. [CrossRef] [PubMed]
88. Fung, T.C.; Artis, D.; Sonnenberg, G.F. Anatomical localization of commensal bacteria in immune cell homeostasis and disease. *Immunol. Rev.* **2014**, *260*, 35–49. [CrossRef]
89. de Kivit, S.; Tobin, M.C.; Forsyth, C.B.; Keshavarzian, A.; Landay, A.L. Regulation of intestinal immune responses through tlr activation: Implications for pro- and prebiotics. *Front. Immunol.* **2014**, *5*, 60. [CrossRef]
90. Geijtenbeek, T.B.; Gringhuis, S.I. Signalling through c-type lectin receptors: Shaping immune responses. *Nat. Rev. Immunol.* **2009**, *9*, 465. [CrossRef]
91. Macpherson, A.J.; Uhr, T. Induction of protective iga by intestinal dendritic cells carrying commensal bacteria. *Science* **2004**, *303*, 1662–1665. [CrossRef]
92. Belkaid, Y.; Hand, T.W. Role of the microbiota in immunity and inflammation. *Cell* **2014**, *157*, 121–141. [CrossRef] [PubMed]
93. Gonzalez-Perez, G.; Lamouse-Smith, E.S. Gastrointestinal microbiome dysbiosis in infant mice alters peripheral CD8(+) T cell receptor signaling. *Front. Immunol.* **2017**, *8*, 265. [CrossRef] [PubMed]
94. Bermudez-Brito, M.; Rosch, C.; Schols, H.A.; Faas, M.M.; de Vos, P. Resistant starches differentially stimulate toll-like receptors and attenuate proinflammatory cytokines in dendritic cells by modulation of intestinal epithelial cells. *Mol. Nutr. Food Res.* **2015**, *59*, 1814–1826. [CrossRef] [PubMed]
95. Vogt, L.; Ramasamy, U.; Meyer, D.; Pullens, G.; Venema, K.; Faas, M.M.; Schols, H.A.; de Vos, P. Immune modulation by different types of beta2->1-fructans is toll-like receptor dependent. *PloS ONE* **2013**, *8*, e68367. [CrossRef] [PubMed]
96. Bermudez-Brito, M.; Faas, M.M.; de Vos, P. Modulation of dendritic-epithelial cell responses against sphingomonas paucimobilis by dietary fibers. *Sci. Rep.* **2016**, *6*, 30277. [CrossRef] [PubMed]
97. Aagaard, K.; Ma, J.; Antony, K.M.; Ganu, R.; Petrosino, J.; Versalovic, J. The placenta harbors a unique microbiome. *Sci. Transl. Med.* **2014**, *6*, 237ra265. [CrossRef] [PubMed]

98. Bager, P.; Wohlfahrt, J.; Westergaard, T. Caesarean delivery and risk of atopy and allergic disesase: Meta-analyses. *Clin. Exp. Allergy* **2008**, *38*, 634–642. [CrossRef] [PubMed]
99. Negele, K.; Heinrich, J.; Borte, M.; von Berg, A.; Schaaf, B.; Lehmann, I.; Wichmann, H.E.; Bolte, G.; LISA Study Group. Mode of delivery and development of atopic disease during the first 2 years of life. *Pediatr. Allergy Immunol.* **2004**, *15*, 48–54. [CrossRef]
100. Sevelsted, A.; Stokholm, J.; Bønnelykke, K.; Bisgaard, H. Cesarean section and chronic immune disorders. *Pediatrics* **2015**, *135*, e92–e98. [CrossRef] [PubMed]
101. Yuan, C.; Gaskins, A.J.; Blaine, A.I.; Zhang, C.; Gillman, M.W.; Missmer, S.A.; Field, A.E.; Chavarro, J.E. Association between cesarean birth and risk of obesity in offspring in childhood, adolescence, and early adulthood. *JAMA Pediatr.* **2016**, *170*, e162385. [CrossRef]
102. Penders, J.; Thijs, C.; Vink, C.; Stelma, F.F.; Snijders, B.; Kummeling, I.; van den Brandt, P.A.; Stobberingh, E.E. Factors influencing the composition of the intestinal microbiota in early infancy. *Pediatrics* **2006**, *118*, 511–521. [CrossRef] [PubMed]
103. Appleman, M.D.; Wormser, G.P. Strict and facultative anaerobes: Medical and environmental aspects edited by michiko m. Nakano and peter zuber wymondham, norfolk, u.K.: Horizon bioscience, 2004 392 pp., illustrated. $139.95 (cloth). *Clin. Infect. Dis.* **2005**, *41*, 132. [CrossRef]
104. Jiménez, E.; Marín, M.L.; Martín, R.; Odriozola, J.M.; Olivares, M.; Xaus, J.; Fernández, L.; Rodríguez, J.M. Is meconium from healthy newborns actually sterile? *Res. Microbiol.* **2008**, *159*, 187–193. [CrossRef] [PubMed]
105. Nagpal, R.; Kurakawa, T.; Tsuji, H.; Takahashi, T.; Kawashima, K.; Nagata, S.; Nomoto, K.; Yamashiro, Y. Evolution of gut bifidobacterium population in healthy japanese infants over the first three years of life: A quantitative assessment. *Sci. Rep.* **2017**, *7*, 10097. [CrossRef] [PubMed]
106. Nagpal, R.; Tsuji, H.; Takahashi, T.; Nomoto, K.; Kawashima, K.; Nagata, S.; Yamashiro, Y. Ontogenesis of the gut microbiota composition in healthy, full-term, vaginally born and breast-fed infants over the first 3 years of life: A quantitative bird's-eye view. *Front. Microbiol.* **2017**, *8*, 1388. [CrossRef]
107. Young, B. Breastfeeding and human milk: Short and long-term health benefits to the recipient infant. In *Early Nutrition and Long-Term Health*; Saavedra, J.M., Dattilo, A.M., Eds.; Elsevier: Amsterdam, The Netherlands, 2017; pp. 25–53.
108. Victora, C.G.; Bahl, R.; Barros, A.J.; França, G.V.; Horton, S.; Krasevec, J.; Murch, S.; Sankar, M.J.; Walker, N.; Rollins, N.C. Breastfeeding in the 21st century: Epidemiology, mechanisms, and lifelong effect. *Lancet* **2016**, *387*, 475–490. [CrossRef]
109. Penders, J.; Thijs, C.; van den Brandt, P.A.; Kummeling, I.; Snijders, B.; Stelma, F.; Adams, H.; van Ree, R.; Stobberingh, E.E. Gut microbiota composition and development of atopic manifestations in infancy: The koala birth cohort study. *Gut* **2006**, *56*, 661–667. [CrossRef] [PubMed]
110. Rinne, M.; Kalliomaki, M.; Arvilommi, H.; Salminen, S.; Isolauri, E. Effect of probiotics and breastfeeding on the bifidobacterium and lactobacillus/enterococcus microbiota and humoral immune responses. *J. Pediatr.* **2005**, *147*, 186–191. [CrossRef] [PubMed]
111. Leder, S.; Hartmeier, W.; Marx, S.P. Alpha-galactosidase of bifidobacterium adolescentis dsm 20083. *Curr. Microbiol.* **1999**, *38*, 101–106. [CrossRef] [PubMed]
112. Smilowitz, J.T.; Lebrilla, C.B.; Mills, D.A.; German, J.B.; Freeman, S.L. Breast milk oligosaccharides: Structure-function relationships in the neonate. *Annu. Rev. Nutr.* **2014**, *34*, 143–169. [CrossRef] [PubMed]
113. Marcobal, A.; Sonnenburg, J. Human milk oligosaccharide consumption by intestinal microbiota. *Clin. Microbiol. Infect.* **2012**, *18*, 12–15. [CrossRef] [PubMed]
114. Asakuma, S.; Hatakeyama, E.; Urashima, T.; Yoshida, E.; Katayama, T.; Yamamoto, K.; Kumagai, H.; Ashida, H.; Hirose, J.; Kitaoka, M. Physiology of the consumption of human milk oligosaccharides by infant-gut associated bifidobacteria. *J. Biol. Chem.* **2011**, *111*, 24583–24592. [CrossRef] [PubMed]
115. Garrido, D.; Kim, J.H.; German, J.B.; Raybould, H.E.; Mills, D.A. Oligosaccharide binding proteins from bifidobacterium longum subsp. Infantis reveal a preference for host glycans. *PloS ONE* **2011**, *6*, e17315. [CrossRef]
116. Wada, J.; Ando, T.; Kiyohara, M.; Ashida, H.; Kitaoka, M.; Yamaguchi, M.; Kumagai, H.; Katayama, T.; Yamamoto, K. Bifidobacterium bifidum lacto-n-biosidase, a critical enzyme for the degradation of human milk oligosaccharides with a type 1 structure. *Appl. Environ. Microbiol.* **2008**, *74*, 3996–4004. [CrossRef] [PubMed]

117. Garrido, D.; Ruiz-Moyano, S.; Lemay, D.G.; Sela, D.A.; German, J.B.; Mills, D.A. Comparative transcriptomics reveals key differences in the response to milk oligosaccharides of infant gut-associated bifidobacteria. *Sci. Rep.* **2015**, *5*, 13517. [CrossRef] [PubMed]
118. Ruiz-Moyano, S.; Totten, S.M.; Garrido, D.; Smilowitz, J.T.; German, J.B.; Lebrilla, C.B.; Mills, D.A. Variation in consumption of human milk oligosaccharides by infant-gut associated strains of bifidobacterium breve. *Appl. Environ. Microbiol.* **2013**, *79*, 6040–6049. [CrossRef] [PubMed]
119. González, R.; Klaassens, E.S.; Malinen, E.; De Vos, W.M.; Vaughan, E.E. Differential transcriptional response of bifidobacterium longum to human milk, formula milk, and galactooligosaccharide. *Appl. Environ. Microbiol.* **2008**, *74*, 4686–4694. [CrossRef] [PubMed]
120. Hugenholtz, F.; Ritari, J.; Nylund, L.; Davids, M.; Satokari, R.; De Vos, W.M. Feasibility of metatranscriptome analysis from infant gut microbiota: Adaptation to solid foods results in increased activity of firmicutes at six months. *Int. J. Microbiol.* **2017**, *2017*. [CrossRef] [PubMed]
121. Fallani, M.; Amarri, S.; Uusijarvi, A.; Adam, R.; Khanna, S.; Aguilera, M.; Gil, A.; Vieites, J.M.; Norin, E.; Young, D.; et al. Determinants of the human infant intestinal microbiota after the introduction of first complementary foods in infant samples from five european centres. *Microbiology* **2011**, *157*, 1385–1392. [CrossRef] [PubMed]
122. Thompson, A.L.; Monteagudo-Mera, A.; Cadenas, M.B.; Lampl, M.L.; Azcarate-Peril, M.A. Milk- and solid-feeding practices and daycare attendance are associated with differences in bacterial diversity, predominant communities, and metabolic and immune function of the infant gut microbiome. *Front. Cell. Infect. Microbiol.* **2015**, *5*, 3. [CrossRef] [PubMed]
123. Scheiwiller, J.; Arrigoni, E.; Brouns, F.; Amado, R. Human faecal microbiota develops the ability to degrade type 3 resistant starch during weaning. *J. Pediatr. Gastroenterol. Nutr.* **2006**, *43*, 584–591. [CrossRef]
124. Birt, D.F.; Boylston, T.; Hendrich, S.; Jane, J.L.; Hollis, J.; Li, L.; McClelland, J.; Moore, S.; Phillips, G.J.; Rowling, M.; et al. Resistant starch: Promise for improving human health. *Adv. Nutr.* **2013**, *4*, 587–601. [CrossRef] [PubMed]
125. Flint, H.J.; Scott, K.P.; Duncan, S.H.; Louis, P.; Forano, E. Microbial degradation of complex carbohydrates in the gut. *Gut Microbes* **2012**, *3*, 289–306. [CrossRef] [PubMed]
126. Kovatcheva-Datchary, P.; Egert, M.; Maathuis, A.; Rajilić-Stojanović, M.; De Graaf, A.A.; Smidt, H.; De Vos, W.M.; Venema, K. Linking phylogenetic identities of bacteria to starch fermentation in an in vitro model of the large intestine by rna-based stable isotope probing. *Environ. Microbiol.* **2009**, *11*, 914–926. [CrossRef] [PubMed]
127. Shipman, J.A.; Berleman, J.E.; Salyers, A.A. Characterization of four outer membrane proteins involved in binding starch to the cell surface of bacteroides thetaiotaomicron. *J. Bacteriol.* **2000**, *182*, 5365–5372. [CrossRef]
128. Crittenden, R.; Laitila, A.; Forssell, P.; Matto, J.; Saarela, M.; Mattila-Sandholm, T.; Myllarinen, P. Adhesion of bifidobacteria to granular starch and its implications in probiotic technologies. *Appl. Environ. Microbiol.* **2001**, *67*, 3469–3475. [CrossRef]
129. Shipman, J.A.; Cho, K.H.; Siegel, H.A.; Salyers, A.A. Physiological characterization of susg, an outer membrane protein essential for starch utilization by bacteroides thetaiotaomicron. *J. Bacteriol.* **1999**, *181*, 7206–7211. [PubMed]
130. Koropatkin, N.M.; Smith, T.J. Susg: A unique cell-membrane-associated alpha-amylase from a prominent human gut symbiont targets complex starch molecules. *Structure* **2010**, *18*, 200–215. [CrossRef]
131. Stewart, M.L.; Timm, D.A.; Slavin, J.L. Fructooligosaccharides exhibit more rapid fermentation than long-chain inulin in an in vitro fermentation system. *Nutr. Res.* **2008**, *28*, 329–334. [CrossRef] [PubMed]
132. Warren, F.J.; Fukuma, N.M.; Mikkelsen, D.; Flanagan, B.M.; Williams, B.A.; Lisle, A.T.; Cuív, P.Ó.; Morrison, M.; Gidley, M.J. Food starch structure impacts gut microbiome composition. *mSphere* **2018**, *3*, e00086-18. [CrossRef]
133. Wong, J.M.; de Souza, R.; Kendall, C.W.; Emam, A.; Jenkins, D.J. Colonic health: Fermentation and short chain fatty acids. *J. Clin. Gastroenterol.* **2006**, *40*, 235–243. [CrossRef]
134. Morrison, D.J.; Preston, T. Formation of short chain fatty acids by the gut microbiota and their impact on human metabolism. *Gut Microbes* **2016**, *7*, 189–200. [CrossRef] [PubMed]
135. Herrmann, E.; Young, W.; Rosendale, D.; Conrad, R.; Riedel, C.U.; Egert, M. Determination of resistant starch assimilating bacteria in fecal samples of mice by in vitro rna-based stable isotope probing. *Front. Microbiol.* **2017**, *8*, 1331. [CrossRef]

136. Boets, E.; Gomand, S.V.; Deroover, L.; Preston, T.; Vermeulen, K.; Preter, V.; Hamer, H.M.; den Mooter, G.; Vuyst, L.; Courtin, C.M. Systemic availability and metabolism of colonic-derived short-chain fatty acids in healthy subjects: A stable isotope study. *J. Physiol.* **2017**, *595*, 541–555. [CrossRef]
137. Koga, Y.; Tokunaga, S.; Nagano, J.; Sato, F.; Konishi, K.; Tochio, T.; Murakami, Y.; Masumoto, N.; Tezuka, J.-I.; Sudo, N.; et al. Age-associated effect of kestose on faecalibacterium prausnitzii and symptoms in the atopic dermatitis infants. *Pediatr. Res.* **2016**, *80*, 844–851. [CrossRef] [PubMed]
138. Bridgman, S.L.; Azad, M.B.; Field, C.J.; Haqq, A.M.; Becker, A.B.; Mandhane, P.J.; Subbarao, P.; Turvey, S.E.; Sears, M.R.; Scott, J.A.; et al. Fecal short-chain fatty acid variations by breastfeeding status in infants at 4 months: Differences in relative versus absolute concentrations. *Front. Nutr.* **2017**, *4*, 11. [CrossRef] [PubMed]
139. Macfarlane, S.; Macfarlane, G.T. Regulation of short-chain fatty acid production. *Proc. Nutr. Soc.* **2003**, *62*, 67–72. [CrossRef]
140. Vinolo, M.A.; Rodrigues, H.G.; Nachbar, R.T.; Curi, R. Regulation of inflammation by short chain fatty acids. *Nutrients* **2011**, *3*, 858–876. [CrossRef]
141. Kalina, U.; Koyama, N.; Hosoda, T.; Nuernberger, H.; Sato, K.; Hoelzer, D.; Herweck, F.; Manigold, T.; Singer, M.V.; Rossol, S. Enhanced production of il-18 in butyrate-treated intestinal epithelium by stimulation of the proximal promoter region. *Eur. J. Immunol.* **2002**, *32*, 2635–2643. [CrossRef]
142. Louis, P.; Flint, H.J. Formation of propionate and butyrate by the human colonic microbiota. *Environ. Microbiol.* **2017**, *19*, 29–41. [CrossRef] [PubMed]
143. Tedelind, S.; Westberg, F.; Kjerrulf, M.; Vidal, A. Anti-inflammatory properties of the short-chain fatty acids acetate and propionate: A study with relevance to inflammatory bowel disease. *World J. Gastroenterol.* **2007**, *13*, 2826. [CrossRef] [PubMed]
144. Fukuda, S.; Toh, H.; Taylor, T.D.; Ohno, H.; Hattori, M. Acetate-producing bifidobacteria protect the host from enteropathogenic infection via carbohydrate transporters. *Gut Microbes* **2012**, *3*, 449–454. [CrossRef]
145. Hosseini, E.; Grootaert, C.; Verstraete, W.; Van de Wiele, T. Propionate as a health-promoting microbial metabolite in the human gut. *Nutr. Rev.* **2011**, *69*, 245–258. [CrossRef]
146. Mariadason, J.M.; Barkla, D.H.; Gibson, P.R. Effect of short-chain fatty acids on paracellular permeability in caco-2 intestinal epithelium model. *Am. J. Physiol.* **1997**, *272*, G705–G712. [CrossRef]
147. Gantois, I.; Ducatelle, R.; Pasmans, F.; Haesebrouck, F.; Hautefort, I.; Thompson, A.; Hinton, J.C.; Van Immerseel, F. Butyrate specifically down-regulates salmonella pathogenicity island 1 gene expression. *Appl. Environ. Microbiol.* **2006**, *72*, 946–949. [CrossRef]
148. Louis, P.; Flint, H.J. Diversity, metabolism and microbial ecology of butyrate-producing bacteria from the human large intestine. *FEMS Microbiol. Lett.* **2009**, *294*, 1–8. [CrossRef]
149. Peng, L.; Li, Z.-R.; Green, R.S.; Holzman, I.R.; Lin, J. Butyrate enhances the intestinal barrier by facilitating tight junction assembly via activation of amp-activated protein kinase in caco-2 cell monolayers. *J. Nutr.* **2009**, *139*, 1619–1625. [CrossRef]
150. Yatsunenko, T.; Rey, F.E.; Manary, M.J.; Trehan, I.; Dominguez-Bello, M.G.; Contreras, M.; Magris, M.; Hidalgo, G.; Baldassano, R.N.; Anokhin, A.P. Human gut microbiome viewed across age and geography. *Nature* **2012**, *486*, 222. [CrossRef] [PubMed]
151. Magnúsdóttir, S.; Ravcheev, D.; de Crécy-Lagard, V.; Thiele, I. Systematic genome assessment of b-vitamin biosynthesis suggests co-operation among gut microbes. *Front. Genet.* **2015**, *6*, 148. [CrossRef]
152. Biesalski, H.K. Nutrition meets the microbiome: Micronutrients and the microbiota. *Ann. N. Y. Acad. Sci.* **2016**, *1372*, 53–64. [CrossRef] [PubMed]
153. Ueland, P.M.; McCann, A.; Midttun, Ø.; Ulvik, A. Inflammation, vitamin b6 and related pathways. *Mol. Aspects Med.* **2017**, *53*, 10–27. [CrossRef] [PubMed]
154. Kunisawa, J.; Hashimoto, E.; Ishikawa, I.; Kiyono, H. A pivotal role of vitamin b9 in the maintenance of regulatory t cells in vitro and in vivo. *PloS ONE* **2012**, *7*, e32094. [CrossRef] [PubMed]
155. Tamura, J.; Kubota, K.; Murakami, H.; Sawamura, M.; Matsushima, T.; Tamura, T.; Saitoh, T.; Kurabayshi, H.; Naruse, T. Immunomodulation by vitamin B12: Augmentation of CD8+ T lymphocytes and natural killer (nk) cell activity in vitamin B12-deficient patients by methyl-B12 treatment. *Clin. Exp. Immunol.* **1999**, *116*, 28–32. [CrossRef]
156. Kjer-Nielsen, L.; Patel, O.; Corbett, A.J.; Le Nours, J.; Meehan, B.; Liu, L.; Bhati, M.; Chen, Z.; Kostenko, L.; Reantragoon, R. Mr1 presents microbial vitamin b metabolites to mait cells. *Nature* **2012**, *491*, 717. [CrossRef] [PubMed]

157. de Verteuil, D.; Granados, D.P.; Thibault, P.; Perreault, C. Origin and plasticity of mhc i-associated self peptides. *Autoimmun. Rev.* **2012**, *11*, 627–635. [CrossRef] [PubMed]
158. Gibson, R.S.; Bailey, K.B.; Gibbs, M.; Ferguson, E.L. A review of phytate, iron, zinc, and calcium concentrations in plant-based complementary foods used in low-income countries and implications for bioavailability. *Food Nutr. Bull.* **2010**, *31*, S134–S146. [CrossRef] [PubMed]

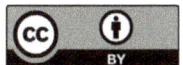

© 2019 by the authors. Licensee MDPI, Basel, Switzerland. This article is an open access article distributed under the terms and conditions of the Creative Commons Attribution (CC BY) license (http://creativecommons.org/licenses/by/4.0/).

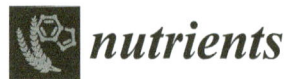

Review

Vitamin D: Nutrient, Hormone, and Immunomodulator

Francesca Sassi, Cristina Tamone and Patrizia D'Amelio *

Department of Medical Science, Gerontology and Bone Metabolic Diseases, University of Turin, 10126 Turin, Italy; francesca.sassi@unito.it (F.S.); cristinatamone78@gmail.com (C.T.)
* Correspondence: patrizia.damelio@unito.it; Tel.: +39-011-6335533

Received: 24 September 2018; Accepted: 31 October 2018; Published: 3 November 2018

Abstract: The classical functions of vitamin D are to regulate calcium-phosphorus homeostasis and control bone metabolism. However, vitamin D deficiency has been reported in several chronic conditions associated with increased inflammation and deregulation of the immune system, such as diabetes, asthma, and rheumatoid arthritis. These observations, together with experimental studies, suggest a critical role for vitamin D in the modulation of immune function. This leads to the hypothesis of a disease-specific alteration of vitamin D metabolism and reinforces the role of vitamin D in maintaining a healthy immune system. Two key observations validate this important non-classical action of vitamin D: first, vitamin D receptor (VDR) is expressed by the majority of immune cells, including B and T lymphocytes, monocytes, macrophages, and dendritic cells; second, there is an active vitamin D metabolism by immune cells that is able to locally convert $25(OH)D_3$ into $1,25(OH)_2D_3$, its active form. Vitamin D and VDR signaling together have a suppressive role on autoimmunity and an anti-inflammatory effect, promoting dendritic cell and regulatory T-cell differentiation and reducing T helper Th 17 cell response and inflammatory cytokines secretion. This review summarizes experimental data and clinical observations on the potential immunomodulating properties of vitamin D.

Keywords: vitamin D; immune system; gut microbiota; autoimmune diseases; T cells

1. Introduction

The role of vitamin D in the regulation of calcium-phosphate homeostasis and in the control of bone turnover is well known. Vitamin D status significantly affects skeletal health during growth and in adult age, its deficiency during growth leads to rickets [1], whereas during adult age it is responsible of osteomalacia and various degree of osteoporo-malacia [2]. Low vitamin D status increases bone turnover, decreases bone density, and is associated with increased fracture risk. In addition to the well-known effect on skeletal health in the last two decades evidence has been accumulated on the pleiotropic effect of vitamin D other than on bone health thanks to the findings that vitamin D receptor (VDR) and the vitamin D activating enzyme 1-α-hydroxylase (CYP27B1) are expressed in several cells outside the bone and kidney, such as in the intestine, platelets, pancreas, and prostate [3]. Several cells involved in the immune function express VDR and CYP27B1, this observation suggests that the active form of vitamin D, $1,25(OH)_2D_3$, is able to control the immune function at different levels. Previous reviews on the role of vitamin D in the regulation of immune system have been published in recent years [4,5]. Here we summarize the recent evidence sexploiting authors' expertise in both experimental and clinical fields.

2. Vitamin D Metabolism

Vitamin D enters the body trough dietary intake (about 20% of vitamin D_3 is assumed with diet) or is synthetized by the skin (80%) from 7-dihydrocholesterol following UVB exposure. Vitamin D_3

becomes biologically active after hydroxylation in the liver by the enzymes cytochrome P450 2R1 (CYP2R1) and cytochrome P450 27 (CYP27A1) becoming 25(OH)D_3. The fully-active metabolite 1,25(OH)$_2D_3$ is hydroxylated in the kidney by the enzyme CYP27B1, parathormone (PTH), and the fibroblast growth factor 23 (FGF-23) control CYP27B1 synthesis and activity [6]. Synthesis of 1,25(OH)$_2D_3$ is strictly regulated in a renal negative feedback loop: high levels of 1,25(OH)$_2D_3$ and FGF-23 inhibit CYP27B1 and induce the cytochrome P45O24A1(CYP24A1), which transforms 1,25(OH)$_2D_3$ into the inactive form 24(OH)D_3 [7].

In addition to the kidney, CYP27B1 is expressed by other cell types, including immune cells. These cells produce 1,25(OH)$_2D_3$ that has autocrine and/or paracrine effects, the high level produced locally is thought to be responsible for immunomodulation. The regulation of CYP27B1 synthesis in immune cells is different than the signals regulating kidney production of 1,25(OH)$_2D_3$. Inflammatory signals, such as lipopolysaccharide (LPS) and cytokines, induce monocyte and macrophage production of CYP27B1 [8–10]. These differences in the regulation of 1,25(OH)$_2D_3$ production point to an autocrine/paracrine effect as immunomodulatory.

3. Vitamin D Status

Vitamin D status is defined by the blood measurement of its hydroxylated form 25(OH)D_3, however, there is no common agreement on the threshold levels to identify desirable vitamin D level. Guidelines from different scientific societies and different countries established 50 nM/L or 75 nM/L to consider vitamin D sufficiency [11–13], however, it is generally accepted that 25(OH)D_3 levels lower than 50 nM/L are associated with bone metabolism alteration, increased risk of falls, and myopathy in adults [14–18]. Experts in the field generally agree to maintain 25(OH)D_3 between 20 and 125 nM/L in order to obtain the certain skeletal effects without toxic effects. Recent literature raises the suspicion that administration of a bolus of vitamin D_3 higher than 50,000 UI may result in an increased risk of falls and fractures [19,20]; moreover, the mortality related to 25(OH)D_3 is a "U shaped curve" and 25(OH)D_3 levels higher than 150 nM/L are associated with increased mortality [21].

4. Vitamin D and the Innate Immune System: Antimicrobial Activity

The innate immune system is the first defense against infection, it is required to rapidly fight against invading pathogens. The innate immune system comprehends components both from the host and resident microbes (microbiota). The host defense comprises physical barriers to infection (as skin, mucous surfaces, mucus, and vascular endothelial cells), enzymes expressed by epithelial and phagocytic cells (as lysozyme), antimicrobial peptides and proteins (as defensins, cathelicidins, and others expressed by phagocytes), inflammatory humoral components (as complement and opsonins), and cell receptors that rapidly recognize pathogens (as toll-like receptors) and cellular components (as mast cells, dendritic cells, macrophages, neutrophils cells and natural killer). Interaction between microbiota a vitamin D will be analyzed in the following paragraph.

Vitamin D is a well-known regulator of innate immunity, the first data on this topic have been generated on the treatment of diseases caused by mycobacteria, such as tuberculosis and leprosy [22,23], however, the mechanisms responsible for these actions have been elucidated in more recent years. 1,25(OH)$_2D_3$ enhances the production of defensin β2 and cathelicidin antimicrobial peptide (CAMP) by macrophage and monocyte keratinocytes increasing their antimicrobial activity [24–26]. Moreover, 1,25(OH)$_2D_3$ increases chemotaxis, autophagy, and phagolysosomal fusion of innate immune cells [27,28]. The exposition of human monocytes to pathogens, such as *M. tuberculosis* and others, up-regulates the expression of CYP27B1 and of VDR, thus enhancing both the cell ability to produce 1,25(OH)$_2D_3$ in the site of infection and to respond to this metabolite. However, macrophages are heterogeneous, with different functions [29]. Macrophages formed after interleukin (IL)-15 stimulus respond to vitamin D stimulus increasing their antimicrobial activity, whereas phagocytic macrophages obtained after stimulus with IL-10 are weakly influenced by vitamin D levels regardless of their high phagocytic activity [10,30].

1,25(OH)$_2$D$_3$ up-regulates CAMP not only by monocytes/macrophages, but also in other cells participating in the innate immune system as first-barrier defenses, such as keratinocytes, epithelial, intestinal, lung and corneal cells, and placenta trophoblasts (see for a comprehensive review Wei and Christakos, 2015) [4].

Data in humans on infections other than mycobacterial have been generated on urinary and respiratory infections and on sepsis. A predisposition to urinary tract infection in children with low vitamin D levels due to the reduced production of CAMP and defensing β2 has been suggested by association studies [31,32]. Additionally, in chronic obstructive pulmonary disease (COPD) patients' levels of CAMP and other antimicrobial peptides were associated with increased risk of acute exacerbations [33]. Consistent with this datum treatment with 1,25(OH)$_2$D$_3$ was effective in reducing respiratory infections in asthma patients thanks to increased CAMP expression and inflammatory cytokine modulation [34]. Data on the role of vitamin D status and vitamin D supplementation in sepsis are also available both in pediatric and in adult patients: in pediatric patients a clear role for 25(OH)D$_3$ and CAMP was not demonstrated [35], whereas in adults lower levels of 25(OH)D$_3$ were found in sepsis [36] and a high-dose of vitamin D3 increases circulating CAMP and reduces inflammatory cytokines as IL-6 and IL-1β [37].

More recently data on a possible role of vitamin D in increasing resistance to HIV infection have been published, in particular HIV-exposed seronegative individuals produced more CAMP in oral-mucosa and peripheral-blood, and have higher CYP24A1 mRNA in vaginal-mucosa; CYP24A1 is considered an indicator of high levels of 1,25(OH)$_2$D$_3$ [38]. Low serum vitamin D has been associated with HIV/AIDS progression and mortality [39].

1,25(OH)$_2$D$_3$ is able to increase the production of other antimicrobial peptides, such as defensing β2-4, this ability has been demonstrated both in vitro by monocytes stimulation [40,41] and in vivo in pediatric patients' blood [32].

Vitamin D is able to modulate innate immune system, also increasing the phagocytic ability on immune cells [42,43] and by reinforcing the physical barrier function of epithelial cells. In particular 1,25(OH)$_2$D$_3$ can enhance corneal [44] and intestinal [45] epithelial barrier function (Figure 1).

Taken together these data point to a role of vitamin D in defending the organism against pathogens suggesting that vitamin D sufficiency has to be granted in patients affected by acute or chronic infection. The ability of immune cells to hydroxylate 25(OH)D$_3$ into its active form 1,25(OH)$_2$D$_3$ suggests administrating vitamin D$_3$ rather than hydroxylated metabolites to patients affected by infections in order to allow the autocrine/paracrine function of 1,25(OH)$_2$D$_3$ without overcoming local hydroxylation and the feedback system.

5. Vitamin D and Microbiota: Increasing Host Defenses

The whole of the commensal, symbiotic, and pathogenic microorganisms living in different areas of the human body has defined microbiota. Microbiota and the host have several relationships, and the perfect balance between microbiota and the host is required for the development, maturation, and properfunction of the immune system [46]. Several papers suggest that vitamin D is one of the actors of the complex relationship between microbiota living in the gut (GM) and immune system modulation. Vitamin D is responsible for the barrier function of the intestinal epithelium and for the modulation of the bowel immune system, hence, low levels may be associated with greater gut permeability and, consequently, with GM-induced metabolic endotoxemia that induces a low-grade inflammation [47]. Moreover, vitamin D administration may influence GM composition, and in vitro data demonstrate that vitamin D enhances macrophages' ability to kill *Escherichia coli*. [48]. In animals with vitamin D depletion and the knockout of the VDR, the GM dysbiosis favors metabolic disorders [49]. Other studies in mice demonstrated that VDR reduces the response to infection of the intestinal epithelium [50].

Elegant studies in transgenic mice demonstrated that over-expression of VDR in the intestinal epithelium induces resistance to colitis [51,52] and decreases mucosal inflammation suppressing epithelial cell apoptosis, boosting tight junction function [51,53]. On the other hand VDR selective deletion in bowel favors a more severe form of colitis characterized by greater Th1 and Th17 mucosal infiltration and inflammatory cytokines production [54]. In humans, observational studies suggest that low levels of 25(OH)D$_3$ are associated with increased risk of inflammatory bowel disease (IBD) [55–57] and that high levels of 25(OH)D$_3$ in these patients protect against *Clostridium difficile* infection [58]. The experimental data on the role of VDR in developing IBD have been confirmed by the finding of a significant reduction of VDR expression (about 50%) in the colon epithelium in patients affected by IBD with respect to healthy controls [51,53]. The reduction in VDR expression by IBD patients may explain the different effect on GM composition of high oral dosages of vitamin D$_3$ demonstrated in a small cohort of patients affected by Crohn's disease with respect to healthy controls [59], however, human data on the effect of vitamin D supplementation on GM in IBD are still controversial, as other studies did not confirm these results [60,61]. In the study by Luthold and coll. [61] dietary intake of vitamin D and 25(OH)D$_3$ were inversely correlated with *Coprococcus* and *Bifidobacterium*, however, thanks to their ability to produce butyrate these bacteria are commonly considered as anti-inflammatory. A possible explanation of these contradictory results may be the different effect of vitamin D on GM according to the different gastro-intestinal tracts considered [62]. Recently, a double-blind placebo-controlled study on patients affected by cystic fibrosis demonstrated that vitamin D insufficiency is associated with different microbiota not only in the gut, but also in the airways, and that the administration of 50,000 IU of oral vitamin D$_3$ weekly significantly affects microbiota composition [63]. Nevertheless, the evaluation of clinical outcomes of microbiota change is still open.

Several data point to an effect of vitamin D on microbiota. Conversely, some recent reports suggest that microbiota, per se, influences vitamin D metabolism mainly through FGF-23; germ-free (GF) mice have low vitamin D and high FGF-23, whereas their colonization with bacteria results in increased levels of tumor necrosis factor-α (TNF-α) and a decrease in FGF-23 with normalization of vitamin D hydroxylated metabolites. Inhibition of FGF-23 in GF mice restores vitamin D metabolism without bacterial colonization of the gut [64] (Figure 1).

The role of GM as an active player in the regulation of bone metabolism in humans is being investigated more and more [46], and the role played by vitamin D is still under debate. Further studies to clarify their interplay are needed.

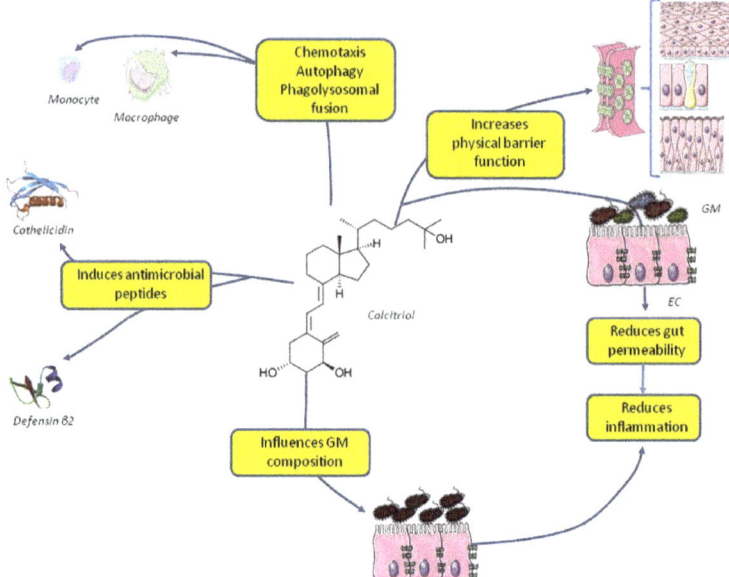

Figure 1. Effects of vitamin D on the innate immune system and gut microbiota. Abbreviations: EC, enteral cells; GM, gut microbiota.

6. Vitamin D and the Adaptive Immune System

The adaptive immune system or acquired immune system is the second defense against infection. It is required to specifically fight against pathogens, is activated by exposure to pathogens, and unlike the innate immune system it is able to learn about the pathogen and enhance the immune response accordingly, thanks to an immunological memory. The adaptive immune system is composed of T and B cells and is also responsible for autoimmune reaction.

$25(OH)D_3$ suppresses adaptive immunity [4,65]. In experimental models it down-regulates the immune responses mediated by T helper (Th) 1 cells, thus inhibiting the production of pro-inflammatory cytokines, such as Interferon-γ IFN-γ, IL-6, IL-2, and TNF-α [66,67]. Although experimental studies in vitro and in animals have yielded encouraging results on the immunomodulatory effect of $1,25(OH)_2D_3$, the same cannot be said about human studies, and few studies have confirmed the suppressive effect of vitamin D on Th1 cells and inflammatory cytokine production in different diseases and spinal tuberculosis [68], uremia [69], and autoimmune thyroiditis [70]; whereas others in IBD [71], dialysis [72], and rheumatoid arthritis [73] do not confirm these results. These discrepancies may be due to the different diseases considered and also to the different type of treatment administered, mainly $1,25(OH)_2D_3$ in vitro and in animals and vitamin D_3 in vivo in humans. Moreover, when considering administration of vitamin D3 different doses were used in different studies. Therefore, it is almost impossible to compare the results.

It has been suggested that $1,25(OH)_2D_3$ acts as an immunomodulatory not only by suppressing Th1 cells activation, but also modulating Th2 cells, T regulatory (Tregs) cells activity, and Th17 cells.

The majority of the in vitro studies assessing the effect of vitamin D on Th2 suggests that $1,25(OH)_2D_3$ upregulates Th2 cells activity [74–76]. Amongst immunomodulatory effects of vitamin D its ability to suppress Th17 and increase Treg cells has been recently demonstrated [77–79]. Th17 cells produce IL-17 and have been implicated in the pathogenesis of several autoimmune diseases, some experimental studies suggest that $1,25(OH)_2D_3$ suppresses Th17 formation and activity [67,80–83] by blocking Nuclear Factor of Activated T-cells (NFAT) and Runt-related Transcription Factor 1

(RUNx1) binding to the IL-17 promoter and inducing Forkhead box P3 (FOXP3) [81], and by inhibiting RAR-related Orphan Receptor Gamma2 (RORγt) which is the transcription factor of IL-17 [84].

More recently our lab showed no effect of the administration of a high bolus of vitamin D_3 (300,000 UI) in the modulation of Th subset in patients affected by early rheumatoid arthritis [73], as well as a study on hemodialysis patients [72].

It has also been suggested that the administration of oral vitamin D_3 increases Tregs function in patients with type 1 diabetes mellitus [85], however, in other diseases, such as early rheumatoid arthritis, this effect was not confirmed [73].

The overall effect of vitamin D on Th cells differentiation may be mediated by its effect on dendritic cells, these cells are antigen-presenting cells (APCs), responsible for T cell differentiation into an effector cell with pro- or anti-inflammatory properties, thus, modulation of APCs is crucial in initiating and maintaining adaptive immune response and self-tolerance [86]. In vitro differentiation of dendritic cells in the presence of $1,25(OH)_2D_3$ induces a "tolerogenic state" characterized by low levels of inflammatory cytokines, such as IL-12 and TNF-α, with increased levels of the anti-inflammatory IL-10, these cells induce the differentiation of Treg cells and induce apoptosis in the autoreactive T cells [87–90] (Figure 2).

Taken together these data are not sufficient to prove a real role for vitamin D in the modulation of adaptive immune system in humans, thus, the therapeutic use of vitamin D and its metabolites in patients aiming to ameliorate the adaptive immune system is not sustained by sufficient data.

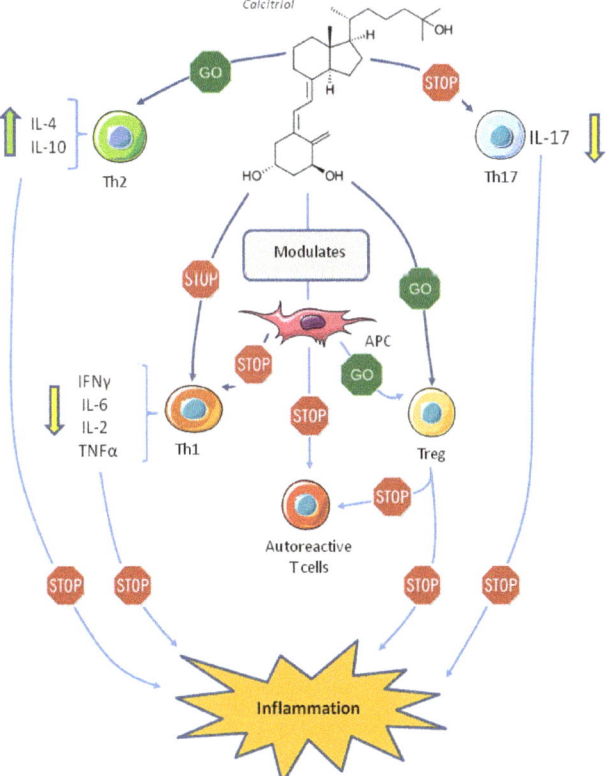

Figure 2. Effect of vitamin D on the adaptive immune system. Abbreviations: APC, antigen presenting cell; IFN, interferon; IL, interleukin; Th1, T helper 1 cell; Th2, T helper 2 cell; Th17, T helper 17 cell; TNF, tumor necrosis factor; Treg, T regulatory cell.

7. Vitamin D and Autoimmune Diseases

Thanks to the evidences of immunomodulatory effect of vitamin D the role of vitamin D deficiency and supplementation in autoimmune diseases has long been studied. Animal studies showed an important role of 1,25(OH)$_2$D$_3$ supplementation in the control of autoimmune diseases, such as experimental autoimmune encephalomyelitis (EAE) and collagen-induced arthritis (CIA). In these two conditions 1,25(OH)$_2$D$_3$ prevents the initiation and reduces the disease progression [91–93]. Similarly, different mouse models of enterocolitis display a more severe phenotype during vitamin D deficiency and reduced inflammation after administration of 1,25(OH)$_2$D$_3$ (see for a review Alhassan et al., 2017) [94]. Despite solid experimental evidence human studies are less convincing: some epidemiological data link increasing latitude and consequent decrease sunlight exposure with higher prevalence of multiple sclerosis [95–97], type I diabetes [98–100], and IBD [101]. It is clear that such differences may be due to genetic and lifestyle factors other than 25(OH)D$_3$ levels. Other epidemiological data reinforcing the hypothesis of a link between sun exposure, vitamin D synthesis, and the risk of developing multiple sclerosis stem from the observation that subjects born in months associated with lower 25(OH)D$_3$ level in the northern hemisphere (April) are at higher risk of developing the disease, whereas patients born in October (higher vitamin D levels) are at lower risk [102].

Some studies correlated vitamin D dietary intake and the prevalence of autoimmune diseases as rheumatoid arthritis [103] and type 1 diabetes mellitus [104,105], however, the correct evaluation of vitamin D intake is challenging as it is based on patient recall. To bypass the challenging measurement of vitamin D intake and sun exposure, levels of 25(OH)D$_3$ in the serum can be useful, and, indeed, low levels of 25(OH)D$_3$ in the serum of patients affected by autoimmune diseases with respect to healthy controls have been found [106–112]. Nevertheless, these studies demonstrated a correlation and not a causal relationship.

Intervention studies with different doses of vitamin D$_3$ in autoimmune diseases lead to different outcomes, recently we demonstrated that a bolus of vitamin D$_3$ (300,000 UI) in patients affected by early rheumatoid arthritis is effective in ameliorating general health, however, we found no effect on disease activity nor on inflammatory markers and T cells subset [73]. In patients affected by type 1 diabetes clinical intervention studies with vitamin D$_3$ or hydroxylated analogs have been disappointing, as no clinical study has demonstrated an effect of vitamin D in ameliorating glucose metabolism and insulin secretion [113,114], however, in a small prospective trial in children with type 1 diabetes autoantibodies 1,25(OH)$_2$D$_3$ administration decreased the serum glutamic acid decarboxylase 65 (GAD65) autoantibody, pointing to some immunomodulation of 1,25(OH)$_2$D$_3$ [115].

In addition to autoimmune diseases vitamin D has also been implicated in the control of other inflammatory conditions, such as cardiovascular diseases: in animal models vitamin D$_3$ administration reduces macrophage production of pro-inflammatory cytokines, and decreases atherosclerosis and inflammation in the epicardial adipose tissue [116,117]. In humans an association between low 25(OH)D$_3$ level and increased activation of inflammatory pathway in epicardial adipose tissue in patients affected by coronary artery disease has been described [118]. Vitamin D deficiency has been linked to cardiovascular disease not only by the modulation of inflammatory pathways, but also through the modulation of endothelial function, the effect on arterial stiffness, and a possible beneficial role on atherosclerotic plaque formation. However, this topic is beyond the scope of this review. For further insight in the role of vitamin D in the pathogenesis of cardiovascular disease see the review by Apostolakis and coll. [119].

8. Conclusions

In summary, several studies point to an important role of vitamin D as an immunomodulator, and strong data demonstrate a role for 1,25(OH)$_2$D$_3$ in increasing the ability of the innate immune system to fight against pathogens, whereas data on the effect of 1,25(OH)$_2$D$_3$ in the modulation of acquired immune system are more controversial. There is no general consensus on the desired level of

25(OH)D$_3$ to achieve immunomodulatory effects, thus, there is no current indication for vitamin D$_3$ supplementation in patients with infections and/or autoimmune diseases. Further studies are needed to clarify the role of vitamin D as immunomodulator in humans.

Author Contributions: All three authors participated in the bibliographic search, discussion and writing of the manuscript. The manuscript was finalized by P.D.

Funding: This research received no external funding

Conflicts of Interest: The authors declare that they have no conflict of interest.

References

1. Antonucci, R.; Locci, C.; Clemente, M.G.; Chicconi, E.; Antonucci, L. Vitamin D deficiency in childhood: Old lessons and current challenges. *J. Pediatr. Endocrinol. Metab.* **2018**, *31*, 247–260. [CrossRef] [PubMed]
2. Uday, S.; Högler, W. Prevention of rickets and osteomalacia in the UK: Political action overdue. *Arch. Dis. Child.* **2018**, *103*, 901–906. [CrossRef] [PubMed]
3. D'Amelio, P.; Cristofaro, M.A.; De Vivo, E.; Ravazzoli, M.; Grosso, E.; Di Bella, S.; Aime, M.; Cotto, N.; Silvagno, F.; Isaia, G.; et al. Platelet vitamin D receptor is reduced in osteoporotic patients. *Panminerva Med.* **2012**, *54*, 225–231. [PubMed]
4. Wei, R.; Christakos, S. Mechanisms Underlying the regulation of innate and adaptive immunity by vitamin D. *Nutrients* **2015**, *7*, 8251–8260. [CrossRef] [PubMed]
5. Altieri, B.; Muscogiuri, G.; Barrea, L.; Mathieu, C.; Vallone, C.V.; Mascitelli, L.; Bizzaro, G.; Altieri, V.M.; Tirabassi, G.; Balercia, G.; et al. Does vitamin D play a role in autoimmune endocrine? A proof of concept. *Rev. Endocr. Metab. Disord.* **2013**, *18*, 335–346. [CrossRef] [PubMed]
6. Borel, P.; Caillaud, D.; Cano, N.J. Vitamin D bioavailability: State of the art. *Crit. Rev. Food Sci. Nutr.* **2015**, *55*, 1193–1205. [CrossRef] [PubMed]
7. Anderson, P.H. Vitamin D Activity and Metabolism in Bone. *Curr. Osteoporos. Rep.* **2017**, *15*, 443–449. [CrossRef] [PubMed]
8. Liu, P.T.; Stenger, S.; Li, H.; Wenzel, L.; Tan, B.H.; Krutzik, S.R.; Ochoa, M.T.; Schauber, J.; Wu, K.; Meinken, C.; et al. Toll-like receptor triggering of a vitamin D-mediated human antimicrobial response. *Science* **2006**, *311*, 1770–1773. [CrossRef] [PubMed]
9. Stoffels, K.; Overbergh, L.; Giulietti, A.; Verlinden, L.; Bouillon, R.; Mathieu, C. Immune regulation of 25-hydroxyvitamin-D$_3$-1alpha-hydroxylase in human monocytes. *J. Bone Miner. Res.* **2006**, *21*, 37–47. [CrossRef] [PubMed]
10. Krutzik, S.R.; Hewison, M.; Liu, P.T.; Robles, J.A.; Stenger, S.; Adams, J.S.; Modlin, R.L. IL-15 links TLR2/1-induced macrophage differentiation to the vitamin D-dependent antimicrobial pathway. *J. Immunol.* **2008**, *181*, 7115–7120. [CrossRef] [PubMed]
11. Ross, A.C.; Manson, J.E.; Abrams, S.A.; Aloia, J.F.; Brannon, P.M.; Clinton, S.K.; Durazo-Arvizu, R.A.; Gallagher, J.C.; Gallo, R.L.; Jones, G.; et al. The 2011 report on dietary reference intakes for calcium and vitamin D from the Institute of Medicine: What clinicians need to know. *J. Clin. Endocrinol. Metab.* **2011**, *96*, 53–58. [CrossRef] [PubMed]
12. Holick, M.F.; Binkley, N.C.; Bischoff-Ferrari, H.A.; Gordon, C.M.; Hanley, D.A.; Heaney, R.P.; Murad, M.H.; Weaver, C.M. Endocrine Society Evaluation, treatment, and prevention of vitamin D deficiency: An Endocrine Society clinical practice guideline. *J. Clin. Endocrinol. Metab.* **2011**, *96*, 1911–1930. [CrossRef] [PubMed]
13. Cesareo, R.; Attanasio, R.; Caputo, M.; Castello, R.; Chiodini, I.; Falchetti, A.; Guglielmi, R.; Papini, E.; Santonati, A.; Scillitani, A.; et al. Italian Association of Clinical Endocrinologists (AME) and Italian chapter of the American Association of Clinical Endocrinologists (AACE) position statement: Clinical management of vitamin D deficiency in adults. *Nutrients* **2018**, *10*, 546. [CrossRef] [PubMed]
14. Valcour, A.; Blocki, F.; Hawkins, D.M.; Rao, S.D. Effects of age and serum 25-OH-vitamin D on serum parathyroid hormone levels. *J. Clin. Endocrinol. Metab.* **2012**, *97*, 3989–3995. [CrossRef] [PubMed]
15. LeBlanc, E.; Chou, R.; Zakher, B.; Daeges, M.; Pappas, M. *Screening for Vitamin D Deficiency: Systematic Review for the U.S. Preventive Services Task Force Recommendation*; Agency for Healthcare Research and Quality: Rockville, MD, USA, 2014.

16. LeBlanc, E.S.; Zakher, B.; Daeges, M.; Pappas, M.; Chou, R. Screening for vitamin D deficiency: A systematic review for the U.S. Preventive Services Task Force. *Ann. Intern. Med.* **2015**, *162*, 109–122. [CrossRef] [PubMed]
17. Gillespie, L.D.; Robertson, M.C.; Gillespie, W.J.; Sherrington, C.; Gates, S.; Clemson, L.M.; Lamb, S.E. Interventions for preventing falls in older people living in the community. *Cochrane Database Syst. Rev.* **2012**. [CrossRef] [PubMed]
18. Bhattoa, H.P.; Konstantynowicz, J.; Laszcz, N.; Wojcik, M.; Pludowski, P. Vitamin D: Musculoskeletal health. *Rev. Endocr. Metab. Disord.* **2017**, *18*, 363–371. [CrossRef] [PubMed]
19. Sanders, K.M.; Stuart, A.L.; Williamson, E.J.; Simpson, J.A.; Kotowicz, M.A.; Young, D.; Nicholson, G.C. Annual high-dose oral vitamin D and falls and fractures in older women: A randomized controlled trial. *JAMA* **2010**, *303*, 1815–1822. [CrossRef] [PubMed]
20. Bischoff-Ferrari, H.A.; Dawson-Hughes, B.; Orav, E.J.; Staehelin, H.B.; Meyer, O.W.; Theiler, R.; Dick, W.; Willett, W.C.; Egli, A. Monthly high-dose vitamin D Treatment for the prevention of functional decline: A randomized clinical trial. *JAMA Intern. Med.* **2016**, *176*, 175–183. [CrossRef] [PubMed]
21. Amrein, K.; Quraishi, S.A.; Litonjua, A.A.; Gibbons, F.K.; Pieber, T.R.; Camargo, C.A.; Giovannucci, E.; Christopher, K.B. Evidence for a U-shaped relationship between prehospital vitamin D status and mortality: A cohort study. *J. Clin. Endocrinol. Metab.* **2014**, *99*, 1461–1469. [CrossRef] [PubMed]
22. Airey, F.S. Vitamin D as a remedy for lupus vulgaris. *Med. World* **1946**, *64*, 807–810. [PubMed]
23. Herrera, G. Vitamin D in massive doses as an adjuvant to the sulfones in the treatment of tuberculoid leprosy. *Int. J. Lepr.* **1949**, *17*, 35–42. [PubMed]
24. Wang, T.-T.; Nestel, F.P.; Bourdeau, V.; Nagai, Y.; Wang, Q.; Liao, J.; Tavera-Mendoza, L.; Lin, R.; Hanrahan, J.W.; Mader, S.; et al. Cutting edge: 1,25-dihydroxyvitamin D_3 is a direct inducer of antimicrobial peptide gene expression. *J. Immunol.* **2004**, *173*, 2909–2912. [CrossRef] [PubMed]
25. Gombart, A.F.; Borregaard, N.; Koeffler, H.P. Human cathelicidin antimicrobial peptide (CAMP) gene is a direct target of the vitamin D receptor and is strongly up-regulated in myeloid cells by 1,25-dihydroxyvitamin D_3. *FASEB J.* **2005**, *19*, 1067–1077. [CrossRef] [PubMed]
26. Dai, X.; Sayama, K.; Tohyama, M.; Shirakata, Y.; Hanakawa, Y.; Tokumaru, S.; Yang, L.; Hirakawa, S.; Hashimoto, K. PPARγ mediates innate immunity by regulating the 1α,25-dihydroxyvitamin D_3 induced hBD-3 and cathelicidin in human keratinocytes. *J. Dermatol. Sci.* **2010**, *60*, 179–186. [CrossRef] [PubMed]
27. Liu, P.T.; Stenger, S.; Tang, D.H.; Modlin, R.L. Cutting edge: Vitamin D-mediated human antimicrobial activity against Mycobacterium tuberculosis is dependent on the induction of cathelicidin. *J. Immunol.* **2007**, *179*, 2060–2063. [CrossRef] [PubMed]
28. White, J.H. Vitamin D as an inducer of cathelicidin antimicrobial peptide expression: Past, present and future. *J. Steroid Biochem. Mol. Biol.* **2010**, *121*, 234–238. [CrossRef] [PubMed]
29. Bursuker, I.; Goldman, R. On the origin of macrophage heterogeneity: A hypothesis. *J. Reticuloendothel. Soc.* **1983**, *33*, 207–220. [PubMed]
30. Kim, E.W.; Teles, R.M.B.; Haile, S.; Liu, P.T.; Modlin, R.L. Vitamin D status contributes to the antimicrobial activity of macrophages against Mycobacterium leprae. *PLoS Negl. Trop. Dis.* **2018**, *12*. [CrossRef] [PubMed]
31. ÖvünçHacıhamdioğlu, D.; Altun, D.; Hacıhamdioğlu, B.; Çekmez, F.; Aydemir, G.; Kul, M.; Müftüoğlu, T.; Süleymanoğlu, S.; Karademir, F. The association between serum 25-hydroxy vitamin D level and urine cathelicidin in children with a urinary tract infection. *J. Clin. Res. Pediatr. Endocrinol.* **2016**, *8*, 325–329. [CrossRef] [PubMed]
32. Georgieva, V.; Kamolvit, W.; Herthelius, M.; Lüthje, P.; Brauner, A.; Chromek, M. Association between vitamin D, antimicrobial peptides and urinary tract infection in infants and young children. *Acta Paediatr.* **2018**. [CrossRef] [PubMed]
33. Persson, L.J.P.; Aanerud, M.; Hardie, J.A.; Miodini Nilsen, R.; Bakke, P.S.; Eagan, T.M.; Hiemstra, P.S. Antimicrobial peptide levels are linked to airway inflammation, bacterial colonisation and exacerbations in chronic obstructive pulmonary disease. *Eur. Respir. J.* **2017**, *49*. [CrossRef] [PubMed]
34. Ramos-Martínez, E.; López-Vancell, M.R.; Fernández de Córdova-Aguirre, J.C.; Rojas-Serrano, J.; Chavarría, A.; Velasco-Medina, A.; Velázquez-Sámano, G. Reduction of respiratory infections in asthma patients supplemented with vitamin D is related to increased serum IL-10 and IFNγ levels and cathelicidin expression. *Cytokine* **2018**, *108*, 239–246. [CrossRef] [PubMed]

35. Mathias, E.; Tangpricha, V.; Sarnaik, A.; Farooqi, A.; Sethuraman, U. Association of vitamin D with cathelicidin and vitamin D binding protein in pediatric sepsis. *J. Clin. Transl. Endocrinol.* **2017**, *10*, 36–38. [CrossRef] [PubMed]
36. Greulich, T.; Regner, W.; Branscheidt, M.; Herr, C.; Koczulla, A.R.; Vogelmeier, C.F.; Bals, R. Altered blood levels of vitamin D, cathelicidin and parathyroid hormone in patients with sepsis-a pilot study. *Anaesth. Intensive Care* **2017**, *45*, 36–45. [PubMed]
37. Quraishi, S.A.; De Pascale, G.; Needleman, J.S.; Nakazawa, H.; Kaneki, M.; Bajwa, E.K.; Camargo, C.A.; Bhan, I. Effect of cholecalciferol supplementation on vitamin D status and cathelicidin levels in sepsis: A randomized, placebo-controlled trial. *Crit. Care Med.* **2015**, *43*, 1928–1937. [CrossRef] [PubMed]
38. Aguilar-Jimenez, W.; Zapata, W.; Rugeles, M.T. Antiviral molecules correlate with vitamin D pathway genes and are associated with natural resistance to HIV-1 infection. *Microbes. Infect.* **2016**, *18*, 510–516. [CrossRef] [PubMed]
39. Coussens, A.K.; Naude, C.E.; Goliath, R.; Chaplin, G.; Wilkinson, R.J.; Jablonski, N.G. High-dose vitamin D3 reduces deficiency caused by low UVB exposure and limits HIV-1 replication in urban Southern Africans. *PNAS* **2015**, *112*, 8052–8057. [CrossRef] [PubMed]
40. Liu, P.T.; Schenk, M.; Walker, V.P.; Dempsey, P.W.; Kanchanapoomi, M.; Wheelwright, M.; Vazirnia, A.; Zhang, X.; Steinmeyer, A.; Zügel, U.; et al. Convergence of IL-1beta and VDR activation pathways in human TLR2/1-induced antimicrobial responses. *PLoS ONE* **2009**, *4*. [CrossRef]
41. Castañeda-Delgado, J.E.; Araujo, Z.; Gonzalez-Curiel, I.; Serrano, C.J.; Rivas Santiago, C.; Enciso-Moreno, J.A.; Rivas-Santiago, B. Vitamin D and l-isoleucine promote antimicrobial peptide hBD-2 production in peripheral blood mononuclear cells from elderly individuals. *Int. J. Vitam. Nutr. Res.* **2016**, *86*, 56–61. [CrossRef] [PubMed]
42. Sly, L.M.; Lopez, M.; Nauseef, W.M.; Reiner, N.E. 1alpha,25-Dihydroxyvitamin D_3-induced monocyte antimycobacterial activity is regulated by phosphatidylinositol 3-kinase and mediated by the NADPH-dependent phagocyte oxidase. *J. Biol. Chem.* **2001**, *276*, 35482–35493. [CrossRef] [PubMed]
43. Shin, D.-M.; Yuk, J.-M.; Lee, H.-M.; Lee, S.-H.; Son, J.W.; Harding, C.V.; Kim, J.-M.; Modlin, R.L.; Jo, E.-K. Mycobacterial lipoprotein activates autophagy via TLR2/1/CD14 and a functional vitamin D receptor signaling. *Cell. Microbiol.* **2010**, *12*, 1648–1665. [CrossRef] [PubMed]
44. Yin, Z.; Pintea, V.; Lin, Y.; Hammock, B.D.; Watsky, M.A. Vitamin D enhances corneal epithelial barrier function. *Invest. Ophthalmol. Vis. Sci.* **2011**, *52*, 7359–7364. [CrossRef] [PubMed]
45. Pálmer, H.G.; González-Sancho, J.M.; Espada, J.; Berciano, M.T.; Puig, I.; Baulida, J.; Quintanilla, M.; Cano, A.; de Herreros, A.G.; Lafarga, M.; et al. Vitamin D_3 promotes the differentiation of colon carcinoma cells by the induction of E-cadherin and the inhibition of beta-catenin signaling. *J. Cell Biol.* **2001**, *154*, 369–387. [CrossRef] [PubMed]
46. D'Amelio, P.; Sassi, F. Gut Microbiota, Immune System, and Bone. *Calcif. Tissue Int.* **2018**, *102*, 415–425. [CrossRef] [PubMed]
47. Caricilli, A.M.; Picardi, P.K.; de Abreu, L.L.; Ueno, M.; Prada, P.O.; Ropelle, E.R.; Hirabara, S.M.; Castoldi, Â.; Vieira, P.; Camara, N.O.S.; et al. Gut microbiota is a key modulator of insulin resistance in TLR 2 knockout mice. *PLoS Biol.* **2011**, *9*. [CrossRef] [PubMed]
48. Flanagan, P.K.; Chiewchengchol, D.; Wright, H.L.; Edwards, S.W.; Alswied, A.; Satsangi, J.; Subramanian, S.; Rhodes, J.M.; Campbell, B.J. Killing of escherichia coli by Crohn's disease monocyte-derived macrophages and its enhancement by hydroxychloroquine and vitamin D. *Inflamm. Bowel Dis.* **2015**, *21*, 1499–1510. [CrossRef] [PubMed]
49. Su, D.; Nie, Y.; Zhu, A.; Chen, Z.; Wu, P.; Zhang, L.; Luo, M.; Sun, Q.; Cai, L.; Lai, Y.; et al. Vitamin D signaling through induction of paneth cell defensins maintains gut microbiota and improves metabolic disorders and hepatic steatosis in animal models. *Front Physiol.* **2016**, *7*. [CrossRef] [PubMed]
50. Wu, S.; Liao, A.P.; Xia, Y.; Li, Y.C.; Li, J.-D.; Sartor, R.B.; Sun, J. Vitamin D receptor negatively regulates bacterial-stimulated NF-kappaB activity in intestine. *Am. J. Pathol.* **2010**, *177*, 686–697. [CrossRef] [PubMed]
51. Liu, W.; Chen, Y.; Golan, M.A.; Annunziata, M.L.; Du, J.; Dougherty, U.; Kong, J.; Musch, M.; Huang, Y.; Pekow, J.; et al. Intestinal epithelial vitamin D receptor signaling inhibits experimental colitis. *JCI* **2013**, *123*, 3983–3996. [CrossRef] [PubMed]

52. Golan, M.A.; Liu, W.; Shi, Y.; Chen, L.; Wang, J.; Liu, T.; Li, Y.C. Transgenic expression of vitamin D receptor in gut epithelial cells ameliorates spontaneous colitis caused by interleukin-10 deficiency. *Dig. Dis. Sci.* **2015**, *60*, 1941–1947. [CrossRef] [PubMed]
53. Du, J.; Chen, Y.; Shi, Y.; Liu, T.; Cao, Y.; Tang, Y.; Ge, X.; Nie, H.; Zheng, C.; Li, Y.C. 1,25-Dihydroxyvitamin D protects intestinal epithelial barrier by regulating the myosin light chain kinase signaling pathway. *Inflamm. Bowel Dis.* **2015**, *21*, 2495–2506. [CrossRef] [PubMed]
54. He, L.; Liu, T.; Shi, Y.; Tian, F.; Hu, H.; Deb, D.K.; Chen, Y.; Bissonnette, M.; Li, Y.C. Gut epithelial vitamin D receptor regulates microbiota-dependent mucosal inflammation by suppressing intestinal epithelial cell apoptosis. *Endocrinology* **2018**, *159*, 967–979. [CrossRef] [PubMed]
55. Loftus, E.V.; Sandborn, W.J. Epidemiology of inflammatory bowel disease. *Gastroenterol. Clin. North Am.* **2002**, *31*, 1–20. [CrossRef]
56. Loftus, E.V. Clinical epidemiology of inflammatory bowel disease: Incidence, prevalence, and environmental influences. *Gastroenterology* **2004**, *126*, 1504–1517. [CrossRef] [PubMed]
57. Lim, W.-C.; Hanauer, S.B.; Li, Y.C. Mechanisms of disease: Vitamin D and inflammatory bowel disease. *Nat. Clin. Pract. Gastroenterol. Hepatol.* **2005**, *2*, 308–315. [CrossRef] [PubMed]
58. Ananthakrishnan, A.N.; Cagan, A.; Gainer, V.S.; Cheng, S.-C.; Cai, T.; Szolovits, P.; Shaw, S.Y.; Churchill, S.; Karlson, E.W.; Murphy, S.N.; et al. Higher plasma vitamin D is associated with reduced risk of Clostridium difficile infection in patients with inflammatory bowel diseases. *Aliment. Pharmacol. Ther.* **2014**, *39*, 1136–1142. [CrossRef] [PubMed]
59. Schäffler, H.; Herlemann, D.P.; Klinitzke, P.; Berlin, P.; Kreikemeyer, B.; Jaster, R.; Lamprecht, G. Vitamin D administration leads to a shift of the intestinal bacterial composition in Crohn's disease patients, but not in healthy controls. *J. Dig. Dis.* **2018**, *19*, 225–234. [CrossRef] [PubMed]
60. Garg, M.; Hendy, P.; Ding, J.N.; Shaw, S.; Hold, G.; Hart, A. The effect of vitamin D on intestinal inflammation and faecal microbiota in patients with ulcerative colitis. *J. Crohns. Colitis.* **2018**, *12*, 963–972. [CrossRef] [PubMed]
61. Luthold, R.V.; Fernandes, G.R.; Franco-de-Moraes, A.C.; Folchetti, L.G.D.; Ferreira, S.R.G. Gut microbiota interactions with the immunomodulatory role of vitamin D in normal individuals. *Metab. Clin. Exp.* **2017**, *69*, 76–86. [CrossRef] [PubMed]
62. Bashir, M.; Prietl, B.; Tauschmann, M.; Mautner, S.I.; Kump, P.K.; Treiber, G.; Wurm, P.; Gorkiewicz, G.; Högenauer, C.; Pieber, T.R. Effects of high doses of vitamin D_3 on mucosa-associated gut microbiome vary between regions of the human gastrointestinal tract. *Eur. J. Nutr.* **2016**, *55*, 1479–1489. [CrossRef] [PubMed]
63. Kanhere, M.; He, J.; Chassaing, B.; Ziegler, T.R.; Alvarez, J.A.; Ivie, E.A.; Hao, L.; Hanfelt, J.; Gewirtz, A.T.; Tangpricha, V. Bolus weekly vitamin D_3 supplementation impacts gut and airway microbiota in adults with cystic fibrosis: A double-blind, randomized, placebo-controlled clinical trial. *J. Clin. Endocrinol. Metab.* **2018**, *103*, 564–574. [CrossRef] [PubMed]
64. Bora, S.A.; Kennett, M.J.; Smith, P.B.; Patterson, A.D.; Cantorna, M.T. The gut microbiota regulates endocrine vitamin D metabolism through fibroblast growth factor 23. *Front Immunol.* **2018**, *9*. [CrossRef] [PubMed]
65. Chun, R.F.; Liu, P.T.; Modlin, R.L.; Adams, J.S.; Hewison, M. Impact of vitamin D on immune function: Lessons learned from genome-wide analysis. *Front Physiol.* **2014**, *5*. [CrossRef] [PubMed]
66. Carvalho, J.T.G.; Schneider, M.; Cuppari, L.; Grabulosa, C.C.; T Aoike, D.Q.; Redublo, B.M.C.; Batista, M.; Cendoroglo, M.; Maria Moyses, R.; Dalboni, M.A. Cholecalciferol decreases inflammation and improves vitamin D regulatory enzymes in lymphocytes in the uremic environment: A randomized controlled pilot trial. *PLoS ONE* **2017**, *12*. [CrossRef] [PubMed]
67. Xie, Z.; Chen, J.; Zheng, C.; Wu, J.; Cheng, Y.; Zhu, S.; Lin, C.; Cao, Q.; Zhu, J.; Jin, T. 1,25-dihydroxyvitamin D_3-induced dendritic cells suppress experimental autoimmune encephalomyelitis by increasing proportions of the regulatory lymphocytes and reducing T helper type 1 and type 17 cells. *Immunology* **2017**, *152*, 414–424. [CrossRef] [PubMed]
68. Zhou, S.-H.; Wang, X.; Fan, M.-Y.; Li, H.-L.; Bian, F.; Huang, T.; Fang, H.-Y. Influence of vitamin D deficiency on T cell subsets and related indices during spinal tuberculosis. *Exp. Ther. Med.* **2018**, *16*, 718–722. [CrossRef] [PubMed]
69. Stubbs, J.R.; Idiculla, A.; Slusser, J.; Menard, R.; Quarles, L.D. Cholecalciferol supplementation alters calcitriol-responsive monocyte proteins and decreases inflammatory cytokines in ESRD. *J. Am. Soc. Nephrol.* **2010**, *21*, 353–361. [CrossRef] [PubMed]

70. Drozdenko, G.; Heine, G.; Worm, M. Oral vitamin D increases the frequencies of CD38+ human B cells and ameliorates IL-17-producing T cells. *Exp. Dermatol.* **2014**, *23*, 107–112. [CrossRef] [PubMed]
71. Bendix-Struve, M.; Bartels, L.E.; Agnholt, J.; Dige, A.; Jørgensen, S.P.; Dahlerup, J.F. Vitamin D_3 treatment of Crohn's disease patients increases stimulated T cell IL-6 production and proliferation. *Aliment. Pharmacol. Ther.* **2010**, *32*, 1364–1372. [CrossRef] [PubMed]
72. Seibert, E.; Heine, G.H.; Ulrich, C.; Seiler, S.; Köhler, H.; Girndt, M. Influence of cholecalciferol supplementation in hemodialysis patients on monocyte subsets: A randomized, double-blind, placebo-controlled clinical trial. *Nephron. Clin. Pract.* **2013**, *123*, 209–219. [CrossRef] [PubMed]
73. Buondonno, I.; Rovera, G.; Sassi, F.; Rigoni, M.M.; Lomater, C.; Parisi, S.; Pellerito, R.; Isaia, G.C.; D'Amelio, P. Vitamin D and immunomodulation in early rheumatoid arthritis: A randomized double-blind placebo-controlled study. *PLoS ONE* **2017**, *12*. [CrossRef] [PubMed]
74. Boonstra, A.; Barrat, F.J.; Crain, C.; Heath, V.L.; Savelkoul, H.F.; O'Garra, A. 1alpha,25-Dihydroxyvitamin D_3 has a direct effect on naive CD4+ T cells to enhance the development of Th2 cells. *J. Immunol.* **2001**, *167*, 4974–4980. [CrossRef] [PubMed]
75. Pichler, J.; Gerstmayr, M.; Szépfalusi, Z.; Urbanek, R.; Peterlik, M.; Willheim, M. 1 alpha,25(OH)$_2$D$_3$ inhibits not only Th1 but also Th2 differentiation in human cord blood T cells. *Pediatr. Res.* **2002**, *52*, 12–18. [PubMed]
76. Staeva-Vieira, T.P.; Freedman, L.P. 1,25-dihydroxyvitamin D3 inhibits IFN-gamma and IL-4 levels during in vitro polarization of primary murine CD4+ T cells. *J. Immunol.* **2002**, *168*, 1181–1189. [CrossRef] [PubMed]
77. Fawaz, L.; Mrad, M.F.; Kazan, J.M.; Sayegh, S.; Akika, R.; Khoury, S.J. Comparative effect of 25(OH)D$_3$ and 1,25(OH)$_2$D$_3$ on Th17 cell differentiation. *Clin. Immunol.* **2016**, *166*, 59–71. [CrossRef] [PubMed]
78. Şıklar, Z.; Karataş, D.; Doğu, F.; Hacıhamdioğlu, B.; İkincioğulları, A.; Berberoğlu, M. Regulatory T cells and vitamin D status in children with chronic autoimmune thyroiditis. *J. Clin. Res. Pediatr. Endocrinol.* **2016**, *8*, 276–281. [CrossRef] [PubMed]
79. Korf, H.; Wenes, M.; Stijlemans, B.; Takiishi, T.; Robert, S.; Miani, M.; Eizirik, D.L.; Gysemans, C.; Mathieu, C. 1,25-Dihydroxyvitamin D$_3$ curtails the inflammatory and T cell stimulatory capacity of macrophages through an IL-10-dependent mechanism. *Immunobiology* **2012**, *217*, 1292–1300. [CrossRef] [PubMed]
80. Mann, E.H.; Ho, T.-R.; Pfeffer, P.E.; Matthews, N.C.; Chevretton, E.; Mudway, I.; Kelly, F.J.; Hawrylowicz, C.M. Vitamin D counteracts an IL-23-dependent IL-17A+IFN-γ+ response driven by urban particulate matter. *Am. J. Respir. Cell Mol. Biol.* **2017**, *57*, 355–366. [CrossRef] [PubMed]
81. Joshi, S.; Pantalena, L.-C.; Liu, X.K.; Gaffen, S.L.; Liu, H.; Rohowsky-Kochan, C.; Ichiyama, K.; Yoshimura, A.; Steinman, L.; Christakos, S.; et al. 1,25-dihydroxyvitamin D$_3$ ameliorates Th17 autoimmunity via transcriptional modulation of interleukin-17A. *Mol. Cell. Biol.* **2011**, *31*, 3653–3669. [CrossRef] [PubMed]
82. Chang, J.-H.; Cha, H.-R.; Lee, D.-S.; Seo, K.Y.; Kweon, M.-N. 1,25-Dihydroxyvitamin D$_3$ inhibits the differentiation and migration of TH17 cells to protect against experimental autoimmune encephalomyelitis. *PLoS ONE* **2010**, *5*. [CrossRef]
83. Colin, E.M.; Asmawidjaja, P.S.; van Hamburg, J.P.; Mus, A.M.C.; van Driel, M.; Hazes, J.M.W.; van Leeuwen, J.P.T.M.; Lubberts, E. 1,25-dihydroxyvitamin D$_3$ modulates Th17 polarization and interleukin-22 expression by memory T cells from patients with early rheumatoid arthritis. *Arthritis Rheum.* **2010**, *62*, 132–142. [CrossRef] [PubMed]
84. Palmer, M.T.; Lee, Y.K.; Maynard, C.L.; Oliver, J.R.; Bikle, D.D.; Jetten, A.M.; Weaver, C.T. Lineage-specific effects of 1,25-dihydroxyvitamin D$_3$ on the development of effector CD4 T cells. *J. Biol. Chem.* **2011**, *286*, 997–1004. [CrossRef] [PubMed]
85. Treiber, G.; Prietl, B.; Fröhlich-Reiterer, E.; Lechner, E.; Ribitsch, A.; Fritsch, M.; Rami-Merhar, B.; Steigleder-Schweiger, C.; Graninger, W.; Borkenstein, M.; et al. Cholecalciferol supplementation improves suppressive capacity of regulatory T-cells in young patients with new-onset type 1 diabetes mellitus—A randomized clinical trial. *Clin. Immunol.* **2015**, *161*, 217–224. [CrossRef] [PubMed]
86. Hu, J.; Wan, Y. Tolerogenic dendritic cells and their potential applications. *Immunology* **2011**, *132*, 307–314. [CrossRef] [PubMed]
87. Penna, G.; Adorini, L. 1 Alpha,25-dihydroxyvitamin D$_3$ inhibits differentiation, maturation, activation, and survival of dendritic cells leading to impaired alloreactive T cell activation. *J. Immunol.* **2000**, *164*, 2405–2411. [CrossRef] [PubMed]

88. Piemonti, L.; Monti, P.; Sironi, M.; Fraticelli, P.; Leone, B.E.; Dal Cin, E.; Allavena, P.; Di Carlo, V. Vitamin D_3 affects differentiation, maturation, and function of human monocyte-derived dendritic cells. *J. Immunol.* **2000**, *164*, 4443–4451. [CrossRef] [PubMed]
89. Unger, W.W.J.; Laban, S.; Kleijwegt, F.S.; van der Slik, A.R.; Roep, B.O. Induction of Treg by monocyte-derived DC modulated by vitamin D_3 or dexamethasone: Differential role for PD-L1. *Eur. J. Immunol.* **2009**, *39*, 3147–3159. [CrossRef] [PubMed]
90. Van Halteren, A.G.S.; Tysma, O.M.; van Etten, E.; Mathieu, C.; Roep, B.O. 1alpha,25-dihydroxyvitamin D3 or analogue treated dendritic cells modulate human autoreactive T cells via the selective induction of apoptosis. *J. Autoimmun.* **2004**, *23*, 233–239. [CrossRef] [PubMed]
91. Lemire, J.M.; Archer, D.C. 1,25-dihydroxyvitamin D_3 prevents the in vivo induction of murine experimental autoimmune encephalomyelitis. *JCI* **1991**, *87*, 1103–1107. [CrossRef] [PubMed]
92. Cantorna, M.T.; Hayes, C.E.; DeLuca, H.F. 1,25-Dihydroxyvitamin D_3 reversibly blocks the progression of relapsing encephalomyelitis, a model of multiple sclerosis. *PNAS* **1996**, *93*, 7861–7864. [CrossRef] [PubMed]
93. Cantorna, M.T.; Hayes, C.E.; DeLuca, H.F. 1,25-Dihydroxycholecalciferol inhibits the progression of arthritis in murine models of human arthritis. *J. Nutr.* **1998**, *128*, 68–72. [CrossRef] [PubMed]
94. Alhassan Mohammed, H.; Mirshafiey, A.; Vahedi, H.; Hemmasi, G.; Moussavi NaslKhameneh, A.; Parastouei, K.; Saboor-Yaraghi, A.A. Immunoregulation of inflammatory and inhibitory cytokines by vitamin D_3 in patients with inflammatory bowel diseases. *Scand. J. Immunol.* **2017**, *85*, 386–394. [CrossRef] [PubMed]
95. Tao, C.; Simpson, S.; van der Mei, I.; Blizzard, L.; Havrdova, E.; Horakova, D.; Shaygannejad, V.; Lugaresi, A.; Izquierdo, G.; Trojano, M.; et al. Higher latitude is significantly associated with an earlier age of disease onset in multiple sclerosis. *J. Neurol. Neurosurg. Psychiatry* **2016**, *87*, 1343–1349. [CrossRef] [PubMed]
96. Laursen, J.H.; Søndergaard, H.B.; Sørensen, P.S.; Sellebjerg, F.; Oturai, A.B. Vitamin D supplementation reduces relapse rate in relapsing-remitting multiple sclerosis patients treated with natalizumab. *Mult. Scler. Relat. Disord.* **2016**, *10*, 169–173. [CrossRef] [PubMed]
97. Jelinek, G.A.; Marck, C.H.; Weiland, T.J.; Pereira, N.; van der Meer, D.M.; Hadgkiss, E.J. Latitude, sun exposure and vitamin D supplementation: Associations with quality of life and disease outcomes in a large international cohort of people with multiple sclerosis. *BMC Neurol.* **2015**, *15*. [CrossRef] [PubMed]
98. Mohr, S.B.; Garland, C.F.; Gorham, E.D.; Garland, F.C. The association between ultraviolet B irradiance, vitamin D status and incidence rates of type 1 diabetes in 51 regions worldwide. *Diabetologia* **2008**, *51*, 1391–1398. [CrossRef] [PubMed]
99. Rosecrans, R.; Dohnal, J.C. Seasonal vitamin D changes and the impact on health risk assessment. *Clin. Biochem.* **2014**, *47*, 670–672. [CrossRef] [PubMed]
100. Van der Rhee, H.J.; de Vries, E.; Coebergh, J.W. Regular sun exposure benefits health. *Med. Hypotheses* **2016**, *97*, 34–37. [CrossRef] [PubMed]
101. Szilagyi, A.; Leighton, H.; Burstein, B.; Xue, X. Latitude, sunshine, and human lactase phenotype distributions may contribute to geographic patterns of modern disease: The inflammatory bowel disease model. *Clin. Epidemiol.* **2014**, *6*, 183–198. [CrossRef] [PubMed]
102. Dobson, R.; Giovannoni, G.; Ramagopalan, S. The month of birth effect in multiple sclerosis: Systematic review, meta-analysis and effect of latitude. *J. Neurol. Neurosurg. Psychiatry* **2013**, *84*, 427–432. [CrossRef] [PubMed]
103. Song, G.G.; Bae, S.-C.; Lee, Y.H. Association between vitamin D intake and the risk of rheumatoid arthritis: A meta-analysis. *Clin. Rheumatol.* **2012**, *31*, 1733–1739. [CrossRef] [PubMed]
104. Zipitis, C.S.; Akobeng, A.K. Vitamin D supplementation in early childhood and risk of type 1 diabetes: A systematic review and meta-analysis. *Arch. Dis. Child.* **2008**, *93*, 512–517. [CrossRef] [PubMed]
105. Dong, J.-Y.; Zhang, W.-G.; Chen, J.J.; Zhang, Z.-L.; Han, S.-F.; Qin, L.-Q. Vitamin D intake and risk of type 1 diabetes: A meta-analysis of observational studies. *Nutrients* **2013**, *5*, 3551–3562. [CrossRef] [PubMed]
106. Shen, L.; Zhuang, Q.-S.; Ji, H.-F. Assessment of vitamin D levels in type 1 and type 2 diabetes patients: Results from metaanalysis. *Mol. Nutr. Food Res.* **2016**, *60*, 1059–1067. [CrossRef] [PubMed]
107. Duan, S.; Lv, Z.; Fan, X.; Wang, L.; Han, F.; Wang, H.; Bi, S. Vitamin D status and the risk of multiple sclerosis: A systematic review and meta-analysis. *Neurosci. Lett.* **2014**, *570*, 108–113. [CrossRef] [PubMed]
108. Lin, J.; Liu, J.; Davies, M.L.; Chen, W. Serum vitamin D Level and rheumatoid arthritis disease activity: Review and meta-analysis. *PLoS ONE* **2016**, *11*. [CrossRef] [PubMed]

109. Del Pinto, R.; Pietropaoli, D.; Chandar, A.K.; Ferri, C.; Cominelli, F. Association between inflammatory bowel disease and vitamin D deficiency: A systematic review and meta-analysis. *Inflamm. Bowel Dis.* **2015**, *21*, 2708–2717. [CrossRef] [PubMed]
110. Lu, C.; Yang, J.; Yu, W.; Li, D.; Xiang, Z.; Lin, Y.; Yu, C. Association between 25(OH)D level, ultraviolet exposure, geographical location, and inflammatory bowel disease activity: A systematic review and meta-analysis. *PLoS ONE* **2015**, *10*. [CrossRef] [PubMed]
111. Sadeghian, M.; Saneei, P.; Siassi, F.; Esmaillzadeh, A. Vitamin D status in relation to Crohn's disease: Meta-analysis of observational studies. *Nutrition* **2016**, *32*, 505–514. [CrossRef] [PubMed]
112. Feng, R.; Li, Y.; Li, G.; Li, Z.; Zhang, Y.; Li, Q.; Sun, C. Lower serum 25 (OH) D concentrations in type 1 diabetes: A meta-analysis. *Diabetes Res. Clin. Pract.* **2015**, *108*, e71–e75. [CrossRef] [PubMed]
113. Pitocco, D.; Crinò, A.; Di Stasio, E.; Manfrini, S.; Guglielmi, C.; Spera, S.; Anguissola, G.B.; Visalli, N.; Suraci, C.; Matteoli, M.C.; et al. The effects of calcitriol and nicotinamide on residual pancreatic beta-cell function in patients with recent-onset Type 1 diabetes (IMDIAB XI). *Diabet. Med.* **2006**, *23*, 920–923. [CrossRef] [PubMed]
114. Walter, M.; Kaupper, T.; Adler, K.; Foersch, J.; Bonifacio, E.; Ziegler, A.-G. No effect of the 1alpha,25-dihydroxyvitamin D_3 on beta-cell residual function and insulin requirement in adults with new-onset type 1 diabetes. *Diabetes Care* **2010**, *33*, 1443–1448. [CrossRef] [PubMed]
115. Papadimitriou, D.T.; Marakaki, C.; Fretzayas, A.; Nicolaidou, P.; Papadimitriou, A. Negativation of type 1 diabetes-associated autoantibodies to glutamic acid decarboxylase and insulin in children treated with oral calcitriol. *J. Diabetes* **2013**, *5*, 344–348. [CrossRef] [PubMed]
116. Gunasekar, P.; Swier, V.J.; Fleegel, J.P.; Boosani, C.S.; Radwan, M.M.; Agrawal, D.K. Vitamin D and macrophage polarization in epicardial adipose tissue of atherosclerotic swine. *PLoS ONE* **2018**, *13*. [CrossRef] [PubMed]
117. Yin, K.; You, Y.; Swier, V.; Tang, L.; Radwan, M.M.; Pandya, A.N.; Agrawal, D.K. Vitamin D protects against atherosclerosis via regulation of cholesterol efflux and macrophage polarization in hypercholesterolemic swine. *Arterioscler. Thromb. Vasc. Biol.* **2015**, *35*, 2432–2442. [CrossRef] [PubMed]
118. Dozio, E.; Briganti, S.; Vianello, E.; Dogliotti, G.; Barassi, A.; Malavazos, A.E.; Ermetici, F.; Morricone, L.; Sigruener, A.; Schmitz, G.; et al. Epicardial adipose tissue inflammation is related to vitamin D deficiency in patients affected by coronary artery disease. *Nutr. Metab. Cardiovasc. Dis.* **2015**, *25*, 267–273. [CrossRef] [PubMed]
119. Apostolakis, M.; Armeni, E.; Bakas, P.; Lambrinoudaki, I. Vitamin D and cardiovascular disease. *Maturitas* **2018**, *115*, 1–22. [CrossRef] [PubMed]

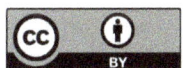

© 2018 by the authors. Licensee MDPI, Basel, Switzerland. This article is an open access article distributed under the terms and conditions of the Creative Commons Attribution (CC BY) license (http://creativecommons.org/licenses/by/4.0/).

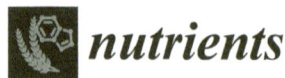

Review

The Immunomodulatory and Anti-Inflammatory Role of Polyphenols

Nour Yahfoufi [1], Nawal Alsadi [1], Majed Jambi [1] and Chantal Matar [1,2,*

[1] Cellular and Molecular Medicine Department, Faculty of Medicine, University of Ottawa, Ottawa, ON K1H8L1, Canada; nyahf074@uottawa.ca (N.Y.); nalsa068@uottawa.ca (N.A.); mjamb055@uottawa.ca (M.J.)
[2] School of Nutrition, Faculty of Health Sciences, University of Ottawa, Ottawa, ON K1H8L1, Canada
* Correspondence: Chantal.matar@uottawa.ca; Tel.: +1-613-562-5406

Received: 30 September 2018; Accepted: 23 October 2018; Published: 2 November 2018

Abstract: This review offers a systematic understanding about how polyphenols target multiple inflammatory components and lead to anti-inflammatory mechanisms. It provides a clear understanding of the molecular mechanisms of action of phenolic compounds. Polyphenols regulate immunity by interfering with immune cell regulation, proinflammatory cytokines' synthesis, and gene expression. They inactivate NF-κB (nuclear factor kappa-light-chain-enhancer of activated B cells) and modulate mitogen-activated protein Kinase (MAPk) and arachidonic acids pathways. Polyphenolic compounds inhibit phosphatidylinositide 3-kinases/protein kinase B (PI3K/AkT), inhibitor of kappa kinase/c-Jun amino-terminal kinases (IKK/JNK), mammalian target of rapamycin complex 1 (mTORC1) which is a protein complex that controls protein synthesis, and JAK/STAT. They can suppress toll-like receptor (TLR) and pro-inflammatory genes' expression. Their antioxidant activity and ability to inhibit enzymes involved in the production of eicosanoids contribute as well to their anti-inflammation properties. They inhibit certain enzymes involved in reactive oxygen species ROS production like xanthine oxidase and NADPH oxidase (NOX) while they upregulate other endogenous antioxidant enzymes like superoxide dismutase (SOD), catalase, and glutathione (GSH) peroxidase (Px). Furthermore, they inhibit phospholipase A2 (PLA2), cyclooxygenase (COX) and lipoxygenase (LOX) leading to a reduction in the production of prostaglandins (PGs) and leukotrienes (LTs) and inflammation antagonism. The effects of these biologically active compounds on the immune system are associated with extended health benefits for different chronic inflammatory diseases. Studies of plant extracts and compounds show that polyphenols can play a beneficial role in the prevention and the progress of chronic diseases related to inflammation such as diabetes, obesity, neurodegeneration, cancers, and cardiovascular diseases, among other conditions.

Keywords: polyphenols; immune system; inflammation; molecular mechanisms; nuclear factor kappa-light-chain-enhancer of activated B cells (NF-κB); arachidonic acid; mitogen-activated protein Kinase (MAPK); cytokines; oxidative stress; reactive oxygen species (ROS); cyclooxygenase (COX); nitric oxide synthase (NOS); lipoxygenase (LOX); superoxide dismutase (SOD); inhibitor of kappa kinase (IKK); extra-cellular signal regulated kinases (ERK); cancer; anti-inflammation; anti-tumorigenic; chronic inflammatory conditions; macrophages; T helper 1 (Th1); Th17; Treg

1. Introduction

Numerous studies have attributed to polyphenols a broad range of biological activities including but not limited to anti-inflammatory, immune-modulatory, antioxidant, cardiovascular protective and anti-cancer actions [1–5]. Polyphenols are ubiquitously made by plants and are present either as glycosides esters or as free aglycones [6]. More than 8000 structural variants exist in the polyphenol family. Polyphenols are bioactive compounds found in fruits and vegetables contributing to their color, flavor, and pharmacological activities [1]. They are classified according to their chemical structures into flavonoids such as flavones, flavonols, isoflavones, neoflavonoids, chalcones, anthocyanidins, and proanthocyanidins and nonflavonoids, such as phenolic acids, stilbenoids, and phenolic amides [7]. The majority of these molecules are metabolites of plants, they are made of several aromatic rings with hydroxyl moieties [8]. Their chemical structures contribute to their classification into different classes. Considering gastrointestinal digestion, some—but not all—polyphenols are absorbed in the small intestine, for example, anthocyanins and the majority of remaining polyphenols except flavonoids are usually stable; these later are unstable in the duodenum. Unabsorbed polyphenols must be hydrolyzed first by digestive enzymes then glycosides with high lipid contents are absorbed by epithelial cells [9,10].

In recent years, consumers prefer using natural food ingredients as additives because of their safety and availability. Applications of phenolic compounds to multiple fresh perishable foods show that they are worthy to be used as preservatives in foods and can be creditable alternatives to synthetic food additives. In this sense, polyphenolic compounds start to substitute chemical additives in food. Different methods like spraying, coating and dipping treatment of food are currently applied in food technology preceding packaging as effective alternatives [11]. Grape seeds and olive oil polyphenols' rich extracts can be used as food additives for their anti-oxidant properties [12]. Various polyphenols like grape polyphenols demonstrate an efficient role as additives in fish and fish products for their anti-oxidant properties in order to prevent lipid oxidation and quality deterioration of polyunsaturated fatty acids [13]. In addition polyphenolic compounds like flavonols, p-coumaric, and caffeic acids can be used as food preservatives for their antimicrobial activity [11].

Back to inflammation, continuous inflammation is known to be a major cause linked to different human disorders involving cancer, diabetes type II, obesity, arthritis, neurodegenerative diseases, and cardiovascular diseases [14,15]. Polyphenols derived from botanic origin have shown anti-inflammatory activity in vitro and in vivo highlighting their beneficial role as therapeutic tools in multiple acute and chronic disorders [16–20]. Accordingly, many epidemiological and experimental researches have been studying the anti-inflammatory and immune modulation activities of dietary polyphenols [15,21]. The ability of these natural compounds to modify the expression of several pro-inflammatory genes like multiple cytokines, lipoxygenase, nitric oxide synthases cyclooxygenase, in addition to their anti-oxidant characteristics such as ROS (reactive oxygen species) scavenging contributes to the regulation of inflammatory signaling [22,23]. This review will discuss the immunomodulatory effects of dietary polyphenols, their anti-inflammatory abilities, the different mechanisms and pathways involved in reducing inflammation and their contribution to protect from different chronic inflammatory diseases with a focus on their anti-cancer activity.

2. Polyphenols and Inflammation

The immune modulation effect of polyphenols is supported by different studies: some polyphenols impact on immune cells populations, modulate cytokines production, and pro-inflammatory genes expression [24,25]. For example, cardioprotective effects of resveratrol present in red wine grape and nuts were mainly attributed to its anti-inflammatory properties. In vivo and in vitro studies demonstrate that resveratrol can inhibit COX, inactivate peroxisome proliferator-activated receptor gamma (PPARγ) and induce eNOS (endothelial nitric oxide synthase) in murine and rat macrophages [26–28]. Likewise, a resveratrol analog, RVSA40, inhibits the pro-inflammatory cytokines TNF-α (Tumor necrosis factor alpha) and IL-6 (interleukin-6) in RAW (Murine macrophages cell line) 264.7 macrophages [29]. Another example is the non-flavonoid curcumin found in turmeric plants and mustard. Curcumin was shown to reduce the expression of inflammatory cytokines: TNF and IL-1, adhesion molecules like ICAM-1 (intercellular adhesion molecule-1) and VCAM-1 (vascular cell adhesion molecule-1) in human umbilical vein endothelial cells and inflammatory mediators like prostaglandins and leukotriens. It also inhibits certain enzymes involved in inflammation like COX in mice (cyclooxygenase), LOX (lipoxygenase) in, human endothelial cells MAPK (mitogen-activated protein Kinase), and IKK (inhibitor of kappa kinase). Moreover, curcumin downregulates NF-κB (nuclear factor kappa-light-chain-enhancer of activated B cells) and STAT3 (signal transducer and activator of transcription) and reduces the expression of TLR-2 (toll-like receptor-2) and 4 while, in vivo, it upregulates PPARγ (Peroxisome proliferator-activated receptor gamma) in male adult rats [30–35]. Caffeic acid phenethyl ester suppresses TLR4 activation and LPS-mediated NF-κB in macrophages, Quercetin was also shown to inhibit leukotriens biosynthesis in human polymorphonuclear leukocytes [36,37]. COX2 expression is also attenuated by ECGC (Epigallocatechin gallate) in colon cancer cell and androgen-independent PC-3 cells of human prostate cancer, gingerol in and piceatannol (EGCG analog found in Norway spruces) leading to NFκ B inactivation [30,38–40]. Furthermore, polyphenols, such as Gingerol and Quercetin can activate the production of adiponectin known for its anti-inflammatory effects [30,39]. Similarily, EGCG blocks NFκ B activation in human epithelial cells and downregulates the expression of iNOS (inducible nitric oxide synthase), NO (nitric oxide) production in macrophages resulting in its immunomodulation [38,40,41]. A series of in vitro studies found that other polyphenols like oleanolic acid, curcumin, kaempferol-3-O-sophoroside, EGCG and lycopene inhibit high mobility group box1 protein, an important chromatin protein that interacts with nucleosomes, transcription factors, and histones regulating transcription and playing a key role in inflammation [35]. All of these examples support the anti-inflammatory effects of polyphenols.

Polyphenols' use is associated with a direct change in the count and differentiation of specific immune cells. An increase in T helper 1(Th1), natural killer (NK), macrophages and dendritic cells (DCs) in Peyer's patches and spleen is associated with oral administration of polyphenols extracted from the fruit date in male C3H/HeN mice [24]. In humans, the count of regulatory T cells (Treg or suppressor T cells) characterized by the (CD4 + CD25 + Foxp3+) phenotype and involved in immune tolerance and autoimmune control can be boosted by polyphenols [42–44]. In vivo, Epigallocatechin-3-gallate, found in green tea and injected to Laboratory inbred strain (BALB)/c mice, rises the number of functional Treg in spleens, pancreatic lymph nodes, and mesentheric lymph nodes [45]. Similarly, in vitro treatment of Jurkat T cells with EGCG or green tea upsurges the expression of Foxp3 and IL10. Baicalin, a flavone, extracted from Huangqin herb, induces Foxp3 expression in HEK 293 T cells and triggers functional Treg from splenic CD4 + CD25− T cells [46]. Additionally, flavonoids show an agonistic effect of aryl hydrocarbon receptor (AhR) and bind xenobiotic-responsive elements in promoter regions of certain genes, including Foxp3 rising its expression [47].

Th1 and Th17 populations are also affected by polyphenols: EGCG reduces the differentiation of Th1 and reduces the numbers of Th17 and Th9 cells in specific pathogen-free C57/BL6 female mice [48]. Other polyphenols like Baicalin show a reduction of Th17 differentiation in vitro and a diminution of IL-17 expression [49].

Macrophages are affected by polyphenols as well. Macrophages are known to be a key player in the inflammatory response. They initiate inflammation by secreting pro-inflammatory mediators and cytokines like IL-6 and TNF-α [50]. Polyphenols repress macrophages by inhibiting cyclooxygenase-2 (COX-2), inducible nitric oxide synthase (iNOS), thus they reduce the production of TNF-α, interleukine-1-beta (IL-1-β) and IL-6 expression [51]. Chinese propolis [52] containing ferulic acid and coumaric acid, an extract of *Lonicera japónica* Thunb [53] or *Kalanchoe gracilis* [54] are a good example in this case as per demonstrated by in vitro studies using RAW 264.7 cells.

3. Polyphenol and Cytokine Modulation

Cytokines are important mediators' proteins, essential in networking communication for immune system. Cytokines can be produced by lymphocytes (lymphokines), or monocytes (monokines) with pro-inflammatory and anti-inflammatory effects. Cytokines with chemotactic activities are termed chemokines. The equilibrum between pro-inflammatory cytokines (IL-1β, IL-2, TNFα, Il-6, IL-8, IFN-γ ...) and anti-inflammatory cytokines (IL-10, IL-4, TGFβ) are thought to be an important parameter in immune response homeostasis and inflammation underlining many disease [55]. In vivo and in vitro studies demonstrate that polyphenols affect macrophages by inhibiting multiple key regulators of inflammatory response such as the inhibition of TNF-α, IL-1-β, and IL-6 [51].

In humans, consumption of bilberries is associated with a decreased inflammation score in patients' blood, reflected by decreasing serum levels of IL-6, IL-12, and high sensitivity C reactive protein [56]. Moreover, clinical trials have shown the ability of polyphenol-enriched extra virgin olive oil to reduce IL-6 and C-reactive protein expression in stable coronary heart disease patients [57].

In lipopolysaccharide (LPS)-treated BALB/c mice, a model system of inflammation olive vegetation water show ability to inhibit the production of tumor necrosis factor-alpha usually activated by inflammation [58]. Flavonoids, as well, play an important anti-inflammatory effect by influencing cytokines' secretion. Several flavonoids are found able to inhibit the expression of various pro-inflammatory cytokines and chemokines like TNFα, IL-1β, IL-6, IL-8, and MCP-1 (monocyte chemoattractant protein-1) in multiple cell types such as LPS-activated mouse primary macrophages, activated human mast cell line, activated human astrocytes, human synovial cells, and human peripheral blood mononuclear cells [59–64]. In murine RAW 264.7 macrophages stimulated by LPS, Chinese propolis as well as extract of *Lonicera japónica* Thunb (*Caprifoliaceae*) or *Kalanchoe gracilis* demonstrated inhibitory effects on TNF-α, IL-1-β, and IL-6 [52–54]. Similarly, certain polyphenol analogs, like curcumin analog EF31, have shown the ability to inhibit the expression and secretion of TNF-α, IL-1-β, and IL-6 in mouse Raw 264.7 macrophages [65].

Likewise, reduction of the secretion of TNF-α and IL-6 without IL-1β modulation is observed with extracts of chamomile, meadowsweet, willow bark, and isolated polyphenols such as quercetin existing in these extracts in THP1 macrophages [66]. Extract of *Cydonia oblonga* inhibits TNF-α and Interleukin 8 while it increases IL-10 and IL-6 in THP-1monocytes stimulated with LPS. The reduction in TNF-α levels limits the acute inflammatory response [67,68]. Other cytokines like IFNγ might also be inhibited by certain polyphenols. For example, kaempferol reduces the production of IFN-γ in a dose-dependent manner in spleen cells and T cell lines [69].

Certain polyphenols exert their effects on the balance between pro- and anti-inflammatory cytokines production such as quercetin and catechins, they enhance IL-10 release while they inhibit TNFα and IL-1β [59,70]. Extract of *Cydonia oblonga* also inhibits the effects of TNF-α and Interleukin 8 (IL-8) while it raises IL-10 in the same type of monocytes [67,68]. Modulation of inflammatory cytokines is one of many common mechanisms by which polyphenols in general exert their immunomodulatory effects.

4. Polyphenols, Inflammation, and Modulation of Different Signaling Pathways

4.1. NFκ B Signaling Pathway

NF-κB or nuclear factor kappa-light-chain-enhancer of activated B cells is a complex protein that plays a key role in deoxyribonucleic acid (DNA) transcription, cytokine production and cell survival. It controls immune, inflammation, stress, proliferation and apoptotic responses of a cell to multiple stimuli [58].

The expression of a large number of genes involved in inflammation is controlled by NF-κB such as COX-2, VEGF (vascular endothelial growth Factor), pro-inflammatory cytokines (IL-1, IL-2, IL-6, and TNFα), chemokines (e.g., IL-8, MIP-1α, and MCP-1), adhesion molecules, immuno-receptors, growth factors, and other agents involved in proliferation and invasion [71].

NFκ B is located in the cytoplasm, it exists as an inactive non-DNA-binding form. Iκ B proteins (Iκ Bs), are inhibitors proteins that are associated with NFκ B resulting in its inactivation. Iκ Bs include Iκ Bα, Iκ Bβ, Iκ Bγ, Iκ Bε, Bcl-3, precursors p100 and p105 [72]. Under stimulatory conditions, Iκ B kinase (IKK) phosphorylate IκB proteins leading to successive ubiquitination, consequent degradation of the inhibitory proteins and release of NFκ B dimer. This later can translocate into the nucleus and prompts the expression of particular genes [72]. Different mechanisms regulate NFκ B activity as per the accumulation and degradation of Iκ B, the phosphorylation of NFκ B, the hyper-phosphorylation of IKK, and the processing of NFκ B precursors [73–75]. Thus, the inhibition of NFκB can be of a great benefit in controlling inflammatory conditions [76]. Several polyphenols modulate NFκ B activation and reduce inflammation [77,78]. Quercetin blocks the nuclear translocation of p50 and p65 subunits of NFκ B and represses the expression of pro-inflammatory associated genes, NOS and COX-2 in RAW264.7 macrophages [79]. It inhibits the phosphorylation of Iκ Bα protein both in vitro (using macrophages) and in vivo (using dextran sulfate sodium (DSS) rat colitis model) leading to inactivation of the NFκ B pathway [80]. In human mast cells, quercetin prevents the degradation of Iκ Bα, as well as the nuclear translocation of p65 resulting in reduction of TNFα, IL-1β, IL-6 and IL-8 [63]. It can modulate chromatin remodeling, for example it blocks the recruitment of a histone acetyl transferase called CBP/p300 to the promoters of interferon-inducible protein 10 (IP-10) and macrophage inflammatory protein-2 (MIP-2) genes in primary murine small intestinal epithelial cell. As a result, it inhibits the expression of these pro-inflammatory cytokines [81]. Quercetin can block the activation of IKK, NFκ B, and it reduces the ability of NFκ B to bind DNA in microglia treated by LPS and IFN-γ in mouse BV-2 microglia [82]. Luteolin, too, blocks NFκ B activation and inhibits pro-inflammatory genes expression and the cytokines production in murine macrophages RAW 264.7 and mouse alveolar macrophages; it also inhibits IKKs in LPS-induced epithelial and dendritic cells [83]. In addition, in co-cultured intestinal epithelial Caco-2 and macrophage RAW 264.7 cells, luteolin represses NF-k B activation and TNF-α secretion [84]. Likewise, Genistein represses LPS-induced activation of NF-k B in monocytes and reduces the inflammation by inhibiting NF-k B activation upon adenosine monophosphate activated protein kinase stimulation in LPS-stimulated macrophages RAW 264.7 [83,85]. Galangin, as well, stops the degradation of Ik Bα and the translocation of p65 NF-k B, repressing the expression of TNF-α, IL-6, IL-1β, and IL-8 in mast cell [86]. EGCG counteracts the activation of IKK and the degradation of Iκ Bα and inhibits NFκ B in culture respiratory epithelial cells and in vivo in male Wistar rats [87,88]. Furthermore, EGCG blocks DNA binding of NFκ B which reduces the expression of IL-12p40 and iNOS in murine peritoneal macrophages [89,90]. Catechin and epichatechin reduce NFκ B activity in PMA-induced Jurkat T cells. Flavonoids can modulate NFκ B activation cascade at early phases by affecting IKK activation and regulation of oxidant levels or at late phases by affecting binding of NF-k B to DNA in jurkat Tcells [91]. Hydroxytyrosol, and resveratrol inhibit NFκ B activation, and the expression of VCAM-1 in LPS-stimulated human umbilical vein endothelial cells [92]. In summary, polyphenols can modulate NFκ B activation cascade at different steps such as by affecting IKK activation and regulating of the oxidant levels or by affecting binding of NF-κ B to DNA leading to an important anti-inflammatory effect responsible for their potential value in treating chronic inflammatory conditions (Figure 1).

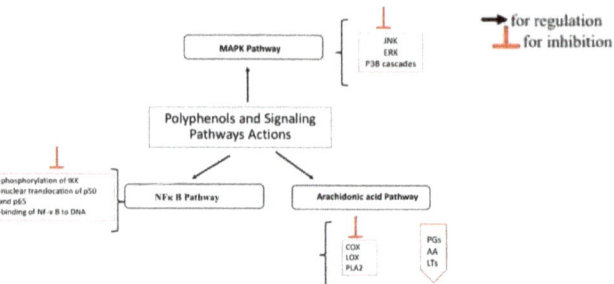

Figure 1. Potential points of action of polyphenols within inflammatory cascade. NF-κ B: nuclear factor kappa-light-chain-enhancer of activated B cells; IKK: IkB-kinase; ERK: extracellular signal-related kinases; JNK: c-Jun amino-terminal kinases; p38 (or p38-MAPK): p38-mitogen-activated protein kinase; COX: cyclooxygenase; LOX: lipoxygenase; AA: arachidonic acid; PLA2: phospholipase A2; PGs: prostaglandins; LTs: leukotriens. For references see the text.

4.2. MAPK Signaling Pathway

The mitogen-activated protein kinases (MAPK) are a highly conserved family of serine/threonine protein kinases. They play a key role in a range of fundamental cellular processes like cell growth, proliferation, death and differentiation. They regulate gene transcription and transcription factor activities involved in inflammation. Extracellular signal-related kinases, like (extracellular signal-related kinases (ERK))-1/2, c-Jun amino-terminal kinases (JNK1/2/3), p38-MAP kinase (α, β, δ, and γ), and ERK5 are different groups of MAPKs expressed in mammals. These are later activated by MAP kinase kinases (MAPKK) which might be triggered by some MAPKK kinases (MAPKKK) [93]. MAPK, in its turn, cross-talks with other pathways such as NFκB, thus the complexity of the MAPK signaling pathway and its interactions. Stress and mitogens activate MAPK signaling: For example, ERK1/2 route is triggered by mitogens and growth factors while JNK and p38 cascade are stimulated by stress [94–97]. Preclinical data propose an anti-inflammatory role of JNK and p38 cascades inhibitors [98,99].

Polyphenols' activity is specific, it depends on the cell types as well as the structure of the polyphenol itself [100]. Polyphenols can block TNF α release by modulating MAPK pathway at different levels of the signaling pathway. Luteolin reduces TNFα liberation by LPS-activated mouse macrophages, it blocks ERK1/2 and p38phosphorylation [100]. In epithelial cells, luteolin, as well as other polyphenols such as chrysin and kaempferol block TNFα triggered ICAM-1 expression by inhibiting ERK, JNK and P38 [100,101]. Quercetin blocks the phosphorylation of ERK, JNK in THP-1 activated human monocytes, while in murine macrophages RAW 246.7 triggered by LPS it blocks the phosphorylation and the activation of JNK/SAPK (stress activated protein kinases), ERK1/2, and p38 leading to a reduction in the transcription and expression of TNF-α expression [102]. EGCG reduces inflammation in various cell types by exerting an anti-MAPK activity. It reduces IL-12 expression in LPS-activated murine macrophages by prohibiting p38 MAPK phosphorylation [89,103]. In addition, EGCG is found to play a protective role in autoimmune-induced tissue damage caused by Sjogren's syndrome: it protects human salivary glands from TNF-α induced cytotoxicity by acting on p38 MAPK1. In vivo, in female ICR mice, EGCG inhibits phorbol ester-induced activation of NFκB and CREB (cAMP response element-binding protein—a cellular transcription factor) in mouse skin by blocking the activation of p38 MAPK [104]. Polyphenols concentration plays as well a role in their modulatory activities on signaling pathways: in human coronary artery endothelial cells, the activation of the MAPKs pathways (p38, ERK1/2, and JNK) and the repression of the plasminogen activator inhibitor by catechin and quercetin is time and dose dependent [105]. The ability of polyphenolic compounds to block MAPK pathways (Figure 1) endowed these bioactive substances with therapeutic potential to protect against inflammation.

4.3. Arachidonic Acid Signaling Pathway

Arachidonic acid (AA) is liberated by membrane phospholipids upon phospholipase A2 (PLA2) cleavage. Cyclooxygenase (COX) or lipoxygenase (LOX) metabolize it and produce, respectively, prostaglandins (PGs) and thromboxane A2 (TXA2) by COX, and hydroxyeicosatetraenoic acids and leukotrienes (LTs) by LOX [106]. The COX family involves different members (COX1, COX-2, and COX-3). COX-2 is responsible of the production of important quantity of prostaglandins, its expression is triggered by lipopolysaccharide and pro-inflammatory cytokines [107]. The ability of polyphenols to reduce the release of arachidonic acid, prostaglandins, and leukotrienes is considered one of their most important anti-inflammatory mechanisms (Figure 1). Their action is mainly realized by their ability to inhibit cellular enzymes, such as PLA2, COX, and LOX [21,108–111]. Quercetin blocks COX and LOX in various cell types such as rat peritoneal leukocyte, murine leukocytes, and guinea pig epidermis [110,112,113]. Similarly, red wine reduces COX-2 expression in old male F344 rats [114]. In LPS activated murine macrophages, green tea polyphenols not only suppress NF-κB and MAPK pathways but also constrain the expression of COX-2 and the release of prostaglandin (PGE2) in RAW 264.7 macrophages [115,116]. Equally, a reduction in the release of PGE2 is observed with other polyphenols, such as kaempferol in culture of LPS-stimulated human whole blood cells [117]. Extra virgin olive oil rich with more than 30 phenolic compounds inhibit 5-LOX in human activated leukocytes reducing leukotriene B4 and suppresses eicosanoids production by animal and human cells in vitro [118,119]. Finally, certain polyphenols show structural and functional similarities with specific anti-inflammatory drugs. A phenolic compound—oleocanthal—demonstrates a natural anti-inflammatory property and exhibits structural similarities to the ibuprofen (a well-known anti-inflammatory drug). Oleocanthal—like ibuprofen—inhibits COX-1 and COX-2 activities in a dose-dependent manner [120].

5. Polyphenols, Oxidative Stress, and Inflammation

Higher production of reactive oxygen species (ROS) is associated with oxidative stress and protein oxidation [121]. In its turn inflammatory molecules and different inflammatory signals (i.e., peroxiredoxin2) are triggered by protein oxidations [122]. Furthermore, overproduction of ROS can prompt tissue injury that might initiates the inflammatory process [123–127]. Therefore, the classical antioxidant actions of polyphenols undoubtedly contribute to their anti-inflammatory roles by interrupting the ROS-inflammation cycle (Figure 2). Polyphenols are known for their antioxidant activities; they scavenge a wide-ranging selection of ROS. Polyphenols can scavenge radicals and chelate metal ions, for example quercetin chelates iron ion [128]. They also inhibit multiple enzymes responsible of ROS generation [129]. In fact, free metal ions, as well as highly reactive hydroxyl radical release, is increased by the formation of ROS. To the opposite, polyphenols are able to chelate metal ions like Fe^{2+}, Cu^{2+}, and free radicals which lead to a reduction of highly oxidizing free radicals [130].

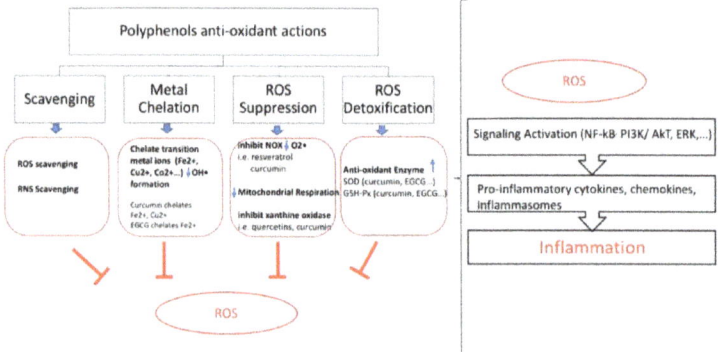

Figure 2. Key polyphenolic anti-oxidant actions in relation to anti-inflammation. Polyphenols scavenge radicals, chelate metal ions, inhibit ROS production and promote ROS detoxification. On the right panel ROS contribution to inflammation. ROS: reactive oxygen species; RNS: reactive nitrogen species; NOX: NADPH oxidase; SOD: superoxide dismutase; GSH-PX: glutathione peroxidase; ERK: extra-cellular signal regulated kinases; PI3K/AkT: phosphatidylinositide 3-kinases/protein kinase B; EGCG: epigallactocatechine gallate.

Transition metal ions, like Fe^{+2}, Cu^{2+}, Co^{2+}, Ti^{3+}, or Cr^{5+}, results in OH• formation from H_2O_2 [131,132]. Curcumin is able to chelate transition metal (Cu^{2+} and Fe^{2+}) ions. Alike, EGCG and quercetin chelate Fe^{2+} (iron ion) [128]. Polyphenols like apocynin, reservatol, and curcumin can inhibit NOX (NADPH oxidase) causing a reduction in the generation of O_2• during infections consecutively in endothelial cells in THP1-monocytes [133–135]. Additionally, polyphenols can attenuate the mitochondrial ATP synthesis by blocking the mitochondrial respiratory chain and ATPase. As a result, ROS production is diminished. Curcumin [136], EGCG [137], phenolic acids [138], capsaicin [139], quercetins [140], anthocyanins [140], and resveratrol analogs [141] inhibit xanthine oxidase. Thus, they reduce ROS production. Polyphenols affect the activity of cyclooxygenase, lipoxygenase, and NOS (nitric oxide synthase) as per found in RAW 264.7 macrophes [142]. These enzymes are known to metabolize arachidonic acid and their inhibition moderates the production of key mediators of inflammation (prostaglandins, leukotrienes, and NO ...) [142]. Polyphenols can also restrain LPS-induced iNOS gene expression in cultured macrophages, decreasing oxidative harm [143]. Finally, they may act by upregulating endogenous antioxidant enzymes. In vivo, curcumin can stimulate antioxidant enzymes like superoxide dismutase (SOD), catalase, and glutathione (GSH) peroxidase (Px) which lead to ROS detoxification [144]. Likewise, EGCG rises SOD and GSH-Px activities with augmented amount of cellular glutathione [145]. In conclusion, polyphenols exert the anti-inflammatory action by different mechanisms: Radical scavenging, metal chelating, NOX inhibition, tempering the mitochondrial respiratory chain, inhibition of certain enzymes involved in ROS production, like xanthine oxidase and upregulation of endogenous antioxidant enzymes.

6. Polyphenols, Chronic Diseases and Cancer

Referring to the previously cited roles of polyphenols in maintaining tissue homeostasis by targeting different signaling pathways and referring to their antioxidant, anti-inflammation, and protection against pro-inflammation properties; polyphenols play a beneficial role in the prevention and the process of chronic diseases related to inflammation.

Various polyphenolic compounds show protective actions in diabetes, obesity, neurodegeneration, cancers, and cardiovascular diseases, among other conditions [30,146–154].

6.1. Polyphenols and Insulin Resistance

Polyphenols reduce insulin resistance. They promote glycolysis by activation of AMPK (AMP-activated protein kinase) or inhibition of mTORC1 and PI3K/AkT in vivo (in rats), ex vivo (in rats' muscles strips) and in vitro (in C2C12 myoblasts and HELA cells) [148,149,155,156]. Additionally, AMPK activation by polyphenols increases glucose uptake by positively affecting eNOS imitating muscle contraction and in vivo activity of insulin [148–150]. Similarly, it is found that polyphenols lower insulin resistance by inhibiting PI3K/AkT and JNK of activation of the AMPK-SirT1-PGC1α axis (i.e., gingerol and anthocyans, and their ability to protect from diabetes and reduce insulin resistance using in vivo, ex vivo and in vitro studies [26–28,148,149,155]. In addition, polyphenols attenuate glucose intake from carbohydrates by inhibiting rats' α-glucosidase [157]. Lastly, polyphenols, like falvonoids, can improve insulin secretion by reducing apoptosis of pancreatic β–cells [145].

6.2. Polyphenols and Inflammatory Cardiovascular Diseases (CVD)

Meta-analysis studies have reported that an intake of three cups of tea per day reduces CVD by 11% [151] while adequate intake of red wine is associated with 32% lower risk of cardiovascular disease (CVD) [158]. Soy and cocoa flavonoids contribute to the prevention of CVD as per meta-analysis of randomized controls trial [159]. Polyphenols exert their protective effects in CVD due to their anti-hypertensive potentials. Resveratrol inhibits ACE (angiotensin converting enzyme) and PDE (phosphodiesterase) and upregulates eNOS (endothelial NOS) resulting in a reduction in high blood pressure as per multiple in vivo and in vitro studies [26–28,155,156,160]. In addition, flavanols and flavonols exert their CVD prevention role by reducing the manifestations of age-related vascular injury. They reduce nicotinamide adenine dinucleotide phosphate (NADPH) oxidase by affecting MAPK signaling and downregulating NF-κB in aged rats [161–163]. At the end, the antioxidant action of polyphenols and their ability to suppress LDL oxidation leads to endothelium-protective activity [164].

Certain polyphenols like resveratrol and anthocyanins protect from CVD by multiple mechanisms; they have (1) antihypertensive properties, they inhibit eNOS, and (2) inhibit NFκB mediated expression of VCAM and ICAM expression as per previously discussed [39,165]. Polyphenols can also reduce LDL oxidation or improve LDL/HDL ratio. For example, flavanones such as hesperetin in orange juice reduce LDL/HDL ratio while quercetin inhibits LDL oxidation with elevated paraoxonase and eliminate atherogenic lesions referring to in vitro and in vivo studies (using human male subjects) [166].

6.3. Polyphenols and Inflammatory Neurological Diseases

Polyphenols show protective effects in neurological disease [152,153]. High flavonoid intake can reduce by 50% dementia and aging. More precisely, it lowers the incidence of Parkinson's and delays the onset of Alzheimer's disease as per different epidemiological studies [167–170]. EGCG has neuroprotective properties due to its antioxidant (SOD, GSHPx) activities and cellular GSH contents and ability to reduce ROS contents. Similarly, anthocyanins neuroprotective characteristics are related to the improvement of oxidative stress and reduction of Aβ deposition [38,171,172]. Other mechanisms of polyphenols protection in neurodegenerative diseases is modulation of neuronal and glial signaling pathways [173]. Polyphenols can downregulate NF-κB related with iNOS generation in glial cells [174–176]. Moreover, their ability to inhibit monoamine oxidase plays a positive role in cognition, depression, and learning ability in vivo in male laca mice [172].

6.4. Polyphenols and Inflammatory Obesity

Polyphenols exert their anti-obesity effect by activation of AMPK (5′ adenosine monophosphate-activated protein kinase) leading to a reduction of cholesterol, fatty acid synthesis, and triglyceride formation by inhibiting HMG-CoA reductase and acetyl CoA carboxylase. Furthermore, they can inhibit genes involved in adipocyte differentiation and triglyceride accumulation. They block mTORC1 and repress specific signals associated with diminished levels of PPARγ and C/EBP α/δ mRNA throughout adipogenesis (in an experimental model of sepsis) and in vitro [30,146]. They can improve energy expenditure, stop the maturation of preadipocytes into adipocytes and increase the expression of adiponectin (a hormonal protein with a role in regulating glucose levels and breaking down fatty acids). For example, capsaicin enhances the energy spending in adipose tissue. Capsaicin diminishes intracellular triglycerides and improves brown adipose tissue thermogenesis. Furthermore, in clinical studies, capsaicin is found able to increase satiety [30,177,178]. EGCG inhibits MEK/ERK and PI3K/AKT pathways leading to inactivation of preadipocytes maturation by downregulating the expression of different genes like PPARγ and C/EBPα that are associated with adipogenesis [38,41,146,179]. Certain polyphenols can increase adiponectin such as gingerol and curcumin in serum of human subjects based on randomized controlled trial [180,181].

6.5. Polyphenols and Cancer

Clinical and epidemiological studies have reported that polyphenols have chemo-preventive and anticancer efficacy [182–184]. Polyphenol compounds have the ability to inhibit the proliferation of different types of cancer such as prostate, bladder, lung, gastrointestinal, breast, and ovarian cancers [154]. For instance, quercetin, resveratrol, green tea polyphenols [185], epigallocatechin-3-gallate [186], and curcumin [187] have demonstrated efficacy as anticancer compounds. Several studies reported that polyphenols are able to prevent cancer initiation (cyto-protective), progression, recurrence, and metastasis to distant organs (cytotoxic) as per different epidemiological, in vitro, and in vivo studie [188–190]. However, a dichotomy exists between polyphenols' antioxidant effects in normal cells, and their potential pro-oxidant effects in cancer cells [154,188].

Recent studies illustrated a direct correlation between ROS in intracellular signaling cascade and carcinogenesis [191]. Oxidative stress targets proteins, lipids, and DNA/RNA causing changes that increase the risks of mutagenesis. ROS/RNS (reactive nitrogen species) overproduction over a prolonged period of time damages cellular structure and functions and causes somatic mutations such as pre-neoplastic and neoplastic transformations that may lead to cell death by necrotic and apoptotic processes [192]. Polyphenols compounds contain hydroxyl groups that donate their protons to reactive oxygen species (ROS) [193]. Moreover, they reduce the activity of phase I enzymes, primarily cytochrome P450 enzymes (CYPs), such as CYP1A1 and CYP1B1 which lead to prevent the formation of reactive and carcinogenic metabolites in human bronchial epithelial cells [194]. They also can induce phase II enzymes that initiate the formation of polar metabolites which are readily excreted from the body [195]. Certain dietary polyphenols such as flavonoids reduce cellular formation of ROS which protects from the oxidation of DNA [193].

In addition to their anti-oxidant properties, pro-oxidant characteristic of polyphenols is important in treating and preventing cancer. Pro-oxidant activity can be initiated by certain conditions such as superoxide leakage [196]. The pro-oxidant activities of polyphenols in cancer cells can result in inducing apoptosis [197], cell cycle arrest [198] and inhibiting the proliferation signaling pathways (i.e., epidermal growth factor receptor/mitogen activated protein kinase, phosphatidylinositide 3-kinases/protein kinase B, as well as NF-kB) [199]. For example, polyphenols from apple are able to inhibit the proliferation of human bladder transitional cell carcinoma (TCC, TSGH-8301 cells), inducing G2/M cell cycle arrest, and promoting apoptosis [200]. In human papilloma virus-18-positive HeLa cervical cancer cells, green tea polyphenols can induce cell cycle arrest at the subG1 phase and apoptosis through caspases activation [201]. Flavonoids, such as quercetin, induce apoptosis in many cancer cells such as leukemic U937 cell [202], prostate cancer cells [203], hepatic cancer cells [204], among other types. A combination of quercetin with resveratrol and catechin inhibits breast cancer progression in vitro and in vivo by inducing apoptosis in carcinogenic breast cells [205]. In addition, polyphenols can reduce cancer metastasis such as quercetin [206,207].

Sufficient studies have reported that NF-κB signaling pathways are closely related to cancer metastasis. Polyphenols can disrupt the metastatic potential of cancer by inhibiting NF-κB activity [208]. Curcumin is a good example [209–211] of decreasing cancer metastasis in mice by suppressing NF-κB expression and down-regulating VEGF (vascular endothelial growth factor), COX-2, and MMP-9 (matrix metallopeptidase-9) expression in tissues of the breast, brain, lung, liver, and spleen [212,213]. Moreover, the strength of metastasis is associated to the epithelial-to-mesenchymal transition (EMT) [214]. There is robust evidence that polyphenols compounds can modulate EMT and its related signaling pathways [215]. For example, EGCG, a flavan-3-ol, induces apoptosis and significantly reduces colony formation and cell migration in nasopharyngeal carcinoma (NPC) and cancer stem cells (CSC) in different cell lines [216]. Luteolin and quercetin reverse the migration and invasiveness of metastatic cells by reducing the expression of mesenchymal markers and transcriptional factors on the cell membrane (i.e., twist, snail, and N-cadherin) and upregulating adhesion molecules such as E-cadherin [217]. Thus, through variable mechanisms, polyphenols broadly downregulate inflammation origination, progression, and evolution to cancers (Figure 3).

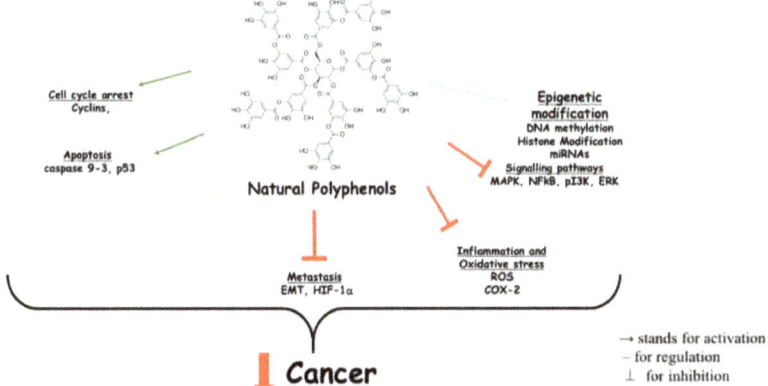

Figure 3. Anti-tumorigenic activities of polyphenols. MAPK: mitogen-activated protein kinase; NFκB: nuclear factor kappa-light-chain-enhancer of activated B cells; PI3K: phosphatidylinositide 3-kinase; ERK: extracellular signal-related kinases; ROS: reactive oxygen species; COX: cyclooxygenase; EMT: epithelial mesenchymal transition; HIF-1α: hypoxia-inducible factor 1-aplha.

In order to emphasize on the beneficial health effects of polyphenols, different medications containing polyphenols are FDA-approved as pharmaceutical drugs. Polyphenon® E, a standardized green tea polyphenol preparation, is an FDA-approved medication to treat genital warts [218]. Another significant event in the use of polyphenols as pharmaceuticals is the FDA approval of crofelemer (a medication rich in oligomeric proanthocyanidin) to manage HIV associated non-infectious diarrhea.

7. Conclusions

In conclusion, the vast number of published studies proved the immunomodulatory role of polyphenols in vivo and in vitro. Different underlying regulatory mechanisms are now well elucidated. These data highlight the promising role of polyphenols in prevention and therapy of diseases with underlining inflammatory conditions, including cancer, neurodegenerative diseases, obesity, type II diabetes, and cardiovascular diseases. However, the role of polyphenols in modulating multiple inflammatory cellular pathways should be further investigated. Many questions remain unanswered about the usage of polyphenols in clinical setting. The role of the microbiota in degrading these polyphenols should be further studied. The notion of bioavailability and its impact on biofunctionality should also be revisited. It is generally believed that polyphenol activity is principally located in the gut where their immunoprotective and anti-inflammatory activities are initiated and subsequently ensuring systemic anti-inflammatory effects. Since different polyphenols can have multiple intracellular targets, additional data is needed to determine the consequences of the interaction or the synergistic effects between multiple polyphenolic compounds or polyphenols and commonly used medications. Moreover, further in vivo and meta-analysis studies in humans are necessary to fully reveal the mechanisms of action of polyphenols in several physiological conditions in order to produce important insights into their prophylactic and therapeutic uses.

Author Contributions: N.Y. wrote all parts of the paper and prepared all Figures as well as the graphabstract except cancer and polyphenol paragraph and Figure 3; N.A. wrote cancer and polyphenol paragraph and prepared Figure 3; M.J. collected some papers and revised the Figures and their design; C.M. revised and guided the work.

Funding: This research received no external funding.

Acknowledgments: Special thanks to uOttawa libraries especially health sciences library and Morisset library and the department of "Nutrition Sciences".

Conflicts of Interest: The authors declare no conflict of interest.

Abbreviations

ROS	Reactive oxygen species
COX	Cyclooxygenase
NOX	NADPH oxidase
SOD	Superoxide dismutase
GSH	Glutathione
Px	Peroxidase
PLA2	Phospholipase A2
PGs	Prostaglandins
LTs	Leukotrienes
MAPK	Mitogen-activated protein Kinase
IKK	Inhibitor of kappa kinase
NFκB	Nuclear factor kappa-light-chain-enhancer of activated B cells
Th1	T helper 1
NK	Natural killer
DCs	Dendritic cells
ECGC	Epigallocatechin gallate
Treg	Regulatory T cells

AhR	Aryl hydrocarbon receptor
iNOS	Inducible nitric oxide synthase
LPS	Lipopolysaccharide
MCP-1	Monocyte chemoattractant protein-1
VEGF	Vascular endothelial growth Factor
IL	Interleukin
JNK	c-Jun amino-terminal kinases
CREB	cAMP response element-binding protein
AA	Arachidonic acid
AMPK	AMP-activated protein kinase
ERK	Extra-cellular signal regulated kinases
ATP	Adenosine triphosphate
CVD	Cardiovascular disease
PI3K	Phosphatidylinositide 3-kinases
Akt	Protein kinase B
LDL	Low density lipoprotein
HDL	High density lipoprotein
RNS	Reactive nitrogen species
PPARγ	Peroxisome proliferator-activated receptor gamma
CYPs	Cytochrome P450 enzymes
MMP-9	Matrix metallopeptidase-9
NPC	Nasopharyngeal carcinoma
CSCs	Cancer stem cells
EMT	Epithelial-to-mesenchymal transition
FDA	Food and drug administration
ICAM	Intercellular adhesion molecule
VCAM	Vascular cell adhesion molecule
HIV	Human immunodeficiency diarrhea
HMG-CoA	3-Hydroxy-3-methyl-glutaryl-coenzyme A
VEGF	Vascular endothelial growth factor
TLR	Toll-like receptor
NO	Nitric oxide
eNOS	Endothelial nitric oxide synthase
PDE	Phosphodiesterase
ACE	Angiotensin converting enzyme

References

1. Recio, M.; Andujar, I.; Rios, J. Anti-Inflammatory Agents from Plants: Progress and Potential. *Curr. Med. Chem.* **2012**, *19*, 2088–2103. [CrossRef] [PubMed]
2. Eberhardt, M.V.; Lee, C.Y.; Liu, R.H. Antioxidant Activity of Fresh Apples. *Nature* **2000**, *405*, 903–904. [CrossRef] [PubMed]
3. Spagnuolo, C.; Russo, M.; Bilotto, S.; Tedesco, I.; Laratta, B.; Russo, G.L. Dietary Polyphenols in Cancer Prevention: The Example of the Flavonoid Quercetin in Leukemia. *Ann. N. Y. Acad. Sci.* **2012**, *1259*, 95–103. [CrossRef] [PubMed]
4. Andriantsitohaina, R.; Auger, C.; Chataigneau, T.; Étenne-Selloum, N.; Li, H.; Martínez, M.C.; Schini-Kerth, V.B.; Laher, I. Molecular Mechanisms of the Cardiovascular Protective Effects of Polyphenols. *Br. J. Nutr.* **2012**, *108*, 1532–1549. [CrossRef] [PubMed]
5. Vauzour, D.; Rodriguez-Mateos, A.; Corona, G.; Oruna-Concha, M.J.; Spencer, J.P.E. Polyphenols and Human Health: Prevention of Disease and Mechanisms of Action. *Nutrients* **2010**, *2*, 1106–1131. [CrossRef] [PubMed]
6. Ma, Y.; Kosinska-Cagnazzo, A.; Kerr, W.L.; Amarowicz, R.; Swanson, R.B.; Pegg, R.B. Separation and Characterization of Soluble Esterified and Glycoside-Bound Phenolic Compounds in Dry-Blanched Peanut Skins by Liquid Chromatography-Electrospray Ionization Mass Spectrometry. *J. Agric. Food Chem.* **2014**, *62*, 11488–11504. [CrossRef] [PubMed]

7. Tsao, R. Chemistry and Biochemistry of Dietary Polyphenols. *Nutrients* **2010**, *2*, 1231–1246. [CrossRef] [PubMed]
8. Cheynier, V. Polyphenols in Food Are More Complex Then Often Thought. *Am. J. Clin. Nutr.* **2005**, *81*, 223–229. [CrossRef] [PubMed]
9. Mosele, J.I.; Macia, A.; Romero, M.-P.; Motilua, M.-J.; Rubio, L. Application of in Vitro Gastrointestinal Digestion and Colonic\nfermentation Models to Pomegranate Products (Juice, Pulp and Peel\nextract) to Study the Stability and Catabolism of Phenolic Compounds. *J. Funct. Food* **2015**, *14*, 529–540. [CrossRef]
10. Correa-Betanzo, J.; Allen-Vercoe, E.; McDonald, J.; Schroeter, K.; Corredig, M.; Paliyath, G. Stability and Biological Activity of Wild Blueberry (Vaccinium Angustifolium) Polyphenols during Simulated in Vitro Gastrointestinal Digestion. *Food Chem.* **2014**, *165*, 522–531. [CrossRef] [PubMed]
11. Martillanes, S.; Rocha-Pimienta, J.; Cabrera-Bañegil, M.; Martín-Vertedor, D.; Delgado-Adámez, J. Application of Phenolic Compounds for Food Preservation: Food Additive and Active Packaging. In *Phenolic Compounds-Biological Activity*; InTech: London, UK, 2017.
12. Maqsood, S.; Benjakul, S.; Shahidi, F. Emerging Role of Phenolic Compounds as Natural Food Additives in Fish and Fish Products. *Crit. Rev. Food Sci. Nutr.* **2013**, *53*, 162–179. [CrossRef] [PubMed]
13. Maestre, R.; Micol, V.; Funes, L.; Medina, I. Incorporation and Interaction of Grape Seed Extract in Membranes and Relation with Efficacy in Muscle Foods. *J. Agric. Food Chem.* **2010**, *58*, 8365–8374. [CrossRef] [PubMed]
14. Kennedy, E.T. Evidence for Nutritional Benefits in Prolonging Wellness. *Am. J. Clin. Nutr.* **2006**, *8*, 16470004. [CrossRef] [PubMed]
15. Bengmark, S. Acute and "Chronic" Phase Reaction-a Mother of Disease. *Clin. Nutr.* **2004**, *23*, 1256–1266. [CrossRef] [PubMed]
16. Visioli, F.; Galli, C. The Effect of Minor Constituents of Olive Oil on Cardiovascular Disease: New Findings. *Nutr. Rev.* **1998**, *56*, 142–147. [CrossRef] [PubMed]
17. Visioli, F.; Galli, C. The Role of Antioxidants in the Mediterranean Diet. *Lipids* **2001**, *36*, S49–S52. [CrossRef] [PubMed]
18. Middleton, E., Jr.; Kandaswami, C.; Theoharides, T.C. The Effects of Plant Flavonoids on Mammalian Cells: Implications for Inflammation, Heart Disease, and Cancer. *Pharmacol. Rev.* **2000**, *52*, 673–751. [PubMed]
19. Urquiaga, I.; Leighton, F. Plant Polyphenol Antioxidants and Oxidative Stress. *Biol. Res.* **2000**, *33*, 55–64. [CrossRef] [PubMed]
20. Scalbert, A.; Manach, C.; Morand, C.; Rémésy, C.; Jiménez, L. Dietary Polyphenols and the Prevention of Diseases. *Crit. Rev. Food Sci. Nutr.* **2005**, *45*, 287–306. [CrossRef] [PubMed]
21. Yoon, J.H.; Baek, S.J. Molecular Targets of Dietary Polyphenols with Anti-Inflammatory Properties. *Yonsei Med. J.* **2005**, *46*, 585–596. [CrossRef] [PubMed]
22. Malireddy, S.; Kotha, S.R.; Secor, J.D.; Gurney, T.O.; Abbott, J.L.; Maulik, G.; Maddipati, K.R.; Parinandi, N.L. Phytochemical Antioxidants Modulate Mammalian Cellular Epigenome: Implications in Health and Disease. *Antioxid. Redox Signal.* **2012**, *17*, 327–339. [CrossRef] [PubMed]
23. Santangelo, C.; Varì, R.; Scazzocchio, B.; Di Benedetto, R.; Filesi, C.; Masella, R. Polyphenols, Intracellular Signalling and Inflammation. *Ann. Ist. Super. Sanita* **2007**, *43*, 394–405. [PubMed]
24. Karasawa, K.; Uzuhashi, Y.; Hirota, M.; Otani, H. A Matured Fruit Extract of Date Palm Tree (*Phoenix dactylifera* L.) Stimulates the Cellular Immune System in Mice. *J. Agric. Food Chem.* **2011**, *59*, 11287–11293. [CrossRef] [PubMed]
25. John, C.M.; Sandrasaigaran, P.; Tong, C.K.; Adam, A.; Ramasamy, R. Immunomodulatory Activity of Polyphenols Derived from Cassia Auriculata Flowers in Aged Rats. *Cell. Immunol.* **2011**, *271*, 474–479. [CrossRef] [PubMed]
26. Mohar, D.; Malik, S. The Sirtuin System: The Holy Grail of Resveratrol? *J. Clin. Exp. Cardiol.* **2012**, *3*, 216. [CrossRef] [PubMed]
27. Speciale, A.; Chirafisi, J.; Saija, A.; Cimino, F. Nutritional Antioxidants and Adaptive Cell Responses: An Update. *Curr. Mol. Med.* **2011**, *11*, 770–789. [CrossRef] [PubMed]
28. Biasutto, L.; Mattarei, A.; Zoratti, M. Resveratrol and Health: The Starting Point. *ChemBioChem* **2012**, *13*, 1256–1259. [CrossRef] [PubMed]
29. Capiralla, H.; Vingtdeux, V.; Venkatesh, J.; Dreses-werringloer, U.; Zhao, H.; Davies, P.; Marambaud, P. Identification of Potent Small? Molecule Inhibitors of STAT3 with Anti? Inflammatory Properties in RAW 264.7 Macrophages. *FEBS J.* **2012**, *279*, 3791–3799. [CrossRef] [PubMed]

30. Leiherer, A.; Mündlein, A.; Drexel, H. Phytochemicals and Their Impact on Adipose Tissue Inflammation and Diabetes. *Vasc. Pharmacol.* **2013**, *58*, 3–20. [CrossRef] [PubMed]
31. Siddiqui, A.M.; Cui, X.; Wu, R.; Dong, W.; Zhou, M.; Hu, M.; Simms, H.H.; Wang, P. The Anti-Inflammatory Effect of Curcumin in an Experimental Model of Sepsis Is Mediated by up-Regulation of Peroxisome Proliferator-Activated Receptor-γ. *Crit. Care Med.* **2006**, *34*, 1874–1882. [CrossRef] [PubMed]
32. Marchiani, A.; Rozzo, C.; Fadda, A.; Delogu, G.; Ruzza, P. Curcumin and Curcumin-like Molecules: From Spice to Drugs. *Curr. Med. Chem.* **2014**, *21*, 204–222. [CrossRef] [PubMed]
33. Noorafshan, A.; Ashkani-Esfahani, S. A Review of Therapeutic Effects of Curcumin. *Curr. Pharm. Des.* **2013**, *19*, 2032–2046. [PubMed]
34. Gupta, S.C.; Prasad, S.; Kim, J.H.; Patchva, S.; Webb, L.J.; Priyadarsini, I.K.; Aggarwal, B.B. Multitargeting by Curcumin as Revealed by Molecular Interaction Studies. *Nat. Prod. Rep.* **2011**, *28*, 1937–1955. [CrossRef] [PubMed]
35. Bae, J. Role of High Mobility Group Box 1 in Inflammatory Disease: Focus on Sepsis. *Arch. Pharm. Res.* **2012**, *35*, 1511–1523. [CrossRef] [PubMed]
36. Tsuda, S.; Egawa, T.; Ma, X.; Oshima, R.; Kurogi, E.; Hayashi, T. Coffee Polyphenol Caffeic Acid but Not Chlorogenic Acid Increases 5′AMP-Activated Protein Kinase and Insulin-Independent Glucose Transport in Rat Skeletal Muscle. *J. Nutr. Biochem.* **2012**, *23*, 1403–1409. [CrossRef] [PubMed]
37. Akyol, S.; Ozturk, G.; Ginis, Z.; Amutcu, F.; Yigitoglu, M.; Akyol, O. In Vivo and in Vitro Antineoplastic Actions of Caffeic Acid Phenethyl Ester (CAPE): Therapeutic Perspectives. *Nutr. Cancer* **2013**, *65*, 1515–1526. [CrossRef] [PubMed]
38. Kanwar, J. Recent Advances on Tea Polyphenols. *Front. Biosci.* **2012**, *E4*, 111–131. [CrossRef]
39. Domitrovic, R. The Molecular Basis for the Pharmacological Activity of Anthocyans. *Curr. Med. Chem.* **2011**, *18*, 4454–4469. [CrossRef] [PubMed]
40. Singh, B.; Shankar, S.; Sriivastava, R. Green Tea Catechin, Epigallocatechin-3-Gallate (EGCG): Mechanisms, Perspectives and Clinical. *Biochem. Pharmacol.* **2011**, *82*, 1807–1821. [CrossRef] [PubMed]
41. Landis-Piwowar, K.; Chen, D.; Foldes, R.; Chan, T.-H.; Dou, Q.P. Novel Epigallocatechin Gallate Analogs as Potential Anticancer Agents: A Patent Review (2009–Present). *Expert Opin. Ther. Pat.* **2013**, *23*, 189–202. [CrossRef] [PubMed]
42. Sakaguchi, S.; Miyara, M.; Costantino, C.M.; Hafler, D.A. FOXP3 + Regulatory T Cells in the Human Immune System. *Nat. Rev. Immunol.* **2010**, *10*, 490–500. [CrossRef] [PubMed]
43. Boissier, M.C.; Assier, E.; Biton, J.; Denys, A.; Falgarone, G.; Bessis, N. Regulatory T Cells (Treg) in Rheumatoid Arthritis. *J. Bone Spine* **2009**, *76*, 10–14. [CrossRef] [PubMed]
44. Robinson, D.S.; Larché, M.; Durham, S.R. Tregs and Allergic Disease. *J. Clin. Investig.* **2004**, *114*, 1389–1397. [CrossRef] [PubMed]
45. Wong, C.P.; Nguyen, L.P.; Noh, S.K.; Bray, T.M.; Bruno, R.S.; Ho, E. Induction of Regulatory T Cells by Green Tea Polyphenol EGCG. *Immunol. Lett.* **2011**, *139*, 7–13. [CrossRef] [PubMed]
46. Yang, J.; Yang, X.; Li, M. Baicalin, a Natural Compound, Promotes Regulatory T Cell Differentiation. *IBMC Complement. Altern. Med.* **2012**, *16*, 64. [CrossRef] [PubMed]
47. Wang, H.K.; Yeh, C.H.; Iwamoto, T.; Satsu, H.; Shimizu, M.; Totsuka, M. Dietary Flavonoid Naringenin Induces Regulatory T Cells via an Aryl Hydrocarbon Receptor Mediated Pathway. *J. Agric. Food Chem.* **2012**, *60*, 2171–2178. [CrossRef] [PubMed]
48. Wang, J.; Pae, M.; Meydani, S.N.; Wu, D. Green Tea Epigallocatechin-3-Gallate Modulates Differentiation of Naïve CD4+T Cells into Specific Lineage Effector Cells. *J. Mol. Med.* **2013**, *91*, 485–495. [CrossRef] [PubMed]
49. Yang, J.; Yang, X.; Chu, Y.; Li, M. Identification of Baicalin as an Immunoregulatory Compound by Controlling TH17 Cell Differentiation. *PLoS ONE* **2011**, *6*, e21359178. [CrossRef] [PubMed]
50. Murray, P.J.; Wynn, T.A. Protective and Pathogenic Functions of Macrophage Subsets. *Nat. Rev. Immunol.* **2011**, *11*, 723–737. [CrossRef] [PubMed]
51. González, R.; Ballester, I.; López-Posadas, R.; Suárez, M.D.; Zarzuelo, A.; Martínez-Augustin, O.; Sánchez de Medina, F. Effects of Flavonoids and Other Polyphenols on Inflammation. *Crit. Rev. Food Sci. Nutr.* **2011**, *51*, 331–362. [CrossRef] [PubMed]
52. Wang, K.; Ping, S.; Huang, S.; Hu, L.; Xuan, H.; Zhang, C.; Hu, F. Molecular Mechanisms Underlying the In Vitro Anti-Inflammatory Effects of a Flavonoid -Rich Ethanol Extract from Chinese Propolis (Poplar Type). *Cell* **2013**, *2013*, 127672.

53. Park, K.I.; Kang, S.R.; Park, H.S.; Lee, D.H.; Nagappan, A.; Kim, J.A.; Shin, S.C.; Kim, E.H.; Lee, W.S.; Chung, H.J.; et al. Regulation of Proinflammatory Mediators via NF-KB and P38 MAPK-Dependent Mechanisms in RAW 264.7 Macrophages by Polyphenol Components Isolated from Korea Lonicera Japonica THUNB. *Evid.-Based Complement. Altern. Med.* **2012**, *2012*, 22611435. [CrossRef] [PubMed]
54. Lai, Z.-R.; Ho, Y.-L.; Huang, S.-C.; Huang, T.-H.; Lai, S.-C.; Tsai, J.-C.; Wang, C.-Y.; Huang, G.-J.; Chang, Y.-S. Antioxidant, Anti-Inflammatory and Antiproliferative Activities of *Kalanchoe gracilis* (L.) DC Stem. *Am. J. Chin. Med.* **2011**, *39*, 1275–1290. [CrossRef] [PubMed]
55. Bohstam, M.; Asgary, S.; Kouhpayeh, S.; Shariati, L.; Khanhamad, H. Aptamers Against Pro- and Anti-Inflammatory Cytokines: A Review. *Inflamm. Febr.* **2017**, *40*, 340–349. [CrossRef] [PubMed]
56. Kolehmainen, M.; Mykkänen, O.; Kirjavainen, P.V.; Leppänen, T.; Moilanen, E.; Adriaens, M.; Laaksonen, D.E.; Hallikainen, M.; Puupponen-Pimiä, R.; Pulkkinen, L.; et al. Bilberries Reduce Low-Grade Inflammation in Individuals with Features of Metabolic Syndrome. *Mol. Nutr. Food Res.* **2012**, *56*, 1501–1510. [CrossRef] [PubMed]
57. Fitó, M.; Cladellas, M.; de la Torre, R.; Martí, J.; Muñoz, D.; Schröder, H.; Alcántara, M.; Pujadas-Bastardes, M.; Marrugat, J.; Ló-Sabater, M.C.; et al. Anti-Inflammatory Effect of Virgin Olive Oil in Stable Coronary Disease Patients: A Randomized, Crossover, Controlled Trial. *Eur. J. Clin. Nutr.* **2008**, *62*, 570–574. [CrossRef] [PubMed]
58. Bitler, C.M.; Viale, T.M.; Damaj, B.; Crea, R. Hydrolyzed Olive Vegetation Water in Mice Has Anti-Inflammatory Activity. *J. Nutr.* **2005**, *135*, 1475–1479. [CrossRef] [PubMed]
59. Comalada, M.; Ballester, I.; Bailon, E.; Sierra, S.; Xaus, J.; de Medina, F.; Zarzuelo, A. Inhibition of pro-Inflammatory Markers in Primary Bone Marrow-Derived Mouse Macrophages by Naturally Occurring Flavonoids: Analysis of the Structure-Activity Relationship. *Biochem. Pharmacol.* **2006**, *72*, 1010–1021. [CrossRef] [PubMed]
60. Blonska, M.; Czuba, Z.P.; Krol, W. Effect of Flavone Derivatives on Interleukin-1beta (IL-1beta) MRNA Expression and IL-1beta Protein Synthesis in Stimulated RAW 264.7 Macrophages. *Scand. J. Immunol.* **2003**, *57*, 162–166. [CrossRef] [PubMed]
61. Sharma, V.; Mishra, M.; Ghosh, S.; Tewari, R.; Basu, A.; Seth, P.; Sen, E. Modulation of Interleukin-1beta Mediated Inflammatory Response in Human Astrocytes by Flavonoids: Implications in Neuroprotection. *Brain Res. Bull.* **2007**, *73*, 55–63. [CrossRef] [PubMed]
62. Sato, M.; Miyazaki, T.; Kambe, F.; Maeda, K.; Seo, H. Quercetin, a Bioflavonoid, Inhibits the Induction of Interleukin 8 and Monocyte Chemoattractant Protein-1 Expression by Tumor Necrosis Factor-Alpha in Cultured Human Synovial Cells. *J. Rheumatol.* **1997**, *24*, 1680–1684. [PubMed]
63. Min, Y.; Choi, C.; Bark, H.; Son, H.; Park, H.; Lee, S.; Park, J.; Park, E.; Shin, H.; Kim, S. Quercetin Inhibits Expression of Inflammatory Cytokines through Attenuation of NFkappaB and P38 MAPK in HMC-1 Human Mast Cell Line. *Inflamm. Res.* **2007**, *56*, 210–215. [CrossRef] [PubMed]
64. Lyu, S.Y.; Park, W.B. Production of Cytokine and NO by RAW 264.7 Macrophages and PBMC in Vitro Incubation with Flavonoids. *Arch. Pharm. Res.* **2005**, *28*, 573–581. [CrossRef] [PubMed]
65. Olivera, A.; Moore, T.W.; Hu, F.; Brown, A.P.; Sun, A.; Liotta, D.C.; Snyder, J.P.; Yoon, Y.; Shim, H.; Marcus, A.I.; et al. Inhibition of the NF-KB Signaling Pathway by the Curcumin Analog, 3,5-Bis(2-Pyridinylmethylidene)-4-Piperidone (EF31): Anti-Inflammatory and Anti-Cancer Properties. *Int. Immunopharmacol.* **2012**, *12*, 368–377. [CrossRef] [PubMed]
66. Drummond, E.M.; Harbourne, N.; Marete, E.; Martyn, D.; Jacquier, J.C.; O'Riordan, D.; Gibney, E.R. Inhibition of Proinflammatory Biomarkers in THP1 Macrophages by Polyphenols Derived from Chamomile, Meadowsweet and Willow Bark. *Phyther. Res.* **2013**, *27*, 588–594. [CrossRef] [PubMed]
67. Schindler, R.; Mancilla, J.; Endres, S.; Ghorbani, R.; Clark, S.C.; Dinarello, C.A. Correlations and Interactions in the Production of Interleukin-6 (IL-6), IL-1, and Tumor Necrosis Factor (TNF) in Human Blood Mononuclear Cells: IL-6 Suppresses IL-1 and TNF. *Blood* **1990**, *75*, 40–47. [PubMed]
68. Essafi-Benkhadir, K.; Refai, A.; Riahi, I.; Fattouch, S.; Karoui, H.; Essafi, M. Quince (*Cydonia oblonga* Miller) Peel Polyphenols Modulate LPS-Induced Inflammation in Human THP-1-Derived Macrophages through NF-KB, P38MAPK and Akt Inhibition. *Biochem. Biophys. Res. Commun.* **2012**, *418*, 180–185. [CrossRef] [PubMed]

69. Okamoto, I.; Iwaki, K.; Koya-Miyata, S.; Tanimoto, T.; Kohno, K.; Ikeda, M.; Kurimoto, M. The Flavonoid Kaempferol Suppresses the Graft-versus-Host Reaction by Inhibiting Type 1 Cytokine Production and CD8+T Cell Engraftment. *Clin. Immunol.* **2002**, *103*, 132–144. [CrossRef] [PubMed]
70. Crouvezier, S.; Powell, B.; Keir, D.; Yaqoob, P. The Effects of Phenolic Components of Tea on the Production of Pro- and Anti-Inflammatory Cytokines by Human Leukocytes in Vitro. *Cytokine* **2001**, *13*, 280–286. [CrossRef] [PubMed]
71. Nam, N. Naturally Occurring NF-kappa B Inhibitors. *Mini Rev. Med. Chem.* **2006**, *6*, 945–951. [CrossRef] [PubMed]
72. Hayden, M.S.; Ghosh, S. Signaling to NF-KappaB. *Genes Dev.* **2004**, *18*, 2195–2224. [CrossRef] [PubMed]
73. Haddad, J.J. Redox Regulation of pro-Inflammatory Cytokines and IkappaB-Alpha/NF-KappaB Nuclear Translocation And. *Biochem. Biophys. Res. Commun.* **2002**, *296*, 847–856. [CrossRef]
74. Karin, M.; Ben-Neriah, Y. Phosphorylation Meets Ubiquitination: The Control of NF-[Kappa]B Activity. *Annu. Rev. Immunol.* **2000**, *18*, 621–663. [CrossRef] [PubMed]
75. Perkins, N.D. Integrating Cell-Signalling Pathways with NF-KB and IKK Function. *Nat. Rev. Mol. Cell Biol.* **2007**, *8*, 49–62. [CrossRef] [PubMed]
76. Karin, M.; Yamamoto, Y.; Wang, Q.M. The IKK NF-KB System: A Treasure Trove for Drug Development. *Nat. Rev. Drug Discov.* **2004**, *3*, 17–26. [CrossRef] [PubMed]
77. Rahman, I.; Biswas, S.; Kirkham, P. Regulation of Inflammation and Redox Signaling by Dietary Polyphenols. *Biochem. Pharmacol.* **2006**, *72*, 1439–1452. [CrossRef] [PubMed]
78. Rahman, I.; Marwick, J.; Kirkham, P. Redox Modulation of Chromatin Remodeling: Impact on Histone Acetylation and Deacetylation, NF-KappaB and pro-Inflammatory Gene Expression. *Biochem. Pharmacol.* **2004**, *68*, 1255–1267. [CrossRef] [PubMed]
79. De Stefano, D.; Maiuri, M.C.; Simeon, V.; Grassia, G.; Soscia, A.; Cinelli, M.P.; Carnuccio, R. Lycopene, Quercetin and Tyrosol Prevent Macrophage Activation Induced by Gliadin and IFN-γ. *Eur. J. Pharmacol.* **2007**, *566*, 192–199. [CrossRef] [PubMed]
80. Comalada, M.; Camuesco, D.; Sierra, S.; Ballester, I.; Xaus, J.; Gálvez, J.; Zarzuelo, A. In Vivo Quercitrin Anti-Inflammatory Effect Involves Release of Quercetin, Which Inhibits Inflammation through down-Regulation of the NF-KB Pathway. *Eur. J. Immunol.* **2005**, *35*, 584–592. [CrossRef] [PubMed]
81. Ruiz, P.A.; Braune, A.; Hölzlwimmer, G.; Quintanilla-Fend, L.; Haller, D. Quercetin Inhibits TNF-Induced NF-KB Transcription Factor Recruitment to Proinflammatory Gene Promoters in Murine Intestinal Epithelial Cells. *J. Nutr.* **2007**, *137*, 1208–1215. [CrossRef] [PubMed]
82. Chen, J.C.; Ho, F.M.; Chao, P.D.L.; Chen, C.P.; Jeng, K.C.G.; Hsu, H.B.; Lee, S.T.; Wen, T.W.; Lin, W.W. Inhibition of INOS Gene Expression by Quercetin Is Mediated by the Inhibition of IκB Kinase, Nuclear Factor-Kappa B and STAT1, and Depends on Heme Oxygenase-1 Induction in Mouse BV-2 Microglia. *Eur. J. Pharmacol.* **2005**, *521*, 9–20. [CrossRef] [PubMed]
83. Gracia-Lafuente, A.; Guillamon, E.; Villares, A.; Rostagno, M.; Martinez, J. Flavonoids as Anti-Inflammatory Agents: Implications in Cancer and Cardiovascular Disease. *Inflamm. Res.* **2009**, *58*, 537–552. [CrossRef] [PubMed]
84. Nishitani, Y.; Yamamoto, K.; Yoshida, M.; Azuma, T.; Kanazawa, K.; Hashimoto, T.; Mizuno, M. Intestinal Anti-Inflammatory Activity of Luteolin: Role of the Aglycone in NF-KB Inactivation in Macrophages Co-Cultured with Intestinal Epithelial Cells. *Biofactors* **2013**, *39*, 522–533. [CrossRef] [PubMed]
85. Ji, G.; Zhang, Y.; Yang, Q.; Cheng, S.; Hao, J.; Zhao, X.; Jiang, Z. Genistein Suppresses LPS-Induced Inflammatory Response through Inhibiting NF-KB Following AMP Kinase Activation in RAW 264.7 Macrophages. *PLoS ONE* **2012**, *7*, e23300870. [CrossRef] [PubMed]
86. Kim, H.H.; Bae, Y.; Kim, S.H. Galangin Attenuates Mast Cell-Mediated Allergic Inflammation. *Food Chem. Toxicol.* **2013**, *57*, 209–216. [CrossRef] [PubMed]
87. Wheeler, D.S.; Catravas, J.D.; Odoms, K.; Denenberg, A.; Malhotra, V.; Wong, H.R. Epigallocatechin-3-Gallate, a Green Tea-Derived Polyphenol, Inhibits IL-1 Beta-Dependent Proinflammatory Signal Transduction in Cultured Respiratory Epithelial Cells. *J. Nutr.* **2004**, *134*, 1039–1044. [CrossRef] [PubMed]
88. Aneja, R.; Hake, P.W.; Burroughs, T.J.; Denenberg, A.G.; Wong, H.R.; Zingarelli, B. Epigallocatechin, a Green Tea Polyphenol, Attenuates Myocardial Ischemia Reperfusion Injury in Rats. *Mol. Med.* **2004**, *10*, 55–62. [CrossRef] [PubMed]

89. Ichikawa, D.; Matsui, A.; Imai, M.; Sonoda, Y.; Kasahara, T. Effect of Various Catechins on the IL-12 p40 Production by Murine Peritoneal Macrophages and A. *Biol. Pharm. Bull.* **2004**, *27*, 1353–1358. [CrossRef] [PubMed]
90. Lin, Y.; Lin, J. Epigallocatechin-3-Gallate Blocks the Induction of Nitric Oxide Synthase by Down-Regulating Lipopolysaccharide-Induced Activity of Transcription Factor Nuclear Factor-κB. *Mol. Pharmacol.* **1997**, *472*, 465–472. [CrossRef]
91. Mackenzie, G.; Carrasquedo, F.; Delfino, J.; Keen, C.; Fraga, C.; Oteiza, P. Epicatechin, Catechin, and Dimeric Procyanidins Inhibit PMA? Induced NF? KappaB Activation at Multiple Steps in Jurkat T Cells. *FASEB J.* **2004**, *18*, 167–169. [CrossRef] [PubMed]
92. Carluccio, M.A.; Siculella, L.; Ancora, M.A.; Massaro, M.; Scoditti, E.; Storelli, C.; Visioli, F.; Distante, A.; De Caterina, R. Olive Oil and Red Wine Antioxidant Polyphenols Inhibit Endothelial Activation: Antiatherogenic Properties of Mediterranean Diet Phytochemicals. *Arterioscler. Thromb. Vasc. Biol.* **2003**, *23*, 622–629. [CrossRef] [PubMed]
93. Chang, L.; Karin, M. Mammalian MAP Kinase Signalling Cascades. *Nature* **2001**, *410*, 37–40. [CrossRef] [PubMed]
94. Khan, N.; Afaq, F.; Saleem, M.; Ahmad, N.; Mukhtar, H. Targeting Multiple Signaling Pathways by Green Tea Polyphenol (−)-Epigallocatechin-3-Gallate. 1 Khan N, Afaq F, Saleem M, Ahmad N, Mukhtar H. Author Information Full. *Cancer Res.* **2006**, *66*, 2500–2505. [CrossRef] [PubMed]
95. Kolch, W. Coordinating ERK/MAPK Signalling through Scaffolds and Inhibitors. *Nat. Rev. Mol. Cell Biol.* **2005**, *6*, 827–837. [CrossRef] [PubMed]
96. Lu, Z.; Xu, S. ERK1/2 MAP Kinases in Cell Survival and Apoptosis. *IUBMB Life* **2006**, *58*, 621–631. [CrossRef] [PubMed]
97. Mayor, F.; Jurado-Pueyo, M.; Campos, P.M.; Murga, C. Interfering with MAP Kinase Docking Interactions: Implications and Perspective for the P38 Route. *Cell Cycle* **2007**, *6*, 528–533. [CrossRef] [PubMed]
98. Kaminska, B. MAPK Signalling Pathways as Molecular Targets for Anti-Inflammatory Therapy—From Molecular Mechanisms to Therapeutic Benefits. *Biochim. Biophys. Acta* **2005**, *1754*, 253–262. [CrossRef] [PubMed]
99. Karin, M. Inflammation-Activated Protein Kinases as Targets for Drug Development. *Proc. Am. Thorac. Soc.* **2005**, *2*, 386–390. [CrossRef] [PubMed]
100. Xagorari, A.; Roussos, C.; Papapetropoulos, A. Inhibition of LPS-Stimulated Pathways in Macrophages by the Flavonoid Luteolin. *Br. J. Pharmacol.* **2002**, *136*, 1058–1064. [CrossRef] [PubMed]
101. Chen, C.; Chow, M.; Huang, W.; Lin, Y.; Chang, Y. Flavonoids Inhibit Tumor Necrosis Factor-Alpha-Induced up-Regulation of Intercellular Adhesion Molecule-1 (ICAM-1) in Respiratory Epithelial Cells through Activator Protein-1 and Nuclear Factor-KappaB: Structure-Activity Relationships. *Mol. Pharmacol.* **2004**, *66*, 683–693. [PubMed]
102. Wadsworth, T.L.; McDonald, T.L.; Koop, D.R. Effects of Ginkgo Biloba Extract (EGb 761) and Quercetin on Lipopolysaccharide-Induced Signaling Pathways Involved in the Release of Tumor Necrosis Factor-Alpha. *Biochem. Pharmacol.* **2001**, *62*, 963–974. [CrossRef]
103. Cho, S.; Park, S.; Kwon, M.; Jeong, T.; Bok, S.; Choi, W.; Jeong, W.; Ryu, S.; Do, S.; Song, C.; et al. Quercetin Suppresses Proinflammatory Cytokines Production through MAP Kinases AndNF-Kappa B Pathway in Lipopolysaccharide-Stimulated Macrophage. *Mol. Cell. Biochem.* **2003**, *243*, 153–160. [CrossRef] [PubMed]
104. Kundu, J.K.; Surh, Y.J. Epigallocatechin Gallate Inhibits Phorbol Ester-Induced Activation of NF-KB and CREB in Mouse Skin Role of P38 MAPK. *Ann. N. Y. Acad. Sci.* **2007**, *1095*, 504–512. [CrossRef] [PubMed]
105. Pasten, C.; Olave, N.; Zhou, L.; Tabengwa, E.; Wolkowicz, P.; Grenett, H. Polyphenols Downregulate PAI-1 Gene Expression in Cultured Human Coronary Artery Endothelial Cells: Molecular Contributor to Cardiovascular Protection. *Thromb. Res.* **2007**, *121*, 59–65. [CrossRef] [PubMed]
106. Chandrasekharan, N.V.; Dai, H.; Roos, K.L.T.; Evanson, N.K.; Tomsik, J.; Elton, T.S.; Simmons, D.L. COX-3, a Cyclooxygenase-1 Variant Inhibited by Acetaminophen and Other Analgesic/Antipyretic Drugs: Cloning, Structure, and Expression. *Proc. Natl. Acad. Sci. USA* **2002**, *99*, 13926–13931. [CrossRef] [PubMed]
107. Needleman, P.; Isakson, P. The Discovery and Function of COX-2. *J. Rheumatol. Suppl.* **2018**, *49*, 6–8.
108. Kim, H.P.; Son, K.H.; Chang, H.W.; Kang, S.S. Anti-Inflammatory Plant Flavonoids and Cellular Action Mechanisms. *J. Pharmacol. Sci.* **2004**, *96*, 229–245. [CrossRef] [PubMed]

109. Welton, A.F.; Tobias, L.D.; Fiedler-Nagy, C.; Anderson, W.; Hope, W.; Meyers, K.; Coffey, J.W. Effect of Flavonoids on Arachidonic Acid Metabolism. *Prog. Clin. Biol. Res.* **1986**, *213*, 231–242. [PubMed]
110. Laughton, M.; Evans, P.; Moroney, M.; Hoult, J.; Halliwell, B. Inhibition of Mammalian 5-Lipoxygenase and Cyclo-Oxygenase by Flavonoids and Phenolic Dietary Additives. Relationship to Antioxidant Activity and to Iron Ion-Reducing Ability. *Biochem. Pharmacol.* **1991**, *42*, 1673–1681. [CrossRef]
111. Aviram, M.; Fuhrman, B. Polyphenolic Flavonoids Inhibit Macrophage-Mediated Oxidation of LDL and Attenuate Atherogenesis. *Atherosclerosis* **1998**, *137*, 9694541. [CrossRef]
112. Ferrandiz, M.L.; Alcaraz, M.J. Ferrandiz 1991-Anti-Inflammatory Activity and Inhibition of Arachidonic Acid Metabolism by Flavonoids. *Agent Action* **1991**, *32*, 283–288. [CrossRef]
113. Kim, H.; Mani, I.; Iversen, L.; Ziboh, V. Effects of Naturally-Occurring Flavonoids and Biflavonoids on Epidermal Cyclooxygenase and Lipoxygenase from Guinea-Pigs. *Prostaglandin Leukot. Essent. Fat. Acid.* **1998**, *58*, 17–24. [CrossRef]
114. Luceri, C.; Caderni, G.; Sanna, A.; Dolara, P. Red Wine and Black Tea Polyphenols Modulate the Expression of Cyclooxygenase-2, Inducible Nitric Oxide Synthase and Glutathione-Related Enzymes in Azoxymethane-Induced F344 Rat Colon Tumors. *J. Nutr.* **2002**, *132*, 1376–1379. [CrossRef] [PubMed]
115. Hou, D.X.; Luo, D.; Tanigawa, S.; Hashimoto, F.; Uto, T.; Masuzaki, S.; Fujii, M.; Sakata, Y. Prodelphinidin B-4 3′-O-Gallate, a Tea Polyphenol, Is Involved in the Inhibition of COX-2 and INOS via the Downregulation of TAK1-NF-KB Pathway. *Biochem. Pharmacol.* **2007**, *74*, 742–751. [CrossRef] [PubMed]
116. Hou, D.; Masuzaki, S.; Hashimoto, F.; Uto, T.; Tanigawa, S.; Fujii, M.; Sakata, Y. Green Tea Proanthocyanidins Inhibit Cyclooxygenase-2 Expression in LPS-Activated Mouse Macrophages: Molecular Mechanisms and Structure? Activity Relationship. *Arch. Biochem. Biophys.* **2007**, *460*, 67–74. [CrossRef] [PubMed]
117. Miles, E.A.; Zoubouli, P.; Calder, P.C. Differential Anti-Inflammatory Effects of Phenolic Compounds from Extra Virgin Olive Oil Identified in Human Whole Blood Cultures. *Nutrition* **2005**, *21*, 389–394. [CrossRef] [PubMed]
118. Tuck, K.L.; Hayball, P.J. Major Phenolic Compounds in Olive Oil: Metabolism and Health Effects. *J. Nutr. Biochem.* **2002**, *13*, 636–644. [CrossRef]
119. De la Puerta, R.; Gutierrez, V.R.; Hoult, J. Inhibition of Leukocyte 5 Lipoxygenase by Phenolics from Virgin Olive Oil. *Biochem. Pharmacol.* **1999**, *57*, 445–449. [CrossRef]
120. Beauchamp, G.K.; Keast, R.S.J.; Morel, D.; Lin, J.; Pika, J.; Han, Q.; Lee, C.H.; Smith, A.B.; Breslin, P.A.S. Ibuprofen-like Activity in Extra-Virgin Olive Oil. *Nature* **2005**, *437*, 45–46. [CrossRef] [PubMed]
121. Berlett, B.S.; Stadtman, E.R.; Berlett, B.S.; Stadtman, E.R. Protein Oxidation in Aging, Disease, and Oxidative Stress. *J. Biol. Chem.* **1997**, *272*, 20313–20316. [CrossRef] [PubMed]
122. Salzano, S.; Checconi, P.; Hanschmann, E.-M.; Lillig, C.H.; Bowler, L.D.; Chan, P.; Vaudry, D.; Mengozzi, M.; Coppo, L.; Sacre, S.; et al. Linkage of Inflammation and Oxidative Stress via Release of Glutathionylated Peroxiredoxin-2, Which Acts as a Danger Signal. *Proc. Natl. Acad. Sci. USA* **2014**, *111*, 12157–12162. [CrossRef] [PubMed]
123. Willcox, J.K.; Ash, S.L.; Catignani, G.L. Antioxidants and Prevention of Chronic Disease. *Crit. Rev. Food Sci. Nutr.* **2004**, *44*, 275–295. [CrossRef] [PubMed]
124. Bryan, N.; Ahswin, H.; Smart, N.; Bayon, Y.; Wohlert, S.; Hunt, J.A. Reactive Oxygen Species (ROS)-A Family of Fate Deciding Molecules Pivotal in Constructive Inflammation and Wound Healing. *Eur. Cells Mater.* **2012**, *24*, 249–265. [CrossRef]
125. Naik, E.; Dixit, V.M. Mitochondrial Reactive Oxygen Species Drive Proinflammatory Cytokine Production: Figure 1. *J. Exp. Med.* **2011**, *208*, 417–420. [CrossRef] [PubMed]
126. Clark, R.A.; Valente, A.J. Nuclear Factor Kappa B Activation by NADPH Oxidases. *Mech. Ageing Dev.* **2004**, *125*, 799–810. [CrossRef] [PubMed]
127. Geiszt, M.; Leto, T.L. The Nox Family of NAD(P)H Oxidases: Host Defense and Beyond. *J. Biol. Chem.* **2004**, *279*, 51715–51718. [CrossRef] [PubMed]
128. Heim, K.E.; Tagliaferro, A.R.; Bobilya, D.J. Flavonoid Antioxidants: Chemistry, Metabolism and Structure-Activity Relationships. *J. Nutr. Biochem.* **2002**, *13*, 572–584. [CrossRef]
129. Mishra, A.; Sharma, A.K.; Kumar, S.; Saxena, A.K.; Pandey, A.K. Bauhinia Variegata Leaf Extracts Exhibit Considerable Antibacterial, Antioxidant, and Anticancer Activities. *Biomed. Res. Int.* **2013**, *2013*, 915436. [CrossRef] [PubMed]

130. Mishra, A.; Kumar, S.; Pandey, A.K. Scientific Validation of the Medicinal Efficacy of Tinospora Cordifolia. *Sci. World J.* **2013**, *2013*, 292934. [CrossRef] [PubMed]
131. Marnett, L.J.; Riggins, J.N.; West, J.D. Endogenous Generation of Reactive Oxidants and Electrophiles and Their Reactions with DNA and Protein. *J. Clin. Investig.* **2003**, *111*, 583–593. [CrossRef] [PubMed]
132. Prousek, J. Fenton Chemistry in Biology and Medicine. *Pure Appl. Chem.* **2007**, *79*, 2007–2010. [CrossRef]
133. Deby-Dupont, G.; Mouithys-Mickalad, A.; Serteyn, D.; Lamy, M.; Deby, C. Resveratrol and Curcumin Reduce the Respiratory Burst of Chlamydia-Primed THP-1 Cells. *Biochem. Biophys. Res. Commun.* **2005**, *333*, 21–27. [CrossRef] [PubMed]
134. Chow, S.E.; Hshu, Y.C.; Wang, J.S.; Chen, J.K. Resveratrol Attenuates OxLDL-Stimulated NADPH Oxidase Activity and Protects Endothelial Cells from Oxidative Functional Damages. *J. Appl. Physiol.* **2007**, *102*, 1520–1527. [CrossRef] [PubMed]
135. Petrônio, M.S.; Zeraik, M.L.; Da Fonseca, L.M.; Ximenes, V.F. Apocynin: Chemical and Biophysical Properties of a NADPH Oxidase Inhibitor. *Molecules* **2013**, *18*, 2821–2839. [CrossRef] [PubMed]
136. Shen, L.; Ji, H.F. Insights into the Inhibition of Xanthine Oxidase by Curcumin. *Bioorg. Med. Chem. Lett.* **2009**, *19*, 5990–5993. [CrossRef] [PubMed]
137. Aucamp, J. Inhibition of Xanthine Oxidase by Tea Catechins (Camellia Sinensis). *Method Mol. Biol.* **1997**, *702*, 47–60.
138. Schmidt, A.; Böhmer, A.E.; Antunes, C.; Schallenberger, C.; Porciuncula, L.; Elisabetsky, E.; Lara, D.; Souza, D. Anti-Nociceptive Properties of the Xanthine Oxidase Inhibitor Allopurinol in Mice: Role of A1 Adenosine Receptors. *Br. J. Pharmacol.* **2009**, *156*, 163–172. [CrossRef] [PubMed]
139. Nguyen, M.T.T.; Nguyen, N.T. Xanthine Oxidase Inhibitors from Vietnamese *Blume balsamifer* L. *Phyther. Res.* **2012**, *26*, 1178–1181. [CrossRef] [PubMed]
140. Bräunlich, M.; Slimestad, R.; Wangensteen, H.; Brede, C.; Malterud, K.E.; Barsett, H. Extracts, Anthocyanins and Procyanidins from Aronia Melanocarpa as Radical Scavengers and Enzyme Inhibitors. *Nutrients* **2013**, *5*, 663–678. [CrossRef] [PubMed]
141. Huang, X.F.; Li, H.Q.; Shi, L.; Xue, J.Y.; Ruan, B.F.; Zhu, H.L. Synthesis of Resveratrol Analogues, and Evaluation of Their Cytotoxic and Xanthine Oxidase Inhibitory Activities. *Chem. Biodivers.* **2008**, *5*, 636–642. [CrossRef] [PubMed]
142. Cheon, B.S.; Kim, Y.H.; Son, K.S.; Chang, H.W.; Kang, S.S.; Kim, H.P. Effects of Prenylated Flavonoids and Biflavonoids on Lipopolysaccharide-Induced Nitric Oxide Production from the Mouse Macrophage Cell Line RAW 264.7. *Planta Med.* **2000**, *66*, 596–600. [CrossRef] [PubMed]
143. Sarkar, A.; Bhaduri, A. Black Tea Is a Powerful Chemopreventor of Reactive Oxygen and Nitrogen Species: Comparison with Its Individual Catechin Constituents and Green Tea. *Biochem. Biophys. Res. Commun.* **2001**, *284*, 173–178. [CrossRef] [PubMed]
144. Sporn, M.B.; Liby, K.T. NRF2 and Cancer: The Good, the Bad and the Importance of Context. *Nat. Rev. Cancer* **2012**, *12*, 564–571. [CrossRef] [PubMed]
145. Chu, A. Antagonism by Bioactive Polyphenols Against Inflammation: A Systematic View. *Inflamm. Allergy Drug Targets* **2014**, *13*, 34–64. [CrossRef] [PubMed]
146. Meydani, M.; Hasan, S.T. Dietary Polyphenols and Obesity. *Nutrients* **2010**, *2*, 737–751. [CrossRef] [PubMed]
147. Yahfoufi, N.; Mallet, J.F.; Graham, E.; Matar, C. Role of Probiotics and Prebiotics in Immunomodulation. *Curr. Opin. Food Sci.* **2018**, *20*, 82–91. [CrossRef]
148. Roy, D.; Perreault, M.; Marette, A. Insulin Stimulation of Glucose Uptake in Skeletal Muscles and Adipose Tissues in Vivo Is NO Dependent. *Am. J. Physiol. Endocrinol. Metab.* **1998**, *274*, E692–E699. [CrossRef]
149. Fryer, L.G.; Hajduch, E.; Rencurel, F.; Salt, I.P.; Hundal, H.S.; Hardie, D.G.; Carling, D. Activation of Glucose Transport by AMP-Activated Protein Kinase via Stimulation of Nitric Oxide Synthase. *Diabetes* **2000**, *49*, 1978–1985. [CrossRef] [PubMed]
150. Roberts, C.K.; Barnard, R.J.; Scheck, S.H.; Balon, T.W. Exercise-Stimulated Glucose Transport in Skeletal Muscle Is Nitric Oxide Dependent. *Am. J. Physiol.* **1997**, *273*, E220–E225. [PubMed]
151. Peters, U.; Poole, C.; Arab, L. Does Tea Affect Cardiovascular Disease? A Meta-Analysis. *Am. J. Epidemiol.* **2001**, *154*, 495–503. [CrossRef] [PubMed]
152. Lindsay, J.; Laurin, D.; Verreault, R.; Hébert, R.; Helliwell, B.; Hill, G.; McDowell, I. Risk Factors for Alzheimer's Disease: A Prospective Analysis from the Canadian Study of Health and Aging. *Am. J. Epidemiol.* **2002**, *156*, 445–453. [CrossRef] [PubMed]

153. Truelsen, T.; Thudium, D.; Grønbaek, M.; Copenhagen City Heart Study. Amount and Type of Alcohol and Risk of Dementia: The Copenhagen City Heart Study. *Neurology* **2002**, *59*, 1313–1319. [CrossRef] [PubMed]
154. Hadi, S.M.; Asad, S.F.; Singh, S.; Ahmad, A. Putative Mechanism for Anticancer and Apoptosis-Inducing Properties of Plant-Derived Polyphenolic Compounds. *IUBMB Life* **2000**, *50*, 167–171. [PubMed]
155. Park, S.; Ahmad, F.; Philip, A.; Baar, K.; William, T.; Luo, H.; Ke, H.; Rehmann, H.; Taussing, R.; Brown, A.; et al. Resveratrol Ameliorates Aging-Related Metabolic Phenotypes by Inhibiting CAMP Phosphodiesterases. *Cell* **2012**, *148*, 421–433. [CrossRef] [PubMed]
156. Wallerath, T.; Deckert, G.; Ternes, T.; Anderson, H.; Li, H.; Witte, K.; Forstermann, U. Resveratrol, a Polyphenolic Phytoalexin Present in Red Wine, Enhances Expression and Activity of Endothelial Nitric Oxide Synthase. *Circulation* **2002**, *106*, 1652–1658. [CrossRef] [PubMed]
157. Kumar, S.; Narwal, S.; Kumar, V.; Prakash, O. α-Glucosidase Inhibitors from Plants: A Natural Approach to Treat Diabetes. *Pharmacogn. Rev.* **2011**, *5*, 19–29. [CrossRef] [PubMed]
158. Di Castelnuovo, A.; Rotondo, S.; Iacoviello, L.; Donati, M.B.; De Gaetano, G. Meta-Analysis of Wine and Beer Consumption in Relation to Vascular Risk. *Circulation* **2002**, *105*, 2836–2844. [CrossRef] [PubMed]
159. Hooper, L.; Kroon, P.A.; Rimm, E.B.; Cohn, J.S.; Harvey, I.; Cornu, K.A.; Le Ryder, J.J.; Hall, W.L.; Cassidy, A. Flavonoids, Flavonoid-Rich Foods, and Cardiovascular Risk: A Meta-Analysis of Randomized Controlled Trials 1, 2. *Am. J. Clin. Nutr.* **2008**, *88*, 38–50. [CrossRef] [PubMed]
160. Shen, M.; Zhao, L.; Wu, R.X.; Yue, S.Q.; Pei, J.M. The Vasorelaxing Effect of Resveratrol on Abdominal Aorta from Rats and Its Underlying Mechanisms. *Vasc. Pharmacol.* **2013**, *58*, 64–70. [CrossRef] [PubMed]
161. Peppa, M.; Raptis, S.A. Advanced Glycation End Products and Cardiovascular Disease. *Curr. Diabete Rev.* **2008**, *4*, 92–100. [CrossRef]
162. Huang, S.M.; Wu, C.H.; Yen, G.C. Effects of Flavonoids on the Expression of the Pro-Inflammatory Response in Human Monocytes Induced by Ligation of the Receptor for AGEs. *Mol. Nutr. Food Res.* **2006**, *50*, 1129–1139. [CrossRef] [PubMed]
163. Kim, J.M.; Lee, E.K.; Kim, D.H.; Yu, B.P.; Chung, H.Y. Kaempferol Modulates Pro-Inflammatory NF-KB Activation by Suppressing Advanced Glycation Endproducts-Induced NADPH Oxidase. *Age* **2010**, *32*, 197–208. [CrossRef] [PubMed]
164. Wilkinson-Berka, J.L.; Rana, I.; Armani, R.; Agrotis, A. Reactive Oxygen Species, Nox and Angiotensin II in Angiogenesis: Implications for Retinopathy. *Clin. Sci.* **2013**, *124*, 597–615. [CrossRef] [PubMed]
165. Thomasset, S.; Teller, N.; Cai, H.; Marko, D.; Berry, D.; Steward, W.; Gescher, A. Do Anthocyanins and Anthocyanidins, Cancer Chemopreventive Pigments in the Diet, Merit Development as Potential Drugs? *Cancer Chemother. Pharmacol.* **2009**, *64*, 201–211. [CrossRef] [PubMed]
166. Aviram, M.; Fuhrman, B. Wine Flavonoids Protect against LDL Oxidation and Atherosclerosis. *Ann. N. Y. Acad. Sci.* **2002**, *957*, 146–161. [CrossRef] [PubMed]
167. Commenges, D.; Scotet, V.; Renaud, S.; Jacqmin-Gadda, H.; Barberger-Gateau, P.; Dartigues, J.F. Intake of Flavonoids and Risk of Dementia. *Eur. J. Epidemiol.* **2000**, *16*, 357–363. [CrossRef] [PubMed]
168. Dai, Q.; Borenstein, A.R.; Wu, Y.; Jackson, J.C.; Larson, E.B. Fruit and Vegetable Juices and Alzheimer's Disease: The Kame Project. *Am. J. Med.* **2006**, *119*, 751–759. [CrossRef] [PubMed]
169. Morris, M.C.; Evans, D.A.; Tangney, C.C.; Bienias, J.L.; Wilson, R.S. Associations of Vegetable and Fruit Consumption with Age-Related Cognitive Change. *Neurology* **2006**, *67*, 1370–1376. [CrossRef] [PubMed]
170. Checkoway, H.; Powers, K.; Smith-Weller, T.; Franklin, G.M.; Longstreth, W.T.; Swanson, P.D. Parkinson's Disease Risks Associated with Cigarette Smoking, Alcohol Consumption, and Caffeine Intake. *Am. J. Epidemiol.* **2002**, *155*, 732–738. [CrossRef] [PubMed]
171. Shehzad, A.; Lee, Y.S. Molecular Mechanisms of Curcumin Action: Signal Transduction. *Biofactors* **2013**, *39*, 27–36. [CrossRef] [PubMed]
172. Gomez-Pinilla, F.; Nguyen, T.T.J. Natural Mood Foods: The Actions of Polyphenols against Psychiatric and Cognitive Disorders. *Nutr. Neurosci.* **2012**, *15*, 127–133. [CrossRef] [PubMed]
173. Vauzour, D.; Vafeiadou, K.; Rice-Evans, C.; Williams, R.J.; Spencer, J.P.E. Activation of Pro-Survival Akt and ERK1/2 Signalling Pathways Underlie the Anti-Apoptotic Effects of Flavanones in Cortical Neurons. *J. Neurochem.* **2007**, *103*, 1355–1367. [CrossRef] [PubMed]
174. Vafeiadou, K.; Vauzour, D.; Lee, H.Y.; Rodriguez-Mateos, A.; Williams, R.J.; Spencer, J.P.E. The Citrus Flavanone Naringenin Inhibits Inflammatory Signalling in Glial Cells and Protects against Neuroinflammatory Injury. *Arch. Biochem. Biophys.* **2009**, *484*, 100–109. [CrossRef] [PubMed]

175. Wang, X.; Chen, S.; Ma, G.; Ye, M.; Lu, G. Genistein Protects Dopaminergic Neurons by Inhibiting Microglial Activation. *Neuroreport* **2005**, *16*, 267–270. [CrossRef] [PubMed]
176. Bhat, N.R.; Feinstein, D.L.; Shen, Q.; Bhat, A.N. P38 MAPK-Mediated Transcriptional Activation of Inducible Nitric-Oxide Synthase in Glial Cells: Roles of Nuclear Factors, Nuclear Factor KB, CAMP Response Element-Binding Protein, CCAAT/Enhancer-Binding Protein-β, and Activating Transcription Factor-2. *J. Biol. Chem.* **2002**, *277*, 29584–29592. [CrossRef] [PubMed]
177. Whiting, S.; Derbyshire, E.; Tiwari, B.K. Capsaicinoids and Capsinoids. A Potential Role for Weight Management? A Systematic Review of the Evidence. *Appetite* **2012**, *59*, 341–348. [CrossRef] [PubMed]
178. Saito, M.; Yoneshiro, T. Capsinoids and Related Food Ingredients Activating Brown Fat Thermogenesis and Reducing Body Fat in Humans. *Curr. Opin. Lipidol.* **2013**, *24*, 71–77. [CrossRef] [PubMed]
179. Higuchi, M.; Dusting, G.J.; Peshavariya, H.; Jiang, F.; Hsiao, S.T.-F.; Chan, E.C.; Liu, G.-S. Differentiation of Human Adipose-Derived Stem Cells into Fat Involves Reactive Oxygen Species and Forkhead Box O1 Mediated Upregulation of Antioxidant Enzymes. *Stem Cell Dev.* **2013**, *22*, 878–888. [CrossRef] [PubMed]
180. Okamoto, M.; Irii, H.; Tahara, Y.; Ishii, H.; Hirao, A.; Udagawa, H.; Hiramoto, M.; Yasuda, K.; Takanishi, A.; Shibata, S.; et al. Synthesis of a New [6]-Gingerol Analogue and Its Protective Effect with Respect to the Development of Metabolic Syndrome in Mice Fed a High-Fat Diet. *J. Med. Chem.* **2011**, *54*, 6295–6304. [CrossRef] [PubMed]
181. Panahi, Y.; Hosseini, M.S.; Khalili, N.; Naimi, E.; Soflaei, S.S.; Majeed, M.; Sahebkar, A. Effects of Supplementation with Curcumin on Serum Adipokine Concentrations: A Randomized Controlled Trial. *Nutrition* **2016**, *32*, 1116–1122. [CrossRef] [PubMed]
182. Yang, C.S.; Landau, J.M.; Huang, M.T.; Newmark, H.L. Inhibition of Carcinogenesis by Dietary Polyphenolic Compounds. *Annu. Rev. Nutr.* **2001**, *21*, 381–406. [CrossRef] [PubMed]
183. Wenzel, U.; Kuntz, S.; Brendel, M.D.; Daniel, H. Dietary Flavone Is a Potent Apoptosis Inducer in Human Colon Carcinoma Cells. *Cancer Res.* **2000**, *60*, 3823–3831. [PubMed]
184. Turrini, E.; Ferruzzi, L.; Fimognari, C. Potential Effects of Pomegranate Polyphenols in Cancer Prevention and Therapy. *Oxid. Med. Cell. Longev.* **2015**, *2015*, 938475. [CrossRef] [PubMed]
185. Wessner, B.; Strasser, E.-M.; Koitz, N.; Schmuckenschlager, C.; Unger-Manhart, N.; Roth, E. Green Tea Polyphenol Administration Partly Ameliorates Chemotherapy-Induced Side Effects in the Small Intestine of Mice. *J. Nutr.* **2007**, *137*, 634–640. [CrossRef] [PubMed]
186. Harper, C.E.; Patel, B.B.; Wang, J.; Eltoum, I.A.; Lamartiniere, C.A. Epigallocatechin-3-Gallate Suppresses Early Stage, but Not Late Stage Prostate Cancer in TRAMP Mice: Mechanisms of Action. *Prostate* **2007**, *67*, 1576–1589. [CrossRef] [PubMed]
187. Chuang, S.E.; Cheng, A.L.; Lin, J.K.; Kuo, M.L. Inhibition by Curcumin of Diethylnitrosamine-Induced Hepatic Hyperplasia, Inflammation, Cellular Gene Products and Cell-Cycle-Related Proteins in Rats. *Food Chem. Toxicol.* **2000**, *38*, 991–995. [CrossRef]
188. Link, A.; Balaguer, F.; Goel, A. Cancer Chemoprevention by Dietary Polyphenols: Promising Role for Epigenetics. *Biochem. Pharmacol.* **2010**, *80*, 1771–1792. [CrossRef] [PubMed]
189. Brenner, D.E.; Gescher, A.J. Cancer Chemoprevention: Lessons Learned and Future Directions. *Br. J. Cancer* **2005**, *93*, 735–739. [CrossRef] [PubMed]
190. Weng, C.-J.; Yen, G.-C. Chemopreventive Effects of Dietary Phytochemicals against Cancer Invasion and Metastasis: Phenolic Acids, Monophenol, Polyphenol, and Their Derivatives. *Cancer Treat. Rev.* **2012**, *38*, 76–87. [CrossRef] [PubMed]
191. Liou, G.-Y.; Storz, P. Reactive Oxygen Species in Cancer. *Free Radic. Res.* **2010**, *44*, 479–496. [CrossRef] [PubMed]
192. Wang, C.; Schuller Levis, G.B.; Lee, E.B.; Levis, W.R.; Lee, D.W.; Kim, B.S.; Park, S.Y.; Park, E. Platycodin D and D3 Isolated from the Root of Platycodon Grandiflorum Modulate the Production of Nitric Oxide and Secretion of TNF-Alpha in Activated RAW 264.7 Cells. *Int. Immunopharmacol.* **2004**, *4*, 1039–1049. [CrossRef] [PubMed]
193. Amararathna, M.; Johnston, M.R.; Rupasinghe, H.P.V. Plant Polyphenols as Chemopreventive Agents for Lung Cancer. *Int. J. Mol. Sci.* **2016**, *17*, 1352. [CrossRef] [PubMed]
194. Tsuji, P.A.; Walle, T. Inhibition of Benzo[a]Pyrene-Activating Enzymes and DNA Binding in Human Bronchial Epithelial BEAS-2B Cells by Methoxylated Flavonoids. *Carcinogenesis* **2006**, *27*, 1579–1585. [CrossRef] [PubMed]

195. Zhai, X.; Lin, M.; Zhang, F.; Hu, Y.; Xu, X.; Li, Y.; Liu, K.; Ma, X.; Tian, X.; Yao, J. Dietary Flavonoid Genistein Induces Nrf2 and Phase II Detoxification Gene Expression via ERKs and PKC Pathways and Protects against Oxidative Stress in Caco-2 Cells. *Mol. Nutr. Food Res.* **2013**, *57*, 249–259. [CrossRef] [PubMed]
196. Lambert, J.D.; Elias, R.J. The Antioxidant and Pro-Oxidant Activities of Green Tea Polyphenols: A Role in Cancer Prevention. *Arch. Biochem. Biophys.* **2010**, *501*, 65–72. [CrossRef] [PubMed]
197. Nakazato, T.; Ito, K.; Ikeda, Y.; Kizaki, M. Green Tea Component, Catechin, Induces Apoptosis of Human Malignant B Cells via Production of Reactive Oxygen Species. *Clin. Cancer Res.* **2005**, *11*, 6040–6049. [CrossRef] [PubMed]
198. Howells, L.M.; Mitra, A.; Manson, M.M. Comparison of Oxaliplatin- and Curcumin-Mediated Antiproliferative Effects in Colorectal Cell Lines. *Int. J. Cancer* **2007**, *121*, 175–183. [CrossRef] [PubMed]
199. Balasubramanian, S.; Efimova, T.; Eckert, R.L. Green Tea Polyphenol Stimulates a Ras, MEKK1, MEK3, and P38 Cascade to Increase Activator Protein 1 Factor-Dependent Involucrin Gene Expression in Normal Human Keratinocytes. *J. Biol. Chem.* **2002**, *277*, 1828–1836. [CrossRef] [PubMed]
200. Kao, Y.-L.; Kuo, Y.-M.; Lee, Y.-R.; Yang, S.-F.; Chen, W.-R.; Lee, H.-J. Apple Polyphenol Induces Cell Apoptosis, Cell Cycle Arrest at G2/M Phase, and Mitotic Catastrophe in Human Bladder Transitional Carcinoma Cells. *J. Funct. Food* **2015**, *14*, 384–394. [CrossRef]
201. Singh, M.; Singh, R.; Bhui, K.; Tyagi, S.; Mahmood, Z.; Shukla, Y. Tea Polyphenols Induce Apoptosis through Mitochondrial Pathway and by Inhibiting Nuclear Factor-KappaB and Akt Activation in Human Cervical Cancer Cells. *Oncol. Res.* **2011**, *19*, 245–257. [CrossRef] [PubMed]
202. Monasterio, A.; Urdaci, M.C.; Pinchuk, I.V.; López-Moratalla, N.; Martínez-Irujo, J.J. Flavonoids Induce Apoptosis in Human Leukemia U937 Cells through Caspase- and Caspase-Calpain-Dependent Pathways. *Nutr. Cancer* **2004**, *50*, 90–100. [CrossRef] [PubMed]
203. Brusselmans, K.; Vrolix, R.; Verhoeven, G.; Swinnen, J.V. Induction of Cancer Cell Apoptosis by Flavonoids Is Associated with Their Ability to Inhibit Fatty Acid Synthase Activity. *J. Biol. Chem.* **2005**, *280*, 5636–5645. [CrossRef] [PubMed]
204. Lee, S.H.; Yumnam, S.; Hong, G.E.; Raha, S.; Saralamma, V.V.G.; Lee, H.J.; Heo, J.D.; Lee, S.J.; Lee, W.-S.; Kim, E.-H.; et al. Flavonoids of Korean *Citrus Aurantium* L. Induce Apoptosis via Intrinsic Pathway in Human Hepatoblastoma HepG2 Cells. *Phyther. Res. PTR* **2015**, *29*, 1940–1949. [CrossRef] [PubMed]
205. Castillo-Pichardo, L.; Dharmawardhane, S.F. Grape Polyphenols Inhibit Akt/Mammalian Target of Rapamycin Signaling and Potentiate the Effects of Gefitinib in Breast Cancer. *Nutr. Cancer* **2012**, *64*, 1058–1069. [CrossRef] [PubMed]
206. Sepporta, M.V.; Fuccelli, R.; Rosignoli, P.; Ricci, G.; Servili, M.; Morozzi, G.; Fabiani, R. Oleuropein Inhibits Tumour Growth and Metastases Dissemination in Ovariectomised Nude Mice with MCF-7 Human Breast Tumour Xenografts. *J. Funct. Food* **2014**, *8*, 269–273. [CrossRef]
207. Rivera, A.R.; Castillo-Pichardo, L.; Gerena, Y.; Dharmawardhane, S. Anti-Breast Cancer Potential of Quercetin via the Akt/AMPK/Mammalian Target of Rapamycin (MTOR) Signaling Cascade. *PLoS ONE* **2016**, *11*, e0157251. [CrossRef] [PubMed]
208. Xia, Y.; Shen, S.; Verma, I.M. NF-KB, an Active Player in Human Cancers. *Cancer Immunol. Res.* **2014**, *2*, 823–830. [CrossRef] [PubMed]
209. Kim, J.-M.; Noh, E.-M.; Kwon, K.-B.; Kim, J.-S.; You, Y.-O.; Hwang, J.-K.; Hwang, B.-M.; Kim, B.-S.; Lee, S.-H.; Lee, S.J.; et al. Curcumin Suppresses the TPA-Induced Invasion through Inhibition of PKCα-Dependent MMP-Expression in MCF-7 Human Breast Cancer Cells. *Phytomed. Int. J. Phyther. Phytopharm.* **2012**, *19*, 1085–1092. [CrossRef] [PubMed]
210. Sarkar, F.H.; Li, Y.; Wang, Z.; Kong, D. The Role of Nutraceuticals in the Regulation of Wnt and Hedgehog Signaling in Cancer. *Cancer Metastasis Rev.* **2010**, *29*, 383–394. [CrossRef] [PubMed]
211. Aggarwal, B.B. Nuclear Factor-KappaB: The Enemy Within. *Cancer Cell* **2004**, *6*, 203–208. [CrossRef] [PubMed]
212. Bachmeier, B.; Nerlich, A.G.; Iancu, C.M.; Cilli, M.; Schleicher, E.; Vené, R.; Dell'Eva, R.; Jochum, M.; Albini, A.; Pfeffer, U. The Chemopreventive Polyphenol Curcumin Prevents Hematogenous Breast Cancer Metastases in Immunodeficient Mice. *Cell. Physiol. Biochem.* **2007**, *19*, 137–152. [CrossRef] [PubMed]
213. Farhangi, B.; Alizadeh, A.M.; Khodayari, H.; Khodayari, S.; Dehghan, M.J.; Khori, V.; Heidarzadeh, A.; Khaniki, M.; Sadeghiezadeh, M.; Najafi, F. Protective Effects of Dendrosomal Curcumin on an Animal Metastatic Breast Tumor. *Eur. J. Pharmacol.* **2015**, *758*, 188–196. [CrossRef] [PubMed]

214. Tsai, J.H.; Yang, J. Epithelial–Mesenchymal Plasticity in Carcinoma Metastasis. *Gene Dev.* **2013**, *27*, 2192–2206. [CrossRef] [PubMed]
215. Kang, J.; Kim, E.; Kim, W.; Seong, K.M.; Youn, H.; Kim, J.W.; Kim, J.; Youn, B. Rhamnetin and Cirsiliol Induce Radiosensitization and Inhibition of Epithelial-Mesenchymal Transition (EMT) by MiR-34a-Mediated Suppression of Notch-1 Expression in Non-Small Cell Lung Cancer Cell Lines. *J. Biol. Chem.* **2013**, *288*, 27343–27357. [CrossRef] [PubMed]
216. Lin, C.-H.; Shen, Y.-A.; Hung, P.-H.; Yu, Y.-B.; Chen, Y.-J. Epigallocatechin Gallate, Polyphenol Present in Green Tea, Inhibits Stem-like Characteristics and Epithelial-Mesenchymal Transition in Nasopharyngeal Cancer Cell Lines. *BMC Complement. Altern. Med.* **2012**, *12*, 201. [CrossRef] [PubMed]
217. Lin, Y.-S.; Tsai, P.-H.; Kandaswami, C.C.; Cheng, C.-H.; Ke, F.-C.; Lee, P.-P.; Hwang, J.-J.; Lee, M.-T. Effects of Dietary Flavonoids, Luteolin, and Quercetin on the Reversal of Epithelial-Mesenchymal Transition in A431 Epidermal Cancer Cells. *Cancer Sci.* **2011**, *102*, 1829–1839. [CrossRef] [PubMed]
218. Hara, Y. Tea Catechins and Their Applications as Supplements and Pharmaceutics. *Pharmacol. Res.* **2011**, *64*, 100–104. [CrossRef] [PubMed]

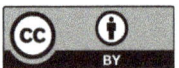

© 2018 by the authors. Licensee MDPI, Basel, Switzerland. This article is an open access article distributed under the terms and conditions of the Creative Commons Attribution (CC BY) license (http://creativecommons.org/licenses/by/4.0/).

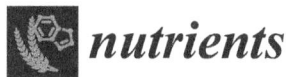

Review

The Role of Vitamin E in Immunity

Ga Young Lee [1,2] and Sung Nim Han [1,2,*]

[1] Department of Food and Nutrition, College of Human Ecology, Seoul National University, Seoul 08826, Korea; lgykiki90@snu.ac.kr
[2] Research Institute of Human Ecology, Seoul National University, Seoul 08826, Korea
* Correspondence: snhan@snu.ac.kr; Tel.: +82-2-880-6836

Received: 30 September 2018; Accepted: 29 October 2018; Published: 1 November 2018

Abstract: Vitamin E is a fat-soluble antioxidant that can protect the polyunsaturated fatty acids (PUFAs) in the membrane from oxidation, regulate the production of reactive oxygen species (ROS) and reactive nitrogen species (RNS), and modulate signal transduction. Immunomodulatory effects of vitamin E have been observed in animal and human models under normal and disease conditions. With advances in understating of the development, function, and regulation of dendritic cells (DCs), macrophages, natural killer (NK) cells, T cells, and B cells, recent studies have focused on vitamin E's effects on specific immune cells. This review will summarize the immunological changes observed with vitamin E intervention in animals and humans, and then describe the cell-specific effects of vitamin E in order to understand the mechanisms of immunomodulation and implications of vitamin E for immunological diseases.

Keywords: vitamin E; macrophages; T cells; dendritic cells; immunomodulation; infection

1. Vitamin E: Definition, Structure, Sources, and Functions

1.1. Definition and Structure

Vitamin E is the collective term for four tocopherols (α-, β-, γ-, and δ-tocopherols) and four tocotrienols (α-, β-, γ-, and δ-tocotrienols) found in food. These forms have antioxidant activities, but cannot be interconverted, and only α-tocopherol meets the human vitamin E requirement [1]. Tocopherols have a chromanol ring and a phytyl tail, while tocotrienols have a chromanol ring and an unsaturated tail. The α-, β-, γ-, and δ- forms differ in the number and position of methyl groups on the chromanol structure. Natural tocopherols have only *RRR* stereochemistry, but synthetic tocopherols are mixtures of eight stereoisomers (*RRR-, RSR-, RRS-, RSS-, SRR-, SSR-, SRS-, SSS-*), because there are three asymmetric carbon atoms (2*R*, 4′*R*, 8′*R*) present in the phytyl tail. The structures of tocopherols and tocotrienols are shown in Figure 1.

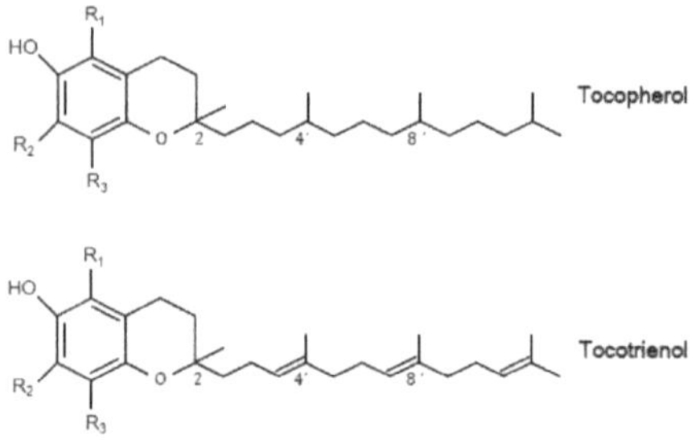

Figure 1. The structures of tocopherol and tocotrienols.

1.2. Sources

The major dietary sources of vitamin E are vegetable oils. Nuts are good sources of vitamin E as well [2]. Soybean, sunflower, corn, walnut, cottonseed, palm, and wheat germ oils contain relatively higher amounts (more than approximately 50 mg vitamin E/100 g oil) of vitamin E than other oils. The proportions of α-, β-, γ-, and δ-tocopherols vary depending on the oil type. Safflower and sunflower oils are high in α-tocopherol, soybean and corn oils contain mainly γ-tocopherol, and cottonseed oil contains similar proportions of α- and γ-tocopherols. Therefore, the types of oils consumed through the diet affect the dietary intake levels of α-tocopherol. Vitamin E supplements are quite popular and contribute considerably to vitamin E intake among some populations. Either natural or synthetic forms of α-tocopherol are used as supplements.

Despite the relatively higher intake of γ-tocopherol from the diet than α-tocopherol, α-tocopherol is the major form of vitamin E in the circulation because α-tocopherol transfer protein (α-TTP) has the preferential binding affinity for α-tocopherol. α-TTP is involved in the transfer of α-tocopherol to the plasma membrane [1].

1.3. Functions

Vitamin E is a major fat-soluble antioxidant that scavenges peroxyl radicals and terminates the oxidation of polyunsaturated fatty acids (PUFAs). In the presence of vitamin E, peroxyl radicals react with α-tocopherol instead of lipid hydroperoxide, the chain reaction of peroxyl radical production is stopped, and further oxidation of PUFAs in the membrane is prevented [1]. Tocopheroxyl radicals—produced from α-tocopherol and peroxyl radicals—are reduced by vitamin C or glutathione, form tocopherol dimers, undergo further oxidation, or act as prooxidants. The antioxidant activity of vitamin E may be responsible for the regulation of several enzymes involved in signal transduction because the activity of signaling enzymes is regulated by the redox state.

Vitamin E inhibits protein kinase C (PKC) activity by increasing PKC-α dephosphorylation through the activation of protein phosphatase 2A. The inhibition of PKC by vitamin E has been reported in various cells, and consequently, the inhibition of platelet aggregation; reduced proliferation of monocytes, macrophages, neutrophils, and vascular smooth muscle cells; and decreased superoxide production in neutrophils and macrophages have been observed [3,4].

Vitamin E may directly bind to the enzymes involved in the generation of lipid mediators or to the transport proteins involved in signal transduction. Vitamin E may affect the membrane protein interaction and translocation of the enzymes to the plasma membrane and therefore change the activity of signal transduction enzymes [4].

2. Modulation of Immune Responses and Infectious Diseases by Vitamin E Supplementation

2.1. Immune Responses in Animals

Dietary interventions of vitamin E at supplemental levels have been shown to enhance cell-mediated and humoral immune responses in various species of animals. Increased lymphocyte proliferation, immunoglobulin levels, antibody responses, natural killer (NK) cell activity, and interleukin (IL)-2 production have been reported with vitamin E supplementation (Table 1).

2.2. Immune Responses in Humans

In humans, many intervention studies have reported increased lymphocyte proliferation in response to mitogenic stimulation, enhanced delayed type hypersensitivity (DTH) response, increased IL-2 production, and decreased IL-6 production with vitamin E supplementation above the recommended levels. However, some studies showed no difference or decreased lymphocyte proliferation responses and decreased chemiluminescence. (Table 2). Differences in dose of vitamin E supplementation used, magnitude of vitamin E level changes with supplementation, age of subjects, and methodology (determination of antibody levels with or without specific vaccination) might have contributed to the different results observed.

2.3. Infectious Diseases in Animals

The immunostimulatory effect of vitamin E has resulted in enhanced resistance against several pathogens. Animal studies in which infectious disease models were used to test the effects of vitamin E supplementation are listed in Table 3.

The mechanisms involved with protection against infectious agents were increased macrophage activity and antibody (Ab) production for *D. pneumoniae* type 1 [5], and higher NK activity and Th1 response for influenza virus [6,7].

2.4. Infectious Diseases in Humans

In humans, the effects of vitamin E on the natural incidence of infectious diseases have been determined in several studies (Table 4). Many studies provided evidence that the immunostimulatory effects of vitamin E confer improved resistance to infections. However, the magnitudes of the effects were rather small, and in some studies, positive effects were only observed in subgroups of subjects.

Table 1. Modulation of immune responses by vitamin E in animal models.

Species	Dosage and Duration	Form of Vitamin E Used	Results	References
Chicks, female broiler (n = 6/group, 6 replicate)	100 mg/kg diet for 21 days	DL-α-tocopheryl acetate	↑Plasma IgM levels at day 21 ↔Splenic expressions of TNF-α, IFN-γ, IL-2, IL-10	Dalia et al. 2018 [8]
Pregnant cows (n = 24/group)	250 IU/day from day 107 of gestation to day 21 of lactation	NA	↑IgG and IgA concentration in sow plasma	Wang et al. 2017 [9]
Domestic cats (39 castrated male and 33 intact female) (n = 8/group)	225, 450 mg/kg diet for 28 days	α-tocopherol	↑Lymphocyte proliferation (ConA, PHA)	O' Brien et al. 2015 [10]
Young and old mice (n = 11–13/group)	500 mg/kg diet for 6 weeks	DL-α-tocotrienol	↑Lymphocyte proliferation in old (ConA, PHA) ↑IL-1β production in young	Ren et al. 2010 [11]
Young rats (n = 6/group)	50, 200 mg/kg diet for 8–10 weeks	DL-α-tocopheryl acetate	↑Lymphocyte proliferation (ConA, LPS)	Bendich et al. 1986 [12]
Old mice (n = 10/group)	500 mg/kg diet for 6 weeks	DL-α-tocopheryl acetate	↑Lymphocyte proliferation (ConA, LPS) ↑DTH response ↑IL-2 production ↓PGE$_2$ production	Meydani et al. 1986 [13]
Young and old mice (n = 5/group)	500 IU (500 mg) for 9 weeks	DL-α-tocopherol acetate	↑Lymphocyte proliferation (ConA) in young ↔Lymphocyte proliferation (ConA) in old ↑IFN-γ in young under restraint stress	Wakikawa et al. 1999 [14]
Young rats (n = 10/group)	50, 100, 250, 500, 2500 mg/kg diet for 7 days	DL-α-tocopheryl acetate	↑Lymphocyte proliferation (>100 mg/kg diet, ConA) (>250 mg/kg diet, LPS) ↑NK activity (>250 mg/kg diet)	Moriguchi et al. 1990 [15]
Old rats (n = 5/group)	585 mg/kg diet for 12 months	DL-α-tocopheryl nicotinate	↑Lymphocyte proliferation (ConA, PHA) ↑IL-2 production	Sakai S & Moriguchi 1997 [16]
Young calves (n = 8/group)	125, 250, 500 IU (125, 250, 500 mg)/day for 24 weeks	DL-α-tocopheryl acetate	↑Lymphocyte proliferation (PHA, ConA, pokeweed mitogen) ↑Antibovine herpesvirus Ab titer to booster in 125 IU/day group	Reddy et al. 1987 [17]
Young mice (n = 8/group)	200 mg/kg diet for 6–12 weeks	α-tocopheryl acetate	↑Ab response ↑Helper T cell activity	Tanake et al. 1979 [18]
Mice (n = 10/group)	500 mg/kg diet for 6 months	α-tocopherol acetate (Tekland, Madison, WI)	↓IL-6 and PGEs (unstimulated) production by macrophages ↓Nitric oxide production (LPS) by macrophages	Beharka et al. 2000 [19]

Ab, antibody; ConA, concanavalin A; IFN-γ, interferon-γ; LPS, lipopolysaccharide; PGE$_2$, prostaglandin E$_2$; PHA, phytohemagglutinin; TNF, Tumor necrosis factor.

Table 2. Modulation of immune responses by vitamin E in humans.

Subjects	Age	Amount and Duration of Supplementation	Form of Vitamin E Used	Effects on Immune Function	References
Young ($n = 5$) and senior athletes ($n = 5$)	18–25, 35–57	4.6 ± 0.3 mg/100 mL of vitamin E-enriched beverage 5 days/week for 5 weeks	α-tocopherol acetate	↑15LOX2, TNF-α expression	Capo et al. 2016 [20]
Healthy women ($n = 108$)	18–25	400 mg TRF/day for 56 days	D-α-tocotrienol D-γ-tocotrienol D-δ-tocotrienol D-α-tocopherol	↑IL-4 (TT vaccine), IFN-γ (ConA) ↓IL-6 (LPS)	Mahalingam et al. 2011 [21]
Healthy men and women ($n = 19, 34$)	20–50	200 mg/day for 56 days	α-tocopherol	↔IL-4, IFN-γ production (ConA)	Radhakrishnan et al. 2009 [22]
Adult males and young boys ($n = 18$)	25–30, 13–18	300 mg/day for 3 weeks	DL-α-tocopheryl acetate	↓Lymphocyte proliferation (PHA) ↔DTH ↓Bactericidal activity	Prasad 1980 [23]
Institutionalized adult males and females ($n = 103$)	24–104	200, 400 mg/day for 6 months	α-tocopherol acetate	↔Ab development to influenza virus	Harman and Miller 1986 [24]
Healthy elderly males and females ($n = 32$)	≥60	800 mg/day for 30 days	DL-α-tocopheryl acetate	↑Lymphocyte proliferation (ConA) ↑DTH ↑IL-2 production (ConA) ↓PGE$_2$ production (PHA)	Meydani et al. 1990 [25]
Eldery males and females ($n = 74$)	≥65	100 mg/day for 3 months	DL-α-tocopheryl acetate	↔Lymphocyte proliferation (ConA, PHA) ↔IgG, IgA levels	De Waart et al. 1997 [26]
Healthy elderly males and females ($n = 88$)	≥65	60, 200, 800 mg/day for 235 days	DL-α-tocopherol	↑DTH and antibody titer to hepatitis B with 200, 800 mg	Meydani et al. 1997 [27]
Healthy elderly males and females ($n = 161$)	65–80	50, 100 mg/day for 6 months	DL-α-tocopheryl acetate	↑No. of positive DTH reaction with 100 mg ↑Diameter of induration of DTH reaction in a subgroup supplemented with 100 mg ↔IL-2 production ↓IFN-γ production	Pallast et al. 1999 [28]
Healthy young adults ($n = 31$) and premature infants ($n = 10$)	24–31	600 mg/day for 3 months 40 mg/kg body weight for 8–14 days		↓Chemiluminescence	Okano et al. 1990 [29]
Cigarette smoker ($n = 60$)	33 ± 4	900 IU/day for 6 weeks		↓Chemiluminescence	Richards et al. 1990 [30]
Healthy males ($n = 40$)	24–57	200 mg/day for 4 months	all-rac-α-tocopherol	Prevented fish-oil-induced suppression of ConA mitogenesis	Kramer et al. 1991 [31]
Healthy elderly ($n = 40$)	>65	100, 200, or 400 mg/day for 3 months	DL-α-tocopherol	↑DTH (maximal diameter) in 100, 200, 400 mg groups ↑Lymphocyte proliferation (ConA) in 200 mg group	Wu et al. 2006 [32]
Sedentary young and elderly males ($n = 21$)	22–29, 55–74	800 IU (727 mg)/day for 48 days	DL-α-tocopherol	↓IL-6 secretion ↓Exercise-enhanced IL-1β secretion	Cannon et al. 1991 [33]

ConA, concanavalin A; DTH, delayed type hypersensitivity; IFN-γ, interferon-γ; 15LOX2, 15-lipoxygenase-2; PGE$_2$, prostaglandin E$_2$; PHA, phytohemagglutinin; TRF, tocotrienol-rich fraction; TT vaccine, tetanous toxoid vaccine.

Table 3. Effects of vitamin E supplementation on infectious diseases in animal models.

Subjects	Age	Dose and Duration of Supplementation	Form of Vitamin E Used	Infection Organism and Route of Infection	Results: Effects of Vitamin E Supplementation	References
Mice BALB/c (n = 3–6/group)	6 months	100 mg/kg for 8 days before MRSA-challenge	δ-, γ-Tocotrienol	MRSA, inoculated onto superficial surgical wounds	Higher NK cytotoxicity; Higher IL-24 mRNA expression levels	Pierpaoli et al. 2017 [34]
Young and aged male mice C57BL/6 (n = 6/group)	2, 22–26 months	500 mg/kg for 4 weeks prior to infection	D-α-tocopheryl acetate	Streptococcus pneumoniae, intra-tracheally injected	1000-fold fewer bacteria in their lung; Age-associated higher production of proinflammatory cytokines (TNF-, IL-6) were reduced; 3-fold reduction in the number of PMNs	Bou Ghanem et al. 2015 [35]
Worm-free lambs (n = 10/group)	28–32 weeks	5.3 IU (3.56 mg)/kg BW for 12 weeks	D-α-tocopherol	H. contortus L3 larvae, route NA	No difference in serum IgG or peripheral mRNA expression of IL-4 or IFN-γ; Lower PCV, FEC, and worm burden	De Wolf et al. 2014 [36]
Male mice BALB/c (n = 6–7/group)	At weaning	Deficient, Adequate (38.4 mg/kg diet), or Supplemented (384 mg/kg diet) for 4 weeks	DL-α-tocopheryl acetate	HSV-1, intranasally	Higher viral titre and IL-β, TNF-α, RANTES in the brain with E deficiency; No difference in expressions of IL-6, TNFα, IL-1β, and IL-10 between adequate and supplemented	Sheridan & Beck. 2008 [37]
Mice C57BL (n = 6–9/group)	22 months	500 mg/kg diet for 8 weeks	DL-α-tocopherol acetate	Influenza by nasal inoculation	Lower viral titer; Higher IL-2 and IFN-γ production	Han et al. 2000 [6]
Mice, C57BL/6 (n = 4–9)	22 months	500mg/kg diet for 6 weeks	DL-α-tocopherol acetate	Influenza A/PC/1/73 (H3N2) by nasal inoculation	Lower viral titre	Hayek et al. 1997 [7]
Mice, C57BL/6 (n = 6)	5 weeks	160 IU/L liquid diet for 4, 8, 12, 16 weeks	all-rac-α-tocopheryl acetate	Murine LP-BM5 leukaemia retrovirus by IP injection	Restored IL-2 and IFN-γ production by splenocytes following infection	Wang et al. 1994 [38]
Calves, Holstein (n = 7)	1d	1400 or 2800 mg orally once per week, 1400 mg injection once per week for 12 weeks	DL-α-tocopheryl acetate	Bovine rhinotracheitis virus, in vitro	Serum from vitamin E-supplemented calves inhibited the replication of bovine rhinotracheitis virus in vitro	Reddy et al. 1986 [39]
Mice, Swiss Webster (n = 10)	4 weeks	180 mg/kg diet for 4 weeks	DL-α-tocopheryl acetate	Diplococcus pneumoniae type I by IP injection	Higher survival	Heinzerling et al. 1974a [5]
Mice, BALB/C (n = 25)	NA	25 or 250 mg/kg bw orally for 4 days, starting 2 days before burn injury	DL-α-tocopheryl acetate	Pseudomonas aeruginosa, subeschar injection to burned mice	Lower mortality rate	Fang et al. 1990 [40]
Mice, BALB/C (NA)	3 weeks	4000mg/kg diet for 2, 4, or 14 weeks	Vitamin E injectable (aqueous)	Listeria monocytogenes by IP injection	No difference in resistance	Watson & Petro 1982 [41]
Rats, Sprague-Dawley (n = 6)	3 weeks	180 mg/kg diet + 6000 IU vitamin A/kg diet for 6 weeks	DL-α-tocopheryl acetate	Mycoplasma pulmonis by aerosol	Higher resistance to infection	Tvedten et al. 1973 [42]
Lambs (n = 10)	NA	1000 IU orally, 300 mg/kg diet for 23 days	DL-α-tocopheryl acetate	Chlamydia by intratracheal inoculation	Faster recovery (higher food intake and weight gains)	Stephens et al. 1979 [43]

Table 3. Cont.

Subjects	Age	Dose and Duration of Supplementation	Form of Vitamin E Used	Infection Organism and Route of Infection	Results: Effects of Vitamin E Supplementation	References
Turkey, broadbreasted white poults ($n = 6$)	1 day	500 mg/kg diet for 14 days before infection and 18–21 days after infection	DL-α-tocopheryl acetate	*Histomonas meleagridis*, oral	No effect on mortality by vitamin E supplementation alone. Lower mortality and lesion score in combination with ipronidazole	Schildknecht & Squibb 1979 [44]
Pigs ($n = 6$)	NA	200 mg/pig per day for 59 days before infection and 22 days after infection	DL-α-tocopheryl acetate	*Treponema hyodysenteriae*, oral	Improved weight gain and recovery rate. No beneficial effect on appetite and diarrhoea	Teige et al. 1982 [45]
Sheep ($n = 12$)	3–6 months	300 mg/kg diet starting 2 weeks before first vaccination	DL-α-tocopheryl acetate	*Clostridium perfringens* type D by IV injection after two IM vaccinations	Higher Ab titre. Fail to prove beneficial effect of vitamin E on protection (none of the vaccinated lambs died)	Tengerdy et al. 1983 [46]
Cows ($n = 20$)	NA	740 mg/cow per day, duration NA	DL-α-tocopheryl acetate	Natural occurrence of clinical mastitis due to *Streptococci*, *Coliform*, *Staphylococci*, *Clostridium bovis*	Lower clinical cases of mastitis	Smith et al. 1984 [47]
Chicks, broiler ($n = 12$–14)	1 day	150 mg or 300mg/kg diet for 2 weeks before infection	DL-α-tocopheryl acetate	*Escherichia coli*, orally and post-thoracic air sac	Lower mortality. Higher Ab titre	Heinzerling et al. 1974b [48]
Chicks, broiler ($n = 10$)	1 day	300 mg/kg diet for 6 weeks, starting 3 weeks before first infection	DL-α-tocopheryl acetate	*E. coli*, post-thoracic air sac	Lower mortality	Tengerdy & Nockels 1975 [49]
Chicks, Leghorn ($n = 22$)	1 day	300 mg/kg diet for 4 weeks before infection	DL-α-tocopheryl acetate	*E. coli* by IV injection	Lower mortality	Likoff et al. 1981 [50]
Pigs ($n = 10$)	6–8 weeks	100, 000 mg/t diet for 10 weeks, starting 2 weeks before infection	Vitamin E; Tompson-Hayward, Minneapolis, MN, USA	*E. coli* by IM injection	Higher serum Ab titre	Ellis & Vorhies 1976 [51]

Ab, antibody; FEC, fecal egg count; HSV, Herpes simplex virus; MRSA, Methicillin-resistant *Staphylococcus aureus*; NK, natural killer; PCV, packed cell volume; PMN, polymorphonuclear leukocyte; RANTES, regulated on activation, normal T cell expressed and secreted; TNF-α, tumor necrosis factor-α. IFN-γ, interferon-γ; IM, intramuscular; IV, intravenous;

Table 4. Effects of vitamin E supplementation on infectious diseases in humans.

Subjects	Age	Dose and Duration of Supplementation	Form of Vitamin E Used	Infection Organism and Route of Infection	Results: Effects of Vitamin E Supplementation	References
Male smoker	50–69	50 mg/d for median of 6 years	DL-α-tocopheryl acetate	Natural incidence of pneumonia	69% Lower incidence of pneumonia among subgroups including participants who smoked 5–19 cigarettes per day at baseline and exercised at leisure time 14% Lower incidence of pneumonia among subgroups including participants who smoked ≥20 cigarettes per day at baseline and did not exercise	Hemila et al. 2016 [52]
HIV-infected pregnant Tanzanian women	25.4	30 mg during pregnancy (multivitamin form with 20 mg vitamins B1, 20 mg B2, 25 mg B6, 100 mg niacin, 50 µg B12, 500 mg C, and 800 µg folic acid)	NA	Natural incidence of malaria after having received malaria prophylaxis during pregnancy	Lower incidence of presumptive clinical malaria, but higher risk of any malaria parasitemia	Olofin et al. 2014 [53]
Patients with HCV-related cirrhosis	54–75	900 IU (604.03 mg for D- or 818.18 mg for DL-)/day for 6 months	α-tocopherol	Natural incidence of cirrhosis	Reduced glutathione (GSH) and glutathione peroxidase, which are significantly lower in cirrhotic patients ($p < 0.05$), were comparably improved by vitamin E regimens	Marotta et al. 2007 [54]
Patients with chronic HCV	18–75	945 IU (634.23 mg)/day for 6 months with 500 mg ascorbic acid and 200 µg of selenium	D-α-tocopherol	Natural incidence of HCV	No difference in median log plasma HCV-RNA	Groenbak et al. 2006 [55]
Nursing home residents	>65	200 IU/day for 1 year	DL-α-tocopherol	Natural incidence of respiratory infections	Fewer numbers of subjects with all and upper respiratory infections Lower incidence of common cold No effect on lower respiratory infection	Meydani et al. 2004 [56]
Male smokers	50–69	50 mg/day during 4-year follow-up	α-tocopherol	Natural incidence of common cold episodes	Lower incidence of common cold Reduction was greatest among older city dwellers who smoked fewer than 15 cigarettes per day	Hemila et al. 2002 [57]
Male smokers	50–69 years	50 mg/day for median of 6.1 years	DL-α-tocopheryl acetate	Natural incidence of pneumonia	No overall effect on the incidence of pneumonia. Lower incidence of pneumonia among the subjects who had initiated smoking at a later age (>21)	Hemila et al. 2004 [58]
Non-institutionalized individuals	>60 years	200 mg/day for median of 441 days	α-tocopherol acetate	Natural incidence and severity of self-reported acute respiratory tract infections	No effect on incidence and severity of acute respiratory tract infections	Graat et al. 2002 [59]

HCV, hepatitis C virus.

3. Vitamin E and Immune Cells

The immunomodulatory mechanisms of α-tocopherol in immune cells are depicted in Figure 2.

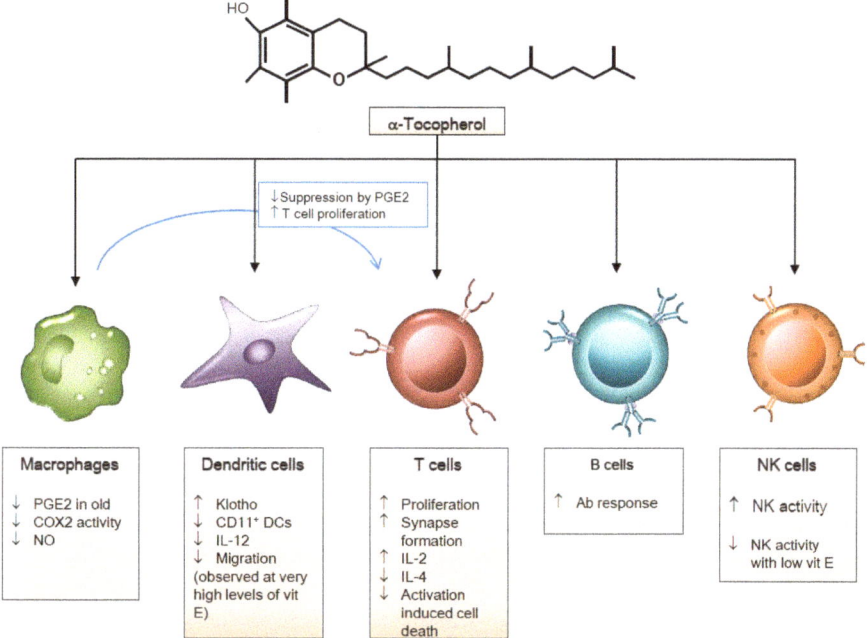

Figure 2. Immunomodulatory effects of vitamin E on immune cells. Abbreviations: PGE_2, prostaglandin E_2; COX2, Cyclooxygenase 2; NO, Nitric oxide; CD, Clusters of Differentiation; DCs, Dendritic cells; IL-12, Interleukin-12; Ab, antibody; NK, Natural killer.

3.1. Macrophages

Macrophages, important effector cells in the innate immune response, serve as antigen presenting cells (APC) and regulate NK cells and T cells by producing cytokines, reactive oxygen species (ROS), reactive nitrogen species (RNS), and prostaglandins. Cytokines produced by T cells and other immune cells can shift the macrophages into different populations with distinct physiologies [60].

The effects of vitamin E on prostaglandin (PG)E_2 production by macrophages from the aged have been suggested as one of the mechanisms by which vitamin E improves the age-associated decrease in the T cell-mediated immune response [61]. In a co-culture experiment in which purified T cells and macrophages from young and old mice were cultured together, T cells from young mice showed suppressed proliferation and IL-2 secretion when cultured with macrophages from old mice. When macrophages from old mice were pre-incubated with 10 μg/mL vitamin E for 4 h, co-cultures of old macrophages and young T cells showed significant improvement in proliferation. Vitamin E pre-incubation of old macrophages improved proliferation and IL-2 production in co-cultures of old macrophages and old T cells [62]. Macrophages from old mice produced significantly higher levels of PGE_2, which was due to higher cyclooxygenase (COX) activity. Macrophages from old mice expressed higher levels of inducible COX2 protein and mRNA [63]. These increases in PGE_2 synthesis and COX activity were lowered by in vivo vitamin E supplementation [64]. Macrophages isolated from old mice fed a diet containing 500 ppm vitamin E for 30 days produced lower amounts of PGE_2 and had lower COX activity than those from old mice fed a control diet containing 30 ppm vitamin E, but the COX2 mRNA levels and protein expression of the control and supplemented groups did not differ. Thus, vitamin E's effect on COX activity seemed to be through post-translational mechanisms rather than through its effect at transcriptome or translational levels. In a subsequent study, it was shown that vitamin E reduced COX activity in macrophages from old mice by decreasing peroxynitrite production [65]. The inhibition of COX activity by vitamin E in old mice disappeared specifically with the addition of a nitric oxide (NO) donor in the presence of a superoxide to elevate peroxynitrite levels in the macrophage culture. There is a complex interplay between the nitric oxide synthase (NOS) and COX pathways and NO increases COX2 activity, which seems to be due to the NO preventing self-deactivation of COX by the superoxide as NO interacts with the superoxide [66].

In vivo supplementation of vitamin E (1500 IU D-α-tocopheryl acetate/day for 16 weeks) in allergic asthmatic patients prevented the suppression of alveolar macrophage nuclear factor (erythroid-derived 2)-like 2 (NRF2) activity after allergen challenge [67]. This study presented the possibility of vitamin E's protective role in allergies and asthmas through regulation of macrophage NRF2 activity, but, further studies are needed to confirm the findings because of the small number of patients (nine mild non-smoking allergic asthmatics) and the lack of appropriate controls.

3.2. Natural Killer Cells

NK activity seems to be related with vitamin E status. The NK activity of a boy with Shwachman syndrome who had a severe vitamin E deficiency was low, but improved after eight weeks of 100 mg/d α-tocopherol supplementation. When α-tocopherol supplementation was stopped, NK activity and $CD16^+$ $CD56^+$ cells decreased. NK activity and $CD16^+$ $CD56^+$ cells were restored upon resuming eight weeks of 100 mg/d α-tocopherol supplementation [68]. In 37 women aged 90–106 years old, NK cell cytotoxicity was positively associated with plasma vitamin E concentration [69]. A two-week supplementation of 750 mg vitamin E in colorectal cancer patients resulted in increased NK activity in six out of seven patients. Vitamin E treatment did not result in changes in perforin expression or IFN-γ production; therefore, mechanisms of improved NK activity by vitamin E could not be determined from the study [70].

NO appears to be involved in the impairment of NK cell function. Co-culture of NK cells and myeloid-derived suppressor cells (MDSCs) showed that NK cell cytotoxicity and IFN-γ were impaired by MDSCs and that the inhibition of inducible nitric oxide synthase (iNOS) rescued the impairment by MDSCs. Exposure of NK cells to NO by treatment with an NO producer caused the nitration of tyrosine residues on $CD16^+$ NK cells. These results suggested that MDSCs impair NK cell function via the production of NO and the nitration of protein tyrosine residues [71]. Vitamin E might exert its effects on NK cell function by modulating NO levels.

3.3. Dendritic Cells

Dendritic cells (DCs) are effective antigen-presenting cells that recognize pathogens and present pathogen-derived antigens to T cells. The interaction of DCs with pathogen-associated molecular patterns (PAMPs) or damage-associated molecular patterns (DAMPs) elicits the activation and maturation of DCs. The increased expression of surface major histocompatibility complex (MHC) molecules and co-stimulatory molecules and the increased production of cytokines occur with the activation of DCs, which allows the effective induction of the T cell response [72–74]. DCs are also involved in tolerance and autoimmunity. DCs might promote tolerance by the generation of Treg cells and/or by the induction of T cell unresponsiveness. DCs might be involved in the pathogenesis of autoimmune disease by promoting the priming or differentiation of self-reactive T cells [72]. Therefore, understanding the regulation of DCs by vitamin E will provide insight into the mechanisms of vitamin E's immune response modulation and implications of vitamin E in immunological diseases.

Several studies have shown that vitamin E could regulate the maturation and functions of DCs. Tan et al. [75] investigated the effects of α-tocopherol and vitamin C, alone or in combination, on the phenotype and functions of human DCs generated from peripheral blood mononuclear cells (PBMCs). During the differentiation of human PBMCs into DCs, various concentrations of α-tocopherol were treated in culture starting from day 2, cells were stimulated on day 5, and then the surface phenotype was determined on day 6. The expression of human leukocyte antigen(HLA)-DR, CD40 CD80, and CD86 appeared to be increased with lower concentrations of α-tocopherol (<0.05 mM), but the combination of vitamin E and C prevented DC activation, as the upregulation of surface markers was not observed. DCs treated with 0.5 mM vitamin E and 10 mM vitamin C showed lower levels of intracellular ROS and inhibition of the nuclear factor (NF)-κB, PKC, and p38 mitogen-activated protein kinase (MAPK) pathways. When bone marrow-derived dendritic cells (BMDCs) from Balb/c mice were treated with 500 μM of α-tocopherol for 2 h, upregulation of phosphorylated inhibitor of κB (IκB) by lipopolysaccharide (LPS)-stimulation was suppressed. Vitamin E treatment for 24 h resulted in a reduced number of $CD11^+CD86^+$ cells and ROS-positive cells, lower production of IL-12p70 and TNF-α, and decreased transwell migration of BMDCs. These effects of vitamin E on BMDCs were partly dependent on Klotho expression. Vitamin E treatment on BMDCs resulted in higher Klotho transcript and protein levels, and silencing of Klotho by transfection of *Klotho* siRNA abolished the inhibitory effects of vitamin E on IL-12p70 production, number of ROS-positive cells, and DC migration [76]. Klotho is a membrane protein that has been shown to mediate calcium transport into the cells; regulate intracellular signaling pathways such as p53/p21, cyclin adenosine monophosphate (cAMP), PKC, and Wnt; and inhibit the NF-κB pathway [77]. Therefore, the upregulation of Klotho by vitamin E could be one of the mechanisms by which vitamin E modulates NF-κB mediated DC function and maturation. However, the level of α-tocopherol used for in vitro treatment (500 μM) was high and, therefore, further research is needed to elucidate the physiological relevance of vitamin E treatment on the expression of Klotho and its involvement in the modulation of DC function.

In vivo supplementation of α-tocopherol at 150, 250, and 500 mg/kg diet in allergic female mice reduced the lung $CD11b^+$ DCs and mRNA levels of IL-4, IL-33, thymic stromal lymphopoietin (TSLP), eotaxin 1 (CCL11), and eotaxin 2 (CCL24) in allergen challenged pups. Furthermore, when BMDCs from 10-day-old neonates born to a control female were treated with 80 μM α-tocopherol for 24 h, the number of $CD45^+$ $CD11b^+$ $CD11^+$ DCs and the number of $CD45^+$ $CD11b^+$ $CD11c^+$ $Ly6c^-$ $MHCII^-$ DCs were reduced. Maternal supplementation with α-tocopherol was effective in decreasing allergic responses in offspring from allergic mothers by affecting the development of subsets of DCs that are critical for allergic responses [78]. On the other hand, γ-tocopherol supplementation exerted an opposite response in the same model. In vivo supplementation of γ-tocopherol at 250 mg/kg diet in allergic female mice resulted in a higher number of lung eosinophils, a higher number of lung $CD11c^+$ $CD11b^+$ DCs, and higher levels of lung lavage CCL11 in the offspring [79].

Modulation of the immune response by vitamin E has been observed in animal and human studies, and DCs play a critical role in bridging innate and adaptive immune systems and initiating adaptive immune responses. Despite the importance of DCs' role in adaptive immune responses and in diseases such as autoimmune diseases, few studies have investigated the DC-specific effect of vitamin E.

3.4. T Cells

The effects of vitamin E on immune cells have been studied the most with T cells. The dysregulation of immune function occurs with aging and the most significant changes are observed in T cells. Age-associated changes in T cells include, but are not limited to, (1) defects in T cell receptor (TCR) signal transduction such as a decrease in linker for the activation of T cells (LAT) phosphorylation by zeta chain of T cell receptor associated protein kinase 70 (ZAP-70), (2) decreased intracellular influx of calcium following stimulation, (3) diminished synapse formation, (4) diminished activation of the mitogen activated protein kinase (MAP kinase) pathway, (5) decreased nuclear factor of activated T-cells (NFAT) binding activity, and (6) a shift of the T cell population toward memory T cells [80]. As a result, diminished production of IL-2 and reduced proliferative capacity of naive T cells are observed and impaired T cell functions contribute to increased susceptibility to infectious diseases and poor response to immunization.

Vitamin E has been shown to increase the cell division and IL-2 producing capacity of naïve T cells, increase the percentage of T cells capable of forming an effective immune synapse, and reverse the age-associated defect in the phosphorylation of LAT in T cells from old animals [81–83].

In vitro pre-incubation with 46 µM vitamin E for 4 h increased proliferation and IL-2 production in T cells purified from old mice stimulated with anti-CD3 and anti-CD28. Increased IL-2 production was due to both an increase in the number of activation-induced IL-2$^+$ cells and an increase in the level of IL-2 accumulated per cell. Vitamin E specifically increased the naive T cells' ability to progress through the cell division cycle in old mice [81]. The gene expression profile of T cells isolated from young and old mice fed a diet supplemented with 500 ppm vitamin E for four weeks provided evidence that vitamin E influences cell cycle-related molecules at the gene expression level. Higher expression of cell cycle-related genes *Ccnb2*, *Cdc2*, and *Cdc6* was observed in stimulated T cells from old mice fed the vitamin E-supplemented diet compared with those fed the control diet, which was not observed in young mice [84]. Cyclin B2, encoded by *Ccnb2*, binds to cyclin-dependent kinase 1 (also known as Cdc2) and regulates the events during both the G_2/M transition and progression through mitosis. Cdc6 is a key regulator in the early steps of DNA replication, as the binding of Cdc6 to chromatin is a necessary and universal step in the acquisition of replication competences [85]. These alterations in the expression of cell cycle-related genes observed with vitamin E might contribute to vitamin E improving the proliferative ability of old T cells.

Marko et al. [82] showed that pre-incubation of CD4+ T cells isolated from old T cells with 46 µM vitamin E for 4 h increased the percentage of CD4$^+$ T cells displaying effective immune synapses. Redistribution of Zap70, LAT, Vav, and phospholipase Cγ (PLCγ) into immune synapse increased significantly with vitamin E treatment. This change was confirmed with in vivo supplementation of vitamin E. In old mice fed a diet containing 500 ppm vitamin E for eight weeks, LAT and Vav showed significantly higher redistribution into the T cell/APC contact area when purified CD4$^+$ T cells were stimulated with murine CD3ε hybridoma. In a subsequent study, it was shown that vitamin E could reverse the age-associated defect in the phosphorylation of LAT on tyrosine 191 [83]. The phosphorylation of LAT is required for the recruitment of adaptor and effector proteins. Therefore, it plays a pivotal role in the assembly of microcluster structures in the initiation of T cell activation signals. This evidence suggests that vitamin E can modulate the early stages of T cell activation.

Vitamin E seems to modulate Th1 and Th2 responses. The polarization of CD4 T cells to T helper (Th)1 or Th2 cells has implications for the protection against different pathogens (intracellular vs. extracellular pathogens) and the development of different types of chronic diseases (inflammatory vs. allergic diseases). PBMCs isolated from allergic donors treated with vitamin E (12.5–50 µM) showed dose-dependent decreases in IL-4 production [86]. IL-4 mRNA levels in activated PBMCs were downregulated by 25 µM vitamin E treatment. Jurkat T cells treated with 50 µM vitamin E exhibited downregulation of IL-4 promoter activity, which might be related to vitamin E blocking the interaction of transcription factors with PRE-1 and P1. In vivo supplementation of vitamin E enhancing the Th1 response has been observed in mice infected with influenza virus and in colorectal cancer patients [6,87]. In colorectal cancer patients, two weeks of supplementation with 750 mg vitamin E led to an increased frequency of IL-2 producing CD4+ T cells and increased IFN-γ production [87]. In old mice infected with influenza virus, 500 ppm vitamin E supplementation for eight weeks prior to infection lowered the viral titer in the lung, and this protective effect of vitamin E was associated with the enhancement of Th1 response. IFN-γ production levels correlated negatively with viral titer, and old mice fed a vitamin E-supplemented diet produced significantly higher levels of IFN-γ and IL-2 [6]. The gene expression profile of T cells isolated from young and old mice fed a diet supplemented with 500 ppm vitamin E for four weeks provided evidence that vitamin E influences the Th1/Th2 balance at the gene expression level. The increase in IL-4 expression following stimulation was lower in T cells from old mice fed the vitamin E-supplemented diet compared with those fed the control diet, and the ratio of IFN-γ and IL-4 expression levels was significantly higher in the vitamin E group than in the control group [84].

Vitamin E can affect activation-induced cell death in T cells. In vitro treatment of primary human T cells with 25 μM vitamin E suppressed CD95L expression and activation-induced cell death [88]. The reduction of CD95L mRNA levels and the proportion of CD95L-positive cells were related to the suppression of NF-κB and AP-1 binding to the CD95L promoter target site by vitamin E. On the other hand, α-tocopheryl succinate was shown to trigger apoptosis in Jurkat cells with caspase-activation involved [89].

3.5. B Cells

Vitamin E supplementation has been reported to enhance humoral responses. Higher antibody responses have been observed in animals and humans [19,27]. However, it is hard to differentiate whether vitamin E's direct effect on B cells or indirect effect through T cells contributes to higher antibody responses.

4. Conclusions

Vitamin E has been shown to enhance immune responses in animal and human models and to confer protection against several infectious diseases. Suggested mechanisms involved with these changes are (1) the reduction of PGE_2 production by the inhibition of COX2 activity mediated through decreasing NO production, (2) the improvement of effective immune synapse formation in naive T cells and the initiation of T cell activation signals, and (3) the modulation of Th1/Th2 balance. Higher NK activity and changes in dendritic function such as lower IL-12 production and migration were observed with vitamin E, but underlying mechanisms need to be further elucidated

Several considerations are warranted for the advancement in our understanding of vitamin E's role in immunity. For in vitro studies to support implications for the regulation of immunological diseases, the physiological relevance of vitamin E levels used for treatment should be considered. Different forms of vitamin E exert differential effects on immune cells. Cell-specific effects of vitamin E provide valuable evidence regarding the immunomodulatory mechanisms of vitamin E, but the interplay between immune cells should not be ignored, because interactions between immune cells are critical in the regulation of immune function.

Author Contributions: Literature search and manuscript preparation were performed by G.Y.L. and S.N.H. The manuscript was revised and finalized by S.N.H.

Funding: This work was supported by the Basic Science Research Program through the National Research Foundation of Korea (NRF) funded by the Ministry of Education (grant number NRF-2018R1D1A1B07049178).

Conflicts of Interest: The author declares no conflicts of interests.

References

1. Traber, M.G. Vitamin E regulatory mechanisms. *Annu. Rev. Nutr.* **2007**, *27*, 347–362. [CrossRef] [PubMed]
2. Sheppard, A.J.; Pennington, J.A.T.; Weihrauch, J.L. Analysis and distribution of vitamin E in vegetable oils and foods. In *Vitamin E in Health and Disease*; Packer, L., Fuchs, J., Eds.; Marcel Dekker: New York, NY, USA, 1980; pp. 7–65.
3. Traber, M.G.; Atkinson, J. Vitamin E, antioxidant and nothing m more. *Free Rad. Biol. Med.* **2007**, *43*, 4–15. [CrossRef] [PubMed]
4. Zingg, J.M. Vitamin E: A role in signal transduction. *Annu. Rev. Nutr.* **2015**, *35*, 135–173. [CrossRef] [PubMed]
5. Heinzerling, R.H.; Tengerdy, R.P.; Wick, L.L.; Lueker, D.C. Vitamin E protects mice against Diplococcus pneumoniae type I infection. *Infect. Immun.* **1974**, *10*, 1292–1295. [PubMed]
6. Han, S.N.; Wu, D.; Ha, W.K.; Beharka, A.; Smith, D.E.; Bender, B.S.; Meydani, S.N. Vitamin E supplementation increases T helper 1 cytokine production in old mice infected with influenza virus. *Immunology* **2000**, *100*, 487–493. [CrossRef] [PubMed]
7. Hayek, M.G.; Taylor, S.F.; Bender, B.S.; Han, S.N.; Meydani, M.; Smith, D.E.; Eghtesada, S.; Meydani, S.N. Vitamin E supplementation decreases lung virus titers in mice infected with influenza. *J. Infect. Dis.* **1997**, *176*, 273–276. [CrossRef] [PubMed]

8. Dalia, A.M.; Loh, T.C.; Sazili, A.Q.; Jahromi, M.F.; Samsudin, A.A. Effects of vitamin E, inorganic selenium, bacterial organic selenium, and their combinations on immunity response in broiler chickens. *BMC Vet. Res.* **2018**, *14*, 249. [CrossRef] [PubMed]
9. Wang, L.; Xu, X.; Su, G.; Shi, B.; Shan, A. High concentration of vitamin E supplementation in sow diet during the last week of gestation and lactation affects the immunological variables and antioxidative parameters in piglets. *J. Dairy Res.* **2017**, *84*, 8–13. [CrossRef] [PubMed]
10. O'Brien, T.; Thomas, D.G.; Morel, P.C.; Rutherfurd-Markwick, K.J. Moderate dietary supplementation with vitamin E enhances lymphocyte functionality in the adult cat. *Res. Vet. Sci.* **2015**, *99*, 63–69. [CrossRef] [PubMed]
11. Ren, Z.; Pae, M.; Dao, M.C.; Smith, D.; Meydani, S.N.; Wu, D. Dietary supplementation with tocotrienols enhances immune function in C57BL/6 mice. *J. Nutr.* **2010**, *140*, 1335–1341. [CrossRef] [PubMed]
12. Bendich, A.; Gabriel, E.; Machlin, L.J. Dietary vitamin E requirement for optimum immune responses in the rat. *J. Nutr.* **1986**, *116*, 675–681. [CrossRef] [PubMed]
13. Meydani, S.N.; Meydani, M.; Verdon, C.P.; Shapiro, A.A.; Blumberg, J.B.; Hayes, K.C. Vitamin E supplementation suppresses prostaglandin E1(2) synthesis and enhances the immune response of aged mice. *Mech. Ageing Dev.* **1986**, *34*, 191–201. [CrossRef]
14. Wakikawa, A.; Utsuyama, M.; Wakabayashi, A.; Kitagawa, M.; Hirokawa, K. Vitamin E enhances the immune functions of young but not old mice under restraint stress. *Exp. Gerontol.* **1999**, *34*, 853–862. [CrossRef]
15. Moriguchi, S.; Kobayashi, N.; Kishino, Y. High dietary intakes of vitamin E and cellular immune functions in rats. *J. Nutr.* **1990**, *120*, 1096–1102. [CrossRef] [PubMed]
16. Sakai, S.; Moriguchi, S. Long-term feeding of high vitamin E diet improves the decreased mitogen response of rat splenic lymphocytes with aging. *J. Nutr. Sci. Vitaminol.* **1997**, *43*, 113–122. [CrossRef] [PubMed]
17. Reddy, P.G.; Morrill, J.L.; Minocha, H.C.; Stevenson, J.S. Vitamin E is Immunostimulatory in calves. *J. Dairy Sci.* **1987**, *70*, 993–999. [CrossRef]
18. Tanaka, J.; Fujiwara, H.; Torisu, M. Vitamin E and immune response. I. Enhancement of helper T cell activity by dietary supplementation of vitamin E in mice. *Immunology* **1979**, *38*, 727–734. [PubMed]
19. Beharka, A.A.; Han, S.N.; Adolfsson, O.; Wu, D.; Lipman, R.; Smith, D.; Cao, G.; Meydani, M.; Meydani, S.N. Long-term dietary antioxidant supplementation reduces production of selected inflammatory mediators by murine macrophages. *Nutr. Res.* **2000**, *20*, 281–296. [CrossRef]
20. Capó, X.; Martorell, M.; Sureda, A.; Riera, J.; Drobnic, F.; Tur, J.A.; Pons, A. Effects of Almond- and Olive Oil-Based Docosahexaenoic- and Vitamin E-Enriched Beverage Dietary Supplementation on Inflammation Associated to Exercise and Age. *Nutrients.* **2016**, *8*, 619. [CrossRef] [PubMed]
21. Mahalingam, D.; Radhakrishnan, A.K.; Amom, Z.; Ibrahim, N.; Nesaretnam, K. Effects of supplementation with tocotrienol-rich fraction on immune response to tetanus toxoid immunization in normal healthy volunteers. *Eur. J. Clin. Nutr.* **2011**, *65*, 63–69. [CrossRef] [PubMed]
22. Radhakrishnan, A.K.; Lee, A.L.; Wong, P.F.; Kaur, J.; Aung, H.; Nesaretnam, K. Daily supplementation of tocotrienol-rich fraction or alpha-tocopherol did not induce immunomodulatory changes in healthy human volunteers. *Br. J. Nutr.* **2009**, *101*, 810–815. [CrossRef] [PubMed]
23. Prasad, J.S. Effect of vitamin E supplementation on leukocyte function. *Am. J. Clin. Nutr.* **1980**, *33*, 606–608. [CrossRef] [PubMed]
24. Harman, D.; Miller, R.W. Effect of vitamin E on the immune response to influenza virus vaccine and the incidence of infectious disease in man. *Age* **1986**, *9*, 21–23. [CrossRef]
25. Meydani, S.N.; Barklund, M.P.; Liu, S.; Meydani, M.; Miller, R.A.; Cannon, J.G.; Morrow, F.D.; Rocklin, R.; Blumberg, J.B. Vitamin E supplementation enhances cell-mediated immunity in healthy elderly subjects. *Am. J. Clin. Nutr.* **1990**, *52*, 557–563. [CrossRef] [PubMed]
26. De Waart, F.G.; Portengen, L.; Doekes, G.; Verwaal, C.J.; Kok, F.J. Effect of 3 months vitamin E supplementation on indices of the cellular and humoral immune response in elderly subjects. *Br. J. Nutr.* **1997**, *78*, 761–774. [CrossRef] [PubMed]
27. Meydani, S.N.; Meydani, M.; Blumberg, J.B.; Leka, L.S.; Siber, G.; Loszewski, R.; Thompson, C.; Pedrosa, M.C.; Diamond, R.D.; Stollar, B.D. Vitamin E supplementation and in vivo immune response in healthy elderly subjects. A randomized controlled trial. *JAMA* **1997**, *277*, 1380–1386. [CrossRef] [PubMed]

28. Pallast, E.G.; Schouten, E.G.; de Waart, F.G.; Fonk, H.C.; Doekes, G.; von Blomberg, B.M.; Kok, F.J. Effect of 50- and 100-mg vitamin E supplements on cellular immune function in noninstitutionalized elderly persons. *Am. J. Clin. Nutr.* **1999**, *69*, 1273–1281. [CrossRef] [PubMed]
29. Okano, T.; Tamai, H.; Mino, M. Superoxide generation in leukocytes and vitamin E. *Int. J. Vitam. Nutr. Res.* **1991**, *61*, 20–26. [PubMed]
30. Richards, G.A.; Theron, A.J.; van Rensburg, C.E.; van Rensburg, A.J.; van der Merwe, C.A.; Kuyl, J.M.; Anderson, R. Investigation of the effects of oral administration of vitamin E and beta-carotene on the chemiluminescence responses and the frequency of sister chromatid exchanges in circulating leukocytes from cigarette smokers. *Am. Rev. Respir. Dis.* **1990**, *142*, 648–654. [CrossRef] [PubMed]
31. Kramer, T.R.; Schoene, N.; Douglass, L.W.; Judd, J.T.; Ballard-Barbash, R.; Taylor, P.R.; Bhagavan, H.N.; Nair, P.P. Increased vitamin E intake restores fish-oil-induced suppressed blastogenesis of mitogen-stimulated T lymphocytes. *Am. J. Clin. Nutr.* **1991**, *54*, 896–902. [CrossRef] [PubMed]
32. Wu, D.; Han, S.N.; Meydani, M.; Meydani, S.N. Effect of concomitant consumption of fish oil and vitamin E on T cell mediated function in the elderly: A randomized double-blind trial. *J. Am. Coll. Nutr.* **2006**, *25*, 300–306. [CrossRef] [PubMed]
33. Cannon, J.G.; Meydani, S.N.; Fielding, R.A.; Fiatarone, M.A.; Meydani, M.; Farhangmehr, M.; Orencole, S.F.; Blumberg, J.B.; Evans, W.J. Acute phase response in exercise. II. Associations between vitamin E, cytokines, and muscle proteolysis. *Am. J. Physiol.* **1991**, *260*, 1235–1240. [CrossRef] [PubMed]
34. Pierpaoli, E.; Orlando, F.; Cirioni, O.; Simonetti, O.; Giacometti, A.; Provinciali, M. Supplementation with tocotrienols from Bixa orellana improves the in vivo efficacy of daptomycin against methicillin-resistant Staphylococcus aureus in a mouse model of infected wound. *Phytomedicine* **2017**, *36*, 50–53. [CrossRef] [PubMed]
35. Bou Ghanem, E.N.; Clark, S.; Du, X.; Wu, D.; Camilli, A.; Leong, J.M.; Meydani, S.N. The α-tocopherol form of vitamin E reverses age-associated susceptibility to streptococcus pneumoniae lung infection by modulating pulmonary neutrophil recruitment. *J. Immunol.* **2015**, *194*, 1090–1099. [CrossRef] [PubMed]
36. De Wolf, B.M.; Zajac, A.M.; Hoffer, K.A.; Sartini, B.L.; Bowdridge, S.; LaRoith, T.; Petersson, K.H. The effect of vitamin E supplementation on an experimental Haemonchus contortus infection in lambs. *Vet. Parasitol.* **2014**, *205*, 140–149. [CrossRef] [PubMed]
37. Sheridan, P.A.; Beck, M.A. The immune response to herpes simplex virus encephalitis in mice is modulated by dietary vitamin E. *J. Nutr.* **2008**, *138*, 130–137. [CrossRef] [PubMed]
38. Wang, Y.; Huang, D.S.; Eskelson, C.D.; Watson, R.R. Long-Term Dietary Vitamin E Retards Development of Retrovirus-Induced Disregulation in Cytokine Production. *Clin. Immunol. Immunopathol.* **1994**, *72*, 70–75. [CrossRef] [PubMed]
39. Reddy, P.G.; Morrill, J.L.; Minocha, H.C.; Morrill, M.B.; Dayton, A.D.; Frey, R.A. Effect of supplemental vitamin E on the immune system of calves. *J. Dairy Sci.* **1986**, *69*, 164–171. [CrossRef]
40. Fang, C.H.; Peck, M.D.; Alexander, J.W.; Babcock, G.F.; Warden, G.D. The effect of free radical scavengers on outcome after infection in burned mice. *J. Trauma* **1990**, *30*, 453–456. [CrossRef] [PubMed]
41. Watson, R.; Petro, T.M. Cellular immune response, corticosteroid levels and resistance to Listeria monocytogenes and murine leukemia in mice fed a high vitamin E diet. *N.Y. Acad. Sci.* **1982**, *393*, 205–210. [CrossRef]
42. Tvedten, H.W.; Whitehair, C.K.; Langham, R.F. Influence of vitamins A and E on gnotobiotic and conventionally maintained rats exposed to Mycoplasma pulmonis. *J. Am. Vet. Med. Assoc.* **1973**, *163*, 605–612. [PubMed]
43. Stephens, L.C.; McChesney, A.E.; Nockels, C.F. Improved recovery of vitamin E-treated lambs that have been experimentally infected with intratracheal Chlamydia. *Br. Vet. J.* **1979**, *135*, 291–293. [CrossRef]
44. Schildknecht, E.G.; Squibb, R.L. The effect of vitamins A, E and K on experimentally induced histomoniasis in turkeys. *Parasitology* **1979**, *78*, 19–31. [CrossRef] [PubMed]
45. Teige, J.; Tollersrud, S.; Lund, A.; Larsen, H.J. Swine dysentery: The influence of dietary vitamin E and selenium on the clinical and pathological effects of Treponema hyodysenteriae infection in pigs. *Res. Vet. Sci.* **1982**, *32*, 95–100. [PubMed]
46. Tengerdy, R.P.; Meyer, D.L.; Lauerman, L.H.; Lueker, D.C.; Nockels, C.F. Vitamin E-enhanced humoral antibody response to Clostridium perfringens type D in sheep. *Br. Vet. J.* **1983**, *139*, 147–152. [CrossRef]

47. Smith, K.L.; Harrison, J.H.; Hancock, D.D.; Todhunter, D.A.; Conrad, H.R. Effect of vitamin E and selenium supplementation on incidence of clinical mastitis and duration of clinical symptoms. *J. Dairy Sci.* **1984**, *67*, 1293–1300. [CrossRef]
48. Heinzerling, R.H.; Nockels, C.F.; Quarles, C.L.; Tengerdy, R.P. Protection of chicks against *E.coli* infection by dietary supplementation with vitamin E. *Proc. Soc. Exp. Biol. Med.* **1974**, *146*, 279–283. [CrossRef] [PubMed]
49. Tengerdy, R.P.; Nockels, C.F. Vitamin E or vitamin A protects chickens against E. coli infection. *Poult. Sci.* **1975**, *54*, 1292–1296. [CrossRef] [PubMed]
50. Likoff, R.O.; Guptill, D.R.; Lawrence, L.M.; McKay, C.C.; Mathias, M.M.; Nockels, C.F.; Tengerdy, R.P. Vitamin E and aspirin depress prostaglandins in protection of chickens against Escherichia coli infection. *Am. J. Clin. Nutr.* **1981**, *34*, 245–251. [CrossRef] [PubMed]
51. Ellis, R.P.; Vorhies, M.W. Effect of supplemental dietary vitamin E on the serologic response of swine to an Escherichia coli bacterin. *J. Am. Vet. Med. Assoc.* **1976**, *168*, 231–232. [PubMed]
52. Hemilä, H. Vitamin E administration may decrease the incidence of pneumonia in elderly males. *Clin. Interv. Aging* **2016**, *11*, 1379–1385. [CrossRef] [PubMed]
53. Olofin, I.O.; Spiegelman, D.; Aboud, S.; Duggan, C.; Danaei, G.; Fawzi, W.W. Supplementation with multivitamins and vitamin A and incidence of malaria among HIV-infected Tanzanian women. *J. Acquir. Immune Defic. Syndr.* **2014**, *67* (Suppl. S4), S173–S178. [CrossRef] [PubMed]
54. Marotta, F.; Yoshida, C.; Barreto, R.; Naito, Y.; Packer, L. Oxidative-inflammatory damage in cirrhosis: Effect of vitamin E and a fermented papaya preparation. *J. Gastroenterol. Hepatol.* **2007**, *22*, 697–703. [CrossRef] [PubMed]
55. Groenbaek, K.; Friis, H.; Hansen, M.; Ring-Larsen, H.; Krarup, H.B. The effect of antioxidant supplementation on hepatitis C viral load, transaminases and oxidative status: A randomized trial among chronic hepatitis C virus-infected patients. *Eur. J. Gastroenterol. Hepatol.* **2006**, *18*, 985–989. [CrossRef] [PubMed]
56. Meydani, S.N.; Leka, L.S.; Fine, B.C.; Dallal, G.E.; Keusch, G.T.; Singh, M.F.; Hamer, D.H. Vitamin E and respiratory tract infections in elderly nursing home residents: A randomized controlled trial. *JAMA* **2004**, *292*, 828–836. [CrossRef] [PubMed]
57. Hemilä, H.; Kaprio, J.; Albanes, D.; Heinonen, O.P.; Virtamo, J. Vitamin C, vitamin E, and beta-carotene in relation to common cold incidence in male smokers. *Epidemiology* **2002**, *13*, 32–37. [CrossRef] [PubMed]
58. Hemilä, H.; Virtamo, J.; Albanes, D.; Kaprio, J. Vitamin E and beta-carotene supplementation and hospital-treated pneumonia incidence in male smokers. *Chest* **2004**, *125*, 557–565. [CrossRef] [PubMed]
59. Graat, J.M.; Schouten, E.G.; Kok, F.J. Effect of daily vitamin E and multivitamin-mineral supplementation on acute respiratory tract infections in elderly persons: A randomized controlled trial. *JAMA* **2002**, *288*, 715–721. [CrossRef] [PubMed]
60. Mosser, D.M.; Edwards, J.P. Exploring the full spectrum of macrophage activation. *Nat. Rev. Immunol.* **2008**, *8*, 958–969. [CrossRef] [PubMed]
61. Meydani, S.N.; Han, S.N.; Wu, D. Vitamin E and immune response in the aged: Molecular mechanisms and clinical implications. *Immunol. Rev.* **2005**, *205*, 269–284. [CrossRef] [PubMed]
62. Beharka, A.A.; We, D.; Han, S.N.; Meydani, S.N. Macrophage prostaglandin production contributes to the age-associated decrease in T cell function which is reversed by the dietary antioxidant vitamin E. *Mech. Age. Dev.* **1997**, *93*, 59–77. [CrossRef]
63. Hayek, M.G.; Mura, C.; Wu, D.; Beharka, A.A.; Han, S.N.; Paulson, K.E.; Hwang, D.; Meydani, S.N. Enhanced expression of inducible cyclooxygenase with age in murine macrophages. *J. Immunol.* **1997**, *159*, 2445–2451. [PubMed]
64. Wu, D.; Mura, C.; Beharka, A.A.; Han, S.N.; Paulson, K.E.; Hwang, D.; Meydani, S.N. Age-associated increase in PGE2 synthesis and COX activity in murine macrophages is reversed by vitamin E. *Am. J. Physiol.* **1998**, *275*, C661–C668. [CrossRef] [PubMed]
65. Beharka, A.A.; Wu, D.; Serafini, M.; Meydani, S.N. Mechanism of vitamin E inhibition of cyclooxygenase activity in macrophages from old mice: Role of peroxynitrite. *Free. Radic. Biol. Med.* **2002**, *32*, 503–511. [CrossRef]
66. Sorokin, A. Nitric Oxide Synthase and Cyclooxygenase Pathways: A Complex Interplay in Cellular Signaling. *Curr. Med. Chem.* **2016**, *23*, 2559–2578. [CrossRef] [PubMed]

67. Dworski, R.; Han, W.; Blackwell, T.S.; Hoskins, A.; Freeman, M.L. Vitamin E prevents NRF2 suppression by allergens in asthmatic alveolar macrophages in vivo. *Free Radic. Biol. Med.* **2011**, *51*, 516–521. [CrossRef] [PubMed]
68. Adachi, N.; Migita, M.; Ohta, T.; Higashi, A.; Matsuda, I. Depressed natural killer cell activity due to decreased natural killer cell population in a vitamin E-deficient patient with Shwachman syndrome: Reversible natural killer cell abnormality by alpha-tocopherol supplementation. *Eur. J. Pediatr.* **1997**, *156*, 444–448. [CrossRef] [PubMed]
69. Ravaglia, G.; Forti, P.; Maioli, F.; Bastagli, L.; Facchini, A.; Mariani, E.; Savarino, L.; Sassi, S.; Cucinotta, D.; Lenaz, G. Effect of micronutrient status on natural killer cell immune function in healthy free-living subjects aged ≥90 y. *Am. J. Clin. Nutr.* **2000**, *71*, 590–598. [CrossRef] [PubMed]
70. Hanson, M.G.; Ozenci, V.; Carlsten, M.C.; Glimelius, B.L.; Frödin, J.E.; Masucci, G.; Malmberg, K.J.; Kiessling, R.V. A short-term dietary supplementation with high doses of vitamin E increases NK cell cytolytic activity in advanced colorectal cancer patients. *Cancer Immunol. Immunother.* **2007**, *56*, 973–984. [CrossRef] [PubMed]
71. Stiff, A.; Trikha, P.; Mundy-Bosse, B.; McMichael, E.; Mace, T.A.; Benner, B.; Kendra, K.; Campbell, A.; Gautam, S.; Abood, D.; et al. Nitric Oxide Production by Myeloid-Derived Suppressor Cells Plays a Role in Impairing Fc Receptor-Mediated Natural Killer Cell Function. *Clin. Cancer Res.* **2018**, *24*, 1891–1904. [CrossRef] [PubMed]
72. Ganguly, D.; Haak, S.; Sisirak, V.; Reizis, B. The role of dendritic cells in autoimmunity. *Nat. Rev. Immunol.* **2013**, *13*, 566–577. [CrossRef] [PubMed]
73. Pearce, E.J.; Everts, B. Dendritic cell metabolism. *Nat. Rev. Immunol.* **2015**, *15*, 18–29. [CrossRef] [PubMed]
74. Alloatti, A.; Kotsias, F.; Magalhaes, J.G.; Amigorena, S. Dendritic cell maturation and cross-presentation: Timing matters! *Immunol. Rev.* **2016**, *272*, 97–108. [CrossRef] [PubMed]
75. Tan, P.H.; Sagoo, P.; Chan, C.; Yates, J.B.; Campbell, J.; Beutelspacher, S.C.; Foxwell, B.M.; Lombardi, G.; George, A.J. Inhibition of NF-kappa B and oxidative pathways in human dendritic cells by antioxidative vitamins generates regulatory T cells. *J. Immunol.* **2005**, *174*, 7633–7644. [CrossRef] [PubMed]
76. Xuan, N.T.; Trang, P.T.; Van Phong, N.; Toan, N.L.; Trung, D.M.; Bac, N.D.; Nguyen, V.L.; Hoang, N.H.; van Hai, N. Klotho sensitive regulation of dendritic cell functions by vitamin E. *Biol. Res.* **2016**, *49*, 45. [CrossRef] [PubMed]
77. Buendía, P.; Ramírez, R.; Aljama, P.; Carracedo, J. Klotho Prevents Translocation of NFκB. *Vitam. Horm.* **2016**, *101*, 119–150. [PubMed]
78. Abdala-Valencia, H.; Berdnikovs, S.; Soveg, F.W.; Cook-Mills, J.M. α-Tocopherol supplementation of allergic female mice inhibits development of CD11c+CD11b+ dendritic cells in utero and allergic inflammation in neonates. *Am. J. Physiol. Lung Cell. Mol. Physiol.* **2014**, *307*, L482–L496. [CrossRef] [PubMed]
79. Abdala-Valencia, H.; Soveg, F.; Cook-Mills, J.M. γ-Tocopherol supplementation of allergic female mice augments development of CD11c+CD11b+ dendritic cells in utero and allergic inflammation in neonates. *Am. J. Physiol. Lung Cell. Mol. Physiol.* **2016**, *310*, L759–L771. [CrossRef] [PubMed]
80. Molano, A.; Meydani, S.N. Vitamin E, signalosomes and gene expression in T cells. *Mol. Aspects. Med.* **2012**, *33*, 55–62. [CrossRef] [PubMed]
81. Adolfsson, O.; Huber, B.T.; Meydani, S.N. Vitamin E-enhanced IL-2 production in old mice: Naive but not memory T cells show increased cell division cycling and IL-2-producing capacity. *J. Immunol.* **2001**, *167*, 3809–3817. [CrossRef] [PubMed]
82. Marko, M.G.; Ahmed, T.; Bunnell, S.C.; Wu, D.; Chung, H.; Huber, B.T.; Meydani, S.N. Age-associated decline in effective immune synapse formation of CD4(+) T cells is reversed by vitamin E supplementation. *J. Immunol.* **2007**, *178*, 1443–1449. [CrossRef] [PubMed]
83. Marko, M.G.; Pang, H.J.; Ren, Z.; Azzi, A.; Huber, B.T.; Bunnell, S.C.; Meydani, S.N. Vitamin E reverses impaired linker for activation of T cells activation in T cells from aged C57BL/6 mice. *J. Nutr.* **2009**, *139*, 1192–1197. [CrossRef] [PubMed]
84. Han, S.N.; Adolfsson, O.; Lee, C.K.; Prolla, T.A.; Ordovas, J.; Meydani, S.N. Age and vitamin E-induced changes in gene expression profiles of T cells. *J. Immunol.* **2006**, *177*, 6052–6061. [CrossRef] [PubMed]
85. Pelizon, C. Down to the origin: Cdc6 protein and the competence to replicate. *Trends Cell Biol.* **2003**, *13*, 110–113. [CrossRef]

86. Li-Weber, M.; Giaisi, M.; Treiber, M.K.; Krammer, P.H. Vitamin E inhibits IL-4 gene expression in peripheral blood T cells. *Eur. J. Immunol.* **2002**, *32*, 2401–2408. [CrossRef]
87. Malmberg, K.J.; Lenkei, R.; Petersson, M.; Ohlum, T.; Ichihara, F.; Glimelius, B.; Frödin, J.E.; Masucci, G. A short-term dietary supplementation of high doses of vitamin E increases T helper 1 cytokine production in patients with advanced colorectal cancer. *Clin. Cancer Res.* **2002**, *8*, 1772–1778. [PubMed]
88. Li-Weber, M.; Weigand, M.A.; Giaisi, M.; Süss, D.; Treiber, M.K.; Baumann, S.; Ritsou, E.; Breitkreutz, R.; Krammer, P.H. Vitamin E inhibits CD95 ligand expression and protects T cells from activation-induced cell death. *J. Clin. Invest.* **2002**, *110*, 681–690. [CrossRef] [PubMed]
89. Neuzil, J.; Svensson, I.; Weber, T.; Weber, C.; Brunk, U.T. α-tocopheryl succinate-induced apoptosis in Jurkat T cells involves caspase-3 activation, and both lysosomal and mitochondrial destabilisation. *FEBS Lett.* **1999**, *445*, 295–300. [CrossRef]

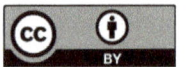 © 2018 by the authors. Licensee MDPI, Basel, Switzerland. This article is an open access article distributed under the terms and conditions of the Creative Commons Attribution (CC BY) license (http://creativecommons.org/licenses/by/4.0/).

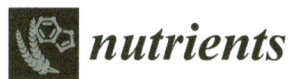

Review

The Microbiotic Highway to Health— New Perspective on Food Structure, Gut Microbiota, and Host Inflammation

Nina Wærling Hansen [1] and Anette Sams [2,*]

1. Molecular Endocrinology Unit (KMEB), Department of Endocrinology, Institute of Clinical Research, University of Southern Denmark, DK-5000 Odense, Denmark; nwhansen@health.sdu.dk
2. Department of Clinical Experimental Research, Glostrup Research Institute, Copenhagen University Hospital, Nordstjernevej 42, DK-2600 Glostrup, Denmark
* Correspondence: anette.nielsen.03@regionh.dk

Received: 28 September 2018; Accepted: 23 October 2018; Published: 30 October 2018

Abstract: This review provides evidence that not only the content of nutrients but indeed the structural organization of nutrients is a major determinant of human health. The gut microbiota provides nutrients for the host by digesting food structures otherwise indigestible by human enzymes, thereby simultaneously harvesting energy and delivering nutrients and metabolites for the nutritional and biological benefit of the host. Microbiota-derived nutrients, metabolites, and antigens promote the development and function of the host immune system both directly by activating cells of the adaptive and innate immune system and indirectly by sustaining release of monosaccharides, stimulating intestinal receptors and secreting gut hormones. Multiple indirect microbiota-dependent biological responses contribute to glucose homeostasis, which prevents hyperglycemia-induced inflammatory conditions. The composition and function of the gut microbiota vary between individuals and whereas dietary habits influence the gut microbiota, the gut microbiota influences both the nutritional and biological homeostasis of the host. A healthy gut microbiota requires the presence of beneficial microbiotic species as well as vital food structures to ensure appropriate feeding of the microbiota. This review focuses on the impact of plant-based food structures, the "fiber-encapsulated nutrient formulation", and on the direct and indirect mechanisms by which the gut microbiota participate in host immune function.

Keywords: carbohydrates; fiber; food structure; formulation; plant; microbiota; inflammation; metabolism; nutrition guidelines

1. Introduction

The gut microbiota is a complex ecosystem residing in the gastro-intestinal (GI) tract and consists of a diverse microbiotic community living in symbiosis with the host. A diverse microbiota is considered a major positive regulator of the interdependent metabolic and immune function of the host. The gut microbiota is shaped alongside the host immune system in a synergistic partnership [1]. Trillions of microorganisms participate in the maturation and regulation of immune function, energy metabolism, and hormonal balance [2], including regulation of intestinal mucosal barriers, fermentation of undigested nutrients, and synthesis of short chain fatty acids (SCFA) [3]. Furthermore, the microbiota releases microbiota-derived antigens [4,5], vitamins [6,7], and other molecules, such as tryptophan metabolites [8,9], that interact with the host biology.

The dynamic relationship between the microbiotic ecosystem and its host is emphasized by the joint utilization of consumed nutrients. Diet is a shared substrate between the host and the gut microbiota and the choice of diet affects host health both directly and indirectly by affecting the abundance and composition of the microbiotic community [10,11].

The structural organization of complex carbohydrates determines the site of digestion and absorption in the GI tract [12], and hence the level of cross feeding [13], community organization, and proliferation of specific microorganisms. Importantly, all plant cell walls consist of complex carbohydrate structures that are digested selectively by microbiotic enzymes and not by host enzymes. Thus, complex polysaccharides in plant cell walls function as both substrate for the microbiota and as a sustained release delivery system of other plant-cell derived nutrients and biomolecules for both microbiotic and host utilization. The structural properties of the cell wall vary between different plant cells [14], and in theory determine the specific site of plant cell wall degradation and nutrient release.

Plant-based foods can be placed on a moving scale from whole foods (unrefined) to fully refined foods, and currently no official distinction based on the degrees of refinement exists. Foods with added refined nutrients (e.g., sugar, starch or oils) or any food, which has been structurally disrupted on the macroscopic level are considered refined. The degree of refinement is thus determined by the degree of macroscopic structural disruption (e.g., intact whole grain vs. ground whole grain vs. sifted flour) and the degree of refined supplementation. When plant-based food structures are completely disrupted requiring no microbiotic interaction for digestion we consider the food fully refined.

Microbiota composition varies greatly among different cultures and individuals [15,16], and specific genera of bacteria are more abundant in healthy individuals as compared to individuals in different disease states, as shown, for example, for *Bifidobacterium* and *Lactobacillus* [17–19], whose functions include carbohydrate fermentation and vitamin synthesis [6,20,21]. The degradation and utilization of complex carbohydrates rely on specific microbiotic enzymes secreted from the microbiota in the lower intestine [22]. The fermentation process yields energy for microbiotic proliferation and metabolites, e.g. SCFA [23] for regulation of inflammatory responses [24] and gut hormone secretion [25] in the host. The latter is of great importance for glucose homeostasis and plays a major role for the metabolic and inflammatory health of the host [26].

Microbiota composition is also closely connected to the integrity of our intestinal mucosal barrier. Upon microbiota dysbiosis mucosal bacteria can impair epithelial function and cause increased gut permeability with consequent immune dysregulation, leading to inflammatory disease states [27]. A number of disorders with an inflammatory component including obesity, inflammatory bowel diseases (IBD), type 2 diabetes (T2D), colorectal cancer, and cardiovascular diseases have been linked with dysbiosis [28–32]. This association presents the gut microbiota as a potentially modifiable factor in the etiology of these conditions. It is therefore of great importance for public and individual health to recognize that microbiota composition may be diversified within days or weeks upon introduction of unrefined plant-based diets [16].

In clinical trials diets are often classified as low carbohydrate vs. high carbohydrate, and low fiber vs. high fiber. These trials lack discrimination between refined and unrefined carbohydrates. Acknowledging the degree of refinement would likely strengthen the reproducibility of diet intervention studies for reasons discussed in the present review [33–35].

This paper analyzes the interplay between structures of plant-based foods or "fiber-encapsulated nutrients", the gut microbiota, and their joint impact on host nutrient bioavailability, immune function, and metabolic function, and proposes a simple tool to select plant-based foods from a nutritional- and microbiota-promoting perspective. The review provides a biological explanation of the health superiority of structurally maintained and unrefined foods compared to nutrient-matched refined foods, combining classic and current scientific knowledge within nutrition, pharmaceutical science, microbiology, and plant biology. In addition, we add the perspective of "fiber as nutrient encapsulation" to the well-established molecular benefits of fiber as microbiotic nutrient (prebiotic). This structural perspective should be included in the current nutritional guidelines, which focus on nutrient and fiber content rather than nutrient and fiber structure.

2. Carbohydrates: Different Structures, Different Properties

The structural characteristics of dietary carbohydrates include the chemical composition, physicochemical properties, and resistance to human digestive enzymes. Dietary polysaccharides display a variety of linkages, branching, and polymerizations and must be broken down into their corresponding monosaccharides (e.g., glucose, galactose, and fructose) before they can be absorbed and metabolized by humans. This carbohydrate breakdown is initiated by α-amylase secreted by salivary glands, continues with pancreatic amylase in the duodenum, and is completed by intestinal enzymes (e.g., sucrase and lactase) located in the brush-border membrane of the enterocytes in the small intestine [22]. Pancreatic amylase hydrolyzes α-linked glucose polymers such as starch and glycogen, but humans lack the enzymes necessary to hydrolyze β-linked glucose polymers like those present in resistant starches and dietary fibers found in plant structures [36].

Resistant starches include starch where (i) the granules are inaccessible to enzymes due to conformation; (ii) the starch is retrograded or (iii) chemically modified. Importantly, starch may also be digestion-resistant due to encapsulation in plant cell fiber matrices [37] and new perspectives on this aspect are the main focus of this review.

Dietary fiber includes a large variety of carbohydrate polymers, e.g., xylans, β-glucans, fructans, β-mannans, celluloses, hemicelluloses, and pectins [38]. Cellulose, hemicellulose, and pectin are major components of plant cell walls, and starch [39] and inulin [40] are heavily represented in plant carbohydrate storage. As such, the above-mentioned molecular carbohydrates are regarded as prebiotics that may stimulate or alter the preferential growth of health-promoting bacterial species already residing in the colon [41].

The microbiota encodes a broad spectrum of enzymes catalyzing the depolymerization and further degradation of polysaccharides [22]. The structural properties of the carbohydrates are important since the ability to utilize different substrates differs between bacterial species, for example, it has been shown in vitro, that *Roseburia* spp. can utilize amylopectin starch and that *Bifidobacterium* spp. cannot [42].

Plant polysaccharides can be separated based on origin (cereals and grains, fruits, vegetables nuts, and legumes), and chemical compositions and physicochemical properties vary depending on origin [14]. The physicochemical properties of plant polysaccharides include fermentability, solubility, and viscosity, each of which impact site and degree of fermentation. Soluble fibers, such as short-chain fructo-oligosaccharides and pectin are depolymerized by bacterial enzymes more proximally in the GI tract, while fibers with a lower solubility, such as cellulose, are partially fermented in the distal colon where transit time is slower and microbiotic density higher [12].

Simple carbohydrates, such as monosaccharides, disaccharides, and oligosaccharides can be classified as host nutrition with direct utilization by host enzymes, whereas complex carbohydrate polymers, such as plant polysaccharides and resistant starches are vital substrates for the microbiota. Thus, a diet that includes a variety of unrefined plant structures can therefore promote proliferation of a broader spectrum of bacteria with specific intrinsic properties. A diet rich in plant structure variety also represents a diverse sustained release device for delivery of various nutrients and bioactive molecules for metabolic and immunological stimulation, as described below.

3. Plant Cell Structure

The plant cell wall is the major difference between animal and plant cells. Except for the cell wall, chloroplasts, and vacuoles, animal and plant cells share intracellular structures and compartmentalization (Figure 1).

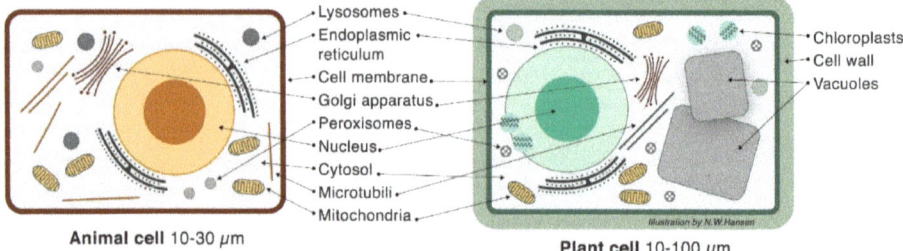

Figure 1. Schematic illustration of an animal and a plant cell. The cell wall (mainly complex carbohydrates), vacuoles (usually starch or lipid storage, depending on cell type), and chloroplasts are plant-cell specific structures that serve as nutrients for the microbiota, whereas the cellular content serves as signal molecules for host metabolic and immune regulation as well as nutrients for both host and microbiota. An intact plant cell is defined as unrefined food whereas the degree of structural disruption (and the supplementation of additives) defines the degree of refinement.

The most characteristic component found in all plant cell walls is the fiber, cellulose [43], which consists of a collection of β-1,4-linked glucan chains that interact with each other via hydrogen bonds to form a crystalline microfibril [44]. In addition to cellulose, the primary plant cell wall contains two categories of matrix polysaccharides-pectins and hemicelluloses, and several proteins and glycoproteins, including various enzymes and structural proteins [45].

Intracellular plant compartments and their relative ratio constitute the macro- and micronutrients in the plant and the dispersion of macronutrients varies from plant to plant, changing during aging with a larger proportion of protein and lipids during early growth [46]. In addition to macronutrients and vitamins, the encapsulated plant cells also contain phytonutrients, such as polyphenols (flavonoids and stilbenes), carotenoids, plant sterols, and poly-unsaturated fatty acids (PUFA), many of which are used as nutraceutical ingredients and exhibit beneficial effects on metabolic and cardiovascular parameters [47].

Although monomers from the cell wall degradation process are absorbed via host transporters, most of the plant-cell wall functions as microbiota substrate [12]. Furthermore, the mixture of macronutrients, vitamins, and phytonutrients encapsulated within the plant cell membrane have a two-tier function, with part of their host-health-promoting effects also benefiting the microbiota. In other words, the microbiota and the host share both host-enzyme-resistant carbohydrates and fiber-encapsulated macro- and micronutrients.

4. Microbiota Composition

In human adults, five bacterial phyla have been reported to be dominant in the gut microbiota of healthy individuals: *Firmicutes, Bacteroidetes, Actinobacteria, Proteobacteria* and *Verrucomicrobia* [48], with more than 90% of the species belonging to *Firmicutes* and *Bacteroidetes*. Representatives of the other phyla comprise from 2 to 10% with great interpersonal variation [49]. Changes in the relative abundance of the two dominant bacterial divisions, *Bacteroidetes* and *Firmicutes*, have been associated with an increased BMI [50]. An overrepresentation of butyrate-producing species, such as *Roseburia* spp. and *Eubacterium* spp. within the *Firmicutes* phylum affects the metabolic potential of the microbiota, i.e., the microbiotic capacity to harvest energy from the diet and produce SCFA available for host consumption [51].

In humans, an abundance and diversity in polysaccharide-fermenting bacteria, such as species within the *Bacteroidetes* phylum, are inversely related to obesity and other metabolic disorders with an inflammatory component [52–55]. Members of *Bacteroidetes* express very large numbers of genes that encode microbiotic enzymes and readily can switch between different energy sources in the gut depending on substrate availability. Within the Bacteroidetes phyla, two genera are particularly dominant and mutual antagonistic; *Bacteroides* and *Prevotella* [56]. The relative ratio between these two genera varies, with the *Bacteroides*-driven type reported as dominant in individuals with a higher intake of protein and animal fat, and *Prevotella* more common in individuals who consume more carbohydrate-rich diets [57,58] These findings represent distinct community composition types—so-called enterotypes—based on genus composition [59], suggesting that such compositional differences both reflect dietary intake and determine an individual's response to different diets [55].

Long-term dietary habits have considerable effect on the gut microbiota as evidence by differences in microbiotic compositions across geographical and/or cultural-dependent diets [28,57,60]. Microbiota composition also respond to short-term macronutrient changes; moreover, functional traits linking enterotypes to diet have been identified [57,58]. Animal and human studies show that an acute dietary switch results in dramatic shifts in the gut microbiota within the course of 24 h [16]. An animal-based diet increases the abundance of bile-tolerant genera (*Alistipes*, *Bilophila*, and *Bacteroides*) and decreases the level of *Firmicutes* species capable of fermenting dietary plant polysaccharides. Microbiotic activity mirrors differences between herbivorous and carnivorous mammals, reflecting trade-offs between carbohydrate and protein fermentation [61]. Analyses of the relative abundance of taxonomic groups have shown that short-term animal-based diets have a greater impact on microbiotic community structure compared to plant-based diets [16], suggesting perhaps a default microbiotic setting favoring plant-based diets.

As mentioned above, bacterial species have varying abilities to degrade fibers from different sources. The ability to degrade a wider variety of complex carbohydrates therefore forms a more diverse bacterial community. Moreover, the biodiversity, function, and abundance of a microbiotic community also depend on cross-feeding among members, which is the process where essential metabolites synthesized by a subset of the community provide substrate for growth of another/other bacterial species [62]. These microbiotic interactions create a complex pattern of interconnected metabolisms and link members of different genera/phyla together in communities.

Biodiversity therefore contributes to the stability and resilience of the bacterial communities. A high level of resilience ensures renewal and reorganization of the community if a species is lost, whereas communities with low biodiversity are more susceptible to loss of individual species. Highly diverse ecosystems most likely contain species with redundant functions, making the loss of a single species tolerable, because other functionally redundant species can take over [63]. Evidently, the microbiotic composition and community organization are reflective of dietary habits and affect host metabolic and immune processes. The distinction between enterotypes with distinct fermentation kinetics should therefore be considered an environmental factor that contributes to both health and disease.

5. Biological Journey and Destiny of Complex and Simple Carbohydrates

Monosaccharides can be absorbed via transporters in the human GI tract whereas polysaccharides that are not encapsulated by a fibrous plant cell wall, undergo digestion in the upper GI tract devoid of the microbiota. The more complex the carbohydrate the more glycosidase activity is necessary for the depolymerization. Thus, the more complex the plant cell wall (nutrient delivery device), the more microbiota interaction is needed. As a result, more caloric harvesting takes place and a larger intestinal area is subject to nutrient absorption, enteroendocrine stimulation, and immunological maturation.

The human gut has the potential to absorb monosaccharides via several transporters located in the absorptive epithelium. Apical sodium-dependent glucose cotransporter 1 (SGLT1) [64], glucose transporter 2 (GLUT2) [65], and glucose transporter 5 (GLUT5) [66] facilitate absorption of glucose and fructose from the intestine, and basolateral GLUT2 and GLUT5 facilitate the basolateral monosaccharide secretion into the host interstitium. Upon ingestion of a sugar-enriched meal, a transient upregulation of the absorptive monosaccharide transporters is induced, perhaps via apical recruitment of GLUT2 [67–69]. Thus, sugar ingestion promotes host absorption and bypasses caloric harvesting by microbiota.

Throughout the GI tract the level of glucose transporters is highly regulated by hexose availability and insulin levels [70–73]. In addition, the expression of glucose transporters has been shown to be increased in e.g., obesity and diabetes [74,75] and as a result, certain individuals experience a larger bioavailability of monosaccharides.

Despite individual differences in host digestive enzyme- and nutrient transporter expression, a general notion must be highlighted: The density and diversity of the microbiota increases with the distance from the stomach. The more complex the carbohydrate, the longer the journey until complete fermentation, and therefore the more likely that carbohydrates are utilized by the microbiota and not by the host.

6. The Plant Cell Wall Viewed as a "Pharmaceutical-Nutrient Formulation"

When applying the drug delivery perspective to unrefined plant-based foods, it is evident that the polysaccharides of plant-cell walls [76,77] are more than just molecular nutrition for the host and microbiota [78]. Unrefined plant-based food structures can be interpreted as a slow release device for nutrients and bioactive molecules in the human GI tract, which has important implications for intestinal absorption and local biological actions. The "device" releases a complex pool of molecules with nutritional value for the host and the microbiota, and with biological effects that trigger the endocrine and immunological maturation of the host. The release of nutrients from the fiber-encapsulated plant cell is thus dependent on microbiota-specific plant cell wall fermentation.

In pharmaceutical drug discovery and development processes, both pharmacokinetic and pharmacodynamic properties are carefully optimized. Whereas the optimized drug molecule determines the specific pharmacological action, the site of action and the duration of action are heavily influenced by the pharmaceutical formulation of the drug molecule. For example, a specific formulation can be used to target sustained or fast absorption from the GI tract. In other words, the drug molecule needs a relevant formulation to reach the relevant site of absorption and to obtain the desired absorption kinetic [79].

Different saccharides (sugars, starches, and fibers) are used as coating material in oral drug formulations to direct drugs through the GI infrastructure and deliver the drug molecule at the desired site of action or absorption [80]. Salicylic acid is, for example, formulated for fast or sustained systemic absorption using different formulation principles. Different cellulose coatings have been used to deliver the drug to distal parts of the gut for local IBD therapy [81,82]. Basically, the microbiota ferments the coating material and releases the drug distally for sustained release (or local treatment). The diversity in fibrous plant cell structures therefore serves as both a saccharide delivery system for bacterial species and as a fiber-encapsulated delivery device of other molecular nutrients (e.g., amino acids, fatty acids, vitamins, and other bioactive molecules). These nutrients are released from the plant cell upon plant-cell-wall fermentation, playing a major role for both host and microbiota biology (Figure 2). Indeed, most bacteria, even *Lactobacillus* and *Bifidobacterium*, express lipid and amino acid transporters [83–86] and regulate the expression dependent on the specific environment.

The biological properties of the microbiota are not solely dependent on the carbohydrate-based prebiotic content, but indeed also on the content of lipids, proteins, amino acids, and vitamins [87]. In vitro studies of bacteria emphasize the perspective that plant-based nutrients beyond fibers are important for microbiotic function. For example, the growth and adhesion properties of specific microbial strains are different in two different media (soy bean media and MRS media) [88] and the growth of *Lactobacillus* and *Bifidobacterium* depends on the media protein content [89,90]. Therefore, a diversity of media is needed to actually culture a diversity of human gut microbiota and study their selective and community properties [91]. Peptides and lipids that are not fiber-encapsulated would most likely only reach the microbiota in limited amounts due to upper-intestinal host absorption. Thus, a major source of amino acids and lipids for the microbiota is formulated in plant cells.

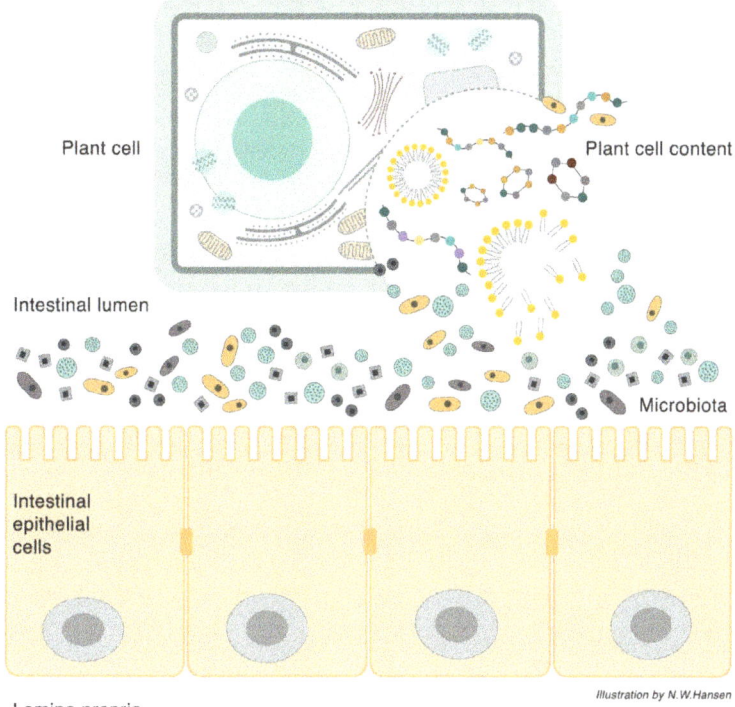

Figure 2. Illustration of interactions between plant cells, microbiota, and the host epithelium. Plant cells are encapsulated by the fibrous cell wall, which is a microbiota-selective nutrient. The cell wall also serves as a transport vehicle for the additional plant cell contents as well as a vehicle for nutrients to be shared between the microbiota and the host upon release from its plant cell structure. The microbiota secretes glycosidases, peptidases, and lipases, thereby releasing molecular nutrients for transport into epithelial or bacterial cells.

If plant cells have been refined, this organization does not remain intact, and even if the fibers reach the microbiota (e.g., fiber supplements), only limited amounts of amino acids and lipids will reach the microbes.

Some bacterial genera e.g., *Bacteroides* [92] and *Lactobacillus* [93] secrete both peptidases and glycosidases and the more distal fiber-fermenting species *Bacteroides thetaiotaomicron* also express dipeptidylpeptidases (DPPs) [94,95]. Interestingly, the DPP4 antagonist vildagliptin, used for the treatment of T2D, induces a higher relative abundance of *Bacteroidetes*, a lower abundance of *Firmicutes*, and thus a reduced ratio of *Firmicutes/Bacteroidetes* in rats [96]. This is one among many examples of anti-diabetic drugs that has recently been shown to induce secondary health promoting actions via the microbiota [97].

Another pharmaceutical exploration of the microbiota is the study of bacterial peptide transporters with the aim to identify new antibiotic targets in virulent bacteria. Since blockage of peptide transporters is a potent antibiotic pathway, specific bacteria are dependent on their endogenous peptide transporters and on amino acid fuel [98]. In both gram negative and gram positive virulent bacteria, two distinct vital types of peptide transporters exist, proton-dependent peptide transporters (PRT or POT) [99] and ATP-binding cassettes (ABC transporters) [100].

As in the case of amino acids, energy dependent fatty acid transporters are also present in both outer and inner membranes of bacterial strains. Even *Lactobacillus* expresses amino acid and fatty acid transporters [83], which supports the bacterial ability and need to consume fatty acids slowly released from plant cells during the microbiotic digestion of the plant cell wall. In specific bacteria, the process requires the outer membrane-bound fatty acid transport protein FadL and the inner membrane associated fatty acyl CoA synthetase (FACS) [101,102].

The diversity in fiber-coated plant cell structures also serves as delivery system for local acting biologically active substances, e.g., taste receptor agonist for distal enterocytes and the microbiota [103], and maturation agents for the immune system [104] which will be discussed below.

7. Pro-Inflammatory Effects of Refined Foods

The consumption of unrefined plant-based foods maintains host health by engaging the microbiota. The immunomodulatory effects of unrefined plant-based foods act through the host-microbiota symbiosis and circumvent the pro-inflammatory effects of refined foods. Mono- and disaccharides in a fibrous sustained release formulation do not produce significant increase in blood glucose because they are partially consumed by the microbiota. The microbiota unwraps molecules from the fibrous formulation in a time-consuming process. In contrast, industrial refinement causes a lack of molecular engagement with the microbiota and distal enterocytes, and polysaccharide molecules are rapidly monomerized and absorbed with the risk of elevated blood glucose levels [26].

Mounting epidemiological evidence suggests that intake of refined sugars and starch is associated with the development and maintenance of several diseases. T2D, for example, is driven by insulin resistance and β-cell dysfunction and manifested by increased risk and severity of hyperglycemic events. The condition is associated with elevated risk of autoimmune and inflammatory diseases, including rheumatoid arthritis [105] asthma [106], psoriasis [107], and cancer [108,109]. Drugs or dietary regiments that normalize hyperglycemia do not surprisingly have a therapeutic effect on immune diseases, e.g., psoriasis [110–112] and rheumatoid arthritis [113].

For diabetics as well as healthy individuals there is a relationship between the ingestion of refined sugars and the risk of developing both obesity [114] and autoimmune/inflammatory diseases, e.g., rheumatoid arthritis [115], asthma [116,117], IBD [118], chronic kidney disease [119], and atherosclerosis [114,120].

Hyperglycemia influences inflammation and immune function through multiple mechanisms. Chemical reactivity of glucose and other reducing sugars (fructose, mannose, galactose) towards proteins [121], lipids, and nucleic acids [122] is important. Non-specific stochastic protein glycations during incidents of hyperglycemia have the potential to initiate and potentiate several inflammatory and immunomodulatory responses, involving activation of pattern recognition receptors (PRR), e.g., RAGE (receptors for advanced glycation end-products) [123,124]. Also, hyperglycemia-induced cytokine release [125], formation of methylglyoxal and other auto-oxidation metabolites, e.g., reactive oxygen species (ROS) and free radicals [126] maintains inflammatory responses. The activity of auto-oxidation metabolites is prevented, for example, by antioxidants, which reduce the oxidative damage induced by glucose metabolites and ROS [127]. The fact that antioxidants are prevalent in plant-based food and synthesized by the microbiota [128] adds to the anti-inflammatory effects of unrefined foods.

8. Anti-Inflammatory Effects of Unrefined Foods

The anti-inflammatory effects of unrefined foods are particularly mediated by their contribution to a high gut biodiversity, which as mentioned above, contributes to the stability and resilience of the bacterial communities. In contrast, the loss of diversity can cause an imbalance between the inflammatory and the immunoregulatory taxa present in a given microbiota. The effects of a complex microbiotic community are ascribed to the additive and synergistic effects of the bacterial species in a microbiotic community. An example of this is monocolonization of a variety of organisms, which cannot reverse the hyper-IgE phenotype in germ-free (GF) mice. However, complex polycolonizations restore normal IgE levels [129].

Imbalances in immunological homeostasis can occur due to the loss of habitat-specific species and symbionts, resulting in an invasion of opportunistic species not normally able to colonize that specific habitat within the intestinal mucosa. Such a mismatch between species and habitat triggers a potentially pathogenic host response [130]. The detection of pathogens by the host is achieved through the families of PRR localized in the intestinal epithelium. PRR recognize conserved molecular structures known as microbe-associated molecular patterns and induce production of innate effector molecules [131,132]. The most well-known PRR are the toll-like receptors (TLR), RAGE, and the NOD-like receptors expressed on the intestinal epithelial cells. Activation of TLR by bacterial products promotes epithelial cell proliferation, secretion of IgA into the gut lumen, and expression of antimicrobial peptides, thereby establishing a microorganism-induced system of epithelial cell homeostasis and repair in the intestine [132].

Bacterial translocation, e.g., infiltration of lipopolysaccharide (LPS) through the intestinal barrier, can promote local and systemic immune responses via PRR. Monocolonization of GF mice by *Escherichia coli* is, for example, sufficient to induce macrophage infiltration, and polarization towards pro-inflammatory phenotype of immune cells in the adipose tissue [133], contributing to a state of low-grade inflammation in the adipose tissue. Disruption of intestinal barrier integrity by viable bacteria has been attributed to various intestinal inflammatory diseases such as IBD, celiac disease, irritable bowel syndrome, and colorectal cancer [32] as well as to diseases in extra-intestinal organs, such as the liver [134].

The major microbiota-derived SCFA, butyrate, acetate, and propionate are implicated in multiple anti-inflammatory mechanisms [135]. Besides being used by colonocytes as a source of ATP, SCFA can act as extracellular signaling molecules that activate cell-surface free fatty acids receptors (FFAR) (G-protein-coupled receptors (GPCR)) or inhibit histone deacetylases (HDAC) [136]. FFAR are differentially expressed on adipocytes, immune cells, and enteroendocrine L-cells. Depending on the location of the receptor and the amount and type of SCFA, the response can have multiple, variable downstream effects [3]. FFAR, expressed on immune cells, such as macrophages, dendritic cells, and neutrophils will upon activation by butyrate inhibit the release of pro-inflammatory cytokines, or stimulate differentiation of T regulatory (Treg) cells [136].

Activation of FFAR2/GPR43 by butyrate on enteroendocrine L-cells of the ileum and colon induces production and secretion of intestinal peptide YY (PYY), glucagon-like peptide 1 (GLP-1) [25,137]. An abundant production of SCFA can therefore indirectly regulate blood glucose levels via the insulinotropic effect of GLP-1 and induce satiety by the anorexigenic effect of PYY on the hypothalamus [138]. In addition, enteroendocrine cells in the duodenum are dependent on microbe-mediated mechanisms to express cholecystokinin (CKK), a gut peptide hormone responsible for stimulating fat absorption. GF mice have exhibited a reduced number of these cells with impact on their fat absorption [139].

SCFA can also act by inhibition of histone deacetylase (HDAC) activity. HDAC is related to a suppression of malignant transformation and a stimulation of apoptosis of precancerous colonic cells [140] as well as to the stimulation of epithelial production of retinoic acid (RA) [141]. RA is involved in many physiological processes, including regulation of IgA [142] and the polarization of specialized mucosal myeloid cells [143].

Specific phytonutrients entail several immunomodulatory functions. Some are mediated by a shift in microbiotic composition favoring the abundance of specific bacteria with health promoting effects or create occupancy resistance to enteric pathogens with pro-inflammatory potential [144]. Others are receptor-mediated, e.g., genistein, a flavonoid compound present in legumes, which can positively effect β-cell mass and mitigate T2D in mice [145,146].

In summary, the biodiversity of the microbiotic community is critical for both inter-microbiotic interactions and host-microbe engagements. In a healthy and proper fed microbiota the inflammatory and immunoregulatory species are in balance and the diverse bacterial communities act together to produce metabolites with direct effect on host health.

9. The Interaction between Food, Microbiota, and Host

In the sections above, we have discussed how ingestion of unrefined plant-based food structures implies that the host shares calories, saccharides, amino acids, fatty acids, and bioactive molecules with the microbiota, which in return shares SCFA, vitamins, antioxidants, and other biomolecules with the host. The microbiota also stimulates mucosal immune function upon ingesting an unrefined diet; a diverse microbiota will express a multitude of different antigens, thereby promoting intestinal bacterial recognition and shaping intestinal immune function.

In contrast, refined foods lack the fiber-encapsulation with the result that the host absorbs most nutrients in a microbiota-independent manner. Refined food is thus directly absorbed through the host GI mucosa without feeding the microbiota and without immunological engagement in the distal gut (Figure 3). Furthermore, when bypassing the microbiota, glucose is rapidly absorbed creating a risk of high blood glucose and associated pro-inflammatory effects.

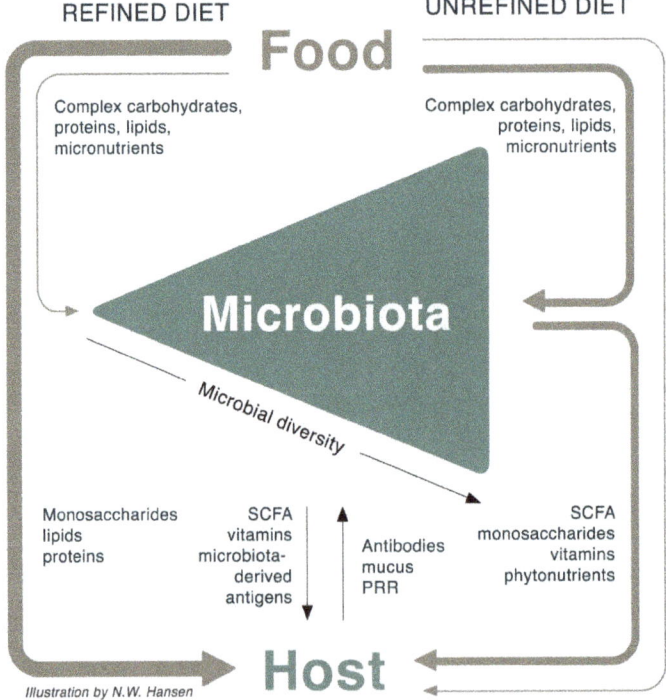

Figure 3. Schematic overview of interactions between food, microbiota, and host. Most of a refined diet bypasses the microbiota, providing a high nutrient bioavailability for the host. In contrast, unrefined, plant-based food structures provide a lower nutrient bioavailability for the host, using the difference to develop and maintain a healthy microbiota. The healthy microbiota provides short chain fatty acids (SCFA), antioxidants, and vitamins for the host along with direct immunomodulatory effects. The high monosaccharide bioavailability in refined foods introduces a risk of hyperglycemia, which cause numerous direct and indirect pro-inflammatory actions [26] (not shown in figure).

10. Implications for Nutritional Guidelines

The mechanisms summarized above underscore the need to consider the microbiota when evaluating human development, nutritional needs, physiological variations, and the impact of diet. Historically, the processing of foods occurred to increase the caloric bioavailability but given the growing prevalence of non-communicable diseases, insulin resistance, overweight, and obesity [147], it is obvious that current nutritional guidelines need to be revisited to re-establish the endogenous microbiota-induced health promotion. The current nutritional guidelines are mainly based on optimal molecular nutrient content for host metabolism, while establishment of synergies between food, host, and microbiotic community are absent.

Nutritional guidelines need to consider both the content and the structure of carbohydrates, because the microbiotic breakdown of carbohydrates strengthens our microbiotic ally in support of host health. Furthermore, it should also reflect that consumption of "fiber-formulated nutrients" is essential to maintain a healthy diverse microbiota to balance our nutritional, immunological, and metabolic health.

We have developed a simple tool to visualize healthy microbiota-engaging food choices (Figure 4). This tool divides foods into four categories depending on their carbohydrate content and the degree of refinement. Healthy, unrefined foods with low relative carbohydrate content (green box) should make up the plant-based bulk of an adult basic diet. These foods interact with the microbiota. Refined foods or foods with high relative carbohydrate content (yellow boxes) should be considered carbohydrate or energy supplementation, while the "comfort" foods in the red box, which are both refined and high in carbohydrate content, should be used sparingly considering their potentially negative health impact and their lack of microbiotic health promotion.

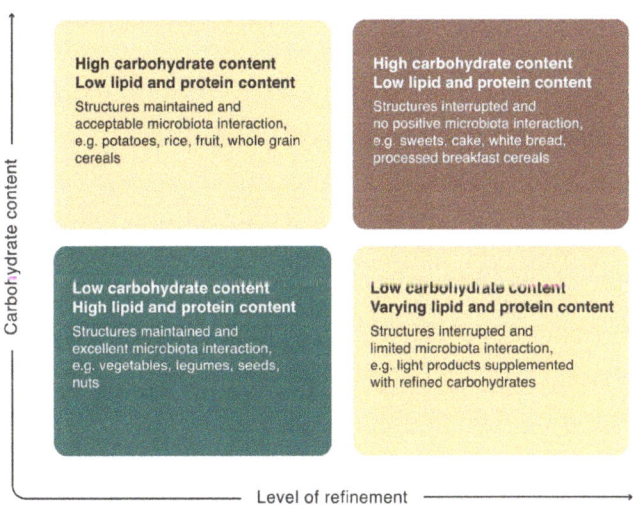

Figure 4. Novel classification of plant-based foods. Plant-based nutrition classified by microbiotic interaction potential and by the potential to induce hyperglycemia. The illustration classifies plant-based foods by the level of refinement and carbohydrate content. The green box represents basic foods for the habitual diet, interacting with our gut microbiota and providing both nutrients and bioactive molecules to microbiota and host. Foods from the green box are health promoting through interaction with the microbiota, and these foods introduce no risk of hyperglycemia. Foods from the green box should be combined to meet the needs for protein and lipid. Food from the yellow boxes can induce hyperglycemia in insulin resistant individuals or be consumed as energy supplementation for children and physically active individuals with a higher energy demand and a low risk of insulin resistance. The yellow square to the left positively interacts with the microbiota whereas the yellow square to the right only have limited microbiota interaction. The red box contains foods, which are high in carbohydrate content and highly refined, introducing the risk of high blood glucose to most people, not only insulin resistant individuals. The contents in the red box should be considered comfort foods with no health promoting effects and with a potential to compromise health.

11. Conclusions

The increasing prevalence of non-communicable diseases with an inflammatory component has led to the understanding of the gut microbiota as an intrinsic regulator of host immune responses. There is a growing awareness of the role of microbiotic communities, microbiota-derived products, and more particularly of the link between these components and disease states in humans. The ability to target immune pathways relies on the understanding of both acute and long-term impacts on the gut microbiota. The microbiotic communities can adapt to host diet in multiple ways by the interaction among different bacterial species, loss or proliferation of specific species, and by interaction with the host. Diet therefore presents itself as a microbiota-modulating factor and hence a health-modulating factor. A revision of the current nutritional guidelines considering both the molecular content and molecular structure of nutrients for insulin resistant and insulin sensitive individuals, could be valuable for the restoration of beneficial bacteria and microbiota diversity, enabling a shift from disease to health promoting states in the individual as well as in the general population.

Author Contributions: Conceptualization, A.S.; Writing-Original Draft Preparation, N.W.H and A.S; Writing-Review & Editing, N.W.H. and A.S.; Visualization, N.W.H and A.S.

Funding: This research received no external funding.

Acknowledgments: We are grateful to Anne Stæhr Johansen, PhD, for her editorial assistance.

Conflicts of Interest: The authors declare no conflict of interest.

References

1. Francino, M.P. Birth Mode-Related Differences in Gut Microbiota Colonization and Immune System Development. *Ann. Nutr. Metab.* **2018**, *73*, 12–16. [CrossRef] [PubMed]
2. Gill, S.R.; Pop, M.; DeBoy, R.T.; Eckburg, P.B.; Turnbaugh, P.J.; Samuel, B.S.; Gordon, J.I.; Relman, D.A.; Fraser-Liggett, C.M.; Nelson, K.E. Metagenomic Analysis of the Human Distal Gut Microbiome. *Science* **2006**, *312*, 1355–1359. [CrossRef] [PubMed]
3. Morrison, D.J.; Preston, T. Formation of short chain fatty acids by the gut microbiota and their impact on human metabolism. *Gut Microbes* **2016**, *7*, 189–200. [CrossRef] [PubMed]
4. Ivanov, I.I.; Atarashi, K.; Manel, N.; Brodie, E.L.; Shima, T.; Karaoz, U.; Wei, D.; Goldfarb, K.C.; Santee, C.A.; Lynch, S.V.; et al. Induction of Intestinal Th17 Cells by Segmented Filamentous Bacteria. *Cell* **2009**, *139*, 485–498. [CrossRef] [PubMed]
5. Ivanov, I.I.; Frutos Rde, L.; Manel, N.; Yoshinaga, K.; Rifkin, D.B.; Sartor, R.B.; Finlay, B.B.; Littman, D.R. Specific microbiota direct the differentiation of IL-17-producing T-helper cells in the mucosa of the small intestine. *Cell. Host Microbe* **2008**, *4*, 337–349. [CrossRef] [PubMed]
6. Rossi, M.; Amaretti, A.; Raimondi, S. Folate Production by Probiotic Bacteria. *Nutrients* **2011**, *3*, 118–134. [CrossRef] [PubMed]
7. LeBlanc, J.G.; Milani, C.; de Giori, G.S.; Sesma, F.; van Sinderen, D.; Ventura, M. Bacteria as vitamin suppliers to their host: A gut microbiota perspective. *Curr. Opin. Biotechnol.* **2013**, *24*, 160–168. [CrossRef] [PubMed]
8. Shimada, Y.; Kinoshita, M.; Harada, K.; Mizutani, M.; Masahata, K.; Kayama, H.; Takeda, K. Commensal bacteria-dependent indole production enhances epithelial barrier function in the colon. *PLoS ONE* **2013**, *8*, e80604. [CrossRef] [PubMed]
9. Bansal, T.; Alaniz, R.C.; Wood, T.K.; Jayaraman, A. The bacterial signal indole increases epithelial-cell tight-junction resistance and attenuates indicators of inflammation. *Proc. Natl. Acad. Sci. USA* **2010**, *107*, 228–233. [CrossRef] [PubMed]
10. Cotillard, A.; Kennedy, S.P.; Kong, L.C.; Prifti, E.; Pons, N.; Le Chatelier, E.; Almeida, M.; Quinquis, B.; Levenez, F.; Galleron, N. Dietary intervention impact on gut microbial gene richness. *Nature* **2013**, *500*, 585–588. [CrossRef] [PubMed]
11. Le Chatelier, E.; Nielsen, T.; Qin, J.J.; Prifti, E.; Hildebrand, F.; Falony, G.; Almeida, M.; Arumugam, M.; Batto, J.M.; Kennedy, S. Richness of human gut microbiome correlates with metabolic markers. *Nature* **2013**, *500*, 541–546. [CrossRef] [PubMed]

12. Koropatkin, N.M.; Cameron, E.A.; Martens, E.C. How glycan metabolism shapes the human gut microbiota. *Nat. Rev. Microbiol.* **2012**, *10*, 323–335. [CrossRef] [PubMed]
13. Falony, G.; De Vuyst, L. *Prebiotics and Probiotics Science and Technology*; Springer: New York, NY, USA, 2009; pp. 639–679.
14. Keegstra, K. Plant cell walls. *Plant. Physiol.* **2010**, *154*, 483–486. [CrossRef] [PubMed]
15. De Filippo, C.; Cavalieri, D.; Di Paola, M.; Ramazzotti, M.; Poullet, J.B.; Massart, S.; Collini, S.; Pieraccini, G.; Lionetti, P. Impact of diet in shaping gut microbiota revealed by a comparative study in children from Europe and rural Africa. *Proc. Natl. Acad. Sci. USA* **2010**, *107*, 14691–14696. [CrossRef] [PubMed]
16. David, L.A.; Maurice, C.F.; Carmody, R.N.; Gootenberg, D.B.; Button, J.E.; Wolfe, B.E.; Ling, A.V.; Devlin, A.S.; Varma, Y.; Fischbach, M.A. Diet rapidly and reproducibly alters the human gut microbiome. *Nature* **2014**, *505*, 559–563. [CrossRef] [PubMed]
17. Clemente, J.C.; Ursell, L.K.; Parfrey, L.W.; Knight, R. The Impact of the Gut Microbiota on Human Health: An Integrative View. *Cell* **2012**, *148*, 1258–1270. [CrossRef] [PubMed]
18. Tojo, R.; Suárez, A.; Clemente, M.G.; de los Reyes-Gavilán, C.G.; Margolles, A.; Gueimonde, M.; Ruas-Madiedo, P. Intestinal microbiota in health and disease: Role of bifidobacteria in gut homeostasis. *World J. Gastroenterol.* **2014**, *20*, 15163–15176. [CrossRef] [PubMed]
19. Marchesi, J.R.; Adams, D.H.; Fava, F.; Hermes, G.D.A.; Hirschfield, G.M.; Hold, G.; Quraishi, M.N.; Kinross, J.; Smidt, H.; Tuohy, K.M. The gut microbiota and host health: A new clinical frontier. *Gut* **2016**, *65*, 330–339. [CrossRef] [PubMed]
20. Bottacini, F.; Ventura, M.; Sinderen, D.; Motherway, M. Diversity, ecology and intestinal function of bifidobacteria. *Microb. Cell. Fact.* **2014**, *13*, S4. [CrossRef] [PubMed]
21. Wells, J.M. Immunomodulatory mechanisms of lactobacilli. *Microb. Cell. Fact.* **2011**, *10*, S17. [CrossRef] [PubMed]
22. El Kaoutari, A.; Armougom, F.; Gordon, J.I.; Raoult, D.; Henrissat, B. The abundance and variety of carbohydrate-active enzymes in the human gut microbiota. *Nat. Rev. Microbiol.* **2013**, *11*, 497–504. [CrossRef] [PubMed]
23. Bach Knudsen, K.E. Microbial Degradation of Whole-Grain Complex Carbohydrates and Impact on Short-Chain Fatty Acids and Health. *Adv. Nutr.* **2015**, *6*, 206–213. [CrossRef] [PubMed]
24. Maslowski, K.M.; Vieira, A.T.; Ng, A.; Kranich, J.; Sierro, F.; Yu, D.; Schilter, H.C.; Rolph, M.S.; Mackay, F.; Artis, D. Regulation of inflammatory responses by gut microbiota and chemoattractant receptor GPR43. *Nature* **2009**, *461*, 1282–1286. [CrossRef] [PubMed]
25. Tolhurst, G.; Heffron, H.; Lam, Y.S.; Parker, H.E.; Habib, A.M.; Diakogiannaki, E.; Cameron, J.; Grosse, J.; Reimann, F.; Gribble, F.M. Short-chain fatty acids stimulate glucagon-like peptide-1 secretion via the G-protein-coupled receptor FFAR2. *Diabetes* **2012**, *61*, 364–371. [CrossRef] [PubMed]
26. Hansen, N.W.; Hansen, A.J.; Sams, A. The endothelial border to health: Mechanistic evidence of the hyperglycemic culprit of inflammatory disease acceleration. *IUBMB Life* **2017**, *69*, 148–161. [CrossRef] [PubMed]
27. Bischoff, S.C.; Barbara, G.; Buurman, W.; Ockhuizen, T.; Schulzke, J.D.; Serino, M.; Tilg, H.; Watson, A.; Wells, J.M. Intestinal permeability—A new target for disease prevention and therapy. *BMC Gastroenterol.* **2014**, *14*, 189. [CrossRef] [PubMed]
28. Ley, R.E.; Turnbaugh, P.J.; Klein, S.; Gordon, J.I. Microbial ecology: Human gut microbes associated with obesity. *Nature* **2006**, *444*, 1022–1023. [CrossRef] [PubMed]
29. Ley, R.E.; Bäckhed, F.; Turnbaugh, P.; Lozupone, C.A.; Knight, R.D.; Gordon, J.I. Obesity alters gut microbial ecology. *Proc. Natl. Acad. Sci. USA* **2005**, *102*, 11070–11075. [CrossRef] [PubMed]
30. Tang, W.H.W.; Kitai, T.; Hazen, S.L. Gut Microbiota in Cardiovascular Health and Disease. *Circ. Res.* **2017**, *120*, 1183–1196. [CrossRef] [PubMed]
31. Serino, M.; Blasco-Baque, V.; Nicolas, S.; Burcelin, R. Managing the manager: Gut microbes, stem cells and metabolism. *Diabetes Metab.* **2014**, *40*, 186–190. [CrossRef] [PubMed]
32. Kang, M.; Martin, A. Microbiome and colorectal cancer: Unraveling host-microbiota interactions in colitis-associated colorectal cancer development. *Semin. Immunol.* **2017**, *32*, 3–13. [CrossRef] [PubMed]

33. Gardner, C.D.; Trepanowski, J.F.; Del Gobbo, L.C.; Hauser, M.E.; Rigdon, J.; Ioannidis, J.P.A.; Desai, M.; King, A.C. Effect of Low-Fat vs Low-Carbohydrate Diet on 12-Month Weight Loss in Overweight Adults and the Association With Genotype Pattern or Insulin Secretion: The DIETFITS Randomized Clinical Trial. *JAMA* **2018**, *319*, 667–679. [CrossRef] [PubMed]
34. Hjorth, M.F.; Ritz, C.; Blaak, E.E.; Saris, W.H.; Langin, D.; Poulsen, S.K.; Larsen, T.M.; Sørensen, T.I.; Zohar, Y.; Astrup, A. Pretreatment fasting plasma glucose and insulin modify dietary weight loss success: Results from 3 randomized clinical trials. *Am. J. Clin. Nutr.* **2017**, *106*, 499–505. [CrossRef] [PubMed]
35. Brouns, F. Overweight and diabetes prevention: Is a low-carbohydrate-high-fat diet recommendable? *Eur. J. Nutr.* **2018**, *57*, 1301–1312. [CrossRef] [PubMed]
36. Dhital, S.; Warren, F.J.; Butterworth, P.J.; Ellis, P.R.; Gidley, M.J. Mechanisms of starch digestion by α-amylase—Structural basis for kinetic properties. *Crit. Rev. Food Sci. Nutr.* **2017**, *57*, 875–892. [CrossRef] [PubMed]
37. Englyst, H.N.; Kingman, S.M.; Cummings, J.H. Classification and measurement of nutritionally important starch fractions. *Eur. J. Clin. Nutr.* **1992**, *46*, S33–S50. [PubMed]
38. Fry, S.C. Primary Cell Wall Metabolism: Tracking the Careers of Wall Polymers in Living Plant. Source *New Phytol.* **2004**, *161*, 641–675. [CrossRef]
39. Preiss, J. Plant starch synthesis. In *Starch Food*, 2nd ed.; Woodhead Publishing: Sawston, Cambridge, UK, 2018; pp. 3–95.
40. Roberfroid, M.B. Introducing inulin-type fructans. *Br. J. Nutr.* **2005**, *93*, S13–S25. [CrossRef] [PubMed]
41. Gibson, G.R.; Scott, K.P.; Rastall, R.A.; Tuohy, K.M.; Hotchkiss, A.; Dubert-Ferrandon, A.; Gareau, M.; Murphy, E.F.; Saulnier, D.; Loh, G. Dietary prebiotics: Current status and new definition. *Food Sci. Technol. Bull. Funct. Foods* **2010**, *7*, 1–19. [CrossRef]
42. Scott, K.P.; Martin, J.C.; Duncan, S.H.; Flint, H.J. Prebiotic stimulation of human colonic butyrate-producing bacteria and bifidobacteria, in vitro. *FEMS Microbiol. Ecol.* **2014**, *87*, 30–40. [CrossRef] [PubMed]
43. Alberts, B.; Johnson, A.; Lewis, J.; Raff, M.; Roberts, K.; Walter, P. The Plant Cell Wall. In *Molecular Biology of the Cell*, 4th ed.; Garland Science: New York, NY, USA, 2002.
44. Somerville, C. Cellulose Synthesis in Higher Plants. *Annu. Rev. Cell. Dev. Biol.* **2006**, *22*, 53–78. [CrossRef] [PubMed]
45. Rose, J.K.C.; Lee, S.J. Straying off the highway: Trafficking of secreted plant proteins and complexity in the plant cell wall proteome. *Plant. Physiol.* **2010**, *153*, 433–436. [CrossRef] [PubMed]
46. Weber, N.; Taylor, D.C.; Underhill, E.W. Biosynthesis of storage lipids in plant cell and embryo cultures. *Adv. Biochem. Eng. Biotechnol.* **1992**, *45*, 99–131. [PubMed]
47. Bagchi, M.; Patel, S.; Zafra-Stone, S.; Bagchi, D. Selected herbal supplements and nutraceuticals. In *Reproductive and Developmental Toxicology*; Academic Press: Cambridge, UK, 2011; pp. 385–393.
48. Tremaroli, V.; Bäckhed, F. Functional interactions between the gut microbiota and host metabolism. *Nature* **2012**, *489*, 242–249. [CrossRef] [PubMed]
49. Turnbaugh, P.J.; Hamady, M.; Yatsunenko, T.; Cantarel, B.L.; Duncan, A.; Ley, R.E.; Sogin, M.L.; Jones, W.J.; Roe, B.A.; Affourtit, J.P. A core gut microbiome in obese and lean twins. *Nature* **2009**, *457*, 480–484. [CrossRef] [PubMed]
50. Koliada, A.; Syzenko, G.; Moseiko, V.; Budovska, L.; Puchkov, K.; Perederiy, V.; Gavalko, Y.; Dorofeyev, A.; Romanenko, M.; Tkach, S. Association between body mass index and Firmicutes/Bacteroidetes ratio in an adult Ukrainian population. *BMC Microbiol.* **2017**, *17*, 120. [CrossRef] [PubMed]
51. Louis, P.; Young, P.; Holtrop, G.; Flint, H.J. Diversity of human colonic butyrate-producing bacteria revealed by analysis of the butyryl-CoA:acetate CoA-transferase gene. *Environ. Microbiol.* **2010**, *12*, 304–314. [CrossRef] [PubMed]
52. InterAct Consortium. Dietary fibre and incidence of type 2 diabetes in eight European countries: The EPIC-InterAct Study and a meta-analysis of prospective studies. *Diabetologia* **2015**, *58*, 1394–1408. [CrossRef] [PubMed]
53. Du, H.; van der, A.D.L.; Boshuizen, H.C.; Forouhi, N.G.; Wareham, N.J.; Halkjaer, J.; Tjønneland, A.; Overvad, K.; Jakobsen, M.U.; Boeing, H.; et al. Dietary fiber and subsequent changes in body weight and waist circumference in European men and women. *Am. J. Clin. Nutr.* **2010**, *91*, 329–336. [CrossRef] [PubMed]
54. Sivaprakasam, S.; Prasad, P.D.; Singh, N. Benefits of short-chain fatty acids and their receptors in inflammation and carcinogenesis. *Pharmacol. Ther.* **2016**, *164*, 144–151. [CrossRef] [PubMed]

55. Hjorth, M.F.; Blædel, T.; Bendtsen, L.Q.; Lorenzen, J.K.; Holm, J.B.; Kiilerich, P.; Roager, H.M.; Kristiansen, K.; Larsen, L.H.; Astrup, A. Prevotella-to-Bacteroides ratio predicts body weight and fat loss success on 24-week diets varying in macronutrient composition and dietary fiber: Results from a post-hoc analysis. *Int. J. Obes.* **2018**. [CrossRef] [PubMed]
56. Chen, T.T.; Long, W.M.; Zhang, C.H.; Liu, S.; Zhao, L.P.; Hamaker, B.R. Fiber-utilizing capacity varies in Prevotella- versus Bacteroides-dominated gut microbiota. *Sci. Rep.* **2017**, *7*, 2594. [CrossRef] [PubMed]
57. Wu, G.D.; Chen, J.; Hoffmann, C.; Bittinger, K.; Chen, Y.Y.; Keilbaugh, S.A.; Bewtra, M.; Knights, D.; Walters, W.A.; Knight, R. Linking long-term dietary patterns with gut microbial enterotypes. *Science* **2011**, *334*, 105–108. [CrossRef] [PubMed]
58. De Moraes, A.C.F.; Fernandes, G.R.; da Silva, I.T.; Almeida-Pititto, B.; Gomes, E.P.; Pereira, A.D.; Ferreira, S.R.G. Enterotype May Drive the Dietary-Associated Cardiometabolic Risk Factors. *Front. Cell. Infect. Microbiol.* **2017**, *7*, 47. [CrossRef] [PubMed]
59. Arumugam, M.; Raes, J.; Pelletier, E.; Le Paslier, D.; Yamada, T.; Mende, D.R.; Fernandes, G.R.; Tap, J.; Bruls, T.; Batto, J.M.; et al. Enterotypes of the human gut microbiome. *Nature* **2011**, *473*, 174–180. [CrossRef] [PubMed]
60. Han, J.-L.; Lin, H.-L. Intestinal microbiota and type 2 diabetes: From mechanism insights to therapeutic perspective. *World J. Gastroenterol.* **2014**, *20*, 17737–17745. [CrossRef] [PubMed]
61. Korpela, K. Diet, Microbiota, and Metabolic Health: Trade-Off Between Saccharolytic and Proteolytic Fermentation. *Annu. Rev. Food Sci. Technol.* **2018**, *9*, 65–84. [CrossRef] [PubMed]
62. Seth, E.C.; Taga, M.E. Nutrient cross-feeding in the microbial world. *Front. Microbiol.* **2014**, *5*, 350. [CrossRef] [PubMed]
63. Loreau, M. Biodiversity and Ecosystem Functioning: Current Knowledge and Future Challenges. *Science* **2001**, *294*, 804–808. [CrossRef] [PubMed]
64. Wright, E.M. The Intestinal Na$^+$/Glucose Cotransporter. *Annu. Rev. Physiol.* **1993**, *55*, 575–589. [CrossRef] [PubMed]
65. Helliwell, P.A.; Richardson, M.; Affleck, J.; Kellett, G.L. Regulation of GLUT5, GLUT2 and intestinal brush-border fructose absorption by the extracellular signal-regulated kinase, p38 mitogen-activated kinase and phosphatidylinositol 3-kinase intracellular signalling pathways: Implications for adaptation to diabetes. *Biochem. J.* **2000**, *350*, 163–169. [PubMed]
66. Burant, C.F.; Takeda, J.; Brot-Laroche, E.; Bell, G.I.; Davidson, N.O. Fructose transporter in human spermatozoa and small intestine is GLUT5. *J. Biol. Chem.* **1992**, *267*, 14523–14526. [PubMed]
67. Miyamoto, K. Differential responses of intestinal glucose transporter mRNA transcripts to levels of dietary sugars. *Biochem. J.* **1993**, *295*, 211–215. [CrossRef] [PubMed]
68. Röder, P.V. The role of SGLT1 and GLUT2 in intestinal glucose transport and sensing. *PLoS ONE* **2014**, *9*, e89977. [CrossRef] [PubMed]
69. Ferraris, R.P. Dietary and developmental regulation of intestinal sugar transport. *Biochem. J.* **2001**, *360*, 265–276. [CrossRef] [PubMed]
70. Gouyon, F. Simple-sugar meals target GLUT2 at enterocyte apical membranes to improve sugar absorption: A study in GLUT2-null mice. *J. Physiol.* **2003**, *552*, 823–832. [CrossRef] [PubMed]
71. Pfannkuche, H.; Gäbel, G. Glucose, epithelium, and enteric nervous system: Dialogue in the dark. *J. Anim. Physiol. Anim. Nutr.* **2009**, *93*, 277–286. [CrossRef] [PubMed]
72. Ferraris, R.P.; Choe, J.-Y.; Patel, C.R. Intestinal Absorption of Fructose. *Annu. Rev. Nutr.* **2018**, *38*, 41–67. [CrossRef] [PubMed]
73. Jones, H.F.; Butler, R.N.; Brooks, D.A. Intestinal fructose transport and malabsorption in humans. *Am. J. Physiol. Gastrointest. Liver Physiol.* **2011**, *2*, 202–206. [CrossRef] [PubMed]
74. Douard, V.; Ferraris, R.P. Regulation of the fructose transporter GLUT5 in health and disease. *Am. J. Physiol. Endocrinol. Metab.* **2008**, *295*, 227–237. [CrossRef] [PubMed]
75. Deal, R.A.; Tang, Y.; Fletcher, R.; Torquati, A.; Omotosho, P. Understanding intestinal glucose transporter expression in obese compared to non-obese subjects. *Surg. Endosc.* **2018**, *32*, 1755–1761. [CrossRef] [PubMed]
76. Pettolino, F.A.; Walsh, C.; Fincher, G.B.; Bacic, A. Determining the polysaccharide composition of plant cell walls. *Nat. Protoc.* **2012**, *7*, 1590–1607. [CrossRef] [PubMed]
77. Valent, B.S.; Albersheim, P. The structure of plant cell walls: On the binding of xyloglucan to cellulose fibers. *Plant. Physiol.* **1974**, *54*, 105–108. [CrossRef] [PubMed]

78. Cummings, J.H. Cellulose and the human gut. *Gut* **1984**, *25*, 805–810. [CrossRef] [PubMed]
79. Meibohm, B.; Derendorf, H. Basic concepts of pharmacokinetic/pharmacodynamic (PK/PD) modelling. *Int. J. Clin. Pharmacol. Ther.* **1997**, *35*, 401–413. [PubMed]
80. Ayorinde, J.; Odeniyi, M.; Balogun-Agbaje, O. Formulation and Evaluation of Oral Dissolving Films of Amlodipine Besylate Using Blends of Starches With Hydroxypropyl Methyl Cellulose. *Polym. Med.* **2016**, *46*, 45–51. [CrossRef] [PubMed]
81. Karrout, Y. In vivo efficacy of microbiota-sensitive coatings for colon targeting: A promising tool for IBD therapy. *J. Control. Release* **2015**, *197*, 121–130. [CrossRef] [PubMed]
82. Chourasia, M.K.; Jain, S.K. Pharmaceutical approaches to colon targeted drug delivery systems. *J. Pharm. Pharm. Sci.* **2003**, *6*, 33–66. [PubMed]
83. Alcantara, C.; Zuniga, M. Proteomic and transcriptomic analysis of the response to bile stress of Lactobacillus casei BL23. *Microbiology* **2012**, *158*, 1206–1218. [CrossRef] [PubMed]
84. Moodley, C.; Reid, S.J.; Abratt, V.R. Molecular characterisation of ABC-type multidrug efflux systems in Bifidobacterium longum. *Anaerobe* **2015**, *32*, 63–69. [CrossRef] [PubMed]
85. Valero, T. Mitochondrial biogenesis: Pharmacological approaches. *Curr. Pharm. Des.* **2014**, *20*, 5507–5509. [CrossRef] [PubMed]
86. Martín, R.; Martín, C.; Escobedo, S.; Suárez, J.E.; Quirós, L.M. Surface glycosaminoglycans mediate adherence between HeLa cells and Lactobacillus salivarius Lv72. *BMC Microbiol.* **2013**, *13*. [CrossRef] [PubMed]
87. Neis, E.; Dejong, C.; Rensen, S. The Role of Microbial Amino Acid Metabolism in Host Metabolism. *Nutrients* **2015**, *7*, 2930–2946. [CrossRef] [PubMed]
88. Grześkowiak, Ł. The effect of growth media and physical treatments on the adhesion properties of canine probiotics. *J. Appl. Microbiol.* **2013**, *115*, 539–545. [CrossRef] [PubMed]
89. Arakawa, K. Lactobacillus gasseri requires peptides, not proteins or free amino acids, for growth in milk. *J. Dairy Sci.* **2015**, *98*, 1593–1603. [CrossRef] [PubMed]
90. Robitaille, G.; Champagne, C.P. Growth-promoting effects of pepsin- and trypsin-treated caseinomacropeptide from bovine milk on probiotics. *J. Dairy Res.* **2014**, *81*, 319–324. [CrossRef] [PubMed]
91. Ito, T.; Sekizuka, T.; Kishi, N.; Yamashita, A.; Kuroda, M. Conventional culture methods with commercially available media unveil the presence of novel culturable bacteria. *Gut Microbes* **2018**, *17*, 1–15. [CrossRef] [PubMed]
92. Elhenawy, W.; Debelyy, M.O.; Feldman, M.F. Preferential packing of acidic glycosidases and proteases into Bacteroides outer membrane vesicles. *mBio* **2014**, *5*, e00909-14. [CrossRef] [PubMed]
93. Gandhi, A.; Shah, N.P. Cell growth and proteolytic activity of Lactobacillus acidophilus, Lactobacillus helveticus, Lactobacillus delbrueckii ssp. bulgaricus, and Streptococcus thermophilus in milk as affected by supplementation with peptide fractions. *Int. J. Food Sci. Nutr.* **2014**, *65*, 937–941. [CrossRef] [PubMed]
94. Nemoto, T.K. Identification of a new subtype of dipeptidyl peptidase 11 and a third group of the S46-family members specifically present in the genus Bacteroides. *Biochimie* **2018**, *147*, 25–35. [CrossRef] [PubMed]
95. Sabljić, I. Crystal structure of dipeptidyl peptidase III from the human gut symbiont Bacteroides thetaiotaomicron. *PLoS ONE* **2017**, *12*, e0187295. [CrossRef] [PubMed]
96. Zhang, Q. Vildagliptin increases butyrate-producing bacteria in the gut of diabetic rats. *PLoS ONE* **2017**, *12*, e0184735. [CrossRef] [PubMed]
97. Meyer, H.W. Extensive Resection of Small and Large Intestine: A Further Twenty-Two Year Follow-Up Report. *Ann. Surg.* **1962**, *168*, 287–289. [CrossRef]
98. Garai, P.; Chandra, K.; Chakravortty, D. Bacterial peptide transporters: Messengers of nutrition to virulence. *Virulence* **2017**, *8*, 297–309. [CrossRef] [PubMed]
99. Steiner, H.Y.; Naider, F.; Becker, J.M. The PTR family: A new group of peptide transporters. *Mol. Microbiol.* **1995**, *16*, 825–834. [CrossRef] [PubMed]
100. Paulsen, I.T.; Skurray, R.A. The POT family of transport proteins. *Trends Biochem. Sci.* **1994**, *19*, 404. [CrossRef]
101. DiRusso, C.C.; Black, P.N. Long-chain fatty acid transport in bacteria and yeast. Paradigms for defining the mechanism underlying this protein-mediated process. *Mol. Cell. Biochem.* **1999**, *192*, 41–52. [CrossRef] [PubMed]
102. Dirusso, C.C.; Black, P.N. Bacterial long chain fatty acid transport: Gateway to a fatty acid-responsive signaling system. *J. Biol. Chem.* **2004**, *279*, 49563–49566. [CrossRef] [PubMed]

103. Englyst, H.N.; Hay, S.; Macfarlane, G.T. Polysaccharide breakdown by mixed populations of human faecal bacteria. *FEMS Microbiol. Lett.* **1987**, *45*, 163–171. [CrossRef]
104. Round, J.L.; Palm, N.W. Causal effects of the microbiota on immune-mediated diseases. *Sci. Immunol.* **2018**, *20*, 1603. [CrossRef] [PubMed]
105. Lu, M.C.; Yan, S.T.; Yin, W.Y.; Koo, M.; Lai, N.-S. Risk of rheumatoid arthritis in patients with type 2 diabetes: A nationwide population-based case-control study. *PLoS ONE* **2014**, *7*, e101528. [CrossRef] [PubMed]
106. Ehrlich, S.F.; Quesenberry, C.P.; Van Den Eeden, S.K.; Shan, J.; Ferrara, A. Patients Diagnosed With Diabetes Are at Increased Risk for Asthma, Chronic Obstructive Pulmonary Disease, Pulmonary Fibrosis, and Pneumonia but Not Lung Cancer. *Diabetes Care* **2010**, *33*, 55–60. [CrossRef] [PubMed]
107. Lønnberg, A.S. Association of Psoriasis With the Risk for Type 2 Diabetes Mellitus and Obesity. *JAMA Dermatology* **2016**, *57*, 645–659. [CrossRef] [PubMed]
108. Wojciechowska, J.; Krajewski, W.; Bolanowski, M.; Kręcicki, T.; Zatoński, T. Diabetes and Cancer: A Review of Current Knowledge. *Exp. Clin. Endocrinol. Diabetes* **2016**, *124*, 263–275. [CrossRef] [PubMed]
109. Holden, S.E. Diabetes and Cancer. *Endocr. Dev.* **2016**, *31*, 135–145. [PubMed]
110. Faurschou, A. Improvement in psoriasis after treatment with the glucagon-like peptide-1 receptor agonist liraglutide. *Acta Diabetol.* **2014**, *51*, 147–150. [CrossRef] [PubMed]
111. Al-Badri, M.R.; Azar, S.T. Effect of glucagon-like peptide-1 receptor agonists in patients with psoriasis. *Ther. Adv. Endocrinol. Metab.* **2014**, *5*, 34–38. [CrossRef] [PubMed]
112. Ahern, T. Glucagon-like peptide-1 analogue therapy for psoriasis patients with obesity and type 2 diabetes: A prospective cohort study. *J. Eur. Acad. Dermatol. Venereol.* **2013**, *27*, 1440–1443. [CrossRef] [PubMed]
113. Schwartz, A.V. Diabetes, bone and glucose-lowering agents: Clinical outcomes. *Diabetologia* **2017**, *7*, 1170–1179. [CrossRef] [PubMed]
114. Malik, V.S.; Popkin, B.M.; Bray, G.A.; Després, J.P.; Hu, F.B. Sugar-Sweetened Beverages, Obesity, Type 2 Diabetes Mellitus, and Cardiovascular Disease Risk. *Circulation* **2010**, *121*, 1356–1364. [CrossRef] [PubMed]
115. Kim, S.C.; Schneeweiss, S.; Glynn, R.J.; Doherty, M.; Goldfine, A.B.; Solomon, D.H. Dipeptidyl peptidase-4 inhibitors in type 2 diabetes may reduce the risk of autoimmune diseases: A population-based cohort study. *Ann. Rheum. Dis.* **2015**, *74*, 1968–1975. [CrossRef] [PubMed]
116. Shi, Z. Association between soft drink consumption and asthma and chronic obstructive pulmonary disease among adults in Australia. *Respirology* **2012**, *17*, 363–369. [CrossRef] [PubMed]
117. DeChristopher, L.R.; Uribarri, J.; Tucker, K.L. Intakes of apple juice, fruit drinks and soda are associated with prevalent asthma in US children aged 2-9 years. *Public Health Nutr.* **2016**, *19*, 123–130. [CrossRef] [PubMed]
118. Legaki, E.; Gazouli, M. Influence of environmental factors in the development of inflammatory bowel diseases. *World J. Gastrointest. Pharmacol. Ther.* **2016**, *7*, 112–125. [CrossRef] [PubMed]
119. Bomback, A.S.; Derebail, V.K.; Shoham, D.A.; Anderson, C.A.; Steffen, L.M.; Rosamond, W.D.K.A. Sugar-sweetened soda consumption, hyperuricemia, and kidney disease. *Kidney Int.* **2012**, *77*, 609–616. [CrossRef] [PubMed]
120. De Koning, L. Sweetened beverage consumption, incident coronary heart disease, and biomarkers of risk in men. *Circulation* **2012**, *125*, 1735–1741. [CrossRef] [PubMed]
121. Bunn, H.F.; Higgins, P.J. Reaction of monosaccharides with proteins: Possible evolutionary significance. *Science* **1981**, *213*, 222–224. [CrossRef] [PubMed]
122. Ahmed, N. Advanced glycation endproducts—Role in pathology of diabetic complications. *Diabetes Res. Clin. Pract.* **2005**, *67*, 3–21. [CrossRef] [PubMed]
123. Ramasamy, R.; Yan, S.F.; Schmidt, A.M. The diverse ligand repertoire of the receptor for advanced glycation endproducts and pathways to the complications of diabetes. *Vascul. Pharmacol.* **2012**, *57*, 160–167. [CrossRef] [PubMed]
124. Chen, Y.-S.; Yan, W.; Geczy, C.L.; Brown, M.A.; Thomas, R. Serum levels of soluble receptor for advanced glycation end products and of S100 proteins are associated with inflammatory, autoantibody, and classical risk markers of joint and vascular damage in rheumatoid arthritis. *Arthritis Res. Ther.* **2009**, *11*, 39. [CrossRef] [PubMed]
125. Rao, R.; Sen, S.; Han, B.; Ramadoss, S.; Chaudhuri, G. Gestational diabetes, preeclampsia and cytokine release: Similarities and differences in endothelial cell function. *Adv. Exp. Med. Biol.* **2014**, *814*, 69–75. [PubMed]

126. Dornadula, S.; Elango, B.; Balashanmugam, P.; Palanisamy, R.; Kunka Mohanram, R. Pathophysiological insights of methylglyoxal induced type-2 diabetes. *Chem. Res. Toxicol.* **2015**, *28*, 1666–1674. [CrossRef] [PubMed]
127. Wu, L.; Juurlink, B.H.J. Increased Methylglyoxal and Oxidative Stress in Hypertensive Rat Vascular Smooth Muscle Cells. *Hypertension* **2002**, *39*, 809–814. [CrossRef] [PubMed]
128. Cardona, F.; Andrés-Lacueva, C.; Tulipani, S.; Tinahones, F.J.; Queipo-Ortuño, M.I. Benefits of polyphenols on gut microbiota and implications in human health. *J. Nutr. Biochem.* **2013**, *24*, 1415–1422. [CrossRef] [PubMed]
129. Cahenzli, J.; Köller, Y.; Wyss, M.; Geuking, M.B.; McCoy, K.D. Intestinal microbial diversity during early-life colonization shapes long-term IgE levels. *Cell. Host Microbe* **2013**, *14*, 559–570. [CrossRef] [PubMed]
130. Palm, N.W.; de Zoete, M.R.; Flavell, R.A. Immune-microbiota interactions in health and disease. *Clin. Immunol.* **2015**, *159*, 122–127. [CrossRef] [PubMed]
131. Williams, A.; Flavell, R.A.; Eisenbarth, S.C. The role of NOD-like Receptors in shaping adaptive immunity. *Curr. Opin. Immunol.* **2010**, *22*, 34–40. [CrossRef] [PubMed]
132. Abreu, M.T. Toll-like receptor signalling in the intestinal epithelium: How bacterial recognition shapes intestinal function. *Nat. Rev. Immunol.* **2010**, *10*, 131–144. [CrossRef] [PubMed]
133. Caesar, R. Gut-derived lipopolysaccharide augments adipose macrophage accumulation but is not essential for impaired glucose or insulin tolerance in mice. *Gut* **2012**, *61*, 1701–1707. [CrossRef] [PubMed]
134. Fouts, D.E.; Torralba, M.; Nelson, K.E.; Brenner, D.A.; Schnabl, B. Bacterial translocation and changes in the intestinal microbiome in mouse models of liver disease. *J. Hepatol.* **2012**, *56*, 1283–1292. [CrossRef] [PubMed]
135. Tan, J. The Role of Short-Chain Fatty Acids in Health and Disease. *Adv. Immunol.* **2014**, *121*, 91–119. [PubMed]
136. Corrêa-Oliveira, R.; Fachi, J.L.; Vieira, A.; Sato, F.T.; Vinolo, M.A.R. Regulation of immune cell function by short-chain fatty acids. *Clin. Transl. Immunol.* **2016**, *5*, e73. [CrossRef] [PubMed]
137. Remely, M. Effects of short chain fatty acid producing bacteria on epigenetic regulation of FFAR3 in type 2 diabetes and obesity. *Gene* **2014**, *537*, 85–92. [CrossRef] [PubMed]
138. Jandhyala, S.M. Role of the normal gut microbiota. *World J. Gastroenterol.* **2015**, *21*, 8787–8803. [CrossRef] [PubMed]
139. Duca, F.A.; Swartz, T.D.; Sakar, Y.; Covasa, M. Increased oral detection, but decreased intestinal signaling for fats in mice lacking gut microbiota. *PLoS ONE* **2012**, *7*, e39748. [CrossRef] [PubMed]
140. Waldecker, M.; Kautenburger, T.; Daumann, H.; Busch, C.; Schrenk, D. Inhibition of histone-deacetylase activity by short-chain fatty acids and some polyphenol metabolites formed in the colon. *J. Nutr. Biochem.* **2008**, *19*, 587–593. [CrossRef] [PubMed]
141. Schilderink, R. The SCFA butyrate stimulates the epithelial production of retinoic acid via inhibition of epithelial HDAC. *Am. J. Physiol. Liver Physiol.* **2016**, *310*, G1138–G1146. [CrossRef] [PubMed]
142. Fagarasan, S.; Honjo, T. Intestinal IgA synthesis: Regulation of front-line body defences. *Nat. Rev. Immunol.* **2003**, *3*, 63–72. [CrossRef] [PubMed]
143. Schey, R.; Danzer, C.; Mattner, J. Perturbations of mucosal homeostasis through interactions of intestinal microbes with myeloid cells. *Immunobiology* **2015**, *220*, 227–235. [CrossRef] [PubMed]
144. Wlodarska, M.; Willing, B.P.; Bravo, D.M.; Finlay, B.B. Phytonutrient diet supplementation promotes beneficial Clostridia species and intestinal mucus secretion resulting in protection against enteric infection. *Sci. Rep.* **2015**, *5*, 9253. [CrossRef] [PubMed]
145. Luo, J. Phytonutrient genistein is a survival factor for pancreatic β-cells via GPR30-mediated mechanism. *J. Nutr. Biochem.* **2018**, *58*, 59–70. [CrossRef] [PubMed]
146. Fu, Z. Genistein Induces Pancreatic β-Cell Proliferation through Activation of Multiple Signaling Pathways and Prevents Insulin-Deficient Diabetes in Mice. *Endocrinology* **2010**, *151*, 3026–3037. [CrossRef] [PubMed]
147. WHO (World Health Organization). *Mortality and Burden of Disease Attributable to Selected Major Risks*; WHO: Geneva, Switzerland, 2009.

© 2018 by the authors. Licensee MDPI, Basel, Switzerland. This article is an open access article distributed under the terms and conditions of the Creative Commons Attribution (CC BY) license (http://creativecommons.org/licenses/by/4.0/).

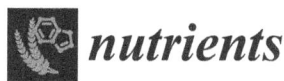

Review

Glutamine: Metabolism and Immune Function, Supplementation and Clinical Translation

Vinicius Cruzat [1,2,*], Marcelo Macedo Rogero [3], Kevin Noel Keane [1], Rui Curi [4] and Philip Newsholme [1,*]

1. School of Pharmacy and Biomedical Sciences, Curtin Health Innovation Research Institute, Biosciences, Curtin University, Perth 6102, Australia; Kevin.Keane@curtin.edu.au
2. Faculty of Health, Torrens University, Melbourne 3065, Australia
3. Department of Nutrition, Faculty of Public Health, University of São Paulo, Avenida Doutor Arnaldo 715, São Paulo 01246-904, Brazil; mmrogero@usp.br
4. Interdisciplinary Post-Graduate Program in Health Sciences, Cruzeiro do Sul University, São Paulo 01506-000, Brazil; ruicuri59@gmail.com
* Correspondence: Vinicius.cruzat@laureate.edu.au (V.C.); Philip.newsholme@curtin.edu.au (P.N.)

Received: 23 September 2018; Accepted: 16 October 2018; Published: 23 October 2018

Abstract: Glutamine is the most abundant and versatile amino acid in the body. In health and disease, the rate of glutamine consumption by immune cells is similar or greater than glucose. For instance, in vitro and in vivo studies have determined that glutamine is an essential nutrient for lymphocyte proliferation and cytokine production, macrophage phagocytic plus secretory activities, and neutrophil bacterial killing. Glutamine release to the circulation and availability is mainly controlled by key metabolic organs, such as the gut, liver, and skeletal muscles. During catabolic/hypercatabolic situations glutamine can become essential for metabolic function, but its availability may be compromised due to the impairment of homeostasis in the inter-tissue metabolism of amino acids. For this reason, glutamine is currently part of clinical nutrition supplementation protocols and/or recommended for immune suppressed individuals. However, in a wide range of catabolic/hypercatabolic situations (e.g., ill/critically ill, post-trauma, sepsis, exhausted athletes), it is currently difficult to determine whether glutamine supplementation (oral/enteral or parenteral) should be recommended based on the amino acid plasma/bloodstream concentration (also known as glutaminemia). Although the beneficial immune-based effects of glutamine supplementation are already established, many questions and evidence for positive in vivo outcomes still remain to be presented. Therefore, this paper provides an integrated review of how glutamine metabolism in key organs is important to cells of the immune system. We also discuss glutamine metabolism and action, and important issues related to the effects of glutamine supplementation in catabolic situations.

Keywords: nutrition; amino acids; leukocytes; skeletal muscle; gut; liver

1. Introduction

At the most basic level, amino acids are the building blocks of proteins in our cells and tissues, and after water are the second most abundant compound in mammals. Amino acids can be obtained from endogenous and/or exogenous (i.e., diet) proteins, and their availability is of fundamental importance for cell survival, maintenance, and proliferation. Mammals, in particular, have developed biochemical and metabolic pathways to control pathogen infection by increasing amino acid catabolism to aid immune responses, thus restricting the availability of nitrogen-containing nutrients to invading microorganisms [1]. This evolutionary mechanism also becomes advantageous for the host to control its own inflammatory responses to infections.

Among the 20 amino acids detailed in the genetic code, glutamine provides the best example of the versatility of amino acid metabolism and immune function. Glutamine is the most abundant and versatile amino acid in the body, and is of fundamental importance to intermediary metabolism, interorgan nitrogen exchange via ammonia (NH_3) transport between tissues, and pH homeostasis. In almost every cell, glutamine can be used as a substrate for nucleotide synthesis (purines, pyrimidines, and amino sugars), nicotinamide adenine dinucleotide phosphate (NADPH), antioxidants, and many other biosynthetic pathways involved in the maintenance of cellular integrity and function [2–4].

Most cells in the body function with a constant turnover and/or supply of nutrients, however, cells of the immune system frequently have to function under nutrient restricted microenvironments [1]. Although glucose is a vital metabolite, and the main fuel for a large number of cells in the body, cells of the immune system, such as lymphocytes, neutrophils, and macrophages, utilize glutamine at high rates similar to or greater than glucose under catabolic conditions, such as sepsis, recovery from burns or surgery, and malnutrition, as well as high intensity/volume physical exercise [5,6]. This theory was first experimentally confirmed in the 1980's by the laboratory of Eric Newsholme (1935–2011, widely accepted now as the origin of hypotheses and evidence for the concept of "immunometabolism") [3,7] in the University of Oxford, and subsequently by many other laboratories worldwide [4,8,9]. For this reason, glutamine is considered as a "fuel for the immune system", where a low blood concentration may impair immune cell function, resulting in poor clinical outcomes and increased risk of mortality [10].

Currently, glutamine is routinely supplied as a component of clinical nutrition supplementation for pre-and post-operative patients, and also for many elite athletes to restore immune functions. Although there is a growing evidence in support of the immune mediating effects of glutamine supplementation, several questions and specific considerations still remain. Therefore, the aim of the present study is to provide an integrated review on how glutamine metabolism in key organs, such as the gut, liver, and skeletal muscles, is important to cells of the immune system. These key organs control glutamine availability and shed light on important considerations in regards to glutaminemia (glutamine concentration into the bloodstream). The immune-enhancing properties and related paradigms of glutamine supplementation in health and disease are also discussed herein.

2. A Brief Overview of Glutamine Metabolism

Glutamine is an L-α-amino acid containing five carbons; its molecular weight is 146.15 kDa and its elemental composition comprises carbon (41.09%), hydrogen (6.90%), oxygen (32.84%), and nitrogen (19.17%). With respect to its physiological pH, glutamine is classified as a neutral amino acid, whereas it is nutritionally classified as a non-essential amino acid. Glutamine has two amino groups, namely the α-amino group and the easily-hydrolysable side-chain amide group, and these features enable the role played by glutamine as a nitrogen transporter and NH_3 carrier. Glutamine is also a proteinogenic amino acid, i.e., amino acids that are incorporated into proteins, and accounts for 5 to 6% of bound amino acids [9].

Healthy individuals weighing about 70 kg have approximately 70 to 80 g of glutamine distributed in the whole body [11]. Using isotopic and pharmacokinetic techniques, it has been estimated that glutamine endogenous production is between 40 to 80 g/day [12,13]. In plasma obtained from blood samples, glutamine concentration varies between ~500 to 800 µM/L (values recorded after 12-h in a fasting state), which represents about 20% of the total free amino acids pool in the blood [9]. In tissues, such as the liver and the skeletal muscles, glutamine concentration is even higher than in plasma, representing about 40% to 60% of the total amino acid pool [14,15]. In both, plasma and tissues, glutamine concentration is 10- to 100-fold in excess of any other amino acid, and for this reason, glutamine is considered the body's most abundant amino acid.

In the whole body, glutamine concentration and availability depends on the balance between its synthesis and/or release, and uptake by human organs and tissues. The lungs, liver, brain, skeletal muscles, and adipose tissue have organ tissue-specific glutamine synthesis activity. On the other hand, primarily glutamine-consuming tissues, such as the intestinal mucosa, leukocytes, and renal tubule cells, have high glutaminase activity and cofactors capable of degrading glutamine. However, the liver may become a glutamine-consuming site, and tissues, such as muscle tissue, may present reduced glutamine synthesis under certain conditions, such as reduced carbohydrate [16] and/or amino acid [17] intake, high catabolic situations, and/or diseases and stress [5]. Many other factors—mainly glucocorticoids [18], thyroid hormones [19], growth hormone [20], and insulin [21]—can modulate the activity performed by glutamine metabolism-regulating enzymes.

Several enzymes are involved in glutamine metabolism; the two main intracellular enzymes are glutamine synthetase (GS, EC 6.3.1.2) and phosphate-dependent glutaminase (GLS, EC 3.5.1.2). GS is responsible for triggering the reaction that synthesizes glutamine from ammonium ion (NH_{4+}), and glutamate through ATP consumption, whereas GLS is responsible for glutamine hydrolysis, which converts it into glutamate and NH_{4+} again [22,23] (Figure 1). With respect to the intracellular location, GS is primarily found in the cytosol, whereas GLS (in its active form) is mainly found within the mitochondria. These locations are compatible with the enzymes' functions: GS produces glutamine for the synthesis of cytoplasmic proteins and nucleotides, whereas GLS catalyses glutamine conversion to glutamate as an important step to the tricarboxylic acid cycle (TCA, also known as the Krebs cycle) entry at 2-oxoglutarate as an energy source or source of metabolic intermediates [3].

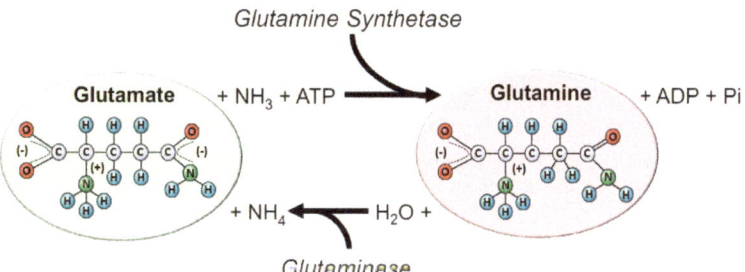

Figure 1. Glutamine synthesis and hydrolysis. Glutamine is mainly synthesized by the enzyme glutamine synthetase (GS) and hydrolysed by the enzyme, glutaminase (GLS). GS catalyses glutamine biosynthesis using glutamate and ammonia (NH_3) as a source. In this reaction, one ATP is consumed. Glutamate can be donated by many amino acids obtained exogenously (i.e., diet) and/or from endogenous amino acids' catabolism. On the other hand, GLS is responsible for glutamine hydrolysis to glutamate and ammonium ion (NH_4). Almost all cells in the body express GS and GLS, and their predominant expression and activity will dictate if the tissue is more likely to produce or consume glutamine in health and disease.

Glutamine synthesis by the GS depends on glutamate availability. Glutamate, in turn, is synthesized from 2-oxoglutarate NH_4, through the action of the glutamate dehydrogenase, or even from the catabolism of other amino acids, such as branched-chain amino acids (BCAAs), mainly leucine [17,24]. Studies conducted with rats reported that BCAAs, such as leucine, can be almost exclusively transaminated with α-ketoglutarate to form glutamate, which in turn can incorporate free NH_3 and under the action of GS form glutamine [6,24] (Figure 2).

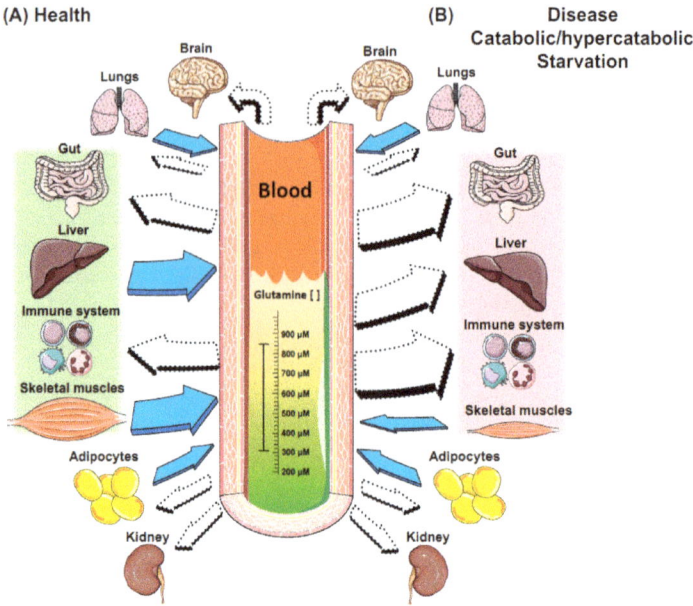

Figure 2. Intertissue glutamine production and utilisation in health and catabolic/hypercatabolic situations. Filled arrows indicate tissues that exhibit GS activity and thus produce glutamine; white arrows indicate tissues that exhibit GLS activity, and thus consume glutamine. In health and/or fed states, glutamine stores are in equilibrium in plasma/bloodstream and tissues, and are maintained constantly mainly by the liver and skeletal muscles, two major stores of glutamine in the body. On the other hand, cells of the immune system are extremely dependent on glucose and glutamine in situation (**A**), and even more in situation (**B**). Although the gut is a major site of glutamine consumption, in situation (**B**), there is a dramatic increase in glutamine consumption from both the luminal and basolateral membrane, when compared to situation (**A**). In addition, the liver switches the role of a major producer to a major glutamine consumer to maintain gluconeogenesis, and the whole body relies on the skeletal muscle's ability/stores to maintain glutamine levels. However, this process is usually accompanied by a dramatic increase in muscle proteolysis, atrophy, and cachexia. The lungs and adipose tissue exhibit both GS and GLS enzymes, and hence can produce and consume glutamine in situations (**A**) and (**B**). The brain and the kidneys do not exhibit GS, only GLS, and hence are mainly dependent on plasma glutamine availability in situations (**A**) and (**B**).

Glutamine tissue and blood concentrations are dependent on GS or GLS activities. Endogenous glutamine synthesis does not meet the human body's demands in catabolic conditions, such as in cancer [25], sepsis [4,26], infections [27,28], surgeries [8], traumas [10], as well as during intense and prolonged physical exercise [29,30]. Glutamine assumes the role of a conditionally essential amino acid in such deficiency conditions by promoting a concomitant increase in GLS expression and inhibiting the GS action [14]. However, it is worth emphasizing that, although plasma glutamine concentration is reduced from its normal concentration (i.e., 500–800 µmol/L) to 300–400 µmol/L, cells depending on this amino acid, such as immune cells, are in fact poorly influenced in terms of proliferation and function [6]. On the other hand, the high tissue catabolism leads to reduced glutamine stock in human tissues, mainly in the muscle and liver (Figure 3). The low glutamine concentration in human tissues affects the whole body since this amino acid provides nitrogen atoms to the synthesis of purines, pyrimidines, and amino sugars [31]. If the high glutamine degradation in these tissues persists, a large number of metabolic pathways and mechanisms that depend on glutamine availability are affected, resulting in immunosuppression. More recently, studies reported that bacterial infections (e.g., *Escherichia coli*) can alter its metabolism and harness glutamine to suppress the effects of acid stress and copper toxicity [32]. Hence, bacterial pathogens can adapt and survive by altering core metabolic pathways important for host-imposed antibacterial strategies.

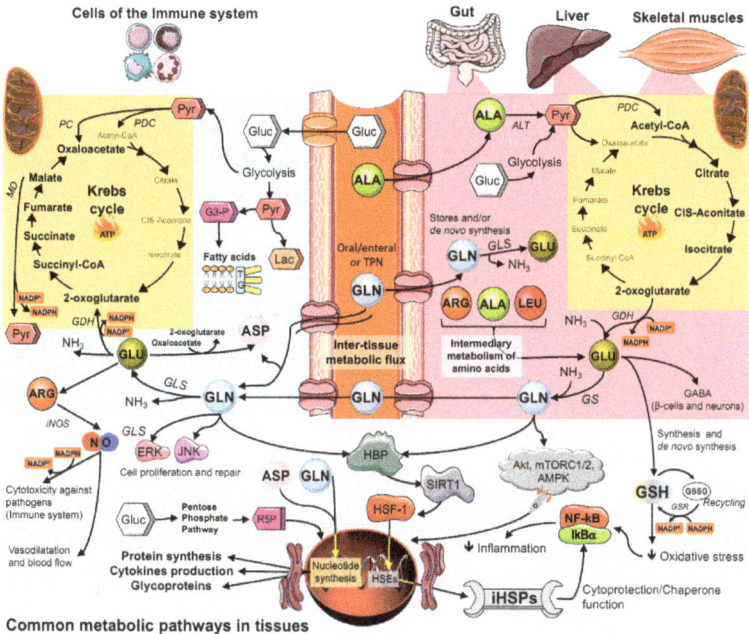

Figure 3. Glutamine inter-tissue metabolic flux starting in skeletal muscle, liver, and gut continues in the immune cells. Abbreviations: Glutamine, GLN; glutamate, GLU; aspartate, ASP; arginine, ARG; leucine, LEU; alanine, ALA; glucose, Gluc; pyruvate, Pyr; pyruvate dehydrogenase; PDC; pyruvate carboxylase, PC; malate dehydrogenase, MD; glyceraldehyde-3-Phosphate, G3-P; lactate, Lac; triacylglycerol, TG; ribose 5-phosphate, R5P; alanine aminotransferase, ALT; glutamate dehydrogenase, GDH; glutamine synthetase, GS; glutaminase, GLS; inducible nitric oxide synthase, iNOS; intracellular heat shock protein, iHSP; heat Shock Factor 1, HSF-1; heat shock elements, HSEs; sirtuin 1, SIRT1; hexosamine biosynthetic pathway, HBP; ammonia, NH_3; glutathione, GSH; oxidized GSH, GSSG; glutathione S-reductase, GSR; protein kinase B, Akt; AMP-activated protein kinase, AMPK; mTOR complex 1 and 2, mTORC1/2, extracellular signal-regulated kinases, ERK; c-Jun N-terminal kinases, JNK; gamma-Aminobutyric acid, GABA.

3. Key Metabolic Organs in Glutamine Homeostasis

3.1. The Gut

Both the small and large intestines are capable of metabolizing large amounts of glutamine supplied by both the diet and/or the bloodstream [33,34]. Glutamine for the gut is quantitatively more relevant than glucose as an energy substrate. For example, in the enterocytes, the glutamine carbon can be metabolized by two main pathways, namely: (i) By forming delta^1-pyrroline-5-carboxylate; (ii) or by conversion to alpha-ketoglutarate as an intermediary in the Krebs cycle. The first pathway enables the formation of proline, ornithine, and citrulline from glutamine carbon by using approximately 10% of the amino acid concentration found in the intestine. Another 10–15% of glutamine is incorporated into the tissue protein; the highest proportion of it (approximately 75%) is metabolized in the Krebs cycle for energy production purposes [14,35].

The glutamine hydrolysis into glutamate, which is catalysed by GLS, corresponds to the first reaction resulting from glutamine consumption [36]. Although the gut is the major site of glutamine consumption, glutamine concentration in the intestinal tissue is low. This is due to the high GLS activity (3–6 µmol/hour/mg of protein), and also high GLS affinity for the substrate, glutamine. Interestingly, there is a correlation between the presence of GSL and the use of glutamine by certain cell types. Almost all GLS found in the intestinal cells is bound to the mitochondrial membrane. The modulation of GLS activity in the intestinal tissue is important to maintain the tissue integrity and enable adequate absorption of nutrients, as well as to prevent bacterial translocation into the bloodstream (i.e., septicaemia) [37]. Prolonged fasting and malnutrition states are associated with reduced GLS activity; on the other hand, GLS activity increases in the postprandial period, after the administration of enteral feeding of branched-chain amino acids and/or L-alanyl-L-glutamine [38].

The ATP-ubiquitin-dependent proteolytic pathway associated with proteasome is known to degrade endogenous short-lived or abnormal proteins/peptides, as well as participating in the regulation of the inflammatory response. The ATP-ubiquitin-dependent proteolytic pathway could be important for the turnover of gut mucosal proteins, which are very short lived. Indeed, the nuclear factor of kappa light polypeptide gene enhancer in B-cells inhibitor (IκB) ubiquitinylation allows the nuclear factor kappa-light-chain-enhancer of activated B cells' (NF-κB) translocation in the nucleus, and thus transcription of proinflammatory genes [17,39,40] (Figure 3). Glutamine stimulates protein synthesis and reduces ubiquitin-dependent proteolysis in the enterocyte since this amino acid reduces ubiquitin gene expression. Glutamine can increase the gene expression of the arginine-succinate synthase enzyme in Caco-2 cells (human colon epithelial-line cell). Glutamine activates the extracellular signal-regulated kinases (ERKs) and the c-Jun N-terminal kinases (JNK) in the enterocyte, and it leads to significant increase in c-Jun gene expression and in the activity of the transcription factor known as activator protein 1 (AP-1) [41,42]. Such glutamine action potentiates the effects of growth factors on cell proliferation and repair. Heat shock (43 °C) induces intestinal epithelial cell death, which can be exacerbated due to the lack of glutamine. However, as it happens with muscle tissues, glutamine supplementation enables a dose-dependent reduction in heat shock-associated cell death. This effect of glutamine partly results from the amino acid capacity of increasing the gene expression of HSP 70 [37].

Dysregulation of cytokine production plays a major role in the pathogenesis of inflammatory bowel disease (IBD). The gut mucosa of patients with IBD (Crohn's disease or ulcerative colitis) has been reported to produce high amounts of proinflammatory cytokines, such as interleukin (IL-)1β, IL-6, IL-8, and tumour necrosis factor-alpha (TNF-α), in contrast to a less marked increase in the production of anti-inflammatory cytokines, such as IL-10. For example, Coeffier, et al. [43] verified that glutamine reduces pro-inflammatory cytokine production by human intestinal mucosa, probably by a posttranscriptional pathway. Glutamine could be useful to modulate inflammatory conditions with imbalanced cytokine production.

3.2. Skeletal Muscles

The body's glutamine availability and metabolism are directly associated with the skeletal muscle tissue. Skeletal muscles are quantitatively the most relevant site of glutamine stock, synthesis, and release despite the relatively-low GS enzyme activity per muscle tissue-unit mass [11]. Thus, skeletal muscles play a fundamental role in glutamine metabolism, since it is one of the most abundant tissues found in the human body [44]. The intramuscular glutamine content corresponds to 50–60% of the total free amino acids found in the skeletal muscle tissue. Approximately 80% of the body glutamine is found in the skeletal muscle, and this concentration is 30 times higher than that recorded for human plasma [45,46]. The free amino acid concentrations in the muscle tissue depend on the muscle fiber type. Studies conducted in the skeletal muscle of rats showed that glutamine concentration was three times higher in slow-twitch muscle fibers (type 1 fibers) than in fast-twitch muscle fibers (type 2 fibers). High glutamine concentration in slow-twitch muscle fibers is due to the high GS enzyme activity and ATP availability for glutamine synthesis [47].

Hormones, such as insulin and insulin-like growth factors (IGFs), stimulate glutamine transport into the intracellular environment, whereas glucocorticoids stimulate glutamine release into the extracellular space. The transmembrane gradient for glutamine through the skeletal muscle is high, a fact that restricts amino acid diffusion through the cell membrane. Glutamine is actively transported into cells through a sodium-dependent channel system, whose outcome is a consumption of ATP. The glutamine transport through the muscle cell membrane is faster than the transport of all other amino acids [48]. Interestingly, the constant maintenance of glutamine availability in the intracellular fluid, as well as the high glutamine concentration gradient across the cell membrane, is supported by many pathways, such as the transport system affinity for the amino acid, its intracellular turnover ratio and the extracellular supply, the intra- and extracellular sodium concentrations, and the influence of other amino acids competing for carrier molecules [49,50].

During the post-absorptive state, approximately 50% of the glutamine synthesis in the skeletal muscle takes place through glutamate uptake from the bloodstream, a fact that characterizes part of the glutamine-glutamate cycle. In addition, muscle protein catabolism directly produces glutamine, although it also leads to BCAAs, glutamate, aspartate, and asparagine release. The carbon skeletons of these amino acids are used for glutamine de novo synthesis [51,52]. Glutamine and alanine correspond, respectively, to 48% and 32% of the amino acids released by the skeletal muscle in the post-absorptive state; the glutamine containing two nitrogen atoms per molecule is the main muscle nitrogen-release source. The glutamine and alanine exchange rates exceed their abundance in the body, and their occurrence in the muscle protein corresponds to 10–15%, thus indicating the constant need of glutamine and alanine de novo synthesis in the skeletal muscle [4]. The glutamine synthesis rate in the skeletal muscle (approximately 50 mmol/h) is higher than that recorded for any other amino acid. Thus, glutamine and alanine should result from the interconversion of amino acids within the cell, in a process that depends on the cell metabolic conditions, which are affected by human nutritional and hormonal status, as well as by physical exercise [53,54].

One of the first studies about muscle glutamine metabolism in catabolic situations has recorded that reduced glutamine concentration in the skeletal muscle is associated with the reduced survival rate of sepsis-state patients. The severe muscle glutamine-concentration decrease in critically-ill patients (80% reduction, on average, in the normal concentration due to protein degradation) is accompanied by increased glutamine synthesis and release from the skeletal muscle. It happens because of the increased messenger RNA (mRNA) and GS enzyme activity in the skeletal muscle during severe catabolic states. Glucocorticoids may increase the amount of GS mRNA in the muscle tissue through a glucocorticoid receptor-dependent process that happens in the cytosol. Once the glucocorticoid is bound to its cytosolic receptor they are translocated to the nucleus, where they bind to regions containing glucocorticoid-response elements, which induce GS gene transcription, among others [55,56].

Although the GS activity increases in response to physiological stress, the protein amount may not increase in parallel to that of the mRNA, thus indicating the activation of post-transcriptional control mechanisms. Thus, the activity of the aforementioned enzyme appears to be controlled through the intracellular glutamine concentration by means of a post-transcriptional control mechanism, which increases the GS enzyme activity when the intracellular glutamine concentration decreases. However, the GS enzyme is relatively unstable in the presence of glutamine; therefore, the increased intracellular glutamine concentration leads to faster GS degradation. In addition, glucocorticoids and intracellular glutamine depletion work synergistically by increasing the GS expression in the skeletal muscle [57].

In vitro studies conducted with several cell types demonstrated that glutamine can also change the gene expression of contractile proteins. According to one study, cardiomyocyte growth and maturation were accompanied by increased mRNA contents in proteins, such as alpha-myosin heavy-chain (α-MHC) and alpha-actin; both parameters were considered non-pathologic hypertrophy [58]. Other studies highlight the relevant role played by glutamine in mediating the activation of pathways, such as the mammalian target of rapamycin (mTOR), which is considered an essential tissue size and mass regulator, either in healthy or ill patients. In fact, the use of amino acids, mainly of leucine, as anabolic inducers in muscle cells has its action compromised via mTOR when glutamine is not available [17]. Despite the essential role played by glutamine in regulating the expression of muscle content-associated genes, there are no in vivo studies supporting the hypothesis that supplementation applied alone can promote muscle mass increase.

Another significant role played by glutamine is associated with its capacity of modulating protective and resistance responses to injuries, which are also known as antioxidant and cytoprotective effects. The high oxidative stress generated in catabolism situations results in several effects that culminate in pro-apoptotic stimuli through classic pathways, such as that of the NF-κB. Reactive oxygen species (ROS), both the radical and the non-radical species, react to minerals, to phospholipid membranes, and to proteins, among other relevant compounds, to cellular homeostasis [59]. Glutamine can modulate the expression of heat shock proteins (HSP). According to a study conducted with acutely-inflamed mice (subjected to endotoxemia, which is a sepsis model), the increased glutamine availability in the animals' tissues helped to keep the HSP expression, mainly in the 70 (the most abundant form), 90, and 27 kDa family. Results concerning skeletal and liver muscles were recorded at protein and gene expression levels. In addition, other genes were highly responsive to glutamine, such as the heat shock factor 1 (HSF-1), which is important for HSP synthesis, and enzymes linked to the antioxidant system (Figure 3). The glutamate resulting from glutamine is an essential substrate for glutathione synthesis, a fact that changes the expression of genes, such as glutathione S-reductase (GSR) and glutathione peroxidase 1 (GPx1). The glutamine cytoprotective and antioxidant properties may be particularly important in high catabolism situations, in which the activity and the expression of inflammatory pathways mediated by NF-κB are modulated [4,39].

3.3. The Liver

The liver is highly metabolic and has many functions, including the detoxification of blood constituents arriving from the digestive tract, production of bile to aid digestion, metabolism of carbohydrates, lipids, proteins, and drugs, blood pH balance, synthesis of plasma proteins, and the storage and synthesis of glycogen and lipids. As indicated already, glutamine is an important precursor for the generation of other metabolites, such as amino acids (glutamate), TCA components (α-ketoglutarate), and nucleotides (AMP, purines, and pyrimidines), along with the activation of the chaperone function (mediated by HSP response) and antioxidant defence (mediated by glutathione, GSH). Therefore, glutamine is crucial for energy metabolism and proliferation of hepatocytes in the liver. In addition, glutamine is an important precursor for gluconeogenesis, the process of glucose production from other non-carbohydrate constituents, which is a central metabolic pathway in the liver that allows maintenance of blood glucose levels in fasting and starvation conditions following depletion of glycogen stores. During severe illness, the skeletal muscle is the major supplier of glutamine, while the liver is a major consumer [28,60]. This consumption supports many of the liver activities listed above, but as a key amino acid involved in nitrogen metabolism, the uptake of glutamine in liver hepatocytes regulates the activity of the urea cycle due to its conversion to glutamate NH_3 by GLS [61]. Consequently, the liver regulates blood pH and the detoxification of NH_3 via the urea cycle using glutamine.

NH_3 and NH_4^+ are toxic metabolic remnants of amino acid catabolism, and blood delivered to the liver from the gut is rich in NH_3/NH_4^+. In hepatocyte mitochondria, the reaction of NH_3 with ATP and the bicarbonate ion (HCO_3^-) leads to the formation of carbamoyl phosphate (CP) by CP synthetase (CPS), a key intermediate in the urea cycle. Under the action of ornithine transcarbamylase, ornithine reacts with CP to form citrulline. This subsequently undergoes various biochemical reactions forming arginine, fumarate, and, ultimately, urea, which is excreted from the hepatocyte cytosol into the blood. In the final urea-forming reaction, ornithine is regenerated to allow the cyclic continuation of the urea cycle with additional NH_3. Importantly, glutamine concentrations in the mitochondria regulate flux through CP generation. High glutamine levels increase glutamate and NH_3 through GLS activity, with the NH_3 reacting with ornithine to form CP. NH_3 is also a co-activator of GLS in the liver [62,63], and since liver GLS is not inhibited by glutamate [61,64], the glutamate produced can form N-acetylglutamate, which is an activator of both GLS and CPS [65,66]. Consequently, both of these biochemical mechanisms result in a high flux toward urea formation due to the elevated levels of NH_3 in the mitochondrial (sourced from digestive tract blood and glutamine degradation), the high affinity of CPS for NH_3, and the increased activity of GLS. However, the ultimate generation of urea appears to be regulated by the sub-cellular level of glutamine and, consequently, its uptake from the extracellular environment.

The intra-, inter-, and extracellular transport of glutamine in hepatocytes is central to the conversion of the NH_3/NH_4^+ to urea, its subsequent excretion, and blood pH balance due to effects on HCO_3^-. The liver architecture is exquisitely designed such that periportal hepatocytes (near the portal vein) receiving blood and nutrients from the gut are primarily responsible for urea production using glutamine as outlined above. However, the distal hepatocytes near the hepatic vein (perivenous), utilise any remaining NH_4^+ from the blood, including that bypassing the periportal hepatocytes, for the re-synthesis and secretion of glutamine into the circulation. In this latter scenario, the NH_3/NH_4^+ enters the perivenous hepatocytes and, using glutamate as a substrate, glutamine is generated by GS. This process scavenges any NH_3/NH_4^+ escaping the periportal process, while also replenishing the glutamine that was used by periportal hepatocytes in the generation of urea and disposal of nitrogen. The different functional regions of the liver were illustrated by the expression status of glutamine-metabolizing enzymes, such that high levels of GLS were found in the portal region [67,68], while only 7% of hepatocytes expressed GS, and these were found specifically around the central hepatic veins [69].

The intercellular or liver compartmentalized cycling of glutamine between these liver regions is also mediated by specific membrane transporters in periportal and perivenous hepatocytes. These transport systems also control intra- and extracellular pH by the antiport translocation of H^+ on the entry of Na^+ and glutamine. Glutamine from the diet is taken up by periportal hepatocytes along with two Na^+ ions, while one H^+ is extruded in the opposite direction from the hepatocyte into the extracellular space. This process is driven by the concentrations of glutamine and Na^+ outside the cell (i.e., in the blood), and also the intracellular concentration of H^+. In essence, this directional transport is also regulated by the relative pH difference between the intracellular and extracellular space, such that periportal hepatic glutamine uptake leads to extracellular acidification and intracellular alkalization, while glutamine export from perivenous hepatocytes leads to intracellular acidification and extracellular alkalization [61]. Experiments in perfused rat livers have shown that a slight alkali increase in extracellular pH (0.4 units) can enhance mitochondrial import of glutamine into hepatocytes, as H^+ is transported externally to possibly reduce extracellular pH and maintain equilibrium. Mitochondrial glutamine concentration increased to about 15–50 mM, while the extracellular (0.6 mM) and cytosolic (6 mM) glutamine concentrations remain unchanged in these perfusion models [70,71]. Therefore, the regulation and flux through GLS in periportal hepatocytes are regulated by the sub-cellular concentration of glutamine, and not just the rate of glutamine entry from extracellular sources. For perivenous hepatocytes, the synthesis and release of glutamine to the blood is facilitated by the increased cytoplasmic, and lower extracellular concentration of glutamine, along with the less acidic intracellular environment, which is countered by the antiport cytosolic influx of H^+ [61].

Importantly, glutamine importation and exportation also affect osmotic balance and therefore influences hepatocyte volume. This has additional consequences for hepatic function, including bile synthesis and release [72], but also regulates anabolic processes, such as glycogen, lipid, and protein synthesis [61]. Largely, glutamine uptake enhances hepatocyte cell swelling and hydration [73], which leads to increased glycogen and fatty acid synthesis [74,75], and reduced proteolysis mediated by P38 mitogen-activated protein kinases (p38 MAPK) signalling [76]. Other amino acids, such as glycine and alanine, along with anabolic hormones, such as insulin, promoted hepatocyte swelling, leading to increased biosynthetic processes [77], while catabolic hormones, like glucagon, reduced intracellular glutamine levels induced hepatocyte shrinkage [78]. Consequently, dehydration due to reduced intracellular glutamine levels is characterized by decreased cell volume, initiation of the catabolic process, and insulin-resistant conditions, and it was recently shown that hypertonic infusion can cause glucose dysregulation in humans [79].

The liver is an insulin-sensitive organ and like skeletal muscle, is responsible for glucose disposal via glycogen synthesis. Development of insulin resistance and subsequent glucotoxic conditions can progress to chronic disorders, such as non-alcoholic fatty liver disease (NAFLD), characterized by excessive lipid accumulation, and non-alcoholic steatohepatitis (NASH), characterized by increased extracellular matrix (ECM) deposition [80,81]. These chronic disorders may lead to further hepatocyte damage, manifesting as liver cirrhosis and possibly hepatocellular carcinoma. The liver can be damaged in various ways, including infection (e.g., hepatitis B and C), alcoholism, metabolic disease, and prolonged unhealthy diets. This damage elicits a pro-inflammatory hepatic environment, which leads to liver tissue fibrosis, causing impaired hepatic function [80]. Untreated fibrosis ultimately progresses to cirrhosis, which is mostly irreversible [80]. A key mediator of liver fibrosis is the hepatic stellate cell (HSC), which is a mesenchymal, fibrogenic cell that resides in the sub-endothelial space of Disse between the hepatocyte epithelium and the sinusoids. While normally in a quiescent state, these cells become activated following liver insult, and they respond to cytokines and proliferate to aid injury repair. However, overactivation or a failure to resolve their activation status (chronic activation from continued exposure to pro-inflammatory stimuli) can lead to the increased ECM deposition in the space of Disse that has a negative consequence for hepatocyte function and normal liver architecture, such as loss of microvilli [80,82]. Kupffer cells, a liver macrophage, are also activated in these conditions, and together with HSCs promote a pro-inflammatory hepatic environment. Pro-inflammatory activators of these cells are beyond the scope of this manuscript, but it has been demonstrated that HSCs require glutamine metabolism to maintain proliferation. It was shown that activated HSC were dependent on glutamine conversion to α-ketoglutarate and non-essential amino acids for proliferation, and reduction of glutamine significantly impaired HSC activation [82]. In addition, glutamine can be used as a precursor for proline synthesis, which is a key component of collagen and ECM formation [82].

At present, there is some evidence to indicate that glutamine supplements slow NAFLD [83] or NASH [84] progression, but most studies have been conducted in rodents. There is no convincing evidence to indicate that glutamine supplements prevent NAFLD or NASH progression in humans, which may be due to the complexity of multiple factors contributing to these disorders. The liver is a remarkable organ and has the ability to regenerate, and some research has indicated that glutamine supplementation may be advantageous for liver growth and repair after resection, but are again limited to animal studies [85]. However, others have suggested that raised glutamine levels are associated with liver failure, and the severity correlated with plasma glutamine [86]. Consequently, the effects of glutamine on liver function beyond urea synthesis have not been fully explored, and the administration of exogenous glutamine to those with compromised hepatic function needs to be considered carefully [86].

4. Glutamine and Immune Cell Function

Glutamine was first considered a biologically important molecule in 1873 when indirect evidence helped to characterize it as a structural component of proteins; then, in 1883, abundant free glutamine was found in certain plants. Interestingly, the number of studies only increased after the research conducted by Sir Hans Adolf Krebs (1900–1981) in the 1930s. At that time, and for the first time in science history, Sir Krebs found that mammalian tissues can hydrolyse and synthesize glutamine [22]. In the 1950s, Eagle, et al. [87] reported that glutamine was utilized by isolated fibroblasts in quantities greater than any other amino acid in the cell incubation medium. Further work at that stage was hampered because glutamine was classified as a non-essential amino acid and it was difficult to measure the levels in plasma and tissues. Throughout the 1960s, 1970s, and 1980s, Hans Krebs, Philip Randle (1926–2006), Derek Williamson (1929–1998), and Eric Newsholme (1935–2011) all worked on metabolic regulation utilizing different research models, from isolated cells in vitro, to human and in vivo experiments. Although glucose is a vital metabolite, and the main fuel for a large number of cells in the body, in the early/mid-1980s, Eric Newsholme was able to advance evidence that glutamine was an important modulator of leukocyte function, such as in lymphocytes [7] and macrophages [88]. One of the authors of this review, Newsholme P et al. (1986; 1987) [88–90], reported for the first time that macrophages utilize glutamine actively. Pithon-Curi et al., in 1997 [91,92] described for the first time the consumption of glutamine by neutrophils. The studies by Eric and Philip Newsholme on glutamine metabolism in lymphocytes and macrophages, respectively, prompted many other publications, which jumped from an average of two or three publications per year in the late 1960s and early 1970s to about 50 publications per year in the last 20 years.

During infection and/or high catabolism, the rate of glutamine consumption by all immune cells is similar or greater than glucose [89,90]. However, the increased demand for glutamine by immune system cells, along with the increased use of this amino acid by other tissues, such as the liver, may lead to a glutamine deficit in the human body. In addition, one of the most important sites of glutamine synthesis, the skeletal muscles, reduce their contribution to maintaining plasma glutamine concentration (Figure 2). This effect, depending on the situation may significantly contribute to worsening diseases and infections, and/or increase the risk of subsequent infection, with possible life-threatening implications [93].

In immune cells, glucose is mainly converted into lactate (glycolysis), whereas glutamine is converted into glutamate, aspartate, and alanine by undergoing partial oxidation to CO_2, in a process called glutaminolysis [3] (Figure 3). This unique conversion plays a key role in the effective functioning of immune system cells. Furthermore, through the pentose phosphate pathway, a metabolic pathway parallel to the glycolysis pathway, cells can produce ribose-5-phosphate (a five-carbon sugar), which is a precursor for the pentose sugars seen in the RNA and DNA structure, as well as glycerol-3-phosphate for phospholipid synthesis [94]. On the other hand, the degradation of glutamine, and thus formation of NH_3, and aspartate leads to the synthesis of purines and pyrimidines of the DNA and RNA. The expression of several genes in immune system cells is largely dependent on glutamine availability [3]. For example, the role glutamine plays in the control of proliferation of immune system cells occurs through activation of proteins, such as ERK and JNK kinases. Both proteins act on the activation of transcription factors, such as JNK and AP-1, and it leads to the transcription of cell proliferation-related genes. For instance, appropriate glutamine concentration leads to the expression of key lymphocyte cells surface markers, such as CD25, CD45RO, and CD71, and the production of cytokines, such as interferon-gamma (IFN-γ), TNF-α, and IL-6 [2,31,95,96]. Thus, glutamine acts as an energy substrate for leukocytes and plays an essential role in cell proliferation, tissue repair process activity, and intracellular pathways associated with pathogen recognition [97].

4.1. Neutrophils

The primary substrate for neutrophil survival endocytosis and ROS generation is glucose. However, glucose is not the only energy metabolite source by these cells. Interestingly, when compared to other leukocytes, such as macrophages and lymphocytes, neutrophils consume glutamine at the highest rates [98,99]. Much of the glutamine is converted to glutamate, aspartate (via Krebs cycle activity), and lactate in neutrophils. Under appropriate conditions, CO_2, glutamine, and glutamate play an important role in the generation of essential compounds for leukocytes' metabolism and function, including GSH. Neutrophils use protein structures composed of uncondensed chromatin and of antimicrobial factors also called neutrophilic extracellular traps (NETs). The action of NETs requires ROS formation, synthesis of enzymes, such as myeloperoxidase (MPO) and elastase, as well as components capable of overriding virulence factors and destroying extracellular bacteria [100]. The process involving ROS depends on the activation of the NADPH oxidase 2 (NOX2) complex.

Based on glutamine, the malate synthesis uses malic enzyme to produce substantial amounts of NADPH, since it is necessary to form the superoxide anion (O_2^-), which presents antimicrobial activity. Similarly, macrophages use glutamine for arginine and thus nitric oxide (NO) synthesis through the action of the inducible NO synthase (iNOS) enzyme, by using NADPH as an energy source. Glutamine increases superoxide generation through NADPH oxidase in neutrophils. 6-Diazo-5-oxo-L-norleucine (DON), an inhibitor of phosphate-dependent glutaminase and thus of glutamine metabolism, causes a significant decrease in superoxide production by neutrophils stimulated with phorbol myristate acetate (PMA). PMA raises mRNA's expression of gp91, p22, and p47, major components of the NADPH oxidase complex. Glutamine increases expressions of these three proteins either in the absence or in the presence of PMA. Glutamine enhances superoxide production in neutrophils, probably via the generation of ATP and regulation of the expression of components of the NADPH oxidase complex [101]. Glutamine plays a role to prevent the changes in NADPH oxidase activity and superoxide production induced by adrenaline in neutrophils [102].

4.2. Macrophages

Metabolism of glucose and glutamine is profoundly affected during the macrophage activation process [103,104]. The effects of thioglycollate (an inflammatory stimulus) and Bacillus Calmette-Guérin—BCG (an activation stimulus) on macrophage glucose and glutamine metabolism have been studied [105]. Either thioglycollate or BCG enhances activities of hexokinase and citrate synthase, and also glucose oxidation whereas BCG markedly increases glutamine metabolism. Lipopolysaccharide (LPS) administration also causes pronounced changes in macrophage metabolism and function (for a review, see Nagy and Haschemi [106]. Glucose and glutamine metabolism is also involved in polarizing signals that up-regulate the transcriptional programs required in the macrophage capacity to perform specialized functions. Protein kinase B (PKB or Akt), mTOR complex 1 (mTORC1), mTORC2, and AMP-activated protein kinase (AMPK) play a critical role in metabolic pathways and associated signalling activation [107,108]. For instance, extracellular glutamine may function as the specific starvation-induced nutrient signal to regulate mTORC1. [17]. Synthesis and secretion of pro-inflammatory cytokines, such as TNF-α, IL-1, and IL-6, by macrophages are also regulated by glutamine availability.

Different populations of macrophages have now been identified, such as M1 and M2 [109–111]. The M1 and M2 are in fact two extremes of a still not completely known spectrum of macrophage activation states [109,111,112]. Reprogramming signalling pathways are involved in the formation of M1 or M2 phenotype macrophages. The metabolic reprogramming of macrophages include key changes in glutamine and glucose metabolism [113]. No reports identified the requirement of fatty acids for human macrophage IL-4 induced polarization [114]. This issue, however, remains controversial. Interestingly, macrophages reprogram their metabolism and function to polarize for pro- or anti-inflammatory cells, and this is a consequence of the environmental conditions and stimuli [115]. Treatment of macrophages with LPS promotes a switch from glucose-dependent oxidative phosphorylation to aerobic glycolysis—the Warburg effect [116]. Pyruvate kinase M2 regulates the hypoxia-inducible factor 1-alpha (Hif-1α) activity and IL-1β expression, being a key molecule to induce the Warburg effect in LPS-activated macrophages [117]. Due to this mechanism, M1 macrophages exhibit a quick increase in ATP formation that is required for the host defence response [113,118,119]. The TCA cycle of M2 macrophages has no metabolic flux escape whereas M1 macrophages (treated with LPS) have two points of substrate flux deviation, one occurring at the isocitrate dehydrogenase step reaction and another one at post succinate formation. As a result, there is an accumulation of TCA cycle intermediates (e.g., succinate, α-ketoglutarate, citrate, and itaconate) that regulates LPS macrophage activation [119]. Itaconate has anti-inflammatory properties through activation of nuclear factor erythroid 2-related factor 2 (Nrf2) via Kelch-like ECH-associated protein 1 (KEAP1) alkylation [97]. The glutamine seems to be fully required for IL-4 induction of macrophage alternative activation [120,121]. Liu, et al. [122] reported α-ketoglutarate, generated through glutaminolysis, promotes M2 macrophage differentiation. PPARγ has been reported to be required for IL-4 induced gene expression and stimulation of macrophage respiration and glutamine oxidation [123]. Macrophage metabolism feature varies with the specific-tissue microenvironment, and this is of critical importance for the tissue-resident macrophage function. The peritoneum is rich in glutamate, a product of glutamine metabolism that is used by resident macrophage to induce specific metabolic changes under microbial sensing [121]. Taken as a whole, glutamine metabolism does play a very important role as a synergistic supporter and modulator of macrophage activation.

4.3. Lymphocytes

Lymphocyte activation is associated with specific metabolic pathways to optimize its function. The integration of multiple extracellular signals affects transcriptional programs and signalling pathways that determine, in CD4+ T cells, for example, multiple events that include modulation of energy metabolism, cell proliferation, and cytokine production. Associated bioenergetic processes are dependent on the activation of AMPK, indicating cross-talk between metabolism and signalling pathways in immune cell differentiation. Greiner, et al. [124] reported in rat thymocytes that the use of the anaerobic glycolytic pathway is strongly increased after antigenic stimulation with Concanavalin (ConA). Eric Newsholme's group was the first to report the utilization of glutamine by lymphocytes [125]. Glutamine plays an important role for the function of these cells in different ways. Pyruvate is a common product of glucose and glutamine metabolism in the cells. Curi, et al. [126] described that mesenteric lymphocytes have increased pyruvate oxidation through pyruvate carboxylase when stimulated with ConA, indicating that both glucose and glutamine are involved in the control of lymphocyte proliferation and function. Mitochondria have been reported to be able to regulate leukocyte activation. Succinate, fumarate, and citrate, metabolites of the Krebs cycle and produced through glucose and glutamine metabolism, participate in the control of immunity and inflammation either in innate and adaptive immune cells [97].

Most glucose molecules are transported via glucose transporter 1 (GLUT1), which is not observed in non-activated lymphocytes [127]. GLUT1 is an important metabolic marker of lymphocyte activation as it migrates rapidly to the cell surface after stimulation. Glucose deprivation causes a lower rate of basal proliferation, as well as increased production of IL-2, TNF-α, INF-γ, and IL-4 by CD4+ T cells [128]. Activation of intracellular signalling by Akt beyond GLUT1 protein levels further increases glucose uptake and T cell activation. mTOR and AMPK play important and distinct roles in metabolism and immunity. The stimulation of lymphoid cells leads to increased GLUT1 uptake of glucose by acting on mTOR protein [129]. This pathway is also involved in the differentiation of CD4+ T-cell subsets since mTOR-deficient mice have a decrease in differentiation for effector T lymphocytes [130,131]. In contrast, the AMPK pathway inhibits mTOR by suppressing the signalling of this protein and promotes activation of mitochondrial oxidative metabolism rather than the glycolytic pathway [132,133]. Glutamine is required for T and B-lymphocytes' proliferation process, as well as for protein synthesis, IL-2 production, and antibody synthesis rates presented by these cells. The evidence has now accumulated that glutamine metabolism plays a key role in the activation of lymphocytes. Glutamine is required for human B lymphocyte differentiation to plasma cell and to lymphoblastic transformation [134].

The cell proliferation process requires both ATP for high-energy expenditure and precursors for the biosynthesis of complex molecules, such as lipids (cholesterol and triglycerides) and nucleotides for RNA and DNA synthesis. To perform rapid proliferation activity under the certain stimulus, lymphocytes switch from oxidative phosphorylation to aerobic glycolysis plus glutaminolysis, and so markedly increase glucose and glutamine utilization. The metabolic transition in a Th0 lymphocyte is crucial for the activation of T cells, since glucose metabolism provides intermediates for the biosynthetic pathways, being a prerequisite for the growth and differentiation of T cells [135]. Glycolysis plays an important role in effector T cell functions associated with the production of inflammatory cytokines, mainly INF-γ and IL-2 [136]. The blockade of glyceraldehyde 3-phosphate dehydrogenase (GAPDH) mRNA by the use of siRNA promotes a reduction of INF-γ in lymphocytes [136]. Therefore, the high glycolytic activity is closely associated with the differentiation of Th0 to Th1 cells [132]. Inhibition of the glycolytic pathway blocks this process whereas it promotes differentiation into Treg cells. Increased glycolysis by proliferating cells is linked to increased uptake of glucose and increased expression and activity of glycolytic enzymes, whereas glucose utilization in the oxidative phosphorylation pathway (OXPHOS) is decreased. Therefore, the "metabolic switch" meets the higher energy requirements, generates metabolic intermediates required for the biosynthesis of macromolecules, and suppresses the metabolic features of rest lymphocytes. Inadequate nutrient delivery or specific metabolic inhibition prevents the activation and proliferation of T cells since the inability to use glucose inhibits T cell differentiation in vitro and in vivo [135,137]. Mitochondrial dynamics are closely associated with T lymphocyte metabolism and function. Activated effector T cells have punctate mitochondria and augmented the activity of anabolic pathways whereas memory T lymphocytes exhibit fused mitochondria and enhanced oxidative phosphorylation activity [138]. HIF1-α plays a central role in the maturation of dendritic cells and the activation of T cells. This factor controls leukocyte metabolism reprogramming, through changes in gene expression, and thus immune cell functions [139].

Glycolysis and glutaminolysis are strongly associated to ensure appropriateness for lymphocyte function. Hexosamine biosynthesis requires glucose and glutamine for the de novo synthesis of uridine diphosphate N-acetylglucosamine (UDP-GlcNAc). This sugar-nucleotide inhibits receptor endocytosis and signalling through promoting N-acetylglucosamine branching of Asn (N)-linked glycans. Araujo, et al. [140] reported that high aerobic glycolysis and glutaminolysis activities in a co-operative way decrease the UDP-GlcNAc synthesis and N-glycan branching in mouse T cell blasts due to the low availability of these metabolites for hexosamine synthesis. As a consequence, growth and pro-inflammatory T_H17 features prevail over anti-inflammatory-induced T regulatory (iTreg) differentiation. The latter process is promoted by IL-2 receptor-α (CD25) loss through endocytosis. The authors then postulated that a primary function of concomitant high aerobic glycolysis and glutaminolysis activities is to limit precursors to N-glycan biosynthesis. This metabolic feature of T lymphocytes has marked implications in autoimmunity and cancer. Glutamine also serves as a precursor for the synthesis of putrescine and the polyamines, spermidine and spermine. High levels of polyamines are reported in tumour cells and in autoreactive B- and T-cells in autoimmune diseases. Polyamines have been described to play a role in the control of normal immune cell function and have been associated with autoimmunity and anti-tumour immune cell properties [141].

5. Immunomodulatory Properties of Glutamine Supplementation

Plasma glutamine concentration may be decreased during intense immune cell activity in patients with critical disease conditions; as occurs in sepsis, burn, and injury. Skeletal muscle is the main source of glutamine in mammals. This tissue synthesizes, stores, and releases this amino acid to be used by several organs and cells, such as lymphoid organs and leukocytes [89], as mentioned above. A decrease in plasma/bloodstream glutamine levels results of either insufficient glutamine production in skeletal muscle or excessive consumption by utilizing-cells or both (Figure 2). The decrease in plasma glutamine availability has been reported to contribute to the impaired immune function in several clinical conditions. In fact, glutamine depletion reduces lymphocyte proliferation, impairs expression of surface activation proteins on and production of cytokines, and induces apoptosis in these cells [9]. Addition of glutamine to the diet increases experimental animal survival to a bacterial challenge. Glutamine given through the parenteral route has been reported to be beneficial for patients after surgery, radiation treatment, bone marrow transplantation, or injury [5,142]. Administration of glutamine before the onset of infection prevents it in animals and humans, possibly by preventing deficiency of this amino acid [143].

Concerning the mechanism of action, glutamine regulates the expression of several genes of cell metabolism, signal transduction proteins, cell defence, and repair regulators, and to activate intracellular signalling pathways [2]. Glutamine action also involves signalling pathways' activation by phosphorylation, such as NF-κB and MAPKs [144]. Thus, the function of glutamine goes beyond that of a metabolic fuel or protein synthesis precursor. This amino acid is also an important regulator of leukocyte function, acting on either gene expression or signalling pathways' activation.

5.1. Glutamine-GSH Axis and the Redox State of the Cell

GSH (γ-L-glutamyl-L-cysteinylglycine) is the most important and concentrated (0.5–10 mmol/L) non-enzymatic antioxidant in mammalian cells. Around 85 to 90% of GSH is found in the cytosol, and about 10 to 15% is located in organelles, such as the mitochondria, nuclear matrix, and peroxisomes. GSH is an antioxidant that can directly react with ROS, generating oxidised GSH (GSSG), and can also donate electrons for peroxide reduction, catalysed by glutathione peroxidase enzyme (GPx) [145]. The redox state of the cell can be obtained from the ratio between the intracellular concentration of glutathione disulphide (GSSG) and GSH, which the ratio is [GSSG]/[GSH], resulting in a reduction of GSH, and an increase in the amounts of GSSG [59]. The redox state of the cells is consequently related to GSH concentrations, which are also influenced by the availability of amino acids. Glutamine (via glutamate), cysteine, and glycine are the precursor amino acids for the synthesis of GSH. However, among these three amino acids, glutamate represents the first and probably the most important step in the synthesis of GSH intermediate compounds. Glutamate synthesis, in turn, is dependent on the glutamine intracellular availability. Thus, a higher glutamine/glutamate ratio reinforces the substrates availability for GSH synthesis [39].

Although all cell types in the human body can synthesize GSH, the liver is quantitatively the main organ for the de novo synthesis of GSH (responsible for ~90% of the circulating GSH in physiological conditions) (Figure 3). The elevated concentration of hepatic GSH is mainly due to the high activity of the enzyme, glutathione reductase, in the γ-glutamyl cycle, also known as Meister's cycle, in honour to Alton Meister (1922–1995) [146]. This cycle provides GSH to be consumed locally by the liver, or under hormonal regulation (e.g., glucagon, vasopressin, and catecholamines), and GSH can be exported into the plasma and other tissues, such as the skeletal muscles. The intracellular and extracellular GSH concentrations are determined by the balance between its synthesis and degradation, as well as by the ability of the cell to transport GSH between the cytosol and the different organelles or the extracellular space [147].

Free radicals and ROS production are essential for cell signalling and immune-mediated oxidative bursts found in phagocytes, such as neutrophils and macrophages. Conversely, there is growing evidence that chronic and/or exaggerated alterations in the redox balance play an important role in many acute and chronic diseases, such as cancer, cardiovascular disease, diabetes, sepsis, and general infections. For instance, in acute inflammatory situations, such as sepsis or viral infection, there is a rise in the intracellular redox state, and all cell compartments are vulnerable to oxidative stress (characterized by increased levels of ROS, and low removal by the antioxidant system) [10,39]. In this situation, glutamine status becomes even more important in dictating the health/recovery outcome, with low glutamine availability, leading to low antioxidant protection via the glutamine-GSH axis. Indeed, many experimental [4,39,148,149] and observational [10,26] studies have already identified that during high catabolism, the low plasma concentration of glutamine is an independent risk factor for mortality [150].

5.2. Heat Shock Protein Response

The ability of all living organisms to respond with rapid and appropriate modifications against physiological challenges is an essential feature for survival. At the most basic cellular level, living organisms respond to unfavourable conditions, such as heat shock, toxins, oxidants, infection, inflammation, and several other stressful situations, by changing the expression of stress-related genes, also known as heat shock genes. This response involves the rapid induction of a specific set of genes encoding for cytoprotective proteins, known as HSP's [94]. HSP's are a family of polypeptide proteins clustered according to their molecular weight, which have many intracellular functions. Possibly, the most important function displayed by HSP's are the action of a molecular chaperone. This function assists protein transport, prevents protein aggregation during folding, and protects newly synthesized polypeptide chains against misfolding and protein denaturation [151]. Although several HSP families have been studied in the last couple of years (e.g., HSP10, HSP25, HSP27; HSP90), the most famous and well described in the literature is the HSP70 (i.e., HSP72 + HSP73) family [29,151,152]. HSP70 acts as anti-inflammatory protein by virtue of turning NF-κB off and attenuating the production of inflammatory mediators [153]. Moreover, HSP70 modulate autophagy by regulating the mTOR/Akt pathway and block signalling pathways associated with protein-degradation [152].

Glutamine found at concentrations similar to those recorded for human plasma leads to a significant HSP72 gene expression increase in peripheral blood mononuclear cells subjected to LPS treatment. On the other hand, reduced glutamine concentration results in reduced HSP72 expression in monocytes; this effect depends on mRNA stability. The preoperative administration of glutamine can modulate HSP70 expression by reducing the activation levels of the cyclic AMP response element binding protein (CREB), which is often associated with exacerbated inflammatory responses. This effect depends on the iNOS activity and leads to an NO production increase. Other studies corroborated the present results and presented similar mechanisms, as well as effects on the expression of other HSP's, such as HSP25, HSP27, and HSP90.

Glutamine plays a crucial role in the modulation of HSP's expression through the hexosamine biosynthetic pathway (HBP, Figure 3) [21,94]. In the HBP, glutamine leads to the production of UDP-GlcNAc and (UDP)-N-acetylgalactosamine (UDP-GalNAc) through the enzyme, fructose-6-phosphate amidotransferase (GFAT, the first and rate-limiting step of HBP). UDP-GlcNAc and UDP-GalNAc, in turn, may be attached to serine or threonine hydroxyl moieties in nuclear and cytoplasmic proteins by the enzymatic action of O-linked-N-acetylglucosaminyl (O-GlcNAc) transferase (a.k.a. OGT) [94]. The main donors for UDP-GlcNAc are glucose, glutamine, and uridine triphosphate (UTP) from the HBP. Interestingly, both nutrients' availability and cell stress affect O-GlcNAc downstream signalling, and, not surprisingly, this mechanism is also altered in several metabolic diseases, infection, and inflammatory processes [154,155]. O-GlcNAc synthesis leads to the activation of many transcriptional factors, for instance, Sp1, phosphorylation of Eukaryotic Initiation Factor 2 (eIF2), and sirtuin-1 (SIRT1) [156]. Both Sp1 and eIF2 are key transcription factors for the induction of the main thermal shock eukaryotic factor, HSF-1 [157]. Alternatively, SIRT1 enhances HSF-1 expression and prolongs its activation by binding to the promoters of HS genes, leading to the HSP's expression [94,158]. Although the O-GlcNAc/Sp1 pathway is considered the main mechanism of the HSP's gene expression and production, glutamine may also act on HBP via p38/MAPK, leading to the HSP's expression in cells, such as neutrophils. This response may explain the reduction in neutrophils' apoptosis after high-intensity physical exercise [144]. Furthermore, by increasing the HBP flux, glutamine stimulates the HSP's expression by blocking the glycogen synthase kinase 3 beta (GSK-3β), an enzyme that constitutively inhibits HSF-1 activation by phosphorylating the transcription factor at Ser303 [94,159].

In vitro [21,160] and in vivo [4,39,161–163] studies demonstrate that glutamine availability maintains cell homeostasis and promotes cell survival against environmental and physiological stress challenges through an enhanced protection mediated by intracellular HSP (iHSP) levels [94]. Interestingly, under severe infection and/or catabolism, low glutamine availability in the body can eventually be accompanied by an aberrant iHSP and lead to the HSP's release to the extracellular space (eHSP) [4]. eHSP have a wide variety of effects on other cells, including impacting on a cell to cell interaction and chemotaxis, and in some cases, act as a signal to the immune and inflammatory responses. On the other hand, eHSP can also function as a stress signalling and pro-inflammatory molecule by interacting with Toll-like receptors 2 (TLR2) and 4 (TLR4) [164]. This effect can down-regulate iHSP in many cells, leading to apoptosis [4], and has also been associated with increased insulin resistance in skeletal muscle cells [165], and β-cell failure in diabetic individuals. Currently, a novel and overall index of immunoinflammatory status, the extracellular to intracellular HSP70 ratio index (H-index), measured in peripheral blood mononuclear cells (PBMCs) [94], has been established.

6. Clinical Translation of Glutamine Delivery

Glutamine is found in relatively high concentrations in vegetable and animal protein-based foods (Table 1). Using a validated food frequency questionnaire (FFQ) of more than 70 thousand participants, Lenders, et al. [166] showed that glutamine (6.85 ± 2.19 g/day), glutamate (7.27 ± 2.44 g/day), and leucine (7.01 ± 2.27 g/day) accounts for the highest intake in protein-based diets. Therefore, a balanced diet provides glutamine, and other essential and non-essential amino acids for homeostasis, growth, and health maintenance. Furthermore, it is also important to state that in healthy individuals with a balanced diet, glutamine supplementation does not increase the efficacy of immune surveillance and/or prevent disease/sickness episodes.

Table 1. Total protein, glutamine, glutamate, and leucine (g/100g food) content in some animal and vegetable foods using the gene sequencing method (adapted from [166]).

g/100g Food	Beef	Skim Milk	White Rice	Corn	Tofu	Egg
Total protein	25.9	3.4	2.7	2.5	6.6	12.6
Glutamine	1.2	0.3	0.3	0.4	0.6	0.6
Glutamate	2.7	0.4	0.2	0.05	0.7	1.0
Leucine	2.2	0.4	0.2	0.4	0.5	0.9

On the contrary, during major and/or critical illness, sepsis, trauma, and post-surgery circumstances, patients suffer from chronic weakness and several nutritional limitations (e.g., state of unconsciousness, gastrointestinal disturbances, and/or chew related problems), which impair homeostasis, and are associated with poor clinical outcomes. Severe disturbances in amino acid metabolism and/or intermediary metabolism followed by skeletal muscle proteolysis are key characteristics of hypermetabolic/hypercatabolic states [167]. During hypercatabolism, some non-essential amino acids, including glutamine, become conditionally essential. As previously mentioned, glutamine is critical for cell homeostasis, and cells cannot survive and/or proliferate in an environment where glutamine is lacking. Therefore, the administration of non-synthetic amino acid supplements, such as glutamine, has been a research target in in the last many years and is currently indicated for hypercatabolic and/or ill patients. However, the efficacy of glutamine supplementation is frequently questioned due to confusing and controversial results [150,168,169].

Glutamine is usually administrated by utilizing its free form (also known as an isolated amino acid), or bond with another amino acid, also known as the dipeptide form (Figure 4). Several glutamine dipeptides with potential recovery health benefits have been described, such as L-glycyl-L-glutamine (Gly-Gln) and L-arginyl-L-glutamine (Arg-Gln); however, the most well-known is possibly L-alanyl-L-glutamine (Ala-Gln) [170]. Given parenterally, many clinical and experimental studies and appropriate systematic reviews [168] have concluded that glutamine dipeptides can reduce the rate of infectious complications [171–174], length of hospital stay [9,175], and mortality of critically ill patients [10,176,177]. The choice for free glutamine or glutamine dipeptides largely depends on the patient's catabolic circumstance and/or the most suitable route of administration (e.g., enteral and parenteral nutrition). For instance, in patients receiving total parenteral nutrition (TPN), glutamine dipeptides offer several advantages, such as stability during sterilization, prolonged storage, and high range of solubility (154 g/L H_2O at 20 °C, 568 g/L H_2O at 20 °C, respectively) when compared to free glutamine (36 g/L H_2O at 20 °C) [170]. Moreover, free glutamine is usually commercially available as a crystalline amino acid powder and can be diluted into commercially available TPN solutions, however, this procedure requires daily preparations at a controlled temperature (i.e., 4 °C), aseptic conditions followed by sterilization through specific membrane filtration, and the concentration should not exceed 1–2%. This is particularly important because, at a low concentration, TPN solutions will increase the patient's fluid intake to meet the daily glutamine recommendation, however, this cannot be feasible for fluid restricted patients.

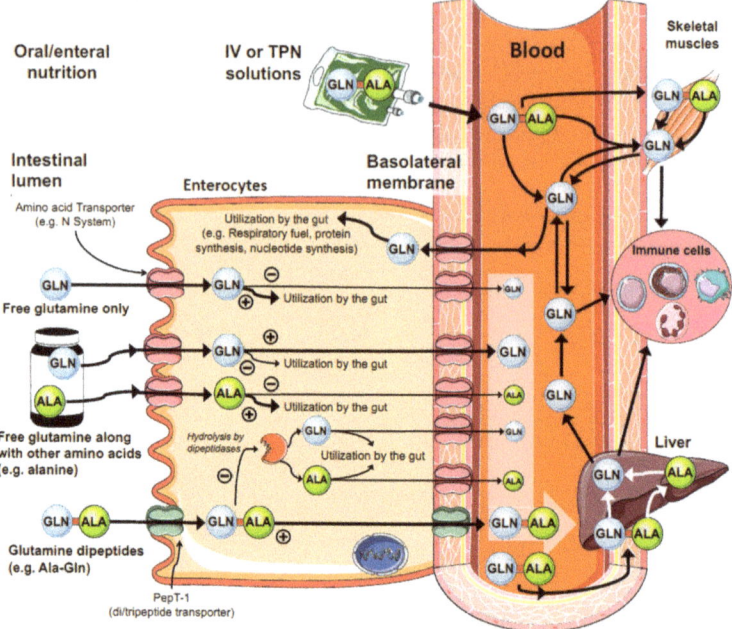

Figure 4. Mechanisms of enteral and parenteral glutamine (GLN) supply. Glutamine is an important substrate for rapidly dividing cells, such as enterocytes. This is a major site of glutamine consumption obtained from both exogenous/diet (luminal membrane) and/or endogenous glutamine synthesis (basolateral membrane). Free glutamine supplementation is mainly metabolized in the gut and poorly contribute to glutaminemia and tissue stores. On the other hand, glutamine dipeptides (e.g., Ala-Gln, Gly-Gln, Arg-Gln) escape from the gut metabolization and quickly supply glutamine to the plasma and target tissues. This effect is mainly attributed to the oligopeptide transporter 1 (Pept-1) located in the luminal membrane of the enterocytes.

In both oral/enteral or parenteral nutrition, the typical glutamine daily administration (free and dipeptide forms) may vary from a fixed dose of 20–35 g/24 h to an adjusted dose of <1.0 g (usually 0.3 g–0.5 g) per kg of body weight [168]. As any other nutrient or medication administrated directly into the bloodstream when free or dipeptide forms of glutamine are given parenterally, the increase in plasma glutamine is superior when compared to oral/enteral feeds [178]. However, it should be noted that although parenteral routes can secure nutrient delivery to target tissues, it is always an invasive route and may increase the risk of infections per se. It is strongly recommended that the decision to use parenteral solutions must be based on several nutritional parameters, such as poor nutritional status, dramatic reduction of body weight and body mass index, low plasma albumin, and/or severe loss of nitrogen and tissue function.

For individuals with regular enteral feeds at home or hospitals, and also elite athletes where glutamine supplementation is eventually recommended, oral or enteral routes are always more physiological. Furthermore, enteral solutions stimulate the intestinal cells to produce other intermediary amino acid derivatives important for immunological functions, and also compromised in hypercatabolic patients, such as arginine and its downstream metabolites (e.g., ornithine and citrulline) [179]. Experimental studies in animal models and humans have shown an increase in glutaminemia between ±30 to ±120 min after oral/enteral free glutamine [50] or Ala-Gln supplementation [50,177]. However, the peak concentration and the area under the curve promoted by Ala-Gln tend to be superior when compared to free glutamine supply. This effect is largely due to the expression of the human oligopeptide transporter 1 (Pept-1) located in the luminal microvilli membrane of the enterocytes [180], and in a lesser extent, through paracellular mechanisms and cell-penetrating peptides' translocation [181,182] (Figure 4). Pept-1 is a high capacity, low-affinity proton-coupled cotransporter of diverse di/tripeptides, which include the glutamine dipeptides. Pept-1 is considered the main route of protein absorption in mammals' intestines since the protein is able to transport about 400 dipeptides and 8000 tripeptides derived from the 20 L-α amino acids [180]. As a result, free glutamine and/or alanine deriving from enteral Ala-Gln administration can be released into the bloodstream, thus making the amino acids available to target tissues, including the liver [183], immune system [39], kidneys [184] and skeletal muscles [53] (Figure 4). Interestingly, the effects promoted by Ala-Gln are also mediated by the presence of the amino acid, alanine, in the peptide formulation. Oral free glutamine along with free alanine promoted similar metabolic, antioxidant, and immunological effects when compared to Ala-Gln supplementation in in vivo animal models submitted to infection [4,39], and exhaustive aerobic [30,45,53] and resistance physical exercise [29,162]. Importantly, in all of these experiments, the supplemented groups received isonitrogenous and isocaloric solutions, i.e., both containing 13.46 g of glutamine/100 mL and 8.20 g of alanine/100 mL. Although the precise mechanisms are still unknown, it is clear that both amino acids work in parallel, especially in absorptive cells (Figure 4). For instance, alanine is rapidly metabolized via alanine aminotransferase to pyruvate, with concomitant production of glutamate from 2-oxoglutarate, which contribute to antioxidant defence mediated by GSH. Although other free amino acid combinations need to be tested, these important discoveries may lead to the design of new formulations for specific hypercatabolic patients.

Oral/enteral or parenteral doses of glutamine supplementation have been tested in hundreds of studies in both animal models and humans, and if offered as a single nutrient supplementation (not combined with other additives), can be considered safe. In addition, there is no scientific evidence demonstrating that glutamine supplementation can suppress and/or inhibit permanently its endogenous production or de novo synthesis. However, as any other amino acid offered in excessive doses, it can promote hyperaminoacidemia and result in poor clinical outcomes. It is considered not to be the best practice to provide glutamine supplementation to patients without a proper evaluation that is supported by a nutritional assessment and biochemical laboratory tests.

Glutamine metabolism and supplementation in cancer has also raised many concerns among the scientific community, and deserve some comments. It is well established that cancer cells are extremely dependent of glutamine metabolism and availability, however, the role played by glutamine in cancer/tumours cells in vivo is still controversial, and thus the effects of the supplementation. Cancer cells take advantage of aerobic glycolysis (also known as the Warburg effect), and therefore glucose to maintain the supraphysiological survival and growth [185,186]. On the other hand, there is an increasing evidence of the role of oncogenes and tumour suppressors in the regulation of nutrient metabolism [187]. Aberrant mutations in these genes lead to altered nutrient metabolism, and can significantly contribute to the development and/or progression of cancer cells [186]. For instance, glucose, glutamine, lipids, and acetate can be utilized as carbon and energy sources [25]. To increase the level of complexity, the nutrient sources may vary among different types of cancer and/or tumour cells and are highly heterogeneous [25,187]. For example, lung cancer cell lines are highly dependent of glutamine supply in vitro, however, in vivo experiments demonstrate that glucose is the preferred source of carbons supplied to the Krebs cycle, through the action of pyruvate carboxylase [188], with little changes in glutamine consumption [187]. Human and mouse gliomas exhibit high rates of glucose catabolism, and use glucose to synthesize glutamine through glutamate-ammonia ligase (GLUL), which in turn promotes nucleotide biosynthesis via the pentose phosphate pathway independently of circulating glutamine [189,190]. Conversely, prostate cancer cell lines exhibit aberrant intracellular lipid metabolism [191], and an increased gene expression of glutaminolitic enzymes and glutamine transporters, thereby stimulating cell growth via glutamine uptake [192].

The variances in cancer cells' nutrient metabolism suggest that different nutritional approaches should be taken into consideration. However, studies have also targeted whether a glutamine exogenous supply may attenuate the side effects promoted by chemotherapy and radiation in cancer patients [193]. In a systematic review, Sayles, et al. [194] reported that in 11 of 15 studies, oral glutamine supplementation (dose range: 30 g/day in 3 divided doses, or 7.5–24 g/day) significantly reduced the grade of mucositis (common in 90% of head/neck cancer patients) [193] and/or attenuated weight loss in cancer patients. In a double-blind, placebo-controlled, randomized trial, colorectal cancer patients undergoing chemotherapy were supplemented with 18 g/day of glutamine (five days before and during the treatment). Glutamine treatment reduced the side-effects induced by chemotherapy, such as intestinal absorption and permeability, diarrhea, and gut mucositis [195]. As a whole, it is important to highlight that glutamine supplementation for cancer patients may also fuel certain types of cancer cells, and have a negative impact on health. However, considering the strong ability of metabolic switching of cancer cells, glucose and/or lipids can also induce similar effects, and therefore it would be difficult for a human to survive and maintain immunity and/or immune surveillance without these nutrients. As mentioned previously, a proper and possibly individualized patient evaluation is required to determine the suitability of glutamine supplementation.

Low plasma glutamine level (hypoglutaminemia) is usually used as a parameter to indicate the need for a glutamine exogenous supply. However, the correlation between the concentration of glutamine in plasma and tissue vary significantly between hypercatabolic patients, and therefore among studies [150]. For instance, muscle glutamine was dramatically reduced in abdominal surgery patients, but no changes were detected in plasma [196]. In critically ill patients, however, there is a profound drop in muscle glutamine, but a variable reduction in plasma [150]. Other important glutamine sites, such as the gut and the liver, may show a concomitant plasma and tissue glutamine reduction, or even an inverse relationship during major illness [86,197,198]. These findings are also in agreement with data obtained in rats [29,45,183] and mice [4,199] submitted to infection and exhaustive exercise.

The variations between plasma and tissue glutamine concentration are due to the fact that only a small fraction of the total body free glutamine is in plasma. To add to the confusion, it is known that cells of the immune system, such as lymphocytes maintained in a low glutamine availability (similar to low plasma glutamine concentration, e.g., ± 400 µM), still proliferate, when compared to resting values (e.g., 600 µM) [4,7,90]. The rate of macrophages' phagocytosis and cytokine production by diverse peripheral blood mononuclear cells (PBMCs) is also dependent on glutamine availability, with decreasing rates at $\pm <600$ µM of glutamine [21,200]. Thus, for some catabolic/hypercatabolic patients, the changes in glutamine concentration, especially in plasma, will not necessarily affect and suppress immune functions, and possibly no significant changes might be observed in data obtained from immune parameters and function, and mortality risk predictors, such as APACHE II or SAPS III. Taken together, hypoglutaminemia can only be interpreted as an independent variable of mortality and/or poor clinical outcome [10,93,168,169,174,201]. More in-depth studies are required to explore the specific relationship between dramatic changes in plasma glutamine and outcomes in critically ill patients. Currently, the decision of glutamine supplementation should be based in a set of immune-inflammatory parameters allied with appropriate nutritional assessment, and eventually, risk predictors. In addition, glutamine supplementation studies cannot be judged on trials where only the very sickest patients (i.e., with two or more organ failures) were eligible for this nutritional intervention, and in these situations, supraphysiologic doses are not an appropriate nutritional solution.

7. Conclusions and Future Perspectives

Immune cells largely depend on glutamine availability to survive, proliferate, and function, and ultimately defend our body against pathogens. During catabolic/hypercatabolic circumstances, the demand for glutamine increases dramatically, a fact that may lead to a glutamine deprivation and severe impairment of the immune function. However, low glutamine availability is not observed in every catabolic/ill or critically ill patient, and thus not all individuals will benefit from glutamine supplementation. It is important to consider that like glycaemia, plasma glutamine and the inter-tissue metabolic flux is maintained at constant levels even during high catabolism by key organs, such as the gut, liver, and skeletal muscles. Not surprisingly, hypoglutaminemia conditions and severity vary significantly between human and animal studies, and by itself do not provide a rational argument for glutamine exogenous supply.

For some catabolic situations, and/or where there is a shortage of glutamine obtained from the diet, amino acid supplementation might be required. In this regard, the immune properties of glutamine supplementation have been extensively studied and new questions and perspectives are formulated. For instance, studies should determine the frequency of nutritional intervention, optimal doses associated with the disease or stress situation, and the concomitant administration with other amino acids or dipeptide combinations. In addition, the evolving metabolomics era has the potential to improve our understanding of the complex regulation of glutamine metabolism, identifying new metabolites (e.g., Itaconate in macrophages) critical for cell function, thus going beyond the concept of "the fuel for the immune system".

Author Contributions: V.C. conceived the idea, and with the help of M.M.R. organised and designed the manuscript. V.C., M.M.R., K.N.K. and R.C. wrote the first draft, which was reviewed and revised by P.N. Figures and Table 1 were designed by V.C. All authors contributed significantly in the manuscript revision and agreed with the final submitted version.

Funding: We thank the Department of Health Science, Torrens University, and the Curtin School of Pharmacy and Biomedical Sciences for financial research support and excellent research facilities, respectively.

Conflicts of Interest: The authors declare no conflict of interest.

References

1. Grohmann, U.; Mondanelli, G.; Belladonna, M.L.; Orabona, C.; Pallotta, M.T.; Iacono, A.; Puccetti, P.; Volpi, C. Amino-acid sensing and degrading pathways in immune regulation. *Cytokine Growth Factor Rev.* **2017**, *35*, 37–45. [CrossRef] [PubMed]
2. Curi, R.; Lagranha, C.J.; Doi, S.Q.; Sellitti, D.F.; Procopio, J.; Pithon-Curi, T.C.; Corless, M.; Newsholme, P. Molecular mechanisms of glutamine action. *J. Cell. Physiol.* **2005**, *204*, 392–401. [CrossRef] [PubMed]
3. Curi, R.; Newsholme, P.; Marzuca-Nassr, G.N.; Takahashi, H.K.; Hirabara, S.M.; Cruzat, V.; Krause, M.; de Bittencourt, P.I.H., Jr. Regulatory principles in metabolism-then and now. *Biochem. J.* **2016**, *473*, 1845–1857. [CrossRef] [PubMed]
4. Cruzat, V.F.; Pantaleao, L.C.; Donato, J., Jr.; de Bittencourt, P.I.H., Jr.; Tirapegui, J. Oral supplementations with free and dipeptide forms of l-glutamine in endotoxemic mice: Effects on muscle glutamine-glutathione axis and heat shock proteins. *J. Nutr. Biochem.* **2014**, *25*, 345–352. [CrossRef] [PubMed]
5. Newsholme, P. Why is l-glutamine metabolism important to cells of the immune system in health, postinjury, surgery or infection? *J. Nutr.* **2001**, *131*, 2514S–2523S. [CrossRef] [PubMed]
6. Cruzat, V.F.; Krause, M.; Newsholme, P. Amino acid supplementation and impact on immune function in the context of exercise. *J. Int. Soc. Sports Nutr.* **2014**, *11*, 61. [CrossRef] [PubMed]
7. Ardawi, M.S.M.; Newsholme, E.A. Maximum activities of some enzymes of glycolysis, the tricarboxylic acid cycle and ketone-body and glutamine utilization pathways in lymphocytes of the rat. *Biochem. J.* **1982**, *208*, 743–748. [CrossRef] [PubMed]
8. Flaring, U.B.; Rooyackers, O.E.; Wernerman, J.; Hammarqvist, F. Glutamine attenuates post-traumatic glutathione depletion in human muscle. *Clin. Sci.* **2003**, *104*, 275–282. [CrossRef] [PubMed]
9. Roth, E. Nonnutritive effects of glutamine. *J. Nutr.* **2008**, *138*, 2025S–2031S. [CrossRef] [PubMed]

10. Rodas, P.C.; Rooyackers, O.; Hebert, C.; Norberg, A.; Wernerman, J. Glutamine and glutathione at icu admission in relation to outcome. *Clin. Sci.* **2012**, *122*, 591–597. [CrossRef] [PubMed]
11. Newsholme, E.A.; Parry-Billings, M. Properties of glutamine release from muscle and its importance for the immune system. *J. Parenter. Enter. Nutr.* **1990**, *14*, 63S–67S. [CrossRef] [PubMed]
12. Wernerman, J. Clinical use of glutamine supplementation. *J. Nutr.* **2008**, *138*, 2040S–2044S. [CrossRef] [PubMed]
13. Berg, A.; Norberg, A.; Martling, C.R.; Gamrin, L.; Rooyackers, O.; Wernerman, J. Glutamine kinetics during intravenous glutamine supplementation in icu patients on continuous renal replacement therapy. *Intensive Care Med.* **2007**, *33*, 660–666. [CrossRef] [PubMed]
14. Labow, B.I.; Souba, W.W.; Abcouwer, S.F. Mechanisms governing the expression of the enzymes of glutamine metabolism—Glutaminase and glutamine synthetase. *J. Nutr.* **2001**, *131*, 2467S–2486S. [CrossRef] [PubMed]
15. Cruzat, V.F.; Newsholme, P. An introduction to glutamine metabolism. In *Glutamine*; CRC Press: Boca Raton, FL, USA, 2017; pp. 1–18.
16. Cooney, G.; Curi, R.; Mitchelson, A.; Newsholme, P.; Simpson, M.; Newsholme, E.A. Activities of some key enzymes of carbohydrate, ketone-body, adenosine and glutamine-metabolism in liver, and brown and white adipose tissues of the rat. *Biochem. Biophys. Res. Commun.* **1986**, *138*, 687–692. [CrossRef]
17. Tan, H.W.S.; Sim, A.Y.L.; Long, Y.C. Glutamine metabolism regulates autophagy-dependent mtorc1 reactivation during amino acid starvation. *Nat. Commun.* **2017**, *8*, 338. [CrossRef] [PubMed]
18. Ardawi, M.S. Glutamine metabolism in the lungs of glucocorticoid-treated rats. *Clin. Sci.* **1991**, *81*, 37–42. [CrossRef] [PubMed]
19. Parry-Billings, M.; Dimitriadis, G.D.; Leighton, B.; Bond, J.; Bevan, S.J.; Opara, E.; Newsholme, E.A. Effects of hyperthyroidism and hypothyroidism on glutamine metabolism by skeletal muscle of the rat. *Biochem. J.* **1990**, *272*, 319–322. [CrossRef] [PubMed]
20. Parry-Billings, M.; Dimitriadis, G.; Leighton, B.; Dunger, D.; Newsholme, E. The effects of growth hormone administration in vivo on skeletal muscle glutamine metabolism of the rat. *Horm. Metab. Res.* **1993**, *25*, 292–293. [CrossRef] [PubMed]
21. Cruzat, V.F.; Keane, K.N.; Scheinpflug, A.L.; Cordeiro, R.; Soares, M.J.; Newsholme, P. Alanyl-glutamine improves pancreatic beta-cell function following ex vivo inflammatory challenge. *J. Endocrinol.* **2015**, *224*, 261–271. [CrossRef] [PubMed]
22. Krebs, H.A. Metabolism of amino-acids: The synthesis of glutamine from glutamic acid and ammonia, and the enzymic hydrolysis of glutamine in animal tissues. *Biochem. J.* **1935**, *29*, 1951–1969. [CrossRef] [PubMed]
23. Neu, J.; Shenoy, V.; Chakrabarti, R. Glutamine nutrition and metabolism: Where do we go from here? *FASEB J.* **1996**, *10*, 829–837. [CrossRef] [PubMed]
24. Holecek, M. Branched-chain amino acids in health and disease: Metabolism, alterations in blood plasma, and as supplements. *Nutr. Metab.* **2018**, *15*, 33. [CrossRef] [PubMed]
25. Altman, B.J.; Stine, Z.E.; Dang, C.V. From krebs to clinic: Glutamine metabolism to cancer therapy. *Nat. Rev. Cancer* **2016**, *16*, 619–634. [CrossRef] [PubMed]
26. Kao, C.; Hsu, J.; Bandi, V.; Jahoor, F. Alterations in glutamine metabolism and its conversion to citrulline in sepsis. *Am. J. Physiol. Endocrinol. Metab.* **2013**, *304*, E1359–E1364. [CrossRef] [PubMed]
27. Rogero, M.M.; Borges, M.C.; Pires, I.S.D.; Borelli, P.; Tirapegui, J. Ffect of glutamine supplementation and in vivo infection with mycobacterium bovis (bacillus calmette-guerin) in the function of peritoneal macrophages in early weaned mice. *Ann. Nutr. Metab.* **2007**, *51*, 173–174.
28. Karinch, A.M.; Pan, M.; Lin, C.M.; Strange, R.; Souba, W.W. Glutamine metabolism in sepsis and infection. *J. Nutr.* **2001**, *131*, 2531S–2550S. [CrossRef] [PubMed]
29. Leite, J.S.; Raizel, R.; Hypolito, T.M.; Rosa, T.D.; Cruzat, V.F.; Tirapegui, J. L-glutamine and l-alanine supplementation increase glutamine-glutathione axis and muscle hsp-27 in rats trained using a progressive high-intensity resistance exercise. *Appl. Physiol. Nutr. Metab.* **2016**, *41*, 842–849. [CrossRef] [PubMed]
30. Cruzat, V.F.; Rogero, M.M.; Tirapegui, J. Effects of supplementation with free glutamine and the dipeptide alanyl-glutamine on parameters of muscle damage and inflammation in rats submitted to prolonged exercise. *Cell Biochem. Funct.* **2010**, *28*, 24–30. [CrossRef] [PubMed]
31. Curi, R.; Lagranha, C.J.; Doi, S.Q.; Sellitti, D.F.; Procopio, J.; Pithon-Curi, T.C. Glutamine-dependent changes in gene expression and protein activity. *Cell Biochem. Funct.* **2005**, *23*, 77–84. [CrossRef] [PubMed]

32. Djoko, K.Y.; Phan, M.D.; Peters, K.M.; Walker, M.J.; Schembri, M.A.; McEwan, A.G. Interplay between tolerance mechanisms to copper and acid stress in *Escherichia coli*. *Proc. Nat. Acad. Sci. USA* **2017**, *114*, 6818–6823. [CrossRef] [PubMed]
33. Wernerman, J. Feeding the gut: How, when and with what—The metabolic issue. *Curr. Opin. Crit. Care* **2014**, *20*, 196–201. [CrossRef] [PubMed]
34. Beutheu, S.; Ouelaa, W.; Guerin, C.; Belmonte, L.; Aziz, M.; Tennoune, N.; Bole-Feysot, C.; Galas, L.; Dechelotte, P.; Coeffier, M. Glutamine supplementation, but not combined glutamine and arginine supplementation, improves gut barrier function during chemotherapy-induced intestinal mucositis in rats. *Clin. Nutr.* **2014**, *33*, 694–701. [CrossRef] [PubMed]
35. Souba, W.W.; Smith, R.J.; Wilmore, D.W. Glutamine metabolism by the intestinal tract. *J. Parenter. Enter. Nutr.* **1985**, *9*, 608–617. [CrossRef] [PubMed]
36. Holecek, M. Side effects of long-term glutamine supplementation. *J. Parenter. Enter. Nutr.* **2013**, *37*, 607–616. [CrossRef] [PubMed]
37. Kim, M.H.; Kim, H. The roles of glutamine in the intestine and its implication in intestinal diseases. *Int. J. Mol. Sci.* **2017**, *18*, 1051. [CrossRef] [PubMed]
38. Souba, W.W.; Herskowitz, K.; Salloum, R.M.; Chen, M.K.; Austgen, T.R. Gut glutamine metabolism. *J. Parenter. Enter. Nutr.* **1990**, *14*, 45S–50S. [CrossRef] [PubMed]
39. Cruzat, V.F.; Bittencourt, A.; Scomazzon, S.P.; Leite, J.S.; de Bittencourt, P.I.H.; Tirapegui, J. Oral free and dipeptide forms of glutamine supplementation attenuate oxidative stress and inflammation induced by endotoxemia. *Nutrition* **2014**, *30*, 602–611. [CrossRef] [PubMed]
40. Aosasa, S.; Wells-Byrum, D.; Alexander, J.W.; Ogle, C.K. Influence of glutamine-supplemented caco-2 cells on cytokine production of mononuclear cells. *J. Parenter. Enter. Nutr.* **2003**, *27*, 333–339. [CrossRef] [PubMed]
41. Coeffier, M.; Claeyssens, S.; Hecketsweiler, B.; Lavoinne, A.; Ducrotte, P.; Dechelotte, P. Enteral glutamine stimulates protein synthesis and decreases ubiquitin mRNA level in human gut mucosa. *Am. J. Physiol. Gastrointest. Liver Physiol.* **2003**, *285*, G266–G273. [CrossRef] [PubMed]
42. Jobin, C.; Hellerbrand, C.; Licato, L.L.; Brenner, D.A.; Sartor, R.B. Mediation by nf-kappa b of cytokine induced expression of intercellular adhesion molecule 1 (icam-1) in an intestinal epithelial cell line, a process blocked by proteasome inhibitors. *Gut* **1998**, *42*, 779–787. [CrossRef] [PubMed]
43. Coeffier, M.; Miralles-Barrachina, O.; Le Pessot, F.; Lalaude, O.; Daveau, M.; Lavoinne, A.; Lerebours, E.; Dechelotte, P. Influence of glutamine on cytokine production by human gut in vitro. *Cytokine* **2001**, *13*, 148–154. [CrossRef] [PubMed]
44. Tirapegui, J.; Cruzat, V. Glutamine and skeletal muscle. In *Glutamine in Clinical Nutrition*; Rajendram, R., Preedy, V.R., Patel, V.B., Eds.; Springer: New York, NY, USA, 2015; pp. 499–511.
45. Cruzat, V.F.; Tirapegui, J. Effects of oral supplementation with glutamine and alanyl-glutamine on glutamine, glutamate, and glutathione status in trained rats and subjected to long-duration exercise. *Nutrition* **2009**, *25*, 428–435. [CrossRef] [PubMed]
46. Walsh, N.P.; Blannin, A.K.; Robson, P.J.; Gleeson, M. Glutamine, exercise and immune function. Links and possible mechanisms. *Sports Med.* **1998**, *26*, 177–191. [CrossRef] [PubMed]
47. Rowbottom, D.G.; Keast, D.; Morton, A.R. The emerging role of glutamine as an indicator of exercise stress and overtraining. *Sports Med.* **1996**, *21*, 80–97. [CrossRef] [PubMed]
48. Curi, R.; Newsholme, P.; Procopio, J.; Lagranha, C.; Gorjao, R.; Pithon-Curi, T.C. Glutamine, gene expression, and cell function. *Front. Biosci.* **2007**, *12*, 344–357. [CrossRef] [PubMed]
49. Rogero, M.M.; Tirapegui, J.; Pedrosa, R.G.; de Castro, I.A.; Pires, I.S.D. Effect of alanyl-glutamine supplementation on plasma and tissue glutamine concentrations in rats submitted to exhaustive exercise. *Nutrition* **2006**, *22*, 564–571. [CrossRef] [PubMed]
50. Rogero, M.M.; Tirapegui, J.; Pedrosa, R.G.; Pires, I.S.D.; de Castro, I.A. Plasma and tissue glutamine response to acute and chronic supplementation with l-glutamine and l-alanyl-l-glutamine in rats. *Nutr. Res.* **2004**, *24*, 261–270. [CrossRef]
51. Wagenmakers, A.J. Muscle amino acid metabolism at rest and during exercise: Role in human physiology and metabolism. *Exerc. Sport Sci. Rev.* **1998**, *26*, 287–314. [CrossRef] [PubMed]
52. Goldberg, A.L.; Chang, T.W. Regulation and significance of amino acid metabolism in skeletal muscle. *Fed. Proc.* **1978**, *37*, 2301–2307. [PubMed]

53. Petry, E.R.; Cruzat, V.F.; Heck, T.G.; Leite, J.S.; Homem de Bittencourt, P.I.H.; Tirapegui, J. Alanyl-glutamine and glutamine plus alanine supplements improve skeletal redox status in trained rats: Involvement of heat shock protein pathways. *Life Sci.* **2014**, *94*, 130–136. [CrossRef] [PubMed]
54. Nieman, D.C.; Pedersen, B.K. Exercise and immune function. Recent developments. *Sports Med.* **1999**, *27*, 73–80. [CrossRef] [PubMed]
55. Anderson, P.M.; Broderius, M.A.; Fong, K.C.; Tsui, K.N.; Chew, S.F.; Ip, Y.K. Glutamine synthetase expression in liver, muscle, stomach and intestine of bostrichthys sinensis in response to exposure to a high exogenous ammonia concentration. *J. Exp. Biol.* **2002**, *205*, 2053–2065. [PubMed]
56. Austgen, T.R.; Chakrabarti, R.; Chen, M.K.; Souba, W.W. Adaptive regulation in skeletal muscle glutamine metabolism in endotoxin-treated rats. *J. Trauma* **1992**, *32*, 600–607. [CrossRef] [PubMed]
57. Labow, B.I.; Souba, W.W.; Abcouwer, S.F. Glutamine synthetase expression in muscle is regulated by transcriptional and posttranscriptional mechanisms. *Am. J. Physiol.* **1999**, *276*, E1136–E1145. [CrossRef] [PubMed]
58. Xia, Y.; Wen, H.Y.; Young, M.E.; Guthrie, P.H.; Taegtmeyer, H.; Kellems, R.E. Mammalian target of rapamycin and protein kinase a signaling mediate the cardiac transcriptional response to glutamine. *J. Biolog. Chem.* **2003**, *278*, 13143–13150. [CrossRef] [PubMed]
59. Galley, H.F. Oxidative stress and mitochondrial dysfunction in sepsis. *Br. J. Anaesth.* **2011**, *107*, 57–64. [CrossRef] [PubMed]
60. Bode, B.P. Recent molecular advances in mammalian glutamine transport. *J. Nutr.* **2001**, *131*, 2475S–2486S. [CrossRef] [PubMed]
61. Haussinger, D.; Schliess, F. Glutamine metabolism and signaling in the liver. *Front. Biosci.* **2007**, *12*, 371–391. [CrossRef] [PubMed]
62. McGivan, J.D.; Bradford, N.M. Characteristics of the activation of glutaminase by ammonia in sonicated rat liver mitochondria. *Biochim. Biophys. Acta* **1983**, *759*, 296–302. [CrossRef]
63. Hoek, J.B.; Charles, R.; De Haan, E.J.; Tager, J.M. Glutamate oxidation in rat-liver homogenate. *Biochim. Biophys. Acta* **1969**, *172*, 407–416. [CrossRef]
64. Halestrap, A.P. The regulation of the matrix volume of mammalian mitochondria in vivo and in vitro and its role in the control of mitochondrial metabolism. *Biochim. Biophys. Acta* **1989**, *973*, 355–382. [CrossRef]
65. Brosnan, J.T.; Brosnan, M.E. Hepatic glutaminase—A special role in urea synthesis? *Nutrition* **2002**, *18*, 455–457. [CrossRef]
66. Meijer, A.J.; Verhoeven, A.J. Regulation of hepatic glutamine metabolism. *Biochem. Soc. Trans.* **1986**, *14*, 1001–1004. [CrossRef] [PubMed]
67. Watford, M.; Smith, E.M. Distribution of hepatic glutaminase activity and mRNA in perivenous and periportal rat hepatocytes. *Biochem. J.* **1990**, *267*, 265–267. [CrossRef] [PubMed]
68. Moorman, A.F.; de Boer, P.A.; Watford, M.; Dingemanse, M.A.; Lamers, W.H. Hepatic glutaminase mRNA is confined to part of the urea cycle domain in the adult rodent liver lobule. *FEBS Lett.* **1994**, *356*, 76–80. [CrossRef]
69. Gebhardt, R.; Mecke, D. Heterogeneous distribution of glutamine synthetase among rat liver parenchymal cells in situ and in primary culture. *EMBO J.* **1983**, *2*, 567–570. [CrossRef] [PubMed]
70. Häussinger, D.; Soboll, S.; Meijer, A.J.; Gerok, W.; Tager, J.M.; Sies, H. Role of plasma membrane transport in hepatic glutamine metabolism. *Eur. J. Biochem.* **1985**, *152*, 597–603. [CrossRef] [PubMed]
71. Lenzen, C.; Soboll, S.; Sies, H.; Haussinger, D. Ph control of hepatic glutamine degradation. Role of transport. *Eur. J. Biochem.* **1987**, *166*, 483–488. [CrossRef] [PubMed]
72. Häussinger, D.; Hallbrucker, C.; Saha, N.; Lang, F.; Gerok, W. Cell volume and bile acid excretion. *Biochem. J.* **1992**, *288*, 681–689. [CrossRef] [PubMed]
73. Haussinger, D.; Lang, F. Cell volume in the regulation of hepatic function: A mechanism for metabolic control. *Biochim. Biophys. Acta* **1991**, *1071*, 331–350. [CrossRef]
74. Gustafson, L.A.; Jumelle-Laclau, M.N.; van Woerkom, G.M.; van Kuilenburg, A.B.P.; Meijer, A.J. Cell swelling and glycogen metabolism in hepatocytes from fasted rats. *Biochim. Biophys. Acta* **1997**, *1318*, 184–190. [CrossRef]
75. Baquet, A.; Gaussin, V.; Bollen, M.; Stalmans, W.; Hue, L. Mechanism of activation of liver acetyl-coa carboxylase by cell swelling. *Eur. J. Biochem.* **1993**, *217*, 1083–1089. [CrossRef] [PubMed]

76. Vom Dahl, S.; Dombrowski, F.; Schmitt, M.; Schliess, F.; Pfeifer, U.; Häussinger, D. Cell hydration controls autophagosome formation in rat liver in a microtubule-dependent way downstream from p38mapk activation. *Biochem. J.* **2001**, *354*, 31–36. [CrossRef] [PubMed]
77. Vom Dahl, S.; Haussinger, D. Nutritional state and the swelling-induced inhibition of proteolysis in perfused rat liver. *J. Nutr.* **1996**, *126*, 395–402. [CrossRef] [PubMed]
78. Häussinger, D.; Kubitz, R.; Reinehr, R.; Bode, J.G.; Schliess, F. Molecular aspects of medicine: From experimental to clinical hepatology. *Mol. Asp. Med.* **2004**, *25*, 221–360. [CrossRef] [PubMed]
79. Jansen, L.T.; Adams, J.; Johnson, E.C.; Kavouras, S.A. Effects of cellular dehydration on glucose regulation in healthy males—A pilot study. *FASEB J.* **2017**, *31*, 1014-2.
80. Friedman, S.L. Molecular regulation of hepatic fibrosis, an integrated cellular response to tissue injury. *J. Biol. Chem.* **2000**, *275*, 2247–2250. [CrossRef] [PubMed]
81. Ghazwani, M.; Zhang, Y.; Gao, X.; Fan, J.; Li, J.; Li, S. Anti-fibrotic effect of thymoquinone on hepatic stellate cells. *Phytomedicine* **2014**, *21*, 254–260. [CrossRef] [PubMed]
82. Li, J.; Ghazwani, M.; Liu, K.; Huang, Y.; Chang, N.; Fan, J.; He, F.; Li, L.; Bu, S.; Xie, W.; et al. Regulation of hepatic stellate cell proliferation and activation by glutamine metabolism. *PLoS ONE* **2017**, *12*, e0182679. [CrossRef] [PubMed]
83. Lin, Z.; Cai, F.; Lin, N.; Ye, J.; Zheng, Q.; Ding, G. Effects of glutamine on oxidative stress and nuclear factor-κb expression in the livers of rats with nonalcoholic fatty liver disease. *Exp. Ther. Med.* **2014**, *7*, 365–370. [CrossRef] [PubMed]
84. Sellmann, C.; Baumann, A.; Brandt, A.; Jin, C.J.; Nier, A.; Bergheim, I. Oral supplementation of glutamine attenuates the progression of nonalcoholic steatohepatitis in c57bl/6j mice. *J. Nutr.* **2017**, *147*, 2041–2049. [CrossRef] [PubMed]
85. Magalhaes, C.R.; Malafaia, O.; Torres, O.J.; Moreira, L.B.; Tefil, S.C.; Pinherio Mda, R.; Harada, B.A. Liver regeneration with l-glutamine supplemented diet: Experimental study in rats. *Rev. Col. Bras. Cir.* **2014**, *41*, 117–121. [CrossRef] [PubMed]
86. Helling, G.; Wahlin, S.; Smedberg, M.; Pettersson, L.; Tjäder, I.; Norberg, Å.; Rooyackers, O.; Wernerman, J. Plasma glutamine concentrations in liver failure. *PLoS ONE* **2016**, *11*, e0150440. [CrossRef] [PubMed]
87. Eagle, H.; Oyama, V.I.; Levy, M.; Horton, C.L.; Fleischman, R. Growth response of mammalian cells in tissue culture to l-glutamine and l glutamic acid. *J. Biol. Chem.* **1956**, *218*, 607–616. [PubMed]
88. Newsholme, P.; Curi, R.; Gordon, S.; Newsholme, E.A. Metabolism of glucose, glutamine, long-chain fatty-acids and ketone-bodies by murine macrophages. *Biochem. J.* **1986**, *239*, 121–125. [CrossRef] [PubMed]
89. Newsholme, E.A.; Newsholme, P.; Curi, R. The role of the citric acid cycle in cells of the immune system and its importance in sepsis, trauma and burns. *Biochem. Soc. Symp.* **1987**, *54*, 145–162. [PubMed]
90. Curi, R.; Newsholme, P.; Newsholme, E.A. Intracellular-distribution of some enzymes of the glutamine utilization pathway in rat lymphocytes. *Biochem. Biophys. Res. Commun.* **1986**, *138*, 318–322. [CrossRef]
91. Curi, T.C.P.; de Melo, M.P.; de Azevedo, R.B.; Curi, R. Glutamine utilisation by rat neutrophils. *Biochem. Soc. Trans.* **1997**, *25*, 249S. [CrossRef] [PubMed]
92. Curi, T.C.P.; DeMelo, M.P.; DeAzevedo, R.B.; Zorn, T.M.T.; Curi, R. Glutamine utilization by rat neutrophils: Presence of phosphate-dependent glutaminase. *Am. J. Physiol. Cell Physiol.* **1997**, *273*, C1124–C1129. [CrossRef]
93. Oudemans-van Straaten, H.M.; Bosman, R.J.; Treskes, M.; van der Spoel, H.J.; Zandstra, D.F. Plasma glutamine depletion and patient outcome in acute icu admissions. *Intensiv. Care Med.* **2001**, *27*, 84–90. [CrossRef]
94. Leite, J.S.M.; Cruzat, V.F.; Krause, M.; Homem de Bittencourt, P.I. Physiological regulation of the heat shock response by glutamine: Implications for chronic low-grade inflammatory diseases in age-related conditions. *Nutrire* **2016**, *41*, 17. [CrossRef]
95. Roth, E.; Oehler, R.; Manhart, N.; Exner, R.; Wessner, B.; Strasser, E.; Spittler, A. Regulative potential of glutamine—Relation to glutathione metabolism. *Nutrition* **2002**, *18*, 217–221. [CrossRef]
96. Hiscock, N.; Petersen, E.W.; Krzywkowski, K.; Boza, J.; Halkjaer-Kristensen, J.; Pedersen, B.K. Glutamine supplementation further enhances exercise-induced plasma il-6. *J. Appl. Physiol.* **2003**, *95*, 145–148. [CrossRef] [PubMed]
97. Mills, E.L.; Kelly, B.; O'Neill, L.A.J. Mitochondria are the powerhouses of immunity. *Nat. Immunol.* **2017**, *18*, 488–498. [CrossRef] [PubMed]

98. Pithon-Curi, T.C.; De Melo, M.P.; Curi, R. Glucose and glutamine utilization by rat lymphocytes, monocytes and neutrophils in culture: A comparative study. *Cell Biochem. Funct.* **2004**, *22*, 321–326. [CrossRef] [PubMed]
99. Pithon-Curi, T.C.; Trezena, A.G.; Tavares-Lima, W.; Curi, R. Evidence that glutamine is involved in neutrophil function. *Cell Biochem. Funct.* **2002**, *20*, 81–86. [CrossRef] [PubMed]
100. Branzk, N.; Lubojemska, A.; Hardison, S.E.; Wang, Q.; Gutierrez, M.G.; Brown, G.D.; Papayannopoulos, V. Neutrophils sense microbe size and selectively release neutrophil extracellular traps in response to large pathogens. *Nat. Immunol.* **2014**, *15*, 1017–1025. [CrossRef] [PubMed]
101. Pithon-Curi, T.C.; Levada, A.C.; Lopes, L.R.; Doi, S.Q.; Curi, R. Glutamine plays a role in superoxide production and the expression of p47(phox), p22(phox) and gp91(phox) in rat neutrophils. *Clin. Sci.* **2002**, *103*, 403–408. [CrossRef] [PubMed]
102. Garcia, C.; Pithon-Curi, T.C.; de Lourdes Firmano, M.; Pires de Melo, M.; Newsholme, P.; Curi, R. Effects of adrenaline on glucose and glutamine metabolism and superoxide production by rat neutrophils. *Clin. Sci.* **1999**, *96*, 549–555. [CrossRef] [PubMed]
103. Newsholme, P.; Costa Rosa, L.F.; Newsholme, E.A.; Curi, R. The importance of fuel metabolism to macrophage function. *Cell Biochem. Funct.* **1996**, *14*, 1–10. [CrossRef] [PubMed]
104. Peres, C.M.; Procopio, J.; Costa, M.; Curi, R. Thioglycolate-elicited rat macrophages exhibit alterations in incorporation and oxidation of fatty acids. *Lipids* **1999**, *34*, 1193–1197. [CrossRef] [PubMed]
105. Costa Rosa, L.F.; Safi, D.A.; Curi, R. Effect of thioglycollate and bcg stimuli on glucose and glutamine metabolism in rat macrophages. *J. Leukoc. Biol.* **1994**, *56*, 10–14. [PubMed]
106. Nagy, C.; Haschemi, A. Time and demand are two critical dimensions of immunometabolism: The process of macrophage activation and the pentose phosphate pathway. *Front. Immunol.* **2015**, *6*, 164. [CrossRef] [PubMed]
107. Langston, P.K.; Shibata, M.; Horng, T. Metabolism supports macrophage activation. *Front. Immunol.* **2017**, *8*, 61. [CrossRef] [PubMed]
108. Vergadi, E.; Ieronymaki, E.; Lyroni, K.; Vaporidi, K.; Tsatsanis, C. Akt signaling pathway in macrophage activation and m1/m2 polarization. *J. Immunol.* **2017**, *198*, 1006–1014. [CrossRef] [PubMed]
109. Martinez, F.O.; Sica, A.; Mantovani, A.; Locati, M. Macrophage activation and polarization. *Front. Biosci.* **2008**, *13*, 453–461. [CrossRef] [PubMed]
110. Gordon, S.; Taylor, P.R. Monocyte and macrophage heterogeneity. *Nat. Rev. Immunol.* **2005**, *5*, 953–964. [CrossRef] [PubMed]
111. Gordon, S.; Martinez, F.O. Alternative activation of macrophages: Mechanism and functions. *Immunity* **2010**, *32*, 593–604. [CrossRef] [PubMed]
112. Mosser, D.M.; Edwards, J.P. Exploring the full spectrum of macrophage activation. *Nat. Rev. Immunol.* **2008**, *8*, 958–969. [CrossRef] [PubMed]
113. O'Neill, L.A.; Pearce, E.J. Immunometabolism governs dendritic cell and macrophage function. *J. Exp. Med.* **2016**, *213*, 15–23. [CrossRef] [PubMed]
114. Namgaladze, D.; Brune, B. Fatty acid oxidation is dispensable for human macrophage il-4-induced polarization. *Biochim. Biophys. Acta* **2014**, *1841*, 1329–1335. [CrossRef] [PubMed]
115. O'Neill, L.A. A broken krebs cycle in macrophages. *Immunity* **2015**, *42*, 393–394. [CrossRef] [PubMed]
116. Warburg, O.; Wind, F.; Negelein, E. The metabolism of tumors in the body. *J. Gen. Physiol.* **1927**, *8*, 519–530. [CrossRef] [PubMed]
117. Palsson-McDermott, E.M.; Curtis, A.M.; Goel, G.; Lauterbach, M.A.; Sheedy, F.J.; Gleeson, L.E.; van den Bosch, M.W.; Quinn, S.R.; Domingo-Fernandez, R.; Johnston, D.G.; et al. Pyruvate kinase M2 regulates hif-1alpha activity and il-1beta induction and is a critical determinant of the warburg effect in lps-activated macrophages. *Cell Metab.* **2015**, *21*, 65–80. [CrossRef] [PubMed]
118. Oren, R.; Farnham, A.E.; Saito, K.; Milofsky, E.; Karnovsky, M.L. Metabolic patterns in three types of phagocytizing cells. *J. Cell Biol.* **1963**, *17*, 487–501. [CrossRef] [PubMed]
119. Tannahill, G.M.; Curtis, A.M.; Adamik, J.; Palsson-McDermott, E.M.; McGettrick, A.F.; Goel, G.; Frezza, C.; Bernard, N.J.; Kelly, B.; Foley, N.H.; et al. Succinate is an inflammatory signal that induces il-1β through hif-1α. *Nature* **2013**, *496*, 238–242. [CrossRef] [PubMed]

120. Jha, A.K.; Huang, S.C.; Sergushichev, A.; Lampropoulou, V.; Ivanova, Y.; Loginicheva, E.; Chmielewski, K.; Stewart, K.M.; Ashall, J.; Everts, B.; et al. Network integration of parallel metabolic and transcriptional data reveals metabolic modules that regulate macrophage polarization. *Immunity* **2015**, *42*, 419–430. [CrossRef] [PubMed]

121. Davies, L.C.; Rice, C.M.; Palmieri, E.M.; Taylor, P.R.; Kuhns, D.B.; McVicar, D.W. Peritoneal tissue-resident macrophages are metabolically poised to engage microbes using tissue-niche fuels. *Nat. Commun.* **2017**, *8*, 2074. [CrossRef] [PubMed]

122. Liu, P.S.; Wang, H.; Li, X.; Chao, T.; Teav, T.; Christen, S.; Di Conza, G.; Cheng, W.C.; Chou, C.H.; Vavakova, M.; et al. Alpha-ketoglutarate orchestrates macrophage activation through metabolic and epigenetic reprogramming. *Nat. Immunol.* **2017**, *18*, 985–994. [PubMed]

123. Nelson, V.L.; Nguyen, H.C.B.; Garcia-Canaveras, J.C.; Briggs, E.R.; Ho, W.Y.; DiSpirito, J.R.; Marinis, J.M.; Hill, D.A.; Lazar, M.A. Ppargamma is a nexus controlling alternative activation of macrophages via glutamine metabolism. *Gen. Dev.* **2018**, *32*, 1035–1044. [CrossRef] [PubMed]

124. Greiner, E.F.; Guppy, M.; Brand, K. Glucose is essential for proliferation and the glycolytic enzyme induction that provokes a transition to glycolytic energy production. *J. Biol. Chem.* **1994**, *269*, 31484–31490. [PubMed]

125. Newsholme, E.A.; Crabtree, B.; Ardawi, M.S. Glutamine metabolism in lymphocytes: Its biochemical, physiological and clinical importance. *Q. J. Exp. Physiol.* **1985**, *70*, 473–489. [CrossRef] [PubMed]

126. Curi, R.; Newsholme, P.; Newsholme, E.A. Metabolism of pyruvate by isolated rat mesenteric lymphocytes, lymphocyte mitochondria and isolated mouse macrophages. *Biochem. J.* **1988**, *250*, 383–388. [CrossRef] [PubMed]

127. Maciolek, J.A.; Pasternak, J.A.; Wilson, H.L. Metabolism of activated t lymphocytes. *Curr. Opin. Immunol.* **2014**, *27*, 60–74. [CrossRef] [PubMed]

128. Tripmacher, R.; Gaber, T.; Dziurla, R.; Haupl, T.; Erekul, K.; Grutzkau, A.; Tschirschmann, M.; Scheffold, A.; Radbruch, A.; Burmester, G.R.; et al. Human cd4(+) T cells maintain specific functions even under conditions of extremely restricted ATP production. *Eur. J. Immunol.* **2008**, *38*, 1631–1642. [CrossRef] [PubMed]

129. Wieman, H.L.; Wofford, J.A.; Rathmell, J.C. Cytokine stimulation promotes glucose uptake via phosphatidylinositol-3 kinase/akt regulation of glut1 activity and trafficking. *Mol. Biol. Cell* **2007**, *18*, 1437–1446. [CrossRef] [PubMed]

130. Delgoffe, G.M.; Kole, T.P.; Zheng, Y.; Zarek, P.E.; Matthews, K.L.; Xiao, B.; Worley, P.F.; Kozma, S.C.; Powell, J.D. The mtor kinase differentially regulates effector and regulatory T cell lineage commitment. *Immunity* **2009**, *30*, 832–844. [CrossRef] [PubMed]

131. Lee, K.; Gudapati, P.; Dragovic, S.; Spencer, C.; Joyce, S.; Killeen, N.; Magnuson, M.A.; Boothby, M. Mammalian target of rapamycin protein complex 2 regulates differentiation of th1 and th2 cell subsets via distinct signaling pathways. *Immunity* **2010**, *32*, 743–753. [CrossRef] [PubMed]

132. Michalek, R.D.; Gerriets, V.A.; Jacobs, S.R.; Macintyre, A.N.; MacIver, N.J.; Mason, E.F.; Sullivan, S.A.; Nichols, A.G.; Rathmell, J.C. Cutting edge: Distinct glycolytic and lipid oxidative metabolic programs are essential for effector and regulatory cd4+ T cell subsets. *J. Immunol.* **2011**, *186*, 3299–3303. [CrossRef] [PubMed]

133. Hardie, D.G.; Hawley, S.A.; Scott, J.W. Amp-activated protein kinas—Development of the energy sensor concept. *J. Physiol.* **2006**, *574*, 7–15. [CrossRef] [PubMed]

134. Crawford, J.; Cohen, H.J. The essential role of l-glutamine in lymphocyte differentiation in vitro. *J. Cell. Physiol.* **1985**, *124*, 275–282. [CrossRef] [PubMed]

135. Matarese, G.; Colamatteo, A.; De Rosa, V. Metabolic fuelling of proper t cell functions. *Immunol. Lett.* **2014**, *161*, 174–178. [CrossRef] [PubMed]

136. Chang, C.H.; Curtis, J.D.; Maggi, L.B., Jr.; Faubert, B.; Villarino, A.V.; O'Sullivan, D.; Huang, S.C.; van der Windt, G.J.; Blagih, J.; Qiu, J.; et al. Posttranscriptional control of t cell effector function by aerobic glycolysis. *Cell* **2013**, *153*, 1239–1251. [CrossRef] [PubMed]

137. Zheng, Y.; Delgoffe, G.M.; Meyer, C.F.; Chan, W.; Powell, J.D. Anergic T cells are metabolically anergic. *J. Immunol.* **2009**, *183*, 6095–6101. [CrossRef] [PubMed]

138. Buck, M.D.; O'Sullivan, D.; Klein Geltink, R.I.; Curtis, J.D.; Chang, C.H.; Sanin, D.E.; Qiu, J.; Kretz, O.; Braas, D.; van der Windt, G.J.; et al. Mitochondrial dynamics controls T cell fate through metabolic programming. *Cell* **2016**, *166*, 63–76. [CrossRef] [PubMed]

139. Corcoran, S.E.; O'Neill, L.A. Hif1alpha and metabolic reprogramming in inflammation. *J. Clin. Investig.* **2016**, *126*, 3699–3707. [CrossRef] [PubMed]
140. Araujo, L.; Khim, P.; Mkhikian, H.; Mortales, C.L.; Demetriou, M. Glycolysis and glutaminolysis cooperatively control T cell function by limiting metabolite supply to n-glycosylation. *eLife* **2017**, *6*, e21330. [CrossRef] [PubMed]
141. Hesterberg, R.S.; Cleveland, J.L.; Epling-Burnette, P.K. Role of polyamines in immune cell functions. *Med. Sci.* **2018**, *6*, 22. [CrossRef] [PubMed]
142. Calder, P.C.; Yaqoob, P. Glutamine and the immune system. *Amino Acids* **1999**, *17*, 227–241. [CrossRef] [PubMed]
143. Wilmore, D.W.; Shabert, J.K. Role of glutamine in immunologic responses. *Nutrition* **1998**, *14*, 618–626. [CrossRef]
144. Lagranha, C.J.; Hirabara, S.M.; Curi, R.; Pithon-Curi, T.C. Glutamine supplementation prevents exercise-induced neutrophil apoptosis and reduces p38 mapk and jnk phosphorylation and p53 and caspase 3 expression. *Cell Biochem. Funct.* **2007**, *25*, 563–569. [CrossRef] [PubMed]
145. Young, V.R.; Ajami, A.M. Glutamine: The emperor or his clothes? *J. Nutr.* **2001**, *131*, 2447S–2486S. [CrossRef] [PubMed]
146. Meister, A.; Anderson, M.E. Glutathione. *Ann. Rev. Biochem.* **1983**, *52*, 711–760. [CrossRef] [PubMed]
147. Gaucher, C.; Boudier, A.; Bonetti, J.; Clarot, I.; Leroy, P.; Parent, M. Glutathione: Antioxidant properties dedicated to nanotechnologies. *Antioxidants* **2018**, *7*, 62. [CrossRef] [PubMed]
148. Liu, N.; Ma, X.; Luo, X.; Zhang, Y.; He, Y.; Dai, Z.; Yang, Y.; Wu, G.; Wu, Z. L-glutamine attenuates apoptosis in porcine enterocytes by regulating glutathione-related redox homeostasis. *J. Nutr.* **2018**, *148*, 526–534. [CrossRef] [PubMed]
149. Da Silva Lima, F.; Rogero, M.M.; Ramos, M.C.; Borelli, P.; Fock, R.A. Modulation of the nuclear factor-kappa b (nf-kappab) signalling pathway by glutamine in peritoneal macrophages of a murine model of protein malnutrition. *Eur. J. Nutr.* **2013**, *52*, 1343–1351. [CrossRef] [PubMed]
150. Smedberg, M.; Wernerman, J. Is the glutamine story over? *Crit. Care* **2016**, *20*, 361. [CrossRef] [PubMed]
151. Heck, T.G.; Scholer, C.M.; de Bittencourt, P.I. Hsp70 expression: Does it a novel fatigue signalling factor from immune system to the brain? *Cell Biochem. Funct.* **2011**, *29*, 215–226. [CrossRef] [PubMed]
152. Singleton, K.D.; Wischmeyer, P.E. Glutamine's protection against sepsis and lung injury is dependent on heat shock protein 70 expression. *Am. J. Physiol. Regul. Integr. Comp. Physiol.* **2007**, *292*, R1839–R1845. [CrossRef] [PubMed]
153. Jordan, I.; Balaguer, M.; Esteban, M.E.; Cambra, F.J.; Felipe, A.; Hernandez, L.; Alsina, L.; Molero, M.; Villaronga, M.; Esteban, E. Glutamine effects on heat shock protein 70 and interleukines 6 and 10: Randomized trial of glutamine supplementation versus standard parenteral nutrition in critically ill children. *Clin. Nutr.* **2016**, *35*, 34–40. [CrossRef] [PubMed]
154. Kim, G.; Meriin, A.B.; Gabai, V.L.; Christians, E.; Benjamin, I.; Wilson, A.; Wolozin, B.; Sherman, M.Y. The heat shock transcription factor hsf1 is downregulated in DNA damage-associated senescence, contributing to the maintenance of senescence phenotype. *Aging Cell* **2012**, *11*, 617–627. [CrossRef] [PubMed]
155. Gabai, V.L.; Meng, L.; Kim, G.; Mills, T.A.; Benjamin, I.J.; Sherman, M.Y. Heat shock transcription factor hsf1 is involved in tumor progression via regulation of hypoxia-inducible factor 1 and RNA-binding protein HUR. *Mol. Cell. Biol.* **2012**, *32*, 929–940. [CrossRef] [PubMed]
156. Dokladny, K.; Zuhl, M.N.; Mandell, M.; Bhattacharya, D.; Schneider, S.; Deretic, V.; Moseley, P.L. Regulatory coordination between two major intracellular homeostatic systems: Heat shock response and autophagy. *J. Biolog. Chem.* **2013**, *288*, 14959–14972. [CrossRef] [PubMed]
157. Martinez, M.R.; Dias, T.B.; Natov, P.S.; Zachara, N.E. Stress-induced o-glcnacylation: An adaptive process of injured cells. *Biochem. Soc. Trans.* **2017**, *45*, 237–249. [CrossRef] [PubMed]
158. Lafontaine-Lacasse, M.; Dore, G.; Picard, F. Hexosamines stimulate apoptosis by altering sirt1 action and levels in rodent pancreatic beta-cells. *J. Endoc.* **2011**, *208*, 41–49. [CrossRef] [PubMed]
159. Kazemi, Z.; Chang, H.; Haserodt, S.; McKen, C.; Zachara, N.E. O-linked beta-n-acetylglucosamine (o-glcnac) regulates stress-induced heat shock protein expression in a gsk-3beta-dependent manner. *J. Biol. Chem.* **2010**, *285*, 39096–39107. [CrossRef] [PubMed]

160. Hamiel, C.R.; Pinto, S.; Hau, A.; Wischmeyer, P.E. Glutamine enhances heat shock protein 70 expression via increased hexosamine biosynthetic pathway activity. *Am. J. Physiol. Cell Physiol.* **2009**, *297*, C1509–1519. [CrossRef] [PubMed]
161. Singleton, K.D.; Serkova, N.; Beckey, V.E.; Wischmeyer, P.E. Glutamine attenuates lung injury and improves survival after sepsis: Role of enhanced heat shock protein expression. *Crit. Care Med.* **2005**, *33*, 1206–1213. [CrossRef] [PubMed]
162. Raizel, R.; Leite, J.S.; Hypolito, T.M.; Coqueiro, A.Y.; Newsholme, P.; Cruzat, V.F.; Tirapegui, J. Determination of the anti-inflammatory and cytoprotective effects of l-glutamine and l-alanine, or dipeptide, supplementation in rats submitted to resistance exercise. *Br. J. Nutr.* **2016**, *116*, 470–479. [CrossRef] [PubMed]
163. Smolka, M.B.; Zoppi, C.C.; Alves, A.A.; Silveira, L.R.; Marangoni, S.; Pereira-Da-Silva, L.; Novello, J.C.; Macedo, D.V. Hsp72 as a complementary protection against oxidative stress induced by exercise in the soleus muscle of rats. *Am. J. Physiol. Regul. Integr. Comp. Physiol.* **2000**, *279*, R1539–R1545. [CrossRef] [PubMed]
164. Gupta, A.; Cooper, Z.A.; Tulapurkar, M.E.; Potla, R.; Maity, T.; Hasday, J.D.; Singh, I.S. Toll-like receptor agonists and febrile range hyperthermia synergize to induce heat shock protein 70 expression and extracellular release. *J. Biolog. Chem.* **2013**, *288*, 2756–2766. [CrossRef] [PubMed]
165. Krause, M.; Keane, K.; Rodrigues-Krause, J.; Crognale, D.; Egan, B.; De Vito, G.; Murphy, C.; Newsholme, P. Elevated levels of extracellular heat-shock protein 72 (ehsp72) are positively correlated with insulin resistance in vivo and cause pancreatic beta-cell dysfunction and death in vitro. *Clin. Sci.* **2014**, *126*, 739–752. [CrossRef] [PubMed]
166. Lenders, C.M.; Liu, S.; Wilmore, D.W.; Sampson, L.; Dougherty, L.W.; Spiegelman, D.; Willett, W.C. Evaluation of a novel food composition database that includes glutamine and other amino acids derived from gene sequencing data. *Eur. J. Clin. Nutr.* **2009**, *63*, 1433–1439. [CrossRef] [PubMed]
167. Hermans, G.; Van den Berghe, G. Clinical review: Intensive care unit acquired weakness. *Crit. Care* **2015**, *19*, 274. [CrossRef] [PubMed]
168. Stehle, P.; Ellger, B.; Kojic, D.; Feuersenger, A.; Schneid, C.; Stover, J.; Scheiner, D.; Westphal, M. Glutamine dipeptide-supplemented parenteral nutrition improves the clinical outcomes of critically ill patients: A systematic evaluation of randomised controlled trials. *Clin. Nutr. ESPEN* **2017**, *17*, 75–85. [CrossRef] [PubMed]
169. Gunst, J.; Vanhorebeek, I.; Thiessen, S.E.; Van den Berghe, G. Amino acid supplements in critically ill patients. *Pharmacol. Res.* **2018**, *130*, 127–131. [CrossRef] [PubMed]
170. Furst, P.; Alteheld, B.; Stehle, P. Why should a single nutrient—Glutamine—Improve outcome? The remarkable story of glutamine dipeptides. *Clin. Nutr. Suppl.* **2004**, *1*, 3–15. [CrossRef]
171. Grau, T.; Bonet, A.; Minambres, E.; Pineiro, L.; Irles, J.A.; Robles, A.; Acosta, J.; Herrero, I.; Palacios, V.; Lopez, J.; et al. The effect of l-alanyl-l-glutamine dipeptide supplemented total parenteral nutrition on infectious morbidity and insulin sensitivity in critically ill patients. *Crit. Care Med.* **2011**, *39*, 1263–1268. [CrossRef] [PubMed]
172. Estivariz, C.F.; Griffith, D.P.; Luo, M.; Szeszycki, E.E.; Bazargan, N.; Dave, N.; Daignault, N.M.; Bergman, G.F.; McNally, T.; Battey, C.H.; et al. Efficacy of parenteral nutrition supplemented with glutamine dipeptide to decrease hospital infections in critically ill surgical patients. *J. Parenter. Enter. Nutr.* **2008**, *32*, 389–402. [CrossRef] [PubMed]
173. Wang, Y.; Jiang, Z.M.; Nolan, M.T.; Jiang, H.; Han, H.R.; Yu, K.; Li, H.L.; Jie, B.; Liang, X.K. The impact of glutamine dipeptide-supplemented parenteral nutrition on outcomes of surgical patients: A meta-analysis of randomized clinical trials. *J. Parenter. Enter. Nutr.* **2010**, *34*, 521–529. [CrossRef] [PubMed]
174. Bollhalder, L.; Pfeil, A.M.; Tomonaga, Y.; Schwenkglenks, M. A systematic literature review and meta-analysis of randomized clinical trials of parenteral glutamine supplementation. *Clin. Nutr.* **2013**, *32*, 213–223. [CrossRef] [PubMed]
175. Dechelotte, P.; Hasselmann, M.; Cynober, L.; Allaouchiche, B.; Coeffier, M.; Hecketsweiler, B.; Merle, V.; Mazerolles, M.; Samba, D.; Guillou, Y.M.; et al. L-alanyl-L-glutamine dipeptide-supplemented total parenteral nutrition reduces infectious complications and glucose intolerance in critically ill patients: The french controlled, randomized, double-blind, multicenter study. *Crit. Care Med.* **2006**, *34*, 598–604. [CrossRef] [PubMed]
176. Weitzel, L.R.; Wischmeyer, P.E. Glutamine in critical illness: The time has come, the time is now. *Crit. Care Clin.* **2010**, *26*, 515–525. [CrossRef] [PubMed]

177. Klassen, P.; Mazariegos, M.; Solomons, N.W.; Furst, P. The pharmacokinetic responses of humans to 20 g of alanyl-glutamine dipeptide differ with the dosing protocol but not with gastric acidity or in patients with acute dengue fever. *J. Nutr.* **2000**, *130*, 177–182. [CrossRef] [PubMed]
178. Melis, G.C.; Boelens, P.G.; van der Sijp, J.R.; Popovici, T.; De Bandt, J.P.; Cynober, L.; van Leeuwen, P.A. The feeding route (enteral or parenteral) affects the plasma response of the dipetide ala-gln and the amino acids glutamine, citrulline and arginine, with the administration of ala-gln in preoperative patients. *Br. J. Nutr.* **2005**, *94*, 19–26. [CrossRef] [PubMed]
179. Krause, M.S.; de Bittencourt, P.I.H.J. Type 1 diabetes: Can exercise impair the autoimmune event? The l-arginine/glutamine coupling hypothesis. *Cell Biochem. Funct.* **2008**, *26*, 406–433. [CrossRef] [PubMed]
180. Adibi, S.A. Regulation of expression of the intestinal oligopeptide transporter (pept-1) in health and disease. *Am. J. Physiol. Gastrointest. Liver Physiol.* **2003**, *285*, G779–G788. [CrossRef] [PubMed]
181. Broer, S. Amino acid transport across mammalian intestinal and renal epithelia. *Physiol. Rev.* **2008**, *88*, 249–286. [CrossRef] [PubMed]
182. Gilbert, E.R.; Wong, E.A.; Webb, K.E. Board-invited review: Peptide absorption and utilization: Implications for animal nutrition and health. *J. Anim. Sci.* **2008**, *86*, 2135–2155. [CrossRef] [PubMed]
183. Petry, E.R.; Cruzat, V.F.; Heck, T.G.; de Bittencourt, P.I.H.; Tirapegui, J. L-glutamine supplementations enhance liver glutamine-glutathione axis and heat shock factor-1 expression in endurance-exercise trained rats. *Int. J. Sport Nutr. Exerc. Metab.* **2015**, *25*, 188–197. [CrossRef] [PubMed]
184. Alba-Loureiro, T.C.; Ribeiro, R.F.; Zorn, T.M.; Lagranha, C.J. Effects of glutamine supplementation on kidney of diabetic rat. *Amino Acids* **2010**, *38*, 1021–1030. [CrossRef] [PubMed]
185. Cheng, T.; Sudderth, J.; Yang, C.; Mullen, A.R.; Jin, E.S.; Mates, J.M.; DeBerardinis, R.J. Pyruvate carboxylase is required for glutamine-independent growth of tumor cells. *Proc. Natl. Acad Sci. USA* **2011**, *108*, 8674–8679. [CrossRef] [PubMed]
186. Hensley, C.T.; Wasti, A.T.; DeBerardinis, R.J. Glutamine and cancer: Cell biology, physiology, and clinical opportunities. *J. Clin. Investig.* **2013**, *123*, 3678–3684. [CrossRef] [PubMed]
187. Hensley, C.T.; Faubert, B.; Yuan, Q.; Lev-Cohain, N.; Jin, E.; Kim, J.; Jiang, L.; Ko, B.; Skelton, R.; Loudat, L.; et al. Metabolic heterogeneity in human lung tumors. *Cell* **2016**, *164*, 681–694. [CrossRef] [PubMed]
188. Davidson, S.M.; Papagiannakopoulos, T.; Olenchock, B.A.; Heyman, J.E.; Keibler, M.A.; Luengo, A.; Bauer, M.R.; Jha, A.K.; O'Brien, J.P.; Pierce, K.A.; et al. Environment impacts the metabolic dependencies of ras-driven non-small cell lung cancer. *Cell Metab.* **2016**, *23*, 517–528. [CrossRef] [PubMed]
189. Choi, C.; Ganji, S.; Hulsey, K.; Madan, A.; Kovacs, Z.; Dimitrov, I.; Zhang, S.; Pichumani, K.; Mendelsohn, D.; Mickey, B.; et al. A comparative study of short- and long-te (1) h mrs at 3 t for in vivo detection of 2-hydroxyglutarate in brain tumors. *NMR Biomed.* **2013**, *26*, 1242–1250. [CrossRef] [PubMed]
190. Tardito, S.; Oudin, A.; Ahmed, S.U.; Fack, F.; Keunen, O.; Zheng, L.; Miletic, H.; Sakariassen, P.O.; Weinstock, A.; Wagner, A.; et al. Glutamine synthetase activity fuels nucleotide biosynthesis and supports growth of glutamine-restricted glioblastoma. *Nat. Cell Biol.* **2015**, *17*, 1556–1568. [CrossRef] [PubMed]
191. Deep, G.; Schlaepfer, I.R. Aberrant lipid metabolism promotes prostate cancer: Role in cell survival under hypoxia and extracellular vesicles biogenesis. *Int. J. Mol. Sci.* **2016**, *17*, 1061. [CrossRef] [PubMed]
192. White, M.A.; Lin, C.; Rajapakshe, K.; Dong, J.; Shi, Y.; Tsouko, E.; Mukhopadhyay, R.; Jasso, D.; Dawood, W.; Coarfa, C.; et al. Glutamine transporters are targets of multiple oncogenic signaling pathways in prostate cancer. *Mol. Cancer Res.* **2017**, *15*, 1017–1028. [CrossRef] [PubMed]
193. Marian, M.J. Dietary supplements commonly used by cancer survivors: Are there any benefits? *Nutr. Clin. Pract.* **2017**, *32*, 607–627. [CrossRef] [PubMed]
194. Sayles, C.; Hickerson, S.C.; Bhat, R.R.; Hall, J.; Garey, K.W.; Trivedi, M.V. Oral glutamine in preventing treatment-related mucositis in adult patients with cancer: A systematic review. *Nutr. Clin. Pract.* **2016**, *31*, 171–179. [CrossRef] [PubMed]
195. Daniele, B.; Perrone, F.; Gallo, C.; Pignata, S.; De Martino, S.; De Vivo, R.; Barletta, E.; Tambaro, R.; Abbiati, R.; D'Agostino, L. Oral glutamine in the prevention of fluorouracil induced intestinal toxicity: A double blind, placebo controlled, randomised trial. *Gut* **2001**, *48*, 28–33. [CrossRef] [PubMed]
196. Hammarqvist, F.; Wernerman, J.; Ali, R.; von der Decken, A.; Vinnars, E. Addition of glutamine to total parenteral nutrition after elective abdominal surgery spares free glutamine in muscle, counteracts the fall in muscle protein synthesis, and improves nitrogen balance. *Ann. Surg.* **1989**, *209*, 455–461. [CrossRef] [PubMed]

197. Souba, W.W.; Herskowitz, K.; Klimberg, V.S.; Salloum, R.M.; Plumley, D.A.; Flynn, T.C.; Copeland, E.M. The effects of sepsis and endotoxemia on gut glutamine metabolism. *Ann. Surg.* **1990**, *211*, 543–551. [CrossRef] [PubMed]
198. Bode, B.P.; Fuchs, B.C.; Hurley, B.P.; Conroy, J.L.; Suetterlin, J.E.; Tanabe, K.K.; Rhoads, D.B.; Abcouwer, S.F.; Souba, W.W. Molecular and functional analysis of glutamine uptake in human hepatoma and liver-derived cells. *Am. J. Physiol. Gastrointest. Liver Physiol.* **2002**, *283*, G1062–G1073. [CrossRef] [PubMed]
199. Rogero, M.M.; Borelli, P.; Fock, R.A.; Borges, M.C.; Vinolo, M.A.R.; Curi, R.; Nakajima, K.; Crisma, A.R.; Ramos, A.D.; Tirapegui, J. Effects of glutamine on the nuclear factor-kappab signaling pathway of murine peritoneal macrophages. *Amino Acids* **2010**, *39*, 435–441. [CrossRef] [PubMed]
200. Parry-Billings, M.; Evans, J.; Calder, P.C.; Newsholme, E.A. Does glutamine contribute to immunosuppression after major burns? *Lancet* **1990**, *336*, 523–525. [CrossRef]
201. Roth, E.; Funovics, J.; Muhlbacher, F.; Schemper, M.; Mauritz, W.; Sporn, P.; Fritsch, A. Metabolic disorders in severe abdominal sepsis: Glutamine deficiency in skeletal muscle. *Clin. Nutr.* **1982**, *1*, 25–41. [CrossRef]

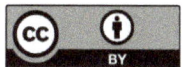

© 2018 by the authors. Licensee MDPI, Basel, Switzerland. This article is an open access article distributed under the terms and conditions of the Creative Commons Attribution (CC BY) license (http://creativecommons.org/licenses/by/4.0/).

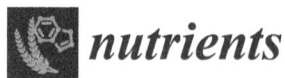

Review

Immune Function and Micronutrient Requirements Change over the Life Course

Silvia Maggini [1,*], Adeline Pierre [1] and Philip C. Calder [2,3]

1   Bayer Consumer Care AG, 4002 Basel, Switzerland; adeline.pierre@bayer.com
2   Human Development & Health, Faculty of Medicine, University of Southampton,
    Southampton SO16 6YD, UK; P.C.Calder@soton.ac.uk
3   NIHR Southampton Biomedical Research Centre, University Hospital Southampton NHS Foundation Trust
    and University of Southampton, Southampton SO16 6YD, UK
*   Correspondence: silvia.maggini@bayer.com; Tel.: +41-582-727-516

Received: 28 September 2018; Accepted: 15 October 2018; Published: 17 October 2018

Abstract: As humans age, the risk and severity of infections vary in line with immune competence according to how the immune system develops, matures, and declines. Several factors influence the immune system and its competence, including nutrition. A bidirectional relationship among nutrition, infection and immunity exists: changes in one component affect the others. For example, distinct immune features present during each life stage may affect the type, prevalence, and severity of infections, while poor nutrition can compromise immune function and increase infection risk. Various micronutrients are essential for immunocompetence, particularly vitamins A, C, D, E, B2, B6, and B12, folic acid, iron, selenium, and zinc. Micronutrient deficiencies are a recognized global public health issue, and poor nutritional status predisposes to certain infections. Immune function may be improved by restoring deficient micronutrients to recommended levels, thereby increasing resistance to infection and supporting faster recovery when infected. Diet alone may be insufficient and tailored micronutrient supplementation based on specific age-related needs necessary. This review looks at immune considerations specific to each life stage, the consequent risk of infection, micronutrient requirements and deficiencies exhibited over the life course, and the available evidence regarding the effects of micronutrient supplementation on immune function and infection.

Keywords: adults; age-related immunity; deficiency; elderly; immunosenescence; infants; infection; micronutrients; older people

1. Introduction

The immune system, which is integrated into all physiological systems, protects the body against infections and other external and internal insults by utilizing three distinct layers, depending on the nature of the threat: physical (e.g., skin, epithelial lining of the gastrointestinal and respiratory tracts) and biochemical barriers (e.g., secretions, mucus, and gastric acid), numerous different immune cells (e.g., granulocytes, CD4 or CD8 T and B cells), and antibodies (i.e., immunoglobulins). The first line of defense is innate immunity, which combines physical and biochemical barriers with a non-specific, leukocyte-mediated cellular response to defend against pathogens [1]. If the pathogen manages to avoid these innate defenses, a more complex, adaptive, antigen-specific response is triggered, mediated by T and B lymphocytes, which produces antibodies to target and destroy the pathogen (Figure 1) [1]. Both systems also protect against native cells that may be harmful, such as cancerous or precancerous cells [2].

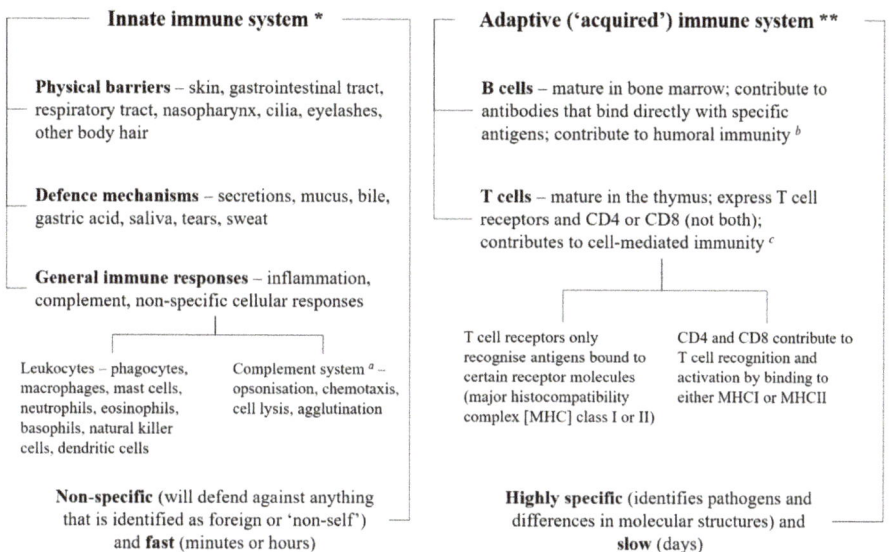

Figure 1. Simple overview of the immune system. The three layers of the immune system (physical and biochemical barriers; cells such as monocytes, granulocytes, lymphocytes, and B and T cells; and antibodies or immunoglobulins) work together to protect the body against pathogens, utilizing the innate and adaptive defense mechanisms. All three layers are involved in the innate and immune systems. * The innate immune system comprises anatomical and biochemical barriers and an unspecific cellular response mediated mainly by monocytes, neutrophils, natural killer cells and dendritic cells; these work together to fight off pathogens before they can start an active infection. ** The adaptive immune system involves an antigen-specific response mediated by T and B lymphocytes that is activated by exposure to pathogens; this works with the innate immune system to reduce the severity of infection. [a] The complement system can work with both the innate and adaptive immune systems; [b] i.e., immunity from serum antibodies produced by plasma cells; [c] i.e., an immune response that does not involve antibodies, but responds to any cells that display aberrant major histocompatibility complex (MHC) markers, such as cells invaded by pathogens.

As humans age, the immune system evolves from the immature and developing immune responses in infants and children, through to immune function that is potentially optimal in adolescents and young adults, followed by a gradual decline in immunity (particularly adaptive processes) in older people [1]. Age-related changes are compounded by certain lifestyle factors (e.g., diet, environmental factors, and oxidative stress) specific to each life stage that can influence and modify, in some cases suppressing, immune function. Accordingly, the risk and severity of infections such as the common cold and influenza (the most common illnesses in humans [3]), pneumonia and diarrheal infections also vary over a lifetime.

Optimal immune function is dependent on a healthy immune system. In turn, adequate nutrition is crucial to ensure a good supply of the energy sources, macronutrients and micronutrients required for the development, maintenance and expression of the immune response [3]. Micronutrients have vital roles throughout the immune system that are independent of life stage (Table 1), and it has been determined that those most needed to sustain immunocompetence include vitamins A, C, D, E, B2, B6 and B12, folic acid, beta carotene, iron, selenium, and zinc [4]. There is a bidirectional interaction among nutrition, infection and immunity: the immune response is compromised when nutrition is poor, predisposing individuals to infections, and a poor nutritional state may be exacerbated by the immune response itself to an infection [5]. It is clear that optimal immunocompetence depends upon nutritional status [6]. It is recognized that micronutrient deficiencies and suboptimal intakes are common worldwide [7], and certain micronutrients may be more likely to be insufficient at different stages of the life course. This can affect the risk and severity of infection, and in fact an individual's nutritional status can predict the clinical course and outcome of certain infections such as diarrhea, pneumonia and measles [4]. Resistance to infection may be enhanced by adding the deficient nutrient back into the diet and restoring immune function [4]. However, it is not always possible to achieve good nutritional status via the diet alone. In developing countries, for example, it may be difficult to find an adequate and varied supply of food. Even in industrialized nations, where it may be presumed that healthy, nutritious food is easier to obtain, social, economic, educational, ethnic and cultural backgrounds influence the diet and may adversely affect an individual's micronutrient status [8].

This review looks at life-stage-specific immunity, risk of infection and micronutrient requirements, from the perspective of industrialized countries where possible. The aim is to highlight the role of tailored supplementation in restoring micronutrients to recommended levels and better supporting immune needs that are specific to each life stage.

Table 1. Overview of key roles played by select micronutrients in the immune system [4,9–14].

Micronutrient/Role	Innate Immunity	Adaptive Immunity
Vitamin C	Effective antioxidant that protects against ROS and RNS produced when pathogens are killed by immune cells [9,14] Regenerates other important antioxidants such as glutathione and vitamin E to their active state [9] Promotes collagen synthesis, thereby supporting the integrity of epithelial barriers [10] Stimulates production, function and movement of leukocytes (e.g., neutrophils, lymphocytes, phagocytes) [9,14] Increases serum levels of complement proteins [14] Has roles in antimicrobial and NK cell activities and chemotaxis [10] Involved in apoptosis and clearance of spent neutrophils from sites of infection by macrophages [12]	Can increase serum levels of antibodies [12,14] Has roles in lymphocyte differentiation and proliferation [10,12]
Vitamin D	Vitamin D receptor expressed in innate immune cells (e.g., monocytes, macrophages, dendritic cells) [14] Increases the differentiation of monocytes to macrophages [10] Stimulates immune cell proliferation and cytokine production and helps protect against infection caused by pathogens [14] 1,25-dihydroxyvitamin D_3, the active form of vitamin D, regulates the antimicrobial proteins cathelicidin and defensin, which can directly kill pathogens, especially bacteria [14]	Mainly inhibitory effect in adaptive immunity [14]; for example, 1,25-dihydroxyvitamin D_3 suppresses antibody production by B cells and inhibits T cell proliferation [14]
Vitamin A	Helps maintain structural and functional integrity of mucosal cells in innate barriers (e.g., skin, respiratory tract, etc.) [14] Important for normal functioning of innate immune cells (e.g., NK cells, macrophages, neutrophils) [14]	Necessary for proper functioning of T and B lymphocytes, and thus for generation of antibody responses to antigen [14] Involved in development and differentiation of Th1 and Th2 cells and supports Th2 anti-inflammatory response [10]
Vitamin E	An important fat-soluble antioxidant [10] Protects the integrity of cell membranes from damage caused by free radicals [14] Enhances IL-2 production and NK cell cytotoxic activity [10]	Enhances T cell-mediated functions and lymphocyte proliferation [10] Optimizes and enhances Th1 and suppresses Th2 response [10]
Vitamin B6	Helps regulate inflammation [13] Has roles in cytokine production and NK cell activity [13,15]	Required in the endogenous synthesis and metabolism of amino acids, the building blocks of cytokines and antibodies [14] Has roles in lymphocyte proliferation, differentiation and maturation [14] Maintains Th1 immune response [10] Has roles in antibody production [13]

Table 1. Cont.

Micronutrient/Role	Innate Immunity	Adaptive Immunity
Vitamin B12	Has roles in NK cell functions [13]	May act as an immunomodulator for cellular immunity, especially with effects on cytotoxic cells (NK cells, CD8+ T-cells) [10] Facilitates production of T lymphocytes [13] Involved in humoral and cellular immunity and one-carbon metabolism (interactions with folate) [13]
Folate	Maintains innate immunity (NK cells) [10]	Has roles in cell-mediated immunity [13] Important for sufficient antibody response to antigens [13] Supports Th 1-mediated immune response [13]
Zinc	Antioxidant effects protect against ROS and RNS [9] Helps modulate cytokine release and induces proliferation of CD8+ T cells [10,16] Helps maintain skin and mucosal membrane integrity [10]	Central role in cellular growth and differentiation of immune cells that have a rapid differentiation and turnover [17] Essential for intracellular binding of tyrosine kinase to T cell receptors, required for T lymphocyte development and activation [9] Supports Th1 response [10]
Iron	Involved in regulation of cytokine production and action [10] Forms highly-toxic hydroxyl radicals, thus involved in the process of killing bacteria by neutrophils [10] Important in the generation of ROS that kill pathogens [14]	Important in the differentiation and proliferation of T lymphocytes [14] Essential for cell differentiation and growth, component of enzymes critical for functioning of immune cells (e.g., ribonucleotide reductase involved in DNA synthesis) [10]
Copper	Free-radical scavenger [4] Antimicrobial properties [14] Accumulates at sites of inflammation, important for IL-2 production and response [13,14] May play a role in the innate immune response to bacterial infections [14]	Has roles in T cell proliferation [13] Has roles in antibody production and cellular immunity [18]
Selenium	Essential for the function of selenium-dependent enzymes (selenoproteins) that can act as redox regulators and cellular antioxidants, potentially counteracting ROS [10,14] Selenoproteins are important for the antioxidant host defense system affecting leukocyte and NK cell function [13]	Involved in T lymphocyte proliferation [4,13] Has roles in the humoral system (e.g, immunoglobulin production) [13]

IL, interleukin; NK, natural killer; RNS, reactive nitrogen species; ROS, reactive oxygen species; Th, helper T cell.

2. The Immune System

2.1. Infants and Children

Prior to birth, babies lack significant antigenic exposure and so have not yet acquired immunological memory and their adaptive immunity is not fully developed [5,10,11,19]. Therefore, immune protection from pathogens such as bacteria and viruses immediately after birth relies on two primary methods of defense, passive immunity and innate immunity. Passive immunity is where maternal antibodies (antigen-specific immunoglobulins) are passed via the placenta before birth, and in maternal colostrum and milk after birth [10]. The primary immunoglobulin (Ig) in human maternal milk is IgA (which plays a crucial role in immune function at mucosal surfaces), but IgG (which provides the majority of antibody-based immunity against invading pathogens) and IgM (which eliminates pathogens in the early stages of B cell-mediated or humoral immunity before there is sufficient IgG) are also present in smaller amounts [20]. Levels of all immunoglobulins in maternal milk decrease in the days following birth [20], and babies and children are more susceptible to infections until they are able to produce sufficient antibodies by themselves. Maternal milk is a rich source of cells and compounds with immunological properties, depending on the stage of lactation, and may facilitate immune development and maturation in infants [21,22]. These include leukocytes (neutrophils, macrophages), cytokines, complement, and long-chain polyunsaturated fatty acids, which variously have antimicrobial, tolerance/priming, immune development, and anti-inflammatory properties [21,22].

The baby's innate immune system is essential to defend against pathogens [10]. The innate system is still functionally immature at birth, to allow the fetus to tolerate non-shared maternal antigens, but also so that it is not constantly triggered by the considerable amount of stress and remodeling that take place during development [19]. The neonatal innate immune system comprises different protective cell populations compared with adults, as well as qualitative differences in the responses by shared cell populations [23]. For example, innate immune cells such as monocytes and dendritic cells produce less of the bioactive form of interleukin (IL)-12 and type 1 interferon in newborns compared with adults, but similar or higher amounts of other interleukins (e.g., IL-6, IL-10, and IL-23) when stimulated by the same pathogen [24]. Neonatal cells are also less able to produce multiple cytokines in response to pathogenic stimulation [24]. Concentrations of NK cells are at their lowest in infants compared with other life-stages [25]. Furthermore, serum concentrations of almost all circulating components of the complement system are much lower (up to 80%) in newborns than in adults, with diminished biological activity [19]. Levels increase after birth, with some complement factors reaching adult concentrations within a month but others evolving much more slowly [19].

An adaptive immune response does occur in newborns, but it is slower and skewed towards T helper-2 (Th-2) reactions against extracellular pathogens [24]. After birth, innate lymphoid cells, which are critical regulators of innate immunity and inflammation at barrier surfaces (e.g., skin, respiratory and gastrointestinal tracts), indirectly modulate adaptive immunity via interactions with stromal cells in lymphoid tissues and epithelial cells at barrier surfaces [26]. Contact with the hostile environment drives cells of the innate and the adaptive mucosal and systemic immune systems to mature and expand, and the immunologic competence of the baby expands rapidly over the first few months of life [11]. Defenses against intracellular pathogens and cell-mediated immunity rely on Th-1 responses, which reach adult levels only after around two years of age [24]. Microbial antigens are essential for the education of the immune system and development of Th-1 type responses and breakdown in such immune education may predispose to allergic, inflammatory and autoimmune diseases [5,10].

As children grow and develop, their immune systems continue to mature and acquire memory after exposure to multiple foreign challenges including from pathogens, food and other environmental components and vaccines [19]. Neutrophil concentrations are increased in children aged 1–6 years compared with infants (but are still only half the adult levels), as are eosinophil and basophil concentrations (both then decrease with age); lymphocyte and platelet counts are lower in children compared with infants and steadily decline with age [25]. Closer analysis of lymphocyte subtypes indicates that the proportion of different lymphocyte subsets changes over time [25]. For example, the percentage of $CD3^+$ T cells (required for activation of $CD4^+$ and $CD8^+$ T cells) is significantly higher in children than in infants. However, the proportion of $CD4^+$ T cells is significantly lower in children than in infants [25]. $CD4^+$ helper T cells recognize peptides presented by major histocompatibility complex (MHC) II molecules found on antigen-presenting cells, and subsequently secrete cytokines that facilitate different immune responses according to the source of the antigen [27]. In contrast, the percentage of $CD8^+$ T cells is significantly higher in children than in infants and steadily increases over time [25]. $CD8^+$ cytotoxic T cells recognize peptides presented by MHC I molecules found on all nucleated cells, and secrete cytokines like tumor-necrosis factor alpha or interferon gamma to help to kill infected or malignant cells [27]. Analysis of B cells indicates that the proportion of $CD19^+$ cells is highest in infants and children and decreases significantly thereafter [25]. CD19 is an antigen that is present on all B cells, is involved in signaling, and is a biomarker for B lymphocyte development [28]. Antibody production increases with age from infancy to childhood. For example, adult levels of IgG (expressed on the surface of mature B cells, and the most prevalent immunoglobulin in serum) are reached by the age of 11–12 years, with a further increase during puberty, while levels of IgA (the second most prevalent immunoglobulin in serum, which can activate the complement pathway) continue to increase past puberty until they reach adult levels; in contrast, adult levels of IgM (the first immunoglobulin made by the fetus and virgin B cells challenged with antigen) are reached by the age of four years [29].

2.2. Adolescents and Adults

After childhood, physical changes occur in lymphoid tissues, which support immune responses and are responsible for producing lymphocytes and antibodies. For example, thymic tissue in the thymus (the organ that is instrumental in the production and maturation of T cells before birth and throughout childhood) is gradually replaced by adipose tissue after puberty and gives the impression of being larger in children and becoming smaller after adolescence [27]. The functional portion of the gland is considerably reduced (known as involution), but the thymus populates secondary lymphatic organs and tissues with T cells [27]. T cells continue to be produced in the thymus throughout a person's lifetime, although to a much smaller extent [27], but it is thought that adults rely on the naïve T cell pool produced mostly before puberty [30]. There is a progressive decline in the percentage of total lymphocytes and absolute numbers of T and B cells in the blood from infancy to adulthood [25]. However, there is a significant increase in all T cell subsets ($CD3^+$, $CD4^+$, and $CD8^+$) in adults compared with children, and a decrease in the biomarker for B lymphocyte development, CD19 [25]. There is also a significant increase in the number of NK cells in adolescents compared with infants and children, as well as in adults compared with infants (but not children) [25].

It should be noted that the immune system reaches maturity by adulthood, and small decreases or increases in single selected markers of immune function may not be clinically important after that. In general, young, non-pregnant adults seem to be well equipped to cope with immune challenges, which may reflect the procreative potential of young adults in the survival of the species [19]. However, there are some sex-specific differences that are evident in the prevalence of certain diseases. For example, autoimmune disorders such as Sjogren syndrome, systemic lupus erythematosus and autoimmune thyroid disease are higher in women [23]. The inflammatory immune response differs between men and women, with females generating higher proinflammatory cytokine and chemokine responses to the influenza virus and experiencing greater morbidity and mortality than males [31]. Women also initiate a higher humoral immune response to the influenza vaccine, and experience more adverse reactions than men [31]. However, the raised immunity in females following vaccination leads to greater cross-protection against novel influenza viruses compared with men [31]. It is thought that women typically mount stronger immune responses than men because of the immunomodulatory effects of estrogen in women and the humoral immunity suppressing effects of testosterone in men; however, the full extent of sex on functional immune responses remains unclear [23].

2.3. Older People

As the body ages, so does the immune system [32] and most older people over the age of 60–65 years (although not all) experience some immune dysregulation that makes them less able to respond to immune challenges [33,34]. There is a loss of lymphoid tissue, particularly in the thymus, with increasing age [25], and the ability to respond to pathogens, antigens and mitogens decreases [5,33]. The development of long-term immune memory is also impaired, with a diminished response to vaccination [5]. This is commonly referred to as immunosenescence, which mostly seems to affect adaptive immunity but also the innate immune system to a lesser extent [32].

Immune cells are constantly renewed from hematopoietic stem cells but these mature with age and become less able to produce lymphocytes; furthermore, the total amount of hematopoietic tissue decreases [34,35]. A loss of immune cells and a decrease in the number of circulating lymphocytes are characteristic in the immune systems of older people [23], consistent with reduced production of T cells in the involuted thymus, as well as diminished function of mature lymphocytes in secondary lymphoid tissues [34,36]. The proportions of naïve T cell subsets also change with age; for example, $CD3^+$ and $CD8^+$ cytotoxic T cells decrease significantly in older people, but $CD4^+$ helper T cells increase from adolescence to adulthood and then stabilize in older people [25], suggesting that $CD4^+$ cells are subject to stricter homeostatic mechanisms given their importance in immune system function [1]. On the other hand, memory T cells accumulate, especially late-stage differentiated $CD8^+$ cells [30]. $CD19^+$ cells decrease significantly from childhood to old age [25]. The total number of naïve B cells remains unchanged with ageing; instead, there is a decrease in memory B cells that may occur secondary to T cell deficiencies [34]. The incidence of autoimmune diseases also increases in later life, as the ageing immune system becomes unable to fully tolerate self-antigens [19,37]. Age-related lymphopenia may lead to a decrease in regulatory T cell function, an increase in T cells with increased affinity to self- or neoantigens, an increased prevalence of autoantibodies, and decreased clearance of apoptotic cells by macrophages [19,33].

Changes in the innate immune system also occur with increasing age. Skin and mucous membranes—the first line of defense against invading pathogens—become less effective as skin cell replacement declines and dermal and subcutaneous atrophy occurs [1]. After 60 years of age, there is a decrease in secretory IgA, which forms part of the first line of defense against pathogens that manage to invade the mucosal surfaces [38]. In older people, functional activity of immune cells such as phagocytes and the intracellular respiratory burst necessary to kill pathogens are reduced [1]. Although healthy ageing does not seem to affect the overall number of dendritic cells, which are responsible for the recognition and phagocytosis of pathogens, processing of antigens, priming of naïve T cells and regulation of the response of B and NK cells [1], they are diminished in certain areas such as Langerhans cells in the skin [39]. However, their ability to recognize invading pathogens is impaired by compromised Toll-like receptors on dendritic cells, for example, which is known to occur in ageing [40]. This reduces their ability to induce proinflammatory cytokine production and regulate antigen presentation to naïve T cells, and to activate antigen-specific adaptive immune responses [41]. The number of NK cells increases significantly in older people compared with younger adults [1,25], which may be the result of an accumulation of long-lived NK cells [42]. However, there is not an accompanying increase in cytotoxicity, but instead a decrease in the functioning of the NK cells, including a slower resolution of inflammatory responses [43].

In fact, a longer inflammatory process is induced in older adults [3]. Increased levels of circulating pro-inflammatory cytokines (e.g., tumor-necrosis factor alpha, IL-1, and IL-6 [1,25]) characterize low-grade chronic inflammation in older people, a process known as inflamm-aging [1]. Inflamm-aging is a physiological response to lifelong antigenic stress and, if kept under control by anti-inflammatory cytokines such as IL-10 [1] represents an efficient defense mechanism in older people. Increased production of anti-inflammatory molecules is an essential counter-regulatory process in ageing, as inflamm-aging would otherwise be damaging [44]. Many of the most common chronic diseases associated with ageing, such as atherosclerosis, Alzheimer's disease, osteoporosis and diabetes [1], are related to low-grade inflammation [32]. Oxidative stress also has a role in inflamm-aging, emphasizing the role of oxidative stress in the complex mechanisms of ageing [44]. Immune cells, which contain a high percentage of polyunsaturated fatty acids in their plasma membrane and so are susceptible to lipid peroxidation, are particularly sensitive to changes in the oxidant–antioxidant balance [10]. Thus, oxidative damage can compromise the integrity of immune cell membranes and alter transmission of signals both within and between different immune cells, leading to an impaired immune response [10]. It has been suggested that, in older people, many immune markers of immunosenescence may actually be more related to prolonged exposure to antigen stimulation and to oxidative stress involving the production of reactive oxygen species (ROS), rather than to "ageing" of the immune system per se [23,35,36]. For example, in modern industrialized populations, the cumulative effect of antigenic exposure may be lower than in less hygienic societies [30]. One individual may experience different environmental factors at different stages of life compared to another, and thus their immune profiles will also differ [23]. Some older people age without any major health problems, known as healthy ageing, and immune system dysfunction appears to be mitigated in this population [1]. Genetic and environmental factors (e.g., good nutritional status) may play a role, but these have yet to be described. It may be that the only truly universal age-related changes in immune markers are the reduction in the numbers and proportions of peripheral blood naïve T cells, due mainly to thymic involution, reflecting the aging of the hematopoietic stem cell system [36].

3. Response to Infection

The nature of the response of the immune system to a pathogen is initially dependent on whether the innate immune defenses can eliminate the infectious organism. If not, previous experience with the pathogen will determine how rapidly T and B cells in the adaptive immune system are able to mount a defense against it, supported by the innate immune system. Certain factors may affect the response of the immune system to infection.

3.1. Infants and Children

The developing immune system is still functionally immature in infants and young children. The innate immune system is relatively susceptible to pathogens, while the adaptive immune system is less able to quickly respond to T-cell-dependent antigens, especially in babies [19]. These factors, combined with their greater potential for exposure to pathogens at nursery and school, means that infants and young children are more susceptible to infections than adolescents and adults [23]. Vaccinations have been developed to combat common but potentially deadly infections (e.g., meningococcal bacteria, diphtheria, polio, pertussis, etc.), administered from around eight weeks after birth (when passive immunity begins to wane) and throughout childhood.

Although most childhood infections happen only once (e.g., chickenpox, measles, and mumps), followed by lifelong protection [19], many rhinoviruses can cause the common cold and reinfection is common. For example, children less than one year old have been noted to experience an average of six colds per year; the frequency decreases with age to about three colds per year in older children (10–14 years) [45]. Males are more often affected than females before three years of age, while the reverse is true in older children [45]. Infection with the seasonal influenza virus, which is caused by a different influenza type each year, is also more common in children under the age of five years [46]. In this age group, symptoms of flu can cause severe illness, complications and even death [46]. Sickness and diarrhea frequently occur in childhood, with many children in industrialized countries experiencing more than one episode of infective gastroenteritis per year, usually caused by rotavirus [47]. The frequency is exacerbated by close contact with other children and often less-than-optimal hygienic practices [47]. Lower respiratory tract infections (e.g., bronchitis and pneumonia) are more common in children under five years old than any other age group worldwide, and risk factors include air pollution and suboptimal breastfeeding [48]. Micronutrient deficiencies also have immunological consequences in infants and young children, and can increase morbidity and mortality from many diseases, including pneumonia, diarrheal disease, and measles [4,49]. Infection and undernutrition have a synergistic relationship, and micronutrient deficiencies cause specific immune impairments that affect both the innate and adaptive immune systems, such as impaired phagocyte and lymphocyte activity with zinc deficiency, or compromised development of neutrophils, macrophages and NK cells with vitamin A deficiency [50].

3.2. Adolescents and Adults

Immunological maturity is achieved by adolescence, and young adults should be well fortified against attack by pathogens [19]. Nevertheless, several lifestyle-related factors affect immune competence in healthy adults and increase their risk of infection (Figure 2). In particular, nutritional status can be compromised by a poor diet, which is often observed in adults with a hectic and stressful lifestyle and ready access to fast food or energy-dense, micronutrient-poor convenience food. Essential micronutrients such as vitamin B12 may be lacking in vegetarians and vegans, while adults in low-income families may be unable to afford fresh, nutritious foods. As outlined in Table 1, micronutrients have essential roles in the immune system and an inadequate intake may have deleterious effects [4]. A poor diet may be combined with a sedentary lifestyle, leading to obesity, suboptimal immune response, and increased risk of infection [51]. However, prolonged and excessive exercise and overtraining are also thought to impair immune function [52–54]. However, this view has recently been disputed; instead, it is suggested that regular physical activities might be beneficial for immunological health and limit or delay age-associated changes to the cellular composition of the adaptive immune system (for example, by countering the expansion of memory T cells that may contribute to systemic inflammation) [55]. Nevertheless, prolonged bouts of exercise and heavy training regimens in adults may create an imbalance between ROS and antioxidant defenses [54], leading to oxidative stress that alters signal transmission in the immune system and impairs the immune response [10]. Pollution and cigarette smoke certainly compromise immune function, particularly when combined with poor nutrition [10]. Reactive oxygen species in, and caused by, pollution can also upset the oxidant–antioxidant balance within the body and cause oxidative stress, which must be counteracted by an adequate supply of antioxidants [10]. Chronic, psychological stress is another factor that can impact immune function, suppressing cellular and humoral responses [56]. Alcohol consumption has variable effects on immunity; moderate amounts of polyphenol-rich alcoholic beverages potentially provide some immune protection while excessive consumption of alcohol can suppress many aspects of immune function and consequently increase the risk of infection [57]. Sleep is an important homeostatic regulator of immune function and plays a specific role in immunological memory [58]. Sleep disturbances and deprivation are therefore likely to have adverse effects on the immune system, including dysregulation of NK cells and pro-inflammatory and anti-inflammatory cytokines [58].

These factors, alone or in combination, weaken the immune system in adults and can increase the risk of infection. The incidence of common cold is lowest in adolescents compared with all other age groups, but increases in adults aged 20–30 years [45]; the risk is likely to be greater in those who come into close contact with children, who are at highest risk. Common cold is also more likely in those suffering from psychological stress [59], while moderate physical exercise may decrease the risk [60]. Infection with influenza viruses other than the seasonal variety (e.g., H1N1) is more prevalent in young to middle-aged, previously healthy adults [61]. In contrast to children, sickness and diarrhea in adults are often caused by norovirus [62] and campylobacter [63]. Worldwide, norovirus causes 685 million cases of acute gastroenteritis every year in adults [64].

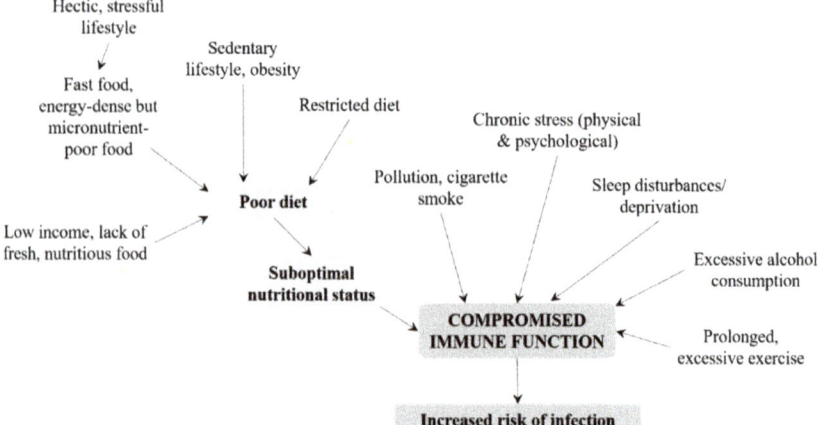

Figure 2. Life-style factors affecting immune function during adulthood. The risk of infection is also influenced by gender, early programming, vaccination history, pathogen exposure, specific health conditions, and diseases.

3.3. Older People

In older people, a lifetime of exposure to antigens and to numerous sources of oxidative stress can cause immune dysregulation that makes them more susceptible to infections than any other age group apart from young children [23,35,36]. Immune memory can be very long lasting, providing protection against many infections for decades; however, people are living much longer than before, and the pool of antigen-specific T cells may diminish over time [36]. In addition, thymic involution and the relative paucity of naïve lymphocytes in older people means that they are less able to mount an adequate defense against neoantigens and thus exposure to them is more hazardous than in younger people [36].

Although certain infections are less likely in older people (for example, the incidence of common cold has been shown to be the lowest those aged over 60 years [45]), the risk of many others such as urinary tract infections, lower respiratory tract infections, skin and soft tissue infections, for example, is greatly increased [65]. Furthermore, this age group is more likely to suffer prolonged infections, severe symptoms and secondary complications [33]. Around two-thirds of older patients with common cold develop lower respiratory illness [66], while older individuals are 2–10 times more likely to die of infection than younger people [11]. In those aged 70 years or older, 1.27 million deaths were thought to be caused by lower respiratory tract infections in 2015 [48]. Infection with seasonal influenza viruses is normally greatest in older people and young children [46]. Although influenza is not a life-threatening illness in most adults [67], in industrialized countries, influenza-associated deaths occur most often among people aged 65 years or older [46]. The greater morbidity and mortality associated with influenza in this age group occur because dysregulation in the immune response predisposes them to secondary bacterial infection of the respiratory tract (e.g., bronchitis and bacterial pneumonia) [68]. Protection against infection is dependent on T-cell-mediated responses and any dysregulation can impair the ability to mount a T-cell response, especially if there is also infection with cytomegalovirus [36]. This is the case in many older people, and these factors may explain why they have a poorer response to vaccines than the young [1,36]. Nevertheless, influenza vaccination can reduce severe illnesses and complications in people aged 65 years or older [46].

4. Micronutrient Requirements and Reported Deficiencies

The development, maintenance and optional functioning of immune cells is dependent on adequate nutrition, evident at all stages of life [4,5,33,49,69]. Key immunomodulatory roles of certain micronutrients are outlined in Table 1. Immune defenses can be impaired by undernutrition, which increases susceptibility to infection [4,5,70]. In turn, infection can cause a significant increase in the demand for micronutrients, met by endogenous or exogenous (i.e., the diet) supplies [5,50]. Vitamins A (and beta carotene), C, D, B2, and B12, folic acid, iron, zinc and selenium are just some micronutrients that have immunomodulatory and/or antioxidant effects and thus influence the susceptibility of a host to infectious diseases, as well as the course and outcome of infection [70].

4.1. Infants and Children

In babies and infants, breast milk is the major nutritional influence and is formulated to ensure that nutritional needs are met [49,71]. Breastmilk contains various immunological components such as antibodies (e.g., antigen-specific IgA), anti-inflammatory cytokines and other antimicrobial factors, but also most of the micronutrients necessary to support neonatal development, including of the immune system [49,71]. The concentrations of certain micronutrients in breastmilk (e.g., calcium, magnesium, and copper) are regulated by maternal homeostatic mechanisms (i.e., independent of maternal nutritional status and diet) to ensure they are sufficient to meet infant needs [72] and to protect them against deficiency or excess [71,73–75]. However, human milk is a poor source of iron and zinc and the needs of the child cannot be met by breast milk alone for zinc, or beyond six months for iron [72]. In contrast, the excretion of fat- and water-soluble micronutrients (e.g., vitamin A, and vitamins B1, B2, B6, B12, and C, respectively) into breast milk is dependent on maternal intake and varies worldwide [71,74,75]. Furthermore, vitamin D content of human milk is low and usually insufficient to meet requirements in exclusively-breastfed infants if the infant's sunlight exposure is limited [72,76]. During weaning and in the first years of life, both vitamin A and zinc play major roles in immunity to infectious disease [77].

Children do not need micronutrients in the same intakes as adults [78] (Table 2), and lower amounts are adequate to fulfill their various roles throughout the body, including within the immune system. Nevertheless, micronutrient deficiencies are prevalent in infants and preschool children in developing and low- to middle-income countries (e.g., [17,79–82]), and this age group is at the highest risk of multiple micronutrient deficiencies [83]. Worldwide, the three most common deficiencies are for iron, vitamin A and iodine [84], but zinc deficiencies are also common [83]. In young children, mainly in industrialized countries, deficiencies may occur because many micronutrients (e.g., vitamin C and B vitamins) are found in fruit and green, leafy vegetables and children are often fussy about what they eat. However, there are few data on micronutrient levels in infants from high-income countries. The available data suggest that, even in industrialized countries, some infants who are breastfed may not be receiving optimal amounts of certain micronutrients, as the levels found in breastmilk, maternal serum or urine did not always reach recommended levels in all women [73,85–95]. Reported micronutrient deficiencies in Europe [96] compared with recommended dietary allowances (RDA) [78] are shown in Table 2. It can be seen from the upper values that some children between the ages of 4 and 14 years had a surfeit of many micronutrients included in the table. However, the lower ranges indicate that there were children who had an insufficient intake of vitamin D (all ages), vitamin A (females 10+ years), vitamin E, folate, zinc (10+ years), iron (all ages) and selenium (all ages). Only the intakes of vitamins C, B6 and B12 and copper were sufficient within this age range.

Table 2. Life-stage-specific micronutrient deficiencies in Europe. Reported micronutrient intakes that are below the recommended dietary allowance are shown in bold. The table also shows the tolerable upper intake levels, the highest level of daily nutrient intake that is likely to pose no risk of adverse health effects in most people.

Select Micronutrients	Recommended Dietary Allowance [78]			Tolerable Upper Intake Levels [78]			Reported Mean Micronutrient Intakes, Min–Max [96]		
	Children [a] 4–8 years 9–13 years 14–18 years: M/F	Adults 19–50 years: M/F [b]	Older age 51 to >70 years: M/F	Children [a] 4–8 years 9–13 years 14–18 years	Adults 19–50 years: [b]	Older age 51 to >70 years	Children 4–6 years: M/F 7–9 years: M/F 10–14 years: M/F 15–18 years: M/F	Adults 19–50 years: M/F	Older age 51 to >70 years: M/F
Vitamin C, mg/day	25 45 75/65	90/75	90/75	650 1200 1800/1800	2000	2000	60–157/61–157 63–172/57–172 73–197/77–222 71–201/67–205	64–153/62–153	59–142/60–160
Vitamin D, µg/day	15	15	15–20	75 100 100/100	100	100	1.8–5.8/1.5–6.5 1.5–6.4/1.5–5.1 1.5–4.8/1.2–4.5 1.8–7.5/1.5–7.1	1.6–10.9/1.2–10.1	0.7–15.0/0.7–12.9
Vitamin A, µg/day	400 600 900/700	900/700	900/700	900 1700 2800/2800	3000	3000	400–1100/400–1200 400–1300/400–1100 400–2400/300–2300 400–1800/300–1600	500–2200/500–2000	500–2500/400–2300
Vitamin E, mg/day	7 11 15	15	15	300 600 800	1000	1000	5.3–9.8/5.1–9.8 6.3–11.2/5.9–13.3 5.9–14.5/5.6–18.1 6.8–20.8/6.0–15.5	3.3–17.7/4.2–16.1	6.3–13.7/6.7–13.7
Vitamin B6, mg/day	0.6 1.0 1.3/1.2	1.3	1.7/1.5	40 60 80	100	100	1.3–1.8/1.0–1.9 1.2–2.5/1.1–1.9 1.2–2.8/1.1–2.7 1.5–3.1/1.2–2.5	1.6–3.5/1.3–2.1	1.2–3.0/1.2–2.9
Vitamin B12, µg/day	1.2 1.8 2.4	2.4	2.4	ND	ND	ND	2.7–5.3/2.6–5.0 3.6–5.5/2.2–5.3 3.2–11.8/2.2–11.1 4.9–7.5/3.5–5.2	1.9–9.3/1.0–8.8	3.1–8.2/2.5–7.5
Folate, µg/day	200 300 400	300–400	400	400 600 800	1000	1000	120–256/109–199 144–290/133–264 149–428/140–360 190–365/154–298	203–494/131–392	139–343/121–335

Table 2. Cont.

Select Micronutrients	Recommended Dietary Allowance [78]			Tolerable Upper Intake Levels [78]			Reported Mean Micronutrient Intakes, Min–Max [96]		
	Children[a] 4–8 years; 9–13 years; 14–18 years: M/F	Adults 19–50 years: M/F[b]	Older age 51 to >70 years: M/F	Children[a] 4–8 years; 9–13 years; 14–18 years	Adults 19–50 years:[b]	Older age 51 to >70 years	Children 4–6 years: M/F; 7–9 years: M/F; 10–14 years: M/F; 15–18 years: M/F	Adults 19–50 years: M/F	Older age 51 to >70 years: M/F
Zinc, mg/day	5 8 11/9	11/8	11/8	12 23 34	40	40	6.0–9.2/5.3–8.9 7.0–10.9/6.4–9.4 7.0–14.6/6.1–13.9 9.3–15.2/6.4–11.0	8.6–14.6/6.7–10.7	7.5–12.3/6.7–11.2
Iron, mg/day	10 8 11/15	8/18	8	40 40 45	45	45	7.3–10.6/6.8–10.6 8.4–11.8/7.7–11.8 9.2–19.4/7.7–14.8 10.2–19.0/7.8–14.0	10.6–26.9/8.2–22.2	10.2–25.2/8.5–20.9
Copper, µg/day	440 700 890	900	900	3000 5000 8000	10,000	10,000	700–2200/700–2000 900–2800/800–2600 800–2900/700–2800 1200–3400/800–2100	1100–2300/1000–2200	1100–1900/900–1900
Selenium, µg/day	30 40 55	55	55	150 280 400	400	400	23–61/24–61 27–41/26–58 29–110/28–104 39–59/30–38	36–73/31–54	39–62/34–55

[a] Although adequate intake values are provided by the Institute of Medicine for infants (0–12 months) and recommended dietary allowances for children (1–3 years) [78], there are few data regarding micronutrient deficiencies in this age groups in industrialized countries and these ages have therefore not been included in this table; [b] values differ in pregnancy and lactation. F, females; M, males; ND, not determined.

4.2. Adolescents and Adults

An adequate amount of all micronutrients is required for optimal immune function in adolescents and adults (and throughout life), but in higher amounts compared with infants and children [78] (Table 2). It is especially important to ensure that antioxidant levels (e.g., vitamins C, E, and A) and micronutrients that are components of antioxidant enzymes (e.g., zinc, copper, iron, and selenium) are sufficient to combat the oxidative stress that is induced by many lifestyle factors common in this group, and which has great impact on immune function [10,23,35,36,44]. An adequate supply of micronutrients that affect the thymus is also important; for example, even marginal zinc deficiency is known to result in thymic atrophy and can increase the risk of infection [97]. Vitamin D intake is usually inadequate in most age groups worldwide, even in countries with mandatory food fortification [98], which can increase the risk of infection, especially respiratory tract infections [71].

Micronutrient deficiencies have been recorded in adolescents and adults in Europe [96] (Table 2). The lower ranges indicate that some adolescents had an insufficient intake of vitamin C (males 15–18 years), vitamin D, vitamin A (males 15–18 years; females 10–18 years), vitamin E, folate, zinc (10–18 years), iron and selenium. Only the intakes of vitamins B6 and B12 and copper were sufficient in all cases. In adults, there were insufficient dietary intakes for all micronutrients shown, apart from vitamin B6 and copper. Intakes were particularly low in female adults for folate, iron and selenium.

4.3. Older People

Although the recommended dietary allowances for older people indicate that their energy needs are lower than their younger counterparts, micronutrient requirements are mostly the same [78] (Table 2). However, micronutrient deficiencies are common in older people; it has been estimated that 35% of those aged 50 years or older in Europe, USA and Canada have a demonstrable deficiency of one or more micronutrients [33]. Many older people have chronic health conditions requiring hospitalization, live in care homes, or tend to eat less and make different food choices (e.g., choosing low nutrient density, often cheaper, and foods) [99,100]. An insufficient intake of micronutrients in older people has been reported both in the community (vitamins A, B12, D and zinc) and at a higher prevalence in long-term care facilities (vitamins A, D, and E) [101], while lower food intake has been associated with lower intakes of calcium, iron, zinc, B vitamins and vitamin E in older people [100]. Overall, data from Europe [96] (Table 2) suggest that there is an insufficient intake of most micronutrients in older people, apart from vitamin B12, iron and copper [96]. In particular, intakes were low for vitamin D (females), vitamin E (males and females) and folate (males and females). Older women, who usually have a longer life expectancy compared to men, are often at higher risk of deficiency, especially for vitamins B12, A, C, and D, iron and zinc [99]. Furthermore, menopause affects utilization of micronutrients; for example, vitamin C gradually decreases as menopause advances, correlated negatively to body mass index [102]. As in younger adults, a sufficient supply of antioxidants (e.g., vitamin C, selenium, and zinc) is required to combat the oxidative stress that is a major factor in immune dysregulation in older people. However, older people lose their ability to produce endogenous antioxidants compared with younger adults [103]. The skin of older adults is less able to synthesize vitamin D, and synthesis is about 75% slower in people aged 65 years than in younger adults [17].

5. Clinical Impact of Micronutrient Deficiencies and Supplementation

An inadequate intake of micronutrients at any stage of life affects various functions within the immune system, manifesting in decreased resistance to infections and an increase in the severity of symptoms (Table 3). For example, zinc deficiency can increase thymic atrophy, decrease lymphocyte number and activity, and increase oxidative stress and inflammation by altering cytokine production [14,97]. As a result, the risk of all types of infection (bacterial, viral, and fungal), but especially diarrhea and pneumonia, is increased [49]. A low vitamin C status also increases susceptibility to infections such as pneumonia [71], possibly because low levels of antioxidants such as vitamin C are unable to counteract the oxidative stress observed in pneumonia [104]. Increased production of ROS during the immune response to pathogens may decrease vitamin C levels further [105]. Vitamin D deficiency increases the risk of infection and autoimmune diseases such as multiple sclerosis and diabetes, probably related to activity of vitamin D receptors, which are found throughout the immune system [106,107].

Considering the importance of micronutrients in immunity, and the fact that many people of all ages have single or multiple micronutrient deficiencies that can have detrimental immunological effects, there is a rationale for micronutrient supplementation to restore concentrations to recommended levels, especially after an infection, and to support immune function and maintenance. To avoid any unwanted side effects, it is of course important to ensure that supplementation does not exceed recommended tolerable upper intake levels (Table 2), the highest level of daily nutrient intake that is likely to pose no risk of adverse health effects in most people [78]. Although this is theoretically possible, the reported micronutrient intake data in Table 2 suggest that over-supplementation is unlikely with most micronutrients, perhaps with the exception of vitamin A in children. It should be noted that the safety margins in micronutrient supplements ensure that proper consumption does not result in over-supplementation, and that food supplement labels should be carefully read to avoid misuse and the potential for over-supplementation.

As no single biomarker exists that accurately reflects the effects of supplementation on the immune response, clinical outcomes are instead used to determine the effectiveness of supplementation [49,69].

Table 3. Impact of micronutrient deficiency and supplementation on immune responses and the risk of infection.

Micronutrient	Impact of Deficiency	Impact of Supplementation
Vitamin C	Increased oxidative damage [104] Increased incidence and severity of pneumonia and other infections [71,104] Decreased resistance to infection and cancer, decreased delayed-type hypersensitivity response, impaired wound healing [49]	Antioxidant properties protect leukocytes and lymphocytes from oxidative stress [14] Older people: possible reduction in incidence and duration of pneumonia [71] Children: reduced duration and severity of common cold symptoms [105]; improved outcomes in pneumonia, malaria and diarrheal symptoms [9]
Vitamin D	Increased susceptibility to infections, especially RTI [71] Increased morbidity and mortality, increased severity of infections, reduced number of lymphocytes, reduced lymphoid organ weight [49] Increased risk of autoimmune diseases (e.g., type 1 diabetes, multiple sclerosis, systemic lupus erythematosus, rheumatoid arthritis) [14]	Reduced acute respiratory tract infections if deficient [71]
Vitamin A	Affects many immune functions, including number and killing activity of NK cells, neutrophil function, macrophage ability to phagocytose pathogens, growth and differentiation of B cells, decreasing number and distribution of T cells, etc. [14] Increased susceptibility to infections (e.g., diarrhea, RTI, measles, malaria) [14,71]	Children: Reduces all-cause mortality, diarrhea incidence and mortality, and measles incidence and morbidity in deficient children (6 month to 5 years) [14,71]; decreased risk of morbidity and mortality from infectious diseases [77] Not beneficial in pneumonia [14]
Vitamin E	Deficiency rare in humans [49] Impairs both humoral and cell-mediated aspects of adaptive immunity, including B and T cell function [14]	Older people: reduced RTI [71]
Vitamin B6	Lymphocytopenia, reduced lymphoid tissue weight, reduced responses to mitogens, general deficiencies in cell-mediated immunity, lowered antibody responses [49]	
Vitamin B12	Depressed immune responses (e.g., delayed-type hypersensitivity response, T-cell proliferation) [49] *	
Folate	Depressed immune responses (e.g., delayed-type hypersensitivity response, T-cell proliferation) [49] *	
Zinc	Decreased lymphocyte number and function, particularly T cells, increased thymic atrophy, altered cytokine production that contributes to oxidative stress and inflammation [14] Increased bacterial, viral and fungal infections (particularly diarrhea and pneumonia) [71] and diarrheal and respiratory morbidity [49] Increased thymic atrophy and consequent risk of infection [97]	Restoration of thymulin activity, increased numbers of cytotoxic T cells, reduced numbers of activated T helper cells (which can contribute to autoimmunity), increased natural killer cell cytotoxicity, reduced incidence of infections [14] Children: reduction in duration of diarrhea and incidence of pneumonia in at-risk children >6 month, but not in children 2–6 month [71]; reduced duration and severity of common cold symptoms [108]; improved outcomes in pneumonia, malaria and diarrheal symptoms [9]

Table 3. Cont.

Micronutrient	Impact of Deficiency	Impact of Supplementation
Iron	Reduced capacity for adequate immune response (decreased delayed-type hypersensitivity response, mitogen responsiveness, NK cell activity), decreased lymphocyte bactericidal activity, lower interleukin-6 levels [49]	May enhance or protect from infection with bacteria, viruses, fungi and protozoa depending on the level of iron [71] May theoretically enhance immunity to infectious diseases, but untargeted supplementation may increase availability of iron for pathogen growth and virulence and increase susceptibility to malaria and bacterial sepsis in particular [71] Children: potential detrimental effects in iron-replete children [14]
Copper	Abnormally low neutrophil levels [14] Potentially increased susceptibility to infection [14]	Children: increased ability of certain white blood cells to engulf pathogens if deficient [14] Reduced antibody production in response to influenza vaccine with chronic high doses in healthy young men [14]
Selenium	Impaired humoral and cell-mediated immunity [14] Increased viral virulence [14,71] Suppression of immune function, increased cancer incidence and cardiomyopathy with chronic deficiency [49] Children: increased risk of respiratory infections in the first 6 weeks of life [71]	Improves cell-mediated immunity and enhances immune response to viruses in deficient individuals, but may worsen allergic asthma and impair the immune response to parasites [14]

* Immune system effects of vitamin B12 deficiency and folate deficiency are clinically indistinguishable [49]. RTI, respiratory tract infections.

5.1. Infants and Children

Micronutrient deficiencies are closely linked to infectious diseases that can cause substantial morbidity and mortality in infants and children [49]. Worldwide, micronutrient supplementation studies have looked at the effects of vitamins D, A and E and minerals such as iron, selenium and zinc [49]. Zinc supplementation reduces morbidity and mortality from infectious diseases among infants and children in developing countries [77]. In low-birthweight infants, supplementary zinc can partly restore cell-mediated immunity [33]. Zinc can also reduce both the risk and duration of pneumonia in children, help to manage infantile diarrhea, lead to fewer episodes of malaria, and reduce the duration of diarrhea [3,17,71]. The duration and severity of common cold symptoms can be reduced by zinc supplementation in children when taken within 24 h of symptom onset [108]. Similar results have been observed with vitamin C, which shortened the duration of a cold in children (especially with higher doses) and reduced the severity of symptoms; a greater effect was observed in children compared with adults, including a greater prophylactic effect of vitamin C [105]. Both zinc and vitamin C may also improve the outcome of pneumonia, malaria and diarrheal infections in children [9]. In children with vitamin A deficiency, supplementation can decrease the risk of morbidity and mortality from infectious diseases [77], and reduce the incidence of diarrhea and measles [14,71].

5.2. Adolescents and Adults

Supplementation with vitamin C reduces the duration and severity of common cold symptoms in adults [105]. In those under physical stress (e.g., at work, during sports, and under extreme temperatures) [104], or in cases where vitamin C levels are slightly below recommended levels, vitamin C supplementation reduces common cold incidence. For example, in young males with marginal vitamin C deficiency, supplementation was shown to reduce the incidence of common cold and the duration of cold symptoms compared with placebo, accompanied by improved activity levels [109]. When used in combination with zinc, vitamin C supplementation can relieve symptoms such as rhinorrhea in common cold [110], which is commonly regarded as the most frequent and troublesome symptoms of the infection (along with nasal congestion) [111]. Supplementation with vitamin D can protect against respiratory tract infections and reduce the risk of acute respiratory illness and influenza, especially with once-daily dosing [112–115]. Benefits are particularly apparent in those who are very vitamin D deficient [115]. In light of their positive effects on respiratory tract infections, it has been suggested that there is a good rationale to combine vitamins C and D with zinc to support immune functions and help minimize the risk of infection [3]. Supplementation with multiple micronutrients has beneficial effects on the symptoms associated with the so-called "sick building syndrome", associated with prolonged contact with environmental factors that act as vehicles for pollutants [10]. Significantly fewer adults who received the micronutrient supplement reported headache, sore eyes, nasal congestion, throat inflammation, tiredness/pain, diarrhea or symptoms associated with an acute respiratory tract infection, such as cough [10].

5.3. Older People

Impaired immunity in older people, often caused by multiple micronutrient deficiencies, is evident in the increased incidence and severity of common infections that affect the upper and lower respiratory tracts, as well as the urinary and genital tracts [33,116]. Supplementation with modest amounts of a combination of micronutrients can have beneficial effects [33]. Higher levels of $CD4^+$ and $CD8^+$ T cells and an increased lymphocyte proliferative response to mitogens have been observed with vitamin A, C and E supplementation [117], while micronutrient supplementation with higher levels of vitamins C, E and beta-carotene increased the number of various subsets of T-cells, enhanced lymphocyte response to mitogen, increased IL-2 production and NK-cell activity, increased the response to the influenza virus vaccine, and led to fewer days of infection [118]. Supplementation with a complex micronutrient formulation in older people increased the number of various types of immune cells, including total lymphocytes, and induced a shift from memory T cells to naïve T cells [119]. Multiple micronutrient supplementation in older people may also reduce antibiotic usage and lead to higher post-vaccination immune responses [33].

Marginal zinc deficiency is common in older people, as their dietary intakes are generally lower and plasma zinc concentrations decline with age, possibly connected to impaired absorption, alterations in cellular uptake, and epigenetic dysregulation of DNA methylation or the methionine/transsulfuration pathway, for example [14]. Supplementation with low to moderate doses of zinc in healthy older people can help to restore thymulin activity, increase the numbers of cytotoxic T cells, reduce the number of activated Th cells (which contribute to autoimmunity) and increase the cytotoxicity of NK cells [14], immunological benefits that help to reduce the incidence of infections such as common cold, cold sores and influenza [120], as well as the incidence and morbidity of pneumonia [121]. There are some reports that an adequate zinc supply could prevent degenerative age-related diseases including infection and cancer [122]. Sufficient vitamin C is also important in older people, who are at risk of vitamin C deficiency, especially females [96]. Adequate vitamin C intakes can optimize cell and tissue levels and help to protect against respiratory and systemic infections (e.g., reduced duration and severity of pneumonia [71]), while higher levels are required during infection to compensate for the increased inflammatory response and metabolic demand induced by the pathogen, and thus help to reduce the duration and severity of symptoms [12]. Supplementation with vitamin E in older people has been shown to significantly improve NK cytotoxic activity, neutrophil chemotaxis and the phagocytic response, and enhance mitogen-induced lymphocyte proliferation and IL-2 production [123]. Vitamin E can also improve T-cell-mediated immunity and increase the production of antibodies in response to the hepatitis B and tetanus vaccines [124]. The risk of upper respiratory tract infections, especially common cold, was significantly lower after vitamin E supplementation in nursing home residents, although there was no apparent effect on lower respiratory tract infections [125]. However, not all studies have reported beneficial effects on respiratory tract infections with vitamin E supplementation in older people [14].

6. Conclusions

The immune system undergoes many changes over the life course—developing and maturing during childhood, potentially achieving peak function in early adulthood, and gradually declining in most people in older age (Figure 3). Distinct immune features are present during each life stage, and specific factors differentially affect immune function, with a resulting difference in the type, prevalence and severity of infections with age. A common factor throughout life is the need for an adequate supply of micronutrients, which play key roles in supporting immune function. Multiple micronutrient deficiencies are common throughout the world, with the likelihood increasing with age. Tailored supplementation based on the specific needs of each age group may help to provide an adequate basis for optimal immune function. The available clinical data suggest that micronutrient supplementation can reduce the risk and severity of infection and support a faster recovery. However, much more research is required into the effects of micronutrient supplementation on immune functions and on clinical outcomes. Nevertheless, current knowledge regarding the importance of micronutrients in immunity, the effects of micronutrient deficiencies on the risk and severity of infection, and the worldwide prevalence of an inadequate micronutrient status form a sound basis for the use of a targeted multiple micronutrient supplement to support immunity over a person's lifetime.

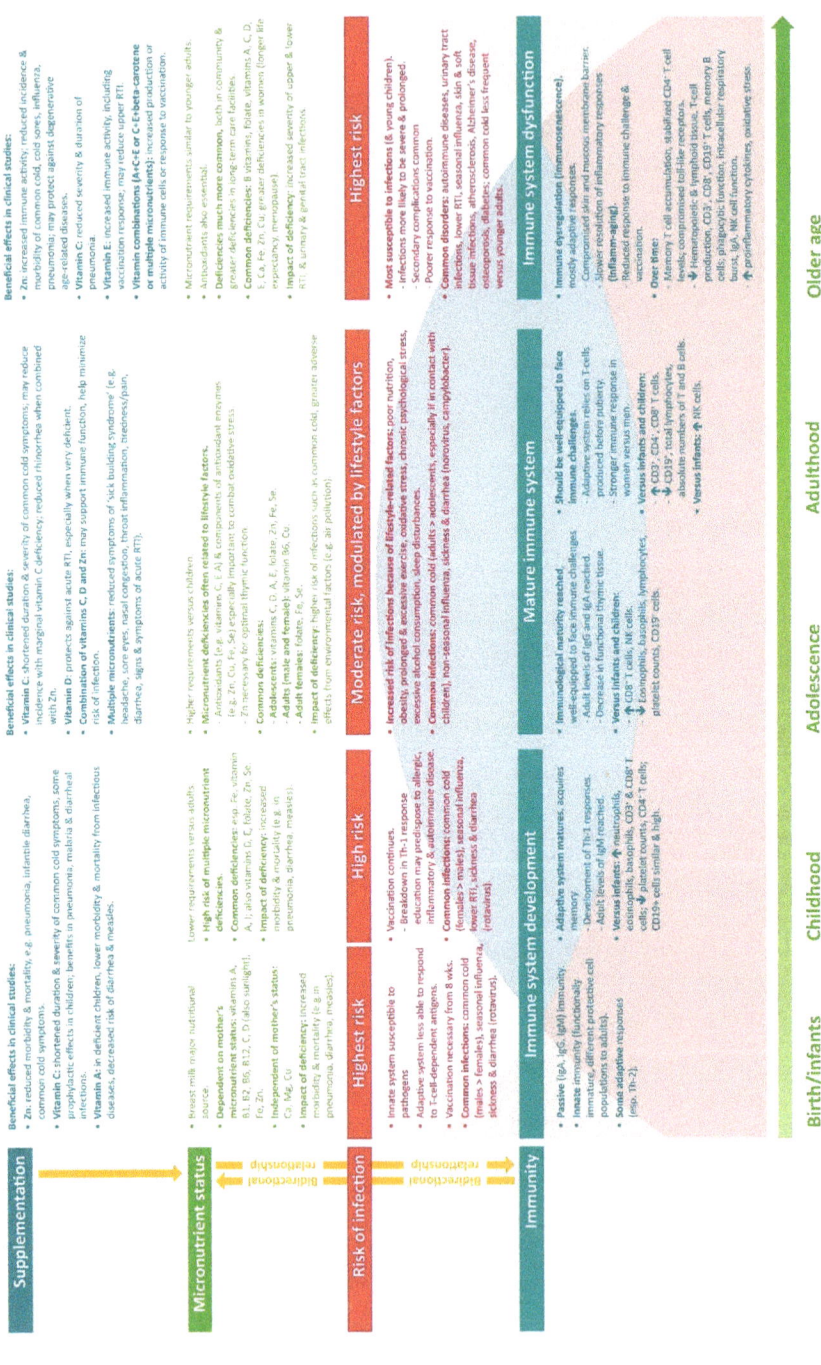

Figure 3. Differences in immunity and nutrition over a lifetime. Ca, calcium; Cu, copper; Fe, iron; I, iodine; Ig, immunoglobulin; Mg, magnesium; NK, natural killer; RTI, respiratory tract infections; Se, selenium; Th, T helper cell; Zn, zinc.

Author Contributions: S.M., A.P. and P.C.C. conceived and co-wrote the review, P.C.C. had primary responsibility for the final content.

Funding: This research received no external funding.

Acknowledgments: A draft of this manuscript was prepared by a professional medical writer (Deborah Nock, Medical WriteAway, UK; funded by Bayer Consumer Care AG), with subsequent full review and approval by all authors.

Conflicts of Interest: S.M. and A.P. are employed by Bayer Consumer Care Ltd., a manufacturer of multivitamins. P.C.C. has received funding, as a Key Opinion Leader, from Bayer Consumer Care Ltd.

References

1. Castelo-Branco, C.; Soveral, I. The immune system and aging: A review. *Gynecol. Endocrinol.* **2014**, *30*, 16–22. [CrossRef] [PubMed]
2. Pandya, P.H.; Murray, M.E.; Pollok, K.E.; Renbarger, J.L. The immune system in cancer pathogenesis: Potential therapeutic approaches. *J. Immunol. Res.* **2016**, *2016*, 4273943. [CrossRef] [PubMed]
3. Maggini, S.; Maldonado, P.; Cardim, P.; Fernandez Newball, C.; Sota Latino, E. Vitamins C., D and zinc: Synergistic roles in immune function and infections. *Vitam. Miner.* **2017**, *6*, 167. [CrossRef]
4. Alpert, P. The role of vitamins and minerals on the immune system. *Home Health Care Manag. Pract.* **2017**, *29*, 199–202. [CrossRef]
5. Calder, P. Conference on 'Transforming the nutrition landscape in Africa'. Plenary Session 1: Feeding the immune system. *Proc. Nutr. Soc.* **2013**, *72*, 299–309. [CrossRef] [PubMed]
6. Watson, R.R.; Zibadi, S.; Preedy, V.R. *Dietary Components and Immune Function*; Springer Science & Business Media: Berlin, Germany, 2010.
7. Biebinger, R.; Hurrell, R.F. 3—Vitamin and mineral fortification of foods. In *Food Fortification and Supplementation*; Ottaway, P.B., Ed.; Woodhead Publishing: Cambridge, UK, 2008; pp. 27–40.
8. Schaefer, E. Micronutrient deficiency in women living in industrialized countries during the reproductive years: Is there a basis for supplementation with multiple micronutrients? *J. Nutr. Disord. Ther.* **2016**, *6*, 199. [CrossRef]
9. Wintergerst, E.; Maggini, S.; Hornig, D. Immune-enhancing role of vitamin C and zinc and effect on clinical conditions. *Ann. Nutr. Metab.* **2006**, *50*, 85–94. [CrossRef] [PubMed]
10. Haryanto, B.; Suksmasari, T.; Wintergerst, E.; Maggini, S. Multivitamin supplementation supports immune function and ameliorates conditions triggered by reduced air quality. *Vitam. Miner.* **2015**, *4*, 1–15.
11. Maggini, S.; Beveridge, S.; Sorbara, J.; Senatore, G. Feeding the immune system: The role of micronutrients in restoring resistance to infections. *CAB Rev.* **2008**, *3*, 1–21. [CrossRef]
12. Carr, A.; Maggini, S. Vitamin C and immune function. *Nutrients* **2017**, *9*, 1211. [CrossRef] [PubMed]
13. Saeed, F.; Nadeem, M.; Ahmed, R.; Nadeem, M.; Arshad, M.; Ullah, A. Studying the impact of nutritional immunology underlying the modulation of immune responses by nutritional compounds—A review. *Food Agric. Immunol.* **2016**, *27*, 205–229. [CrossRef]
14. Micronutrient Information Center. Immunity in Depth. Available online: http://lpi.oregonstate.edu/mic/health-disease/immunity (accessed on 17 April 2018).
15. Meydani, S.; Ribaya-Mercado, J.; Russell, R.; Sahyoun, N.; Morrow, F.; Gershoff, S. Vitamin B-6 deficiency impairs interleukin 2 production and lymphocyte proliferation in elderly adults. *Am. J. Clin. Nutr.* **1991**, *53*, 1275–1280. [CrossRef] [PubMed]
16. Wintergerst, E.; Maggini, S.; Hornig, D. Contribution of selected vitamins and trace elements to immune function. *Nutr. Metab.* **2007**, *51*, 301–323. [CrossRef] [PubMed]
17. World Health Organization; Food and Agricultural Organization of the United Nations. Part 2. Evaluating the public health significance of micronutrient malnutrition. In *Guidelines on Food Fortification with Micronutrients*; World Health Organization: Geneva, Switzerland, 2006.
18. Maggini, S.; Wintergerst, E.S.; Beveridge, S.; Hornig, D.H. Selected vitamins and trace elements support immune function by strengthening epithelial barriers and cellular and humoral immune responses. *Br. J. Nutr.* **2007**, *98*, S29–S35. [CrossRef] [PubMed]
19. Simon, A.; Hollander, G.; McMichael, A. Evolution of the immune system in humans from infancy to old age. *Proc. R. Soc. B* **2015**, *282*, 20143085. [CrossRef] [PubMed]

20. Butler, E.; Kehrli, M. Immunoglobulins and immunocytes in the mammary gland and its secretions. In *Mucosal Immunology*; Mestecky, J., Lamm, M., Ogra, P., Strober, W., Bienenstock, J., McGhee, J., Mayer, L., Eds.; Elsevier: Amsterdam, The Netherlands, 2005; pp. 1763–1793.
21. Field, C.J. The immunological components of human milk and their effect on immune development in infants. *J. Nutr.* 2005, *135*, 1–4. [CrossRef] [PubMed]
22. Witkowska-Zimny, M.; Kaminska-El-Hassan, E. Cells of human breast milk. *Cell. Mol. Biol. Lett.* 2017, *22*, 11. [CrossRef] [PubMed]
23. Brodin, P.; Davis, M. Human immune system variation. *Nat. Rev. Immunol.* 2017, *17*, 21–29. [CrossRef] [PubMed]
24. MacGillivray, D.; Kollmann, T. The role of environmental factors in modulating immune responses in early life. *Front. Immunol.* 2014, *5*, 434. [CrossRef] [PubMed]
25. Valiathan, R.; Ashman, M.; Asthana, D. Effects of ageing on the immune system: Infants to elderly. *Scand. J. Immunol.* 2016, *83*, 255–266. [CrossRef] [PubMed]
26. Hepworth, M.; Sonnenberg, G. Regulation of the adaptive immune system by innate lymphoid cells. *Curr. Opin. Immunol.* 2014, *27*, 75–82. [CrossRef] [PubMed]
27. Tortura, G.J.; Derrickson, B. Metabolism and nutrition. In *Principles of Anatomy and Physiology*, 8th ed.; John Wiley & Sons, Inc.: Hoboken, NJ, USA, 2014; pp. 940–978.
28. Wang, K.; Wei, G.; Liu, D. CD19: A biomarker for B cell development, lymphoma diagnosis and therapy. *Exp. Hematol. Oncol.* 2012, *1*, 36. [CrossRef] [PubMed]
29. Berg, T.; Johansson, S. Immunoglobulin levels during childhood, with special regard to IgE. *Acta Paediatr.* 1969, *58*, 513–524. [CrossRef]
30. Pawelec, G. Hallmarks of human "immunosenescence": Adaptation or dysregulation? *Immun. Ageing* 2012, *9*, 15. [CrossRef] [PubMed]
31. Klein, S.; Hodgson, A.; Robinson, D. Mechanisms of sex disparities in influenza pathogenesis. *J. Leukoc. Biol.* 2012, *92*, 67–73. [CrossRef] [PubMed]
32. Fulop, T.; Witkowski, J.; Pawelec, G.; Alan, C.; Larbi, A. On the immunological theory of aging. In *Aging: Facts and Theories*; Robert, L., Fulop, T., Eds.; Karger: Basel, Switzerland, 2014; Volume 39, pp. 163–176.
33. Chandra, R. Nutrition and the immune system from birth to old age. *Eur. J. Clin. Nutr.* 2002, *56*, S73–S76. [CrossRef] [PubMed]
34. Montecino-Rodriguez, E.; Berent-Maoz, B.; Dorshkind, K. Causes, consequences, and reversal of immune system aging. *J. Clin. Investig.* 2013, *123*, 958–965. [CrossRef] [PubMed]
35. Ventura, M.; Casciaro, M.; Gangemi, S.; Buquicchio, R. Immunosenescence in aging: Between immune cells depletion and cytokines up-regulation. *Clin. Mol. Allergy* 2017, *15*, 21. [CrossRef] [PubMed]
36. Pawelec, G. Does the human immune system ever really become "senescent"? *F1000Research* 2017, *6*, 1323. [CrossRef] [PubMed]
37. Goronzy, J.; Weyand, C. Immune aging and autoimmunity. *Cell. Mol. Life Sci.* 2012, *69*, 1615–1623. [CrossRef] [PubMed]
38. Jafarzadeh, A.; Sadeghi, M.; Karam, G.A.; Vazirinejad, R. Salivary IgA and IgE levels in healthy subjects: Relation to age and gender. *Braz. Oral Res.* 2010, *24*, 21–27. [CrossRef] [PubMed]
39. Grewe, M. Chronological ageing and photoageing of dendritic cells. *Clin. Exp. Dermatol.* 2001, *26*, 608–612. [CrossRef] [PubMed]
40. Pand, A.A.; Qian, F.; Mohanty, S.; van Duin, D.; Newman, F.K.; Zhang, L.; Chen, S.; Towle, V.; Belshe, R.B.; Fikrig, E.; et al. Age-associated decrease in TLR function in primary human dendritic cells predicts influenza vaccine response. *J. Immunol.* 2010, *184*, 2518–2527. [CrossRef] [PubMed]
41. Hemmi, H.; Akira, S. TLR signalling and the function of dendritic cells. *Chem. Immunol. Allergy* 2005, *86*, 120–135. [PubMed]
42. Zhang, Y.; Wallace, D.; de Lara, C.; Ghattas, H.; Asquith, B.; Worth, A.; Griffin, G.; Taylor, G.; Tough, D.; Beverley, P.; et al. In vivo kinetics of human natural killer cells: The effects of ageing and acute and chronic viral infection. *Immunology* 2007, *121*, 258–265. [CrossRef] [PubMed]
43. Hazeldine, J.; Lord, J. The impact of ageing on natural killer cell function and potential consequences for health in older adults. *Ageing Res. Rev.* 2013, *12*, 1069–1078. [CrossRef] [PubMed]

44. Fulop, T.; Larbi, A.; Dupuis, G.; Le Page, A.; Frost, E.; Cohen, A.; Witkowski, J.; Franceschi, C. Immunosenescence and inflamm-aging as two sides of the same coin: Friends or foes? *Front. Immunol.* **2017**, *8*, 1960. [CrossRef] [PubMed]
45. Monto, A.; Ullman, B. Acute respiratory illness in an American community: The Tecumseh study. *JAMA* **1974**, *227*, 164–169. [CrossRef] [PubMed]
46. World Health Organization. Influenza (Seasonal). Fact Sheet. Available online: http://www.who.int/mediacentre/factsheets/fs211/en/ (accessed on 28 April 2018).
47. National Institute for Health and Care Excellence Diarrhoea and Vomiting Caused by Gastroenteritis in under 5s: Diagnosis and Management. Clinical Guideline [CG84]. Available online: https://www.nice.org.uk/guidance/cg84 (accessed on 28 April 2018).
48. GBD 2015 LRI Collaborators. Estimates of the global, regional, and national morbidity, mortality, and aetiologies of lower respiratory tract infections in 195 countries: A systematic analysis for the Global Burden of Disease Study 2015. *Lancet Infect. Dis.* **2017**, *17*, 1133–1161. [CrossRef]
49. Calder, P.; Prescott, S.; Caplan, M. *Scientific Review: The Role of Nutrients in Immune Function of Infants and Young Children*; Emerging Evidence for Long-Chain Polyunsaturated Fatty Acids; Mead Johnson & Company: Glenview, IL, USA, 2007.
50. Bresnahan, K.; Tanumihardjo, S. Undernutrition, the acute phase response to infection, and its effects on micronutrient status indicators. *Adv. Nutr.* **2014**, *5*, 702–711. [CrossRef] [PubMed]
51. Milner, J.; Beck, M. Micronutrients, immunology and inflammation. The impact of obesity on the immune response to infection. *Proc. Nutr. Soc.* **2012**, *71*, 298–306. [CrossRef] [PubMed]
52. Gleeson, M. Effects of exercise on immune function. *Sports Sci. Exch.* **2015**, *28*, 1–6.
53. Gleeson, M. Immunological aspects of sports nutrition. *Immunol. Cell Biol.* **2016**, *94*, 117–123. [CrossRef] [PubMed]
54. Nieman, D. Immunonutrition support for athletes. *Nutr. Rev.* **2008**, *66*, 310–320. [CrossRef] [PubMed]
55. Campbell, J.; Turner, J. Debunking the myth of exercise-induced immune suppression: Redefining the impact of exercise on immunological health across the lifespan. *Front. Immunol.* **2018**, *9*, 648. [CrossRef] [PubMed]
56. Segerstrom, S.; Miller, G. Psychological stress and the human immune system: A meta-analytic study of 30 years of inquiry. *Psychol. Bull.* **2004**, *130*, 601–630. [CrossRef] [PubMed]
57. Romeo, J.; Wärnberg, J.; Nova, E.; Díaz, L.E.; Gómez-Martinez, S.; Marcos, A. Moderate alcohol consumption and the immune system: A review. *Br. J. Nutr.* **2007**, *98*, S111–S115. [CrossRef] [PubMed]
58. Besedovsky, L.; Lange, T.; Born, J. Sleep and immune function. *Eur. J. Physiol.* **2012**, *163*, 121–137. [CrossRef] [PubMed]
59. Cohen, S.; Tyrrell, D.; Smith, A. Psychological stress and susceptibility to the common cold. *N. Engl. J. Med.* **1991**, *325*, 606–612. [CrossRef] [PubMed]
60. Nieman, D. Exercise, upper respiratory tract infection, and the immune system. *Med. Sci. Sports Exerc.* **1994**, *26*, 128–139. [CrossRef] [PubMed]
61. Risk Management Solutions. Learning from the 2009 H1N1 Influenza Pandemic. RMS Special Report. Available online: http://static.rms.com/email/documents/liferisks/reports/learning-from-the-2009-h1n1-influenza-pandemic.pdf (accessed on 28 April 2018).
62. Marshall, J.A.; Bruggink, L.D. The dynamics of norovirus outbreak epidemics: Recent insights. *Int. J. Environ. Res. Public Health* **2011**, *8*, 1141–1149. [CrossRef] [PubMed]
63. Man, S. The clinical importance of emerging Campylobacter species. *Nat. Rev. Gastroenterol. Hepatol.* **2011**, *8*, 669–685. [CrossRef] [PubMed]
64. Centers for Disease Control and Prevention. Norovirus Worldwide. Available online: https://www.cdc.gov/norovirus/worldwide.html (accessed on 29 July 2018).
65. Yoshikawa, T. Epidemiology and unique aspects of aging and infectious diseases. *Clin. Infect. Dis.* **2000**, *30*, 931–933. [CrossRef] [PubMed]
66. Heikkinen, T.; Jarvinen, A. The common cold. *Lancet* **2003**, *361*, 51–59. [CrossRef]
67. Eccles, R. Mechanisms of symptoms of common cold and flu. In *Common Cold*; Eccles, R., Weber, O., Eds.; Birkhauser Verlag: Basel, Switzerland, 2009; pp. 23–45.
68. Ballinger, M.; Standiford, T. Postinfluenza bacterial pneumonia: Host defenses gone awry. *J. Interferon Cytokine Res.* **2010**, *30*, 643–652. [CrossRef] [PubMed]

69. Albers, R.; Bourdet-Sicard, R.; Braun, D.; Calder, P.; Herz, U.; Lambert, C.; Lenoir-Wijnkoop, I.; Meheurst, A.; Ouwehand, A.; Phothirath, P.; et al. Monitoring immune modulation by nutrition in the general population: Identifying and substantiating effects on human health. *Br. J. Nutr.* **2013**, S110–S130. [CrossRef] [PubMed]
70. Bhaskaram, P. Micronutrient malnutrition, infection, and immunity: An overview. *Nutr. Rev.* **2002**, *60*, S40–S45. [CrossRef] [PubMed]
71. Prentice, S. They are what you eat: Can nutritional factors during gestation and early infancy modulate the neonatal immune response? *Front. Immunol.* **2017**, *8*, 1641. [CrossRef] [PubMed]
72. Butte, N.; Lopez-Alarcon, M.; Garza, C. Nutrient Adequacy of Exclusive Breastfeeding for the Term Infant during the First Six Months of Life. Available online: http://apps.who.int/iris/handle/10665/42519 (accessed on 12 December 2017).
73. Björklund, K.; Vahter, M.; Palm, B.; Grandér, M.; Lignell, S.; Berglund, M. Metals and trace element concentrations in breast milk of first time healthy mothers: A biological monitoring study. *Environ. Health* **2012**, *11*, 1–8. [CrossRef] [PubMed]
74. Hall Moran, V.; Lowe, N.; Crossland, N.; Berti, C.; Cetin, I.; Hermoso, M.; Koletzko, B.; Dykes, F. Nutritional requirements during lactation. Towards European alignment of reference values: The EURRECA network. *Matern. Child Health* **2010**, *6*, 39–54. [CrossRef] [PubMed]
75. Kominiarek, M.; Rajan, P. Nutrition recommendations in pregnancy and lactation. *Med. Clin. N. Am.* **2016**, *100*, 1199–1215. [CrossRef] [PubMed]
76. Dawodu, A.; Tsang, R. Maternal vitamin D status: Effect on milk vitamin D content and vitamin D status of breastfeeding infants. *Adv. Nutr.* **2012**, *3*, 353–361. [CrossRef] [PubMed]
77. Semba, R. Impact of micronutrient deficiencies on immune function. In *Micronutrient Deficiencies during the Weaning Period and the First Years of Life, Proceedings of the 54th Nestlé Nutrition Workshop, Pediatric Program, São Paulo, Brazil, 26–30 October 2003*; Pettifor, J., Zlotkin, S., Eds.; Nestlé Nutrition Institute Workshop Series: Lausanne, Switzerland, 2004.
78. Institute of Medicine. *Dietary Reference Intakes for Calcium and Vitamin D*; The National Academies Press: Washington, DC, USA, 2011.
79. Marasinghe, E.; Chackrewarthy, S.; Abeysena, C.; Rajindrajith, S. Micronutrient status and its relationship with nutritional status in preschool children in urban Sri Lanka. *Asia Pac. J. Clin. Nutr.* **2015**, *24*, 144–151. [PubMed]
80. Luo, R.; Shi, Y.; Zhou, H.; Yue, A.; Zhang, L.; Sylvia, S.; Medina, A.; Rozelle, S. Micronutrient deficiencies and developmental delays among infants: Evidence from a cross-sectional survey in rural China. *BMJ Open* **2015**, *5*, e008400. [CrossRef] [PubMed]
81. Özden, T.A.; Gökçay, G.; Cantez, M.S.; Durmaz, Ö.; İşsever, H.; Ömer, B.; Saner, G. Copper, zinc and iron levels in infants and their mothers during the first year of life: A prospective study. *BMC Pediatr.* **2015**, *15*, 157. [CrossRef] [PubMed]
82. Jardim-Botelho, A.; Queiroz Gurgel, R.; Simeone Henriques, G.; Dos Santos, C.B.; Afonso Jordão, A.; Nascimento Faro, F.; Silveira Souto, F.M.; Rodrigues Santos, A.P.; Eduardo Cuevas, L. Micronutrient deficiencies in normal and overweight infants in a low socio-economic population in north-east Brazil. *Paediatr. Int. Child Health* **2016**, *36*, 198–202. [CrossRef] [PubMed]
83. Bailey, R.; West, K.J.; Black, R. The epidemiology of global micronutrient deficiencies. *Ann. Nutr. Metab.* **2015**, *66*, 22–33. [CrossRef] [PubMed]
84. World Health Organization. Food and Agricultural Organization of the United Nations. Part I. The role of food fortification in the control of micronutrient malnutrition. In *Guidelines on Food Fortification with Micronutrients*; Allen, L., de Benoist, B., Dary, O., Hurrell, R., Eds.; World Health Organization: Geneva, Switzerland, 2006.
85. Mackey, A.; Picciano, M. Maternal folate status during extended lactation and the effect of supplemental folic acid. *Am. J. Clin. Nutr.* **1999**, *69*, 285–292. [CrossRef] [PubMed]
86. Houghton, L.; Sherwood, K.; O'Connor, D. How well do blood folate concentrations predict dietary folate intakes in a sample of Canadian lactating women exposed to high levels of folate? An observational study. *BMC Pregnancy Childbirth* **2007**, *7*, 1–8. [CrossRef] [PubMed]
87. Gellert, S.; Ströhle, A.; Hahn, A. Breastfeeding woman are at higher risk of vitamin D deficiency than nonbreastfeeding women - insights from the German VitaMinFemin study. *Int. Breastfeed. J.* **2017**, *12*, 1–10. [CrossRef] [PubMed]

88. Milman, N.; Hvas, A.-M.; Bergholt, T. Vitamin D status during normal pregnancy and postpartum. A longitudinal study in 141 Danish women. *J. Perinat. Med.* **2012**, *40*, 57–61. [CrossRef] [PubMed]
89. Dawodu, A.; Zalla, L.; Woo, J.G.; Herbers, P.M.; Davidson, B.S.; Heubi, J.E.; Morrow, A.L. Heightened attention to supplementation is needed to improve the vitamin D status of breastfeeding mothers and infants when sunshine exposure is restricted. *Matern. Child Health* **2014**, *10*, 383–397. [CrossRef] [PubMed]
90. Hannan, M.; Faraji, B.; Tanguma, J.; Longoria, N.; Rodriguez, R. Maternal milk concentration of zinc, iron, selenium, and iodine and its relationship to dietary intakes. *Biol. Trace Elem. Res.* **2009**, *127*, 6–15. [CrossRef] [PubMed]
91. Charlton, K.; Yeatman, H.; Lucas, C.; Axford, S.; Gemming, L.; Houweling, F.; Goodfellow, A.; Ma, G. Poor knowledge and practices related to iodine nutrition during pregnancy and lactation in australian women: Pre- and post-iodine fortification. *Nutrients* **2012**, *4*, 1317–1327. [CrossRef] [PubMed]
92. Mulrine, H.M.; Skeaff, S.A.; Ferguson, E.L.; Gray, A.R.; Valeix, P. Breast-milk iodine concentration declines over the first 6 mo postpartum in iodine-deficient women. *Am. J. Clin. Nutr.* **2010**, *92*, 849–856. [CrossRef] [PubMed]
93. Valent, F.; Horvat, M.; Mazej, D.; Stibilj, V.; Barbone, F. Maternal diet and selenium concentration in human milk from an Italian population. *J. Epidemiol.* **2011**, *21*, 285–292. [CrossRef] [PubMed]
94. Brenna, J.T.; Varamini, B.; Jensen, R.G.; Diersen-Schade, D.A.; Boettcher, J.A.; Arterburn, L.M. Docosahexaenoic and arachidonic acid concentrations in human breast milk worldwide. *Am. J. Clin. Nutr.* **2007**, *85*, 1457–1464. [CrossRef] [PubMed]
95. Podzolkova, N.; Schaefer, E. Micronutrient intakes and status are frequently insufficient in breastfeeding women. *BMC Pregnancy Childbirth* **2018**, submitted for publication.
96. Elmadfa, I.; Meyer, A.; Nowak, V.; Hasenegger, V.; Putz, P.; Verstraeten, R.; Remaut-DeWinter, A.M.; Kolsteren, P.; Dostálová, J.; Dlouhý, P.; et al. European Nutrition and Health Report. *Forum Nutr.* **2009**, *62*, 1–405. [PubMed]
97. Savino, W.; Dardenne, M. Nutritional imbalances and infections affect the thymus: Consequences on T-cell-mediated immune responses. *Proc. Nutr. Soc.* **2010**, *69*, 636–643. [CrossRef] [PubMed]
98. Palacios, C.; Gonzalez, L. Is vitamin D deficiency a major global public health problem? *J. Steroid Biochem. Mol. Biol.* **2014**, *144PA*, 138–145. [CrossRef] [PubMed]
99. Montgomery, S.; Streit, S.; Beebe, M.; Maxwell IV, P. Micronutrient needs of the elderly. *Nutr. Clin. Pract.* **2014**, *29*, 435–444. [CrossRef] [PubMed]
100. Drenowski, A.; Shultz, J. Impact of aging on eating behaviors, food choices, nutrition, and health status. *J. Nutr. Health Aging* **2001**, *5*, 75–79.
101. High, K. Nutritional strategies to boost immunity and prevent infection in elderly individuals. *Clin. Infect. Dis.* **2001**, *33*, 1892–1900. [CrossRef] [PubMed]
102. Wiacek, M.; Zubrzycki, I.; Bojke, O.; Kim, H. Menopause and age-driven changes in blood level of fat- and water-soluble vitamins. *Climacteric* **2013**, *16*, 689–699. [CrossRef] [PubMed]
103. Karaouzenea, N.; Merzouka, H.; Aribib, M.; Merzoukc, S.; Yahia Berrouiguet, A.; Tessiere, C.; Narce, M. Effects of the association of aging and obesity on lipids, lipoproteins and oxidative stress biomarkers: A comparison of older with young men. *Nutr. Metab. Cardiovasc. Dis.* **2011**, *21*, 792–799. [CrossRef] [PubMed]
104. Hemilä, H. Vitamin C and infections. *Nutrients* **2017**, *9*, 339. [CrossRef] [PubMed]
105. Hemilä, H.; Chalker, E. Vitamin C for preventing and treating the common cold. *Cochrane Database Syst. Rev.* **2013**. Available online: https://www.cochranelibrary.com/cdsr/doi/10.1002/14651858.CD000980.pub4/full (accessed on 17 October 2018).
106. Aranow, C. Vitamin D and the immune system. *J. Investig. Med.* **2011**, *59*, 881–886. [CrossRef] [PubMed]
107. Mangin, M.; Sinha, R.; Fincher, K. Inflammation and vitamin D: The infection connection. *Inflamm. Res.* **2014**, *63*, 803–819. [CrossRef] [PubMed]
108. Hemilä, H. Zinc lozenges may shorten the duration of colds: A systematic review. *Open Respir. Med. J.* **2011**, *5*, 51–58. [PubMed]
109. Johnston, C.; Barkyoumb, G.M.; Schumacher, S.S. Vitamin C supplementation slightly improves physical activity levels and reduces cold incidence in men with marginal vitamin C status: A randomized controlled trial. *Nutrients* **2014**, *6*, 2572–2583. [CrossRef] [PubMed]
110. Maggini, S.; Beveridge, S.; Suter, M. A combination of high-dose vitamin C plus zinc for the common cold. *J. Int. Med. Res.* **2012**, *40*, 28–42. [CrossRef] [PubMed]

111. Graf, P.; Eccles, R.; Chen, S. Efficacy and safety of intranasal xylometazoline and ipratropium in patients with common cold. *Expert Opin. Pharmacother.* **2009**, *10*, 889–908. [CrossRef] [PubMed]
112. Yamshchikov, A.; Desai, N.; Blumberg, H.; Ziegler, T.; Tangpricha, V. Vitamin D for treatment and prevention of infectious diseases: A systematic review of randomized controlled trials. *Endocr. Pract.* **2009**, *15*, 438–449. [CrossRef] [PubMed]
113. Charan, J.; Goyal, J.; Saxena, D.; Yadav, P. Vitamin D for prevention of respiratory tract infections: A systematic review and meta-analysis. *J. Pharmacol. Pharmacother.* **2012**, *3*, 300–303. [CrossRef] [PubMed]
114. Bergman, P.; Lindh, Å.; Björkhem-Bergman, L.; Lindh, J. Vitamin D and respiratory tract infections: A systematic review and meta-analysis of randomized controlled trials. *PLoS ONE* **2013**, *8*, e65835. [CrossRef] [PubMed]
115. Martineau, A.; Jolliffe, D.; Hooper, R.; Greenberg, L.; Aloia, J.; Bergman, P.; Dubnov-Raz, G.; Esposito, S.; Ganmaa, D.; Ginde, A.A.; et al. Vitamin D supplementation to prevent acute respiratory infections: Systematic review and meta-analysis of individual participant data. *BMJ* **2017**, *356*, i6583. [CrossRef] [PubMed]
116. Hamer, D.; Sempértegui, F.; Estrella, B.; Tucker, K.; Rodríguez, A.; Egas, J.; Dallal, G.; Selhub, J.; Griffiths, J.; Meydani, S. Micronutrient deficiencies are associated with impaired immune response and higher burden of respiratory infections in elderly Ecuadorians. *J. Nutr.* **2009**, *139*, 113–119. [CrossRef] [PubMed]
117. Penn, N.D.; Purkins, L.; Kelleher, J.; Heatley, R.V.; Mascie-Taylor, B.H.; Belfield, P.W. The effect of dietary supplementation with vitamins A, C, and E on cell-mediated immune function in elderly log-stay patients: A randomized controlled trial. *Age Ageing* **1991**, *20*, 169–174. [CrossRef] [PubMed]
118. Chandra, R. Effect of vitamin and trace-element supplementation on immune responses and infection in elderly subjects. *Lancet* **1992**, *340*, 1124–1127. [CrossRef]
119. Schmoranzer, F.; Fuchs, N.; Markolin, G.; Carlin, E.; Sakr, L.; Sommeregger, U. Influence of a complex micronutrient supplement on the immune status of elderly individuals. *Int. J. Vitam. Nutr. Res.* **2009**, *79*, 308–318. [CrossRef] [PubMed]
120. Prasad, A. Zinc: Mechanisms of host defense. *J. Nutr.* **2007**, *137*, 1345–1349. [CrossRef] [PubMed]
121. Meydani, S.; Barnett, J.; Dallal, G.; Fine, B.; Jacques, P.; et al. Serum zinc and pneumonia in nursing home elderly. *Am. J. Clin. Nutr.* **2007**, *86*, 1167–1173. [CrossRef] [PubMed]
122. Mocchegiani, E.; Romeo, J.; Malavolta, M.; Costarelli, L.; Giacconi, R.; Diaz, L.; Marcos, A. Zinc: Dietary intake and impact of supplementation on immune function in elderly. *Age (Dordr.)* **2013**, *35*, 839–860. [CrossRef] [PubMed]
123. De la Fuente, M.; Hernanz, A.; Guayerbas, N.; Victor, V.; Arnalich, F. Vitamin E ingestion improves several immune functions in elderly men and women. *Free Radic. Res.* **2008**, *42*, 272–280. [CrossRef] [PubMed]
124. Meydani, S.; Meydani, M.; Blumberg, J.; Leka, L.; Siber, G.; Loszewski, R.; Thompson, C.; Pedrosa, M.; Diamond, R.; Stollar, B. Vitamin E supplementation and in vivo immune response in healthy elderly subjects. A randomized controlled trial. *JAMA* **1997**, *277*, 1380–1386. [CrossRef] [PubMed]
125. Meydani, S.; Leka, L.; Fine, B.; Dallal, G.; Keusch, G.; Singh, M.; Hamer, D. Vitamin E and respiratory tract infections in elderly nursing home residents: A randomized controlled trial. *JAMA* **2004**, *292*, 828–836. [CrossRef] [PubMed]

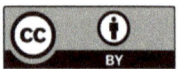

© 2018 by the authors. Licensee MDPI, Basel, Switzerland. This article is an open access article distributed under the terms and conditions of the Creative Commons Attribution (CC BY) license (http://creativecommons.org/licenses/by/4.0/).

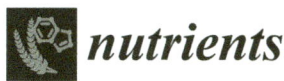

Review
Selenium, Selenoproteins, and Immunity

Joseph C. Avery and Peter R. Hoffmann *

Department of Cell and Molecular Biology, John A. Burns School of Medicine, University of Hawaii, 651 Ilalo Street, Honolulu, HI 96813, USA; jcavery@hawaii.edu
* Correspondence: peterrh@hawaii.edu; Tel.: +1-808-692-1510; Fax: +808-692-1968

Received: 6 August 2018; Accepted: 30 August 2018; Published: 1 September 2018

Abstract: Selenium is an essential micronutrient that plays a crucial role in development and a wide variety of physiological processes including effect immune responses. The immune system relies on adequate dietary selenium intake and this nutrient exerts its biological effects mostly through its incorporation into selenoproteins. The selenoproteome contains 25 members in humans that exhibit a wide variety of functions. The development of high-throughput omic approaches and novel bioinformatics tools has led to new insights regarding the effects of selenium and selenoproteins in human immuno-biology. Equally important are the innovative experimental systems that have emerged to interrogate molecular mechanisms underlying those effects. This review presents a summary of the current understanding of the role of selenium and selenoproteins in regulating immune cell functions and how dysregulation of these processes may lead to inflammation or immune-related diseases.

Keywords: selenocysteine; macrophage; T cell; antibody; inflammation; cancer

1. Introduction

Selenium was discovered by the Swedish chemist Jöns Jakob Berzelius in 1817 and was considered a toxic element for humans and livestock for nearly 150 years [1]. However, in 1957, the benefits of selenium for humans and other mammals were revealed in landmark studies by Klaus Schwartz and Calvin Foltz who demonstrated that dietary selenium protected rats against liver necrosis [2]. Since then, the role of selenium as a trace mineral nutrient in human health and the mechanisms by which it exerts its biological effects have become better understood. Adequate levels of bioavailable selenium are functionally important for several aspects of human biology including the central nervous system, the male reproductive biology, the endocrine system, muscle function, the cardiovascular system, and immunity [3,4]. Many pathological conditions involving the immune system can be affected by the selenium status in an individual, which can be influenced by several factors such as the levels and forms of selenium ingested, the conversion of selenium compounds into metabolites, and genetic characteristics that can impact the use of these metabolites. Selenium deficiency is rare in the United States and Canada [5], but regions of China, New Zealand, and parts of Europe and Russia have low levels of selenium in soil and food [6]. The extent to which immune-related diseases are impacted by differences in selenium intake and how supplementation approaches may be utilized to mitigate these health issues is not entirely clear. However, the development of new high-throughput omic approaches and bioinformatics tools have improved our understanding of the effects of selenium immuno-biology in humans. Additionally, novel experimental systems have provided valuable insight into mechanisms underlying those effects.

The U.S. recommended dietary allowance for selenium for adults is 55 µg/day and most individuals achieve this level while several other countries have higher recommended allowances due to a lower average selenium status in their populations [7]. For example, adults in the U.K. are recommended to ingest 60 µg/day for adult women and 75 µg/day for lactating women and adult men [8]. Commonly used measures of a selenium status include plasma and serum selenium concentrations as well as selenoprotein P levels and glutathione peroxidase activity [9,10]. The average plasma selenium concentration in the U.S. is 70 ng/mL, which is relatively high with selenium intake found to be lower in areas within China and Europe, in New Zealand, and in other parts of the world [11,12]. Dietary selenium is obtained through a wide variety of foods including grains, vegetables, seafood, meat, dairy products, and nuts [13]. The predominant form of selenium ingested by humans is selenomethionine. However, other forms of selenium are also present in foods. Selenium gets metabolized into various small molecular weight seleno-compounds including some that may exert biological effects through redox reactions that can affect cellular processes like DNA repair and epigenetics [14,15]. These bioactive metabolites include hydrogen selenide and methylated selenium compounds like methylseleninic acid, which exerts chemo-preventive effects [16]. Most of the effects of dietary selenium on immune functions are attributable to the insertion of this element into a family of proteins called seleno-proteins. What separates selenium from other nutritional elements is the fact that it is incorporated directly into proteins as the 21st amino acid, selenocysteine (Sec). The synthesis of selenoproteins within cells requires a dedicated set of protein and tRNA factors assembled on ribosomes along with the selenoprotein mRNA, which contains unique structural elements. The coordinated interaction of these elements leads to co-translational insertion of Sec into the nascent polypeptide when the ribosome encounters a uridine-guanosine-adenosine (UGA) codon, which is typically used as a stop codon in other mRNAs [17]. Under conditions of low selenium status, this translational process stalls at the UGA codon and both the mRNA and truncated protein may get degraded through two separate processes called nonsense-mediated decay (NMD) and destruction via C-end degrons (DesCEND), respectively [18,19]. Certain mRNA characteristics potentially play a role in NMD sensitivity such as the location of the Sec codon (UGA) relative to exon–exon junctions [18]. Therefore, the selenium status is directly related to levels of different selenoproteins in different tissues. Given the combined effects of NMD and DesCEND, there appears to be a hierarchy of selenoprotein synthesis that results in some family members having a higher priority of expression under selenium-limiting conditions [20]. In addition, certain tissues like the brain, endocrine tissues, and testes retain selenium under deficient conditions shed light on the priorities given to different physiological systems when selenium levels are low.

In humans, 25 selenoproteins have been identified and 24 of those exist as Sec-containing proteins in rodents [21], which highlights the value of rodent models for determining roles for members of this protein family in immune responses. Selenoproteins exhibit a wide variety of tissue distribution and functions [17]. While many members of the selenoprotein family function as enzymes involved in redox reactions, some are likely not enzymes themselves and functions are gradually becoming better understood for these non-enzymatic members. The most completely characterized selenoprotein enzymes related to immune functions include glutathione peroxidases (GPXs), thioredoxin reductases (TXNRDs), iodothyronine deiodinases (DIOs), methionine-R-sulfoxide reductase B1 (MSRB1), and selenophosphate synthetase 2 (SPS2). For non-enzymatic selenoproteins, the best characterized in terms of immune cell function is selenoprotein K (SELENOK). Table 1 lists selenoproteins and their functions and a more detailed discussion of roles for individual selenoproteins in different immune cells and tissues is provided below.

Table 1. Summary of Selenoprotein Functions.

Selenoprotein	Abbreviations	Functions (References)
Glutathione peroxidase 1	GPX1, cytosolic glutathione peroxidase	Reduces cellular H_2O_2 [22,23].
Glutathione peroxidase 2	GPX2, intestinal glutathione peroxidase	Reduces peroxide in gut [24,25].
Glutathione peroxidase 3	GPX3, Plasma glutathione peroxidase	Reduces peroxide in blood [26,27].
Glutathione peroxidase 4	GPX4, Phospholipid hydroperoxide glutathione peroxidase	Anti-oxidative lipid repair enzyme localized to cytosol, mitochondria, and nucleus, which reduces hydrogen peroxide radicals and lipid peroxides to water and lipid alcohols and prevents iron-induced cellular ferroptosis [28,29].
Glutathione peroxidase 6	GPX6	Importance unknown [30].
Thioredoxin reductase 1	TXNRD1, TR1	Localized to cytoplasm and nucleus and regenerates reduced thioredoxin [31].
Thioredoxin reductase 2	TXNRD2, TR3	Localized to mitochondria and regenerates reduced thioredoxin [32].
Thioredoxin-glutathione reductase	TXNRD3, TR2, TGR	Testes-specific expression, which regenerates reduced thioredoxin [33].
Iodothyronine deiodinase 1	DIO1, D1	Important for systemic active thyroid hormone levels [34].
Iodothyronine deiodinase 2	DIO2, D2	ER enzyme important for local active thyroid hormone levels [34].
Iodothyronine deiodinase 3	DIO3, D3	Inactivates thyroid hormone [34].
Methionine-R-sulfoxide reductase B1	MSRB1, SELR, SELX	Regulator of F-actin repolymerization in macrophages during innate immune response, which works in concert with MICA1s to reduce oxidized methionine (R)-sulfoxide (Met-RO) back to methionine [35,36].
Selenoprotein F	SELENOF, Selenoprotein 15, SEP15	ER-resident thioredoxin-like oxidoreductase that complexes with uridine-guanosine-guanosine-thymidine (UGGT) and improves protein quality control by correcting misglycosylated/misfolded glycoproteins via the calnexin-calreticulin- endoplasmic reticulum proten 57 (ERp57) axis and pH-dependent endoplasmic reticulum proten 44 (ERp44)system [37,38].
Selenoprotein H	SELENOH, SELH, C11orf31	Nuclear localization, which is involved in redox sensing and transcription [39,40].
Selenoprotein I	SELENOI, SELI, EPT1	Involved in phospholipid biosynthesis [41].
Selenoprotein K	SELENOK, SELK	Transmembrane protein localized to the endoplasmic reticulum (ER) and involved in calcium flux in immune cells and ER associated degradation in cell lines [42,43].
Selenoprotein M	SELENOM, SELM, SEPM	Thioredoxin-like ER-resident protein that may be involved in the regulation of body weight and energy metabolism [44].
Selenoprotein N	SELENON, SELN, SEPN1	Transmembrane protein localized to ER. Mutations lead to multiminicore disease and other myopathies [45,46].
Selenoprotein O	SELENOO, SELO	Mitochondrial protein that contains a C-X-X-U (where C is cytosine, X is any nucleotide, and U is uridine) motif suggestive of the redox function [47].
Selenoprotein P	SELENOP, SEPP1, SeP, SELP, SEPP	Secreted into plasma for selenium transport to tissues [20,48].
Selenoprotein S	SELENOS, SELS, SEPS1, VIMP	Transmembrane protein found in ER involved in ER associated degradation [49,50].
Selenoprotein T	SELENOT, SELT	Oxidoreductase localized to the Golgi complex and ER and manifests a thioredoxin-like fold and is involved in redox regulation and cell anchorage. Complexes with UGGTs to improve PQC. Deficiency leads to early embryonic lethality [51].
Selenoprotein V	SELENOV, SELV	Testes-specific expression [21].
Selenoprotein W	SELENOW, SELW, SEPW1	Putative antioxidant role, which may be important in muscle growth [52].
Selenophosphate synthetase 2	SEPHS2, SPS2	Involved in synthesis of all selenoproteins including itself [53].

As mentioned above, nearly all tissues are affected by changes in the selenium status or selenoprotein expression. While the focus of this review is on the immune system, it is important to first touch on other physiological systems impacted by the levels of selenium and selenoproteins. Embryonic lethality arising from deletion of the *trsp* gene encoding the Sec-tRNA required for translation [54] demonstrates the essential nature of selenoproteins. In fact, there have been four individual selenoprotein knockout mice in which gene ablation was shown to result in embryonic lethality: GPX4, TXNRD1 and 2, and Selenoprotein T (SELENOT) [32,51,55,56]. An essential role for one of these selenoproteins in the area of development was demonstrated by the recent study, which showed that GPX4 protects a critical population of interneurons from ferroptotic cell death [29]. In the muscular system, genetic maladies involving selenoproteins include multi-minicore diseases (MmD) such as rigid spine syndrome (RSS) resulting from mutations in the human gene encoding Selenoprotein N (SELENON) [57,58] and an associative dysfunction of the ryanodine receptor 1 (RyR1) receptor [59]. Transgenic overexpression of some selenoproteins potentially regenerates wasted muscle in mice [60]. Thyroid hormone metabolism is dependent upon the combined actions of the three selenoproteins known as iodothyronine deiodinases 1-3 (DIO1-3) [61]. Thus, selenium deficiencies can affect thyroid gland function and the many physiological systems impacted by thyroid hormone activity. In the hepatic system, selenium is absorbed from the gastrointestinal tract and utilized for biosynthesis of selenoproteins including Selenoprotein P (SELENOP), which is the primary plasma selenium transport protein [62]. Several groups have observed that SELENOP inactivation results in normal hepatic selenium levels while selenium content in other tissues decreases significantly. This reduces the total GPX and TXNRD pools [63,64]. Consequently, those organs that rely on SELENOP-mediated selenium delivery become deficient when some tissues are given 'priority' over others for retention of this element since delivery through SELENOP decreases.

The central nervous system is appreciably dependent on an adequate selenium supply and, as mentioned above, diets that are slightly deficient in selenium do not elicit neurological deficits due to the preservation of selenium content in the central nervous tissue during dietary selenium restriction [65]. On the other hand, a targeted reduction in brain selenium reduces SELENOP bioavailability and causes spontaneous neurological deficits [66], which are reversed by selenium supplementation [67,68]. Additionally, overexpression of TRX1 has been found to mitigate oxidative challenges in the brain [69]. GPX1 was the first mammalian selenoprotein to be discovered [70,71] and has been shown to protect the brain from oxidative insults. Like GPX1, GPX4 protects cortical neurons from exogenous oxidative stress-inducing agents [72,73]. Importantly, the protein oxidation product methionine-*R*-sulfoxide contributes to neurodegenerative diseases and can be repaired by thioredoxin-dependent selenoenzyme MSRB1, which reduces methionine-*R*-sulfoxide back to methionine [36]. Inactivation of MSRB1, however, does not produce neurological deficits [36]. In the kidney, several studies have identified the expression of DIOs, thioredoxin reductases (TRs), and GPXs, but their respective roles have not been fully elucidated. Burk et al. demonstrated that glutathione (GSH) deprivation causes severe pathogenic nephropathy [74] while podocyte-specific ablation of the *trsp* gene in diabetic mice did not enhance markers of nephropathic disease. Moreover, murine renal expression of GPX1 has been reported not to be protective against diabetic nephropathy.

For clinically diagnosed disorders, Keshan disease (KD) is perhaps the most firmly established selenium deficiency-based pathology. This cardiomyopathy was first described in rural areas of China due to low selenium content in foods [75]. There is evidence in mouse models that selenium deficiency promotes the conversion of nonvirulent coxsackievirus B3 strains into a more virulent strain due to an increased oxidative stress [76], which suggests that this infectious agent may be a cofactor. Selenoprotein deficiency may also promote osteochondral diseases including Kashin-Beck disease (KBD). This disease is a poly-pathogenic, degenerative osteochondropathy leading to chondrocyte necrosis [77] and apoptosis [78–80], which results in growth retardation and secondary osteoarthrosis [81]. KBD is mainly endemic to Tibet, China, Siberia, and North Korea and is caused in part by poor selenium levels in soil that usually affects children between the ages of 5 to 15 [81,82].

In 1998, Moreno-Reyes et al. established the relationship between this osteoarthropathy and selenium deficiency in rural Tibet [82].

2. Selenium and Immunobiology

The importance of adequate levels of dietary selenium and its efficient incorporation into selenoproteins in immunity has been demonstrated in cell culture models, in rodent models, in livestock and poultry studies, and in humans. Selenium deficiency can give rise to immune-incompetence that leads to increased susceptibility to infections and possibly to cancers. There is some evidence that selenium can modulate the pathology that accompanies chronic inflammatory diseases in the gut and liver as well as in inflammation-associated cancers [83,84]. Selenium deficiency and suppressed selenoprotein expression have been implicated in higher levels of inflammatory cytokines in a variety of tissues including the gastrointestinal tract [85,86], the uterus [87], mammary gland tissues [88], and others. However, some inflammatory processes actually increase when selenium intake changes from deficient to sufficient levels. For example, a mouse model of allergic asthma showed that selenium deficiency reduced airway inflammation while adequate selenium intake produced higher levels of inflammation that were then decreased when supra-nutritional levels of selenium were used [89]. In addition, increasing the selenium status through dietary delivery of sodium selenite raised expression levels and translation of mRNAs encoding stress-related selenoproteins as well as genes involved in inflammation and interferon γ IFNγ responses [90].

Selenium supplementation, for the most part, is immuno-stimulatory, which is measured by a wide range of parameters including T cell proliferation, NK cell activity, innate immune cell functions, and many others [91]. This depends on the baseline selenium status and the strongest effects can be seen when supplementation boosts selenium levels from inadequate to adequate while the benefits of increasing an adequate selenium level to supra-nutritional levels is less clear. The activation of human blood leukocytes has been shown to increase in response to selenium-enriched foods [92]. Vaccine responses against pathogens such as poliovirus have been shown to improve with selenium supplementation [93] even though results were mixed when analyzing the influenza vaccine in older adults [94]. Similarly, integrated-omics analyses of pathways affected by the selenium status in rectal biopsies from 22 healthy adults showed reduced inflammatory and immune responses and cytoskeleton remodeling in the suboptimal selenium status group [95]. Similarly, selenium supplementation was shown to modulate the inflammatory response in respiratory distress syndrome patients by restoring the antioxidant capacity of the lungs, which moderated the inflammatory responses through interleukin (IL)-1β and IL-6 levels and meaningfully improved the respiratory mechanics [96].

There have been few definitive reports of selenium and selenoprotein levels affecting hematopoiesis and the development of the immune system. The deletion of the essential selenoprotein, TXNRD2, does not impair lymphocyte development and maintenance [97]. However, a T cell-specific knockout of all selenoproteins was found to reduce the number of mature T cells emerging from lymphoid tissues [98]. Autoimmunity is an important issue related to immune system development and there have been reports in humans of an increase in the prevalence of autoimmune thyroiditis in low-selenium regions that are consistent with studies in mice [99,100]. While selenium is vital for many immune cell functions (Figure 1), the benefits of applying wide scale selenium supplementation as an approach to boost immunity in the general population have lacked definitive support over the years. This suggests a need for a more refined evaluation of how selenium affects different types of immune responses along with a deeper mechanistic understanding. In the following sections, the effects of selenium on various aspects of immunity and its mechanisms of action will be discussed in further detail.

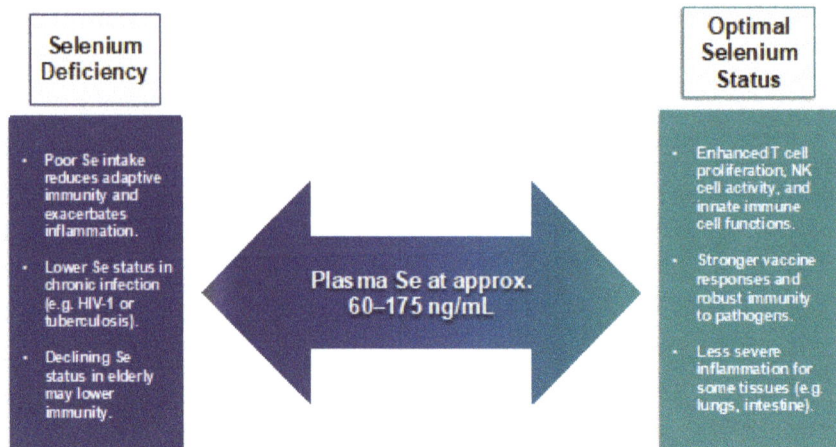

Figure 1. A summary of selenium and immune responses.

3. Leukocyte Functions

Adaptive immunity is affected by selenium intake including the activation and functions of T and B cells. One immunological feature of selenium levels in vivo is the positive effect that higher selenium has on the proliferation and differentiation of cluster of differentiation(CD)4$^+$ T helper (Th) cells. There are several reports of the skewing of T cell immunity toward Th1 phenotypes. For example, our laboratory used a mouse model of viral antigen vaccination to test effects of low (0.087 ppm), medium (0.25 ppm), and high (1.0 ppm) selenium diets and found that Th1 immunity was enhanced along with the T cell receptor signal strength [101]. In a separate study, oral administration of synthetic selenium nanoparticles induced a robust Th1 cytokine pattern after a hepatitis B surface antigen vaccination in a mouse model [102]. Less information is available regarding the effects of selenium on cytotoxic CD8$^+$ T cells even though cytotoxic T cells from aged mice (24 months old) showed enhanced mitogen-induced proliferation when treated with selenium supplementation [103]. Mouse knockout models have shown roles for selenoproteins in antibody production. In particular, T cell deletion of the *trsp* gene responsible for the synthesis of all selenoproteins not only affected T cell maturation and activation but reduced the T cell 'help' provided to B cells for secreting antibodies, which is determined by low levels of serum immunoglobulin [98]. A small study in humans showed a positive effect on antibody titers against the diphtheria vaccine with selenium supplementation that correspond to increased lymphocyte counts [104]. In a more recent study involving Selenoprotein F (SELENOF) knockout mice, elevated levels of immunoglobulins were detected in the sera that were nonfunctional [38]. The authors of this study concluded that SELENOF functions as a gatekeeper of immunoglobulins in the endoplasmic reticulum (ER), which supports the redox quality control of these proteins and likely other proteins.

Innate immune cell functions have also been shown to be impacted by selenium levels. Macrophages are affected by selenium levels in terms of their inflammatory signaling capacity and anti-pathogen activities. Activation of macrophages through pathogen-associated molecular patterns like lipopolysaccharide (LPS) generates an oxidative burst. Additionally, macrophage activation involves the release of cytokine mediators and arachidonic acid-derived prostaglandins like prostaglandin E2 (PGE2), thromboxane A2 (TXA2), and prostaglandin D2 (PGD2) as well as its metabolite 15-Deoxy-Delta-12,14-prostaglandin J2 (15d-PGJ2). It was shown that selenium induces a phenotypic switch in macrophage activation from a classically activated, pro-inflammatory phenotype (M1) toward an alternatively activated, anti-inflammatory phenotype (M2) [105]. Regarding the latter phenotype, selenium was shown to be pivotal for cyclooxygenase-dependent 15d-PGJ2 generation and M2-mediated clearance of helminthic parasite infections [106]. Evidence from several studies demonstrated that selenium levels and selenoproteins regulate migration and phagocytosis functions in macrophages [107,108]. Experiments involving golden Syrian hamster macrophages and *Staphylococcus aureus* showed that higher levels of selenium in culture media led to significant increases in macrophage phagocytic activity, nitric oxide production, and *S. aureus* killing [109]. Furthermore, pre-treatment of RAW264.7 mouse macrophages with selenium supplementation prior to exposure to *S. aureus* led to lower levels of nuclear factor kappa-light-chain-enhancer of activated B cells (NF-κB) activation and downstream inflammatory cytokine release [110]. Less information is available regarding selenium levels and neutrophil function. However, one study demonstrated that increased selenium intake may protect neutrophils from endogenous oxidative stress [111]. Natural Killer (NK) cells are impacted by dietary selenium intake both directly and indirectly. Serum selenium concentration was positively associated with peripheral CD16$^+$ NK cells in older humans [112]. However, functional capacity of these NK cells, e.g., cytotoxicity, was not determined. A separate study in mice showed that selenium supplementation increased the cytotoxic functions of NK cells [113]. The inhibitory receptor, CD94/Natural Killer G2A (NKG2A), was found to be sensitive to selenite treatment, which indicated that NK cell activity may be indirectly increased using this form of selenium [114]. The use of selenium to increase innate immunity may be enhanced when provided along with other nutritional antioxidants. This was demonstrated in prematurely aging mice that exhibited improved macrophage and NK cell functions with a cocktail of antioxidants that included selenium [115].

4. Immune Responses to Pathogens

Innate and adaptive immune responses against bacterial and parasitic infections rely on sufficient selenium for eliminating these pathogens. For example, selenium deficiency in mice was shown to impair innate immunity and induce susceptibility to *Listeria monocytogenes* infection [116]. In this study, C57BL/6 mice fed adequate or deficient selenium diets were infected with *L. monocytogenes* and it was found that mice maintained on a selenium deficient diet produced less IFNγ when compared to mice that were fed the control diet. In addition, selenium supplementation decreased the parasitemia of pregnant Wistar rats infected with *Trypanosoma cruzi* [117]. Selenium intake also affects the plasticity of macrophages during immune responses to helminthic parasite infections. For example, a mouse model of infection with *Nippostrongylus brasiliensis*, which is a gastrointestinal nematode parasite, showed that higher levels of dietary selenium led to optimal expression of selenoproteins and selenium-dependent production of cyclooxygenase (COX)-derived endogenous prostanoids crucial for eliminating *N. brasiliensis* infection [118]. Similarly, mice infected with *Heligmosomoides bakeri* required sufficient selenium intake to eliminate these helminthic pathogens and this correlated with increased local expression of Th2-associated genes in infected small intestinal tissues [119].

Bacterial infections in neonates may be a particularly important outcome related to maternal selenium status, which is suggested by studies in humans and rodent models [120–122]. These studies do not necessarily distinguish between the effects of the selenium on the immune system and other effects that selenium can have on infant health. In addition to the role of the selenium status on the immune system, one must keep in mind the direct effects that selenium has on bacterial pathogens as well the fact that many bacterial species express selenoproteins [123].

Selenium is one of many nutrients implicated in the severity and progression of tuberculosis (TB) caused by the bacterium *Mycobacterium tuberculosis* [124]. Pulmonary TB patients have lower selenium statuses when compared to healthy controls [125]. Interestingly, investigators also observed that TB patients with concomitant HIV infection exhibited a significantly lower concentration of serum selenium along with augmented wasting versus those without HIV infection. Intensified wasting in TB patients was positively correlated with the severity of lung disease and was associated with low serum selenium levels [126]. Following a two-month intervention study, selenium plus vitamin E supplementation enhanced total antioxidant capacity in patients with pulmonary TB even though the effects on the immune system were not determined [127]. However, several researchers have pointed out that some trace nutrients that may be used as supplements to restore immunity and lung function may also be exploited by *M. tuberculosis* to promote growth of the pathogen [128]. This has been supported by data involving the growth of this bacteria under different selenium concentrations [129].

The beneficial effects of a higher selenium status have been supported for some viral infections even though there are some studies that do not conclusively demonstrate effective improvements in anti-viral immunity [130]. Moreover, the antioxidant properties of some selenoproteins have been suggested to contribute to boosting anti-viral immunity [131]. However, some selenoproteins that have not been established as antioxidant enzymes like SELENOK can also play key roles in protecting against viruses [42]. The chronic hepatitis C virus (HCV) has been shown to influence oxidative stress levels in humans and an association between HCV load and the selenium status has been associated with a documented selenium status [132]. Oxidative stress can have genomic altering effects on RNA viruses that can lead to higher virulence of certain viruses themselves and this has been shown to involve the selenium status in the case of coxsackievirus B3 [133]. Thus, the effects of selenium on the virus in some cases may compound the influence of this micronutrient on the immune system. Targeting individuals with low selenium intake or the elderly with a declining selenium status with selenium supplementation may be an effective public health initiative for increasing vaccine responses to viruses [134]. There is evidence to support a positive effect on adaptive immune responses to vaccination against viral pathogens. This causes polio and influenza in populations with a low baseline selenium status [93,135].

The most compelling data available regarding the role of selenium in anti-viral immunity are those related to HIV infection, which is a global pandemic that particularly afflicts persons with inadequate nutrition and directly impairs immunity [136]. Selenium is one micronutrient implicated in disease progression. Low selenium intake has been associated with HIV prevalence [137,138] and the status of CD4$^+$ T cell numbers has been correlated with selenium levels in HIV$^+$ patients [139]. There is some evidence that selenium malabsorption or overutilization in Acquired immune deficiency syndrome (AIDS) patients may affect or be affected by disease progression [140,141]. In particular, selenium-deficient HIV$^+$ patients tend to present with disrupted hemodynamics such as depressed selenium plasma and erythrocyte levels, diminished glutathione peroxidase activity, and stunted cardiac selenium bioavailability. A plasma selenium status is conventionally assessed by SELENOP levels and GPX activity as well as selenium levels, which respond differently to changes in selenium consumption [142]. Thus, it is difficult to directly compare studies using different selenium status readouts [143]. Anti-retroviral therapies may also confound the selenium status [144,145]. However, some studies have not supported this notion [146]. Additionally, selenium is often combined with other nutrients for intervention studies, which makes assessment of its impact difficult to distinguish from other nutritional components. Several cohort studies have illustrated an association between selenium deficiency and progression to AIDS-related mortality [147]. Remarkably, randomized controlled trials demonstrated that selenium supplementation minimized hospitalizations and diarrheal morbidity and improved CD4$^+$ T cell counts [141,148]. Similarly, an inhibitory effect of selenium on HIV in vitro due to the radical scavenger effects of glutathione peroxidase has been reported [141]. Glutathione peroxidase and other antioxidant selenoenzymes along with catalase have been implicated in decreasing a viral activation impact on redox control [141,149]. Thus, the potential benefits of selenium supplementation for HIV infection likely resides in the redox regulating selenoenzymes and resides less with the pro-oxidant seleno-metabolites that are found to affect cancer.

5. Selenium and Its Effects on a Shift toward Anti-Cancer Immunity

The effects of the selenium status on carcinogenesis or tumor progression have been intensely studied and results have led to a wide variety of conclusions. In humans, there have been several epidemiological studies as well as intervention studies involving different types of cancer, which suggests beneficial effects of higher selenium status [150–152]. On the other hand, the selenium status was not found to be a factor in cancer progression in a number of other studies [153–156]. From the perspective of research in humans, it has proven difficult to separate the direct effects that selenium has on carcinogenesis from its impact on the growth of established tumors as well as its influence on cancer immunity. One of the direct anti-cancer effects of selenium is related to the ability of seleno-compounds to induce oxidative stress and DNA damage accumulation and, consequently, apoptosis [15]. Other direct effects of selenium on established tumors in humans are less clear and this is particularly true for those effects that are exerted through the immune system. For example, there is some evidence from one human study suggesting an inhibitory effect of selenium on the epithelial-to-mesenchymal transition (EMT) that drives metastasis [157]. This was accompanied by the capacity of higher levels of selenium to down-regulate expression of genes involved in wound healing and inflammation, which are both related to EMT. The idea that selenium supplementation may be used to support the immune system during cancer treatment has been supported by some studies including those related to childhood leukemia and neutropenia [158,159]. Intervention studies showed positive effects of selenium on mitigating neutropenia in children suffering from leukemia/lymphomas as well as solid tumors [160].

There is evidence that GPX4 modulates hepatocellular carcinoma (HCC) in both humans and rodent models. In humans, GPX4 expression in tumors positively correlated with patient survival and was linked to pathways that regulate cell proliferation, motility, tissue remodeling, and immune responses with a particular effect on M1 macrophage polarization [161]. Corroborative results demonstrate that overexpression of GPX4 decreased the growth of human HCC cell lines using xenotransplantation into immune-deficient non-diabetic (NOD) mice. These findings are consistent with previous studies showing that inhibition of GPX4 expression by siRNA in HCC cells increased the formation of Vascular endothelial growth factor (VEGF) and IL-8 cytokines [162], which are both clinically relevant adverse prognostic factors in HCC patients [162,163]. However, since NOD mice do not include a competent immune system, it is difficult to interpret how the immune relevant data from the human gene arrays can be related to the rodent studies.

The polarization of tumor-associated macrophages away from tolerogenic phenotypes and toward anti-tumor M1 macrophages suggested in the above experiments with GPX4 overexpression was also supported in selenium nanoparticle studies [164]. However, how selenium levels affect macrophage polarization in the tumor microenvironment in human cancers remains to be determined. As discussed in a previous review [165], higher levels of selenium can increase NK cell activity by preventing the non-enzymatic formation of parafibrin that surrounds tumor cells and hinders immune surveillance and by activating the NK cell population in the tumor microenvironment. The anti-tumoral activity of NK cells requires the expression of the activating receptor natural killer group 2 member D (NKG2D) on NK cell surfaces [166]. The selenium metabolite known as methylselenol was found to upregulate two NKG2D ligands on the surface of tumor cells [167]. However, it was not determined if this led to increased NK cell killing of tumor cells. This feature is important for the detection of tumor cells by $CD8^+$ T cells since these cells also express NKG2D. In fact, major histocompatibility-I (MHC-I) present tumor antigens to $CD8^+$ T cells to activate their cytotoxic activities, which is also affected by methylselenol in cancer cells. In particular, this selenium metabolite was shown to alter redox metabolism in melanoma cells and lead to increased levels of MHC-I cell surface antigens [168]. This study showed that the actions of methylselenol mimic IFNγ signaling by also upregulating members of IFNγ responsive genes. However, one must consider the detrimental effects of inducing oxidative stress in some tissues such as the gut where this can promote tumorigenesis and tumor progression [85].

Due to the ability to control experimental conditions, rodent models of selenium and cancer have provided data that may be easier to interpret. However, unless specifically built into the study design, it is difficult if not impossible to distinguish between the effects of the bioavailable selenium on the cancer cells themselves versus the immune cells that are either trying to facilitate tumor progression or trying to eradicate the cancer cells. The mixed results for rodent cancer studies when tumor growth is the primary endpoint for mouse studies highlight this confounding issue. For example, in our mouse model study of syngeneic mesothelioma tumors that utilized immune competent animals, we expected that increasing dietary selenium would hinder tumor progression due to enhanced anti-cancer immunity. However, the tumors progressed at an accelerated rate in mice that were fed higher selenium diets due to the pro-reducing capacity in the tumor cells themselves [169]. Other rodent studies focused on melanoma or breast cancer found different results with higher selenium intake leading to lower tumor growth concurrent with immune enhancing effects [170]. When immune responses have been analyzed, the predominant effect is an enhancement of Th1 immunity and a reduction in regulatory T cells (Tregs) and myeloid-derived suppressor cells that suppress anti-tumor immunity [171,172]. There are many factors to consider when analyzing the results of the rodent cancer studies including the type of cancer, strain, and immune status of the rodents, dose and form of selenium used, and endpoints used for analyses. The generation of new xenograft models as well as humanized rodents will facilitate these studies when the research field moves forward.

6. Specific Mechanisms by Which Selenoproteins Regulate Immunity

There have been some investigations into molecular mechanisms underlying the effects of selenium on the immune system. Because selenium can impact so many cellular functions, it is very difficult to dissect out the many different pathways and individual molecules regulated by this micronutrient. Despite these caveats, the generation of transgenic and knockout mouse models has revealed some intriguing mechanisms involving individual selenoproteins. Two examples shown below involve roles elucidated for two selenoproteins in regulating immune cell functions.

MSRB1 is the lone Sec-containing member of the methionine sulfoxide reductase (MSR) family of proteins, which also includes MSRA, MSRB2, and MSRB3. Reactive oxygen species (ROS) can oxidize methionine residues in proteins to produce a mixture of *S*-stereoisomers and *R*-stereoisomers of methionine sulfoxide, which are reduced by MSRA and MSRB enzymes, respectively [173]. The first report of MSRB1 in macrophage biology described its role in regulating actin polymerization during cellular activation that promoted functions like phagocytosis and cytokine secretion [174]. Two methionine residues in actin are specifically converted to methionine-R-sulfoxide by monooxygenase enzymes called Mical1 and Mical2 and are reduced back to methionine by selenoprotein MSRB1, which supports actin disassembly and assembly, respectively. In this manner, macrophages utilize a system of redox reactions during cellular activation by stimulating MSRB1 expression and activity as a part of innate immunity. There are two intriguing aspects of this regulatory process. First, lipopolysaccharide (LPS) induces expression of MSRB1, but not other MSRs, which suggests stereo-specificity in the reactions. Second, a follow-up study found that MSRB1 controls immune responses by promoting anti-inflammatory cytokine expression in macrophages [35]. It must be noted that bacteria have their own versions of MSRs and the importance of this was shown in the case of *Francisella tularensis*, which replicates within macrophages during infection. The *F. tularensis* MSRB (the only B isoform in bacteria) was crucial in promoting replication while MSRA was not as important [175]. In fact, the roles of MSRB in the pathogenesis of several bacteria have been investigated, but it must be noted that the bacterial enzyme contains cysteine (Cys) in place of Sec and, therefore, these MSRBs are not selenoproteins. Overall, it remains to be determined how the regulated expression of MSRB1 in humans affects infection with this bacterium or other pathogens that replicate within macrophages, but this selenoprotein appears to be quite important in shaping innate immune responses.

Our laboratory has studied SELENOK in the immune system for a number of years starting with the finding that levels of this selenoprotein were relatively high in immune tissues of mice and its expression increased with higher selenium intake [42]. SELENOK knockout mice showed no overt phenotype and were fertile, but we found ~50% reduction in most immune cell functions when the immune system was challenged [42]. We subsequently identified its role in promoting calcium flux during immune cell activation by SELENOK complexing with the enzyme DHHC6 (letters represent the amino acids aspartic acid, histidine, histidine, and cysteine in the catalytic domain and 6 represents the 6th member of the family) to palmitoylate to the endoplasmic reticulum (ER) calcium channel protein inositol-1,4,5-trisphosphate receptor (IP3R) [176]. SELENOK itself does not function as an enzyme but instead binds to DHHC6 to stabilize the acylated intermediate of this enzyme so that it is not hydrolyzed by water, which does not hydrolyze the thioester bond between the acyl group and the cysteine residue in DHHC6 before it can transfer the acyl group to target proteins like IP3R [177]. Other proteins involved in immune functions also depend on SELENOK/DHHC6 for palmitoylation to carry out their activities including CD36 and Arf-GAP with SH3 domain, ANK repeat and PH domain-containing protein 2 (ASAP2) [178,179]. Overall, SELENOK plays an important, non-enzymatic role in regulating immunity by functioning as a cofactor for an enzyme involved in critical post-translational modifications of proteins.

7. Conclusions

The immune system is one aspect of human health that is impacted by dietary selenium levels and selenoprotein expression. Under conditions of selenium deficiency, innate and adaptive immune responses are impaired. The benefits of selenium supplementation to boost immunity against pathogens, vaccinations, or cancers have been explored and have not provided entirely clear results. Some of the issues lie in the fact that some pathogens or tumor cells may themselves benefit from higher levels of selenium. Manipulation of individual selenoproteins may offer a more precise approach for enhancing the immune system or mitigating chronic inflammation. This approach will require a comprehensive characterization of the roles for selenoproteins and an unmasking of molecular mechanisms by which they regulate immune cell functions.

Author Contributions: J.C.A. and P.R.H. wrote the paper.

Funding: This work was supported by the NIAID/NIH grant R01 AI089999.

Conflicts of Interest: The authors declare no conflicts of interest.

References

1. Franke, K.W. A New Toxicant Occurring Naturally in Certain Samples of Plant Foodstuffs: I. Results Obtained in Preliminary Feeding Trials: Eight Figures. *J. Nutr.* **1934**, *8*, 597–608. [CrossRef]
2. Schwarz, K.; Foltz, C.M. Selenium as an integral part of factor 3 against dietary necrosis liver degeneration. *J. Am. Chem. Soc.* **1957**, *79*, 3292–3293. [CrossRef]
3. Roman, M.; Jitaru, P.; Barbante, C. Selenium biochemistry and its role for human health. *Metallomics* **2014**, *6*, 25–54. [CrossRef] [PubMed]
4. Rayman, M.P. Selenium and human health. *Lancet* **2012**, *379*, 1256–1268. [CrossRef]
5. Chun, O.K.; Floegel, A.; Chung, S.J.; Chung, C.E.; Song, W.O.; Koo, S.I. Estimation of antioxidant intakes from diet and supplements in U.S. adults. *J. Nutr.* **2010**, *140*, 317–324. [CrossRef] [PubMed]
6. Kipp, A.P.; Strohm, D.; Brigelius-Flohe, R.; Schomburg, L.; Bechthold, A.; Leschik-Bonnet, E.; Heseker, H.; German Nutrition Society (DGE). Revised reference values for selenium intake. *J. Trace Elem. Med. Biol.* **2015**, *32*, 195–199. [CrossRef] [PubMed]
7. Institute of Medicine, Food and Nutrition Board Staff. *Vitamin C, Vitamin E, Selenium, and Carotenoids*; National Academy Press: Washington, DC, USA, 2000.
8. Dietary reference values for food energy and nutrients for the United Kingdom. Report of the Panel on Dietary Reference Values of the Committee on Medical Aspects of Food Policy. *Rep. Health Soc. Subj. (Lond.)* **1991**, *41*, 1–210.
9. Sunde, R.A. Selenium. In *Modern Nutrition in Health and Disease*, 11th ed.; Ross, A.C., Caballero, B., Cousins, R.J., Tucker, K.L., Ziegler, T.R., Eds.; Lippincott Williams & Wilkins: Philadelphia, PA, USA, 2012; pp. 225–237.
10. Ashton, K.; Hooper, L.; Harvey, L.J.; Hurst, R.; Casgrain, A.; Fairweather-Tait, S.J. Methods of assessment of selenium status in humans: A systematic review. *Am. J. Clin. Nutr.* **2009**, *89*, 2025S–2039S. [CrossRef] [PubMed]

11. Combs, G.F., Jr. Biomarkers of selenium status. *Nutrients* **2015**, *7*, 2209–2236. [CrossRef] [PubMed]
12. Stoffaneller, R.; Morse, N.L. A review of dietary selenium intake and selenium status in Europe and the Middle East. *Nutrients* **2015**, *7*, 1494–1537. [CrossRef] [PubMed]
13. Finley, J.W. Bioavailability of selenium from foods. *Nutr. Rev.* **2006**, *64*, 146–151. [CrossRef] [PubMed]
14. Kassam, S.; Goenaga-Infante, H.; Maharaj, L.; Hiley, C.T.; Juliger, S.; Joel, S.P. Methylseleninic acid inhibits HDAC activity in diffuse large B-cell lymphoma cell lines. *Cancer Chemother. Pharmacol.* **2011**, *68*, 815–821. [CrossRef] [PubMed]
15. Bera, S.; De Rosa, V.; Rachidi, W.; Diamond, A.M. Does a role for selenium in DNA damage repair explain apparent controversies in its use in chemoprevention? *Mutagenesis* **2013**, *28*, 127–134. [CrossRef] [PubMed]
16. Ip, C.; Thompson, H.J.; Zhu, Z.; Ganther, H.E. In vitro and in vivo studies of methylseleninic acid: Evidence that a monomethylated selenium metabolite is critical for cancer chemoprevention. *Cancer Res.* **2000**, *60*, 2882–2886. [PubMed]
17. Reeves, M.A.; Hoffmann, P.R. The human selenoproteome: Recent insights into functions and regulation. *Cell. Mol. Life Sci.* **2009**, *66*, 2457–2478. [CrossRef] [PubMed]
18. Seyedali, A.; Berry, M.J. Nonsense-mediated decay factors are involved in the regulation of selenoprotein mRNA levels during selenium deficiency. *RNA* **2014**, *20*, 1248–1256. [CrossRef] [PubMed]
19. Lin, H.C.; Yeh, C.W.; Chen, Y.F.; Lee, T.T.; Hsieh, P.Y.; Rusnac, D.V.; Lin, S.Y.; Elledge, S.J.; Zheng, N.; Yen, H.S. C-Terminal End-Directed Protein Elimination by CRL2 Ubiquitin Ligases. *Mol. Cell.* **2018**, *70*, 602–613 e603. [CrossRef] [PubMed]
20. Burk, R.F.; Hill, K.E. Regulation of Selenium Metabolism and Transport. *Annu. Rev. Nutr.* **2015**, *35*, 109–134. [CrossRef] [PubMed]
21. Kryukov, G.V.; Castellano, S.; Novoselov, S.V.; Lobanov, A.V.; Zehtab, O.; Guigo, R.; Gladyshev, V.N. Characterization of mammalian selenoproteomes. *Science* **2003**, *300*, 1439–1443. [CrossRef] [PubMed]
22. Lubos, E.; Loscalzo, J.; Handy, D.E. Glutathione peroxidase-1 in health and disease: From molecular mechanisms to therapeutic opportunities. *Antioxid. Redox Signal.* **2011**, *15*, 1957–1997. [CrossRef] [PubMed]
23. Lei, X.G.; Cheng, W.H.; McClung, J.P. Metabolic regulation and function of glutathione peroxidase-1. *Annu. Rev. Nutr.* **2007**, *27*, 41–61. [CrossRef] [PubMed]
24. Brigelius-Flohe, R.; Kipp, A. Glutathione peroxidases in different stages of carcinogenesis. *Biochim. Biophys. Acta* **2009**, *1790*, 1555–1568. [CrossRef] [PubMed]
25. Wingler, K.; Brigelius-Flohe, R. Gastrointestinal glutathione peroxidase. *Biofactors* **1999**, *10*, 245–249. [CrossRef] [PubMed]
26. Koyama, H.; Omura, K.; Ejima, A.; Kasanuma, Y.; Watanabe, C.; Satoh, H. Separation of selenium-containing proteins in human and mouse plasma using tandem high-performance liquid chromatography columns coupled with inductively coupled plasma-mass spectrometry. *Anal. Biochem.* **1999**, *267*, 84–91. [CrossRef] [PubMed]
27. Chu, F.F.; Esworthy, R.S.; Doroshow, J.H.; Doan, K.; Liu, X.F. Expression of plasma glutathione peroxidase in human liver in addition to kidney, heart, lung, and breast in humans and rodents. *Blood* **1992**, *79*, 3233–3238. [PubMed]
28. Conrad, M.; Schneider, M.; Seiler, A.; Bornkamm, G.W. Physiological role of phospholipid hydroperoxide glutathione peroxidase in mammals. *Biol. Chem.* **2007**, *388*, 1019–1025. [CrossRef] [PubMed]
29. Ingold, I.; Berndt, C.; Schmitt, S.; Doll, S.; Poschmann, G.; Buday, K.; Roveri, A.; Peng, X.; Porto Freitas, F.; Seibt, T.; et al. Selenium Utilization by GPX4 Is Required to Prevent Hydroperoxide-Induced Ferroptosis. *Cell* **2018**, *172*, 409–422 e421. [CrossRef] [PubMed]
30. Brigelius-Flohe, R. Glutathione peroxidases and redox-regulated transcription factors. *Biol. Chem.* **2006**, *387*, 1329–1335. [CrossRef] [PubMed]
31. Crosley, L.K.; Meplan, C.; Nicol, F.; Rundlof, A.K.; Arner, E.S.; Hesketh, J.E.; Arthur, J.R. Differential regulation of expression of cytosolic and mitochondrial thioredoxin reductase in rat liver and kidney. *Arch. Biochem. Biophys.* **2007**, *459*, 178–188. [CrossRef] [PubMed]
32. Conrad, M.; Jakupoglu, C.; Moreno, S.G.; Lippl, S.; Banjac, A.; Schneider, M.; Beck, H.; Hatzopoulos, A.K.; Just, U.; Sinowatz, F.; et al. Essential role for mitochondrial thioredoxin reductase in hematopoiesis, heart development, and heart function. *Mol. Cell. Biol.* **2004**, *24*, 9414–9423. [CrossRef] [PubMed]

33. Su, D.; Novoselov, S.V.; Sun, Q.A.; Moustafa, M.E.; Zhou, Y.; Oko, R.; Hatfield, D.L.; Gladyshev, V.N. Mammalian selenoprotein thioredoxin-glutathione reductase. Roles in disulfide bond formation and sperm maturation. *J. Biol. Chem.* **2005**, *280*, 26491–26498. [CrossRef] [PubMed]
34. Darras, V.M.; Van Herck, S.L. Iodothyronine deiodinase structure and function: From ascidians to humans. *J. Endocrinol.* **2012**, *215*, 189–206. [CrossRef] [PubMed]
35. Lee, B.C.; Lee, S.G.; Choo, M.K.; Kim, J.H.; Lee, H.M.; Kim, S.; Fomenko, D.E.; Kim, H.Y.; Park, J.M.; Gladyshev, V.N. Selenoprotein MsrB1 promotes anti-inflammatory cytokine gene expression in macrophages and controls immune response in vivo. *Sci. Rep.* **2017**, *7*, 5119. [CrossRef] [PubMed]
36. Fomenko, D.E.; Novoselov, S.V.; Natarajan, S.K.; Lee, B.C.; Koc, A.; Carlson, B.A.; Lee, T.H.; Kim, H.Y.; Hatfield, D.L.; Gladyshev, V.N. MsrB1 (methionine-R-sulfoxide reductase 1) knock-out mice: Roles of MsrB1 in redox regulation and identification of a novel selenoprotein form. *J. Biol. Chem.* **2009**, *284*, 5986–5993. [CrossRef] [PubMed]
37. Labunskyy, V.M.; Hatfield, D.L.; Gladyshev, V.N. The Sep15 protein family: Roles in disulfide bond formation and quality control in the endoplasmic reticulum. *IUBMB Life* **2007**, *59*, 1–5. [CrossRef] [PubMed]
38. Yim, S.H.; Everley, R.A.; Schildberg, F.A.; Lee, S.G.; Orsi, A.; Barbati, Z.R.; Karatepe, K.; Fomenko, D.E.; Tsuji, P.A.; Luo, H.R.; et al. Role of Selenof as a Gatekeeper of Secreted Disulfide-Rich Glycoproteins. *Cell. Rep.* **2018**, *23*, 1387–1398. [CrossRef] [PubMed]
39. Panee, J.; Stoytcheva, Z.R.; Liu, W.; Berry, M.J. Selenoprotein H is a redox-sensing high mobility group family DNA-binding protein that up-regulates genes involved in glutathione synthesis and phase II detoxification. *J. Biol. Chem.* **2007**, *282*, 23759–23765. [CrossRef] [PubMed]
40. Novoselov, S.V.; Kryukov, G.V.; Xu, X.M.; Carlson, B.A.; Hatfield, D.L.; Gladyshev, V.N. Selenoprotein H is a nucleolar thioredoxin-like protein with a unique expression pattern. *J. Biol. Chem.* **2007**, *282*, 11960–11968. [CrossRef] [PubMed]
41. Horibata, Y.; Hirabayashi, Y. Identification and characterization of human ethanolaminephosphotransferase1. *J. Lipid Res.* **2007**, *48*, 503–508. [CrossRef] [PubMed]
42. Verma, S.; Hoffmann, F.W.; Kumar, M.; Huang, Z.; Roe, K.; Nguyen-Wu, E.; Hashimoto, A.S.; Hoffmann, P.R. Selenoprotein K knockout mice exhibit deficient calcium flux in immune cells and impaired immune responses. *J. Immunol.* **2011**, *186*, 2127–2137. [CrossRef] [PubMed]
43. Fredericks, G.J.; Hoffmann, P.R. Selenoprotein K and protein palmitoylation. *Antioxid. Redox Signal.* **2015**, *23*, 854–862. [CrossRef] [PubMed]
44. Pitts, M.W.; Reeves, M.A.; Hashimoto, A.C.; Ogawa, A.; Kremer, P.; Seale, L.A.; Berry, M.J. Deletion of selenoprotein M leads to obesity without cognitive deficits. *J. Biol. Chem.* **2013**, *288*, 26121–26134. [CrossRef] [PubMed]
45. Lescure, A.; Rederstorff, M.; Krol, A.; Guicheney, P.; Allamand, V. Selenoprotein function and muscle disease. *Biochim. Biophys. Acta* **2009**, *1790*, 1569–1574. [CrossRef] [PubMed]
46. Castets, P.; Lescure, A.; Guicheney, P.; Allamand, V. Selenoprotein N in skeletal muscle: From diseases to function. *J. Mol. Med. (Berl.)* **2012**, *90*, 1095–1107. [CrossRef] [PubMed]
47. Han, S.J.; Lee, B.C.; Yim, S.H.; Gladyshev, V.N.; Lee, S.R. Characterization of mammalian selenoprotein o: A redox-active mitochondrial protein. *PLoS ONE* **2014**, *9*, e95518. [CrossRef] [PubMed]
48. Burk, R.F.; Hill, K.E. Selenoprotein P-expression, functions, and roles in mammals. *Biochim. Biophys. Acta* **2009**, *1790*, 1441–1447. [CrossRef] [PubMed]
49. Ye, Y.; Shibata, Y.; Yun, C.; Ron, D.; Rapoport, T.A. A membrane protein complex mediates retro-translocation from the ER lumen into the cytosol. *Nature* **2004**, *429*, 841–847. [CrossRef] [PubMed]
50. Turanov, A.A.; Shchedrina, V.A.; Everley, R.A.; Lobanov, A.V.; Yim, S.H.; Marino, S.M.; Gygi, S.P.; Hatfield, D.L.; Gladyshev, V.N. Selenoprotein S is involved in maintenance and transport of multiprotein complexes. *Biochem. J.* **2014**, *462*, 555–565. [CrossRef] [PubMed]
51. Boukhzar, L.; Hamieh, A.; Cartier, D.; Tanguy, Y.; Alsharif, I.; Castex, M.; Arabo, A.; El Hajji, S.; Bonnet, J.J.; Errami, M.; et al. Selenoprotein T Exerts an Essential Oxidoreductase Activity That Protects Dopaminergic Neurons in Mouse Models of Parkinson's Disease. *Antioxid. Redox Signal.* **2016**, *24*, 557–574. [CrossRef] [PubMed]
52. Jeon, Y.H.; Park, Y.H.; Lee, J.H.; Hong, J.H.; Kim, I.Y. Selenoprotein W enhances skeletal muscle differentiation by inhibiting TAZ binding to 14-3-3 protein. *Biochim. Biophys. Acta* **2014**, *1843*, 1356–1364. [CrossRef] [PubMed]

53. Xu, X.M.; Carlson, B.A.; Irons, R.; Mix, H.; Zhong, N.; Gladyshev, V.N.; Hatfield, D.L. Selenophosphate synthetase 2 is essential for selenoprotein biosynthesis. *Biochem. J.* **2007**, *404*, 115–120. [CrossRef] [PubMed]
54. Bosl, M.R.; Takaku, K.; Oshima, M.; Nishimura, S.; Taketo, M.M. Early embryonic lethality caused by targeted disruption of the mouse selenocysteine tRNA gene (Trsp). *Proc. Natl. Acad. Sci. USA* **1997**, *94*, 5531–5534. [CrossRef] [PubMed]
55. Yant, L.J.; Ran, Q.; Rao, L.; Van Remmen, H.; Shibatani, T.; Belter, J.G.; Motta, L.; Richardson, A.; Prolla, T.A. The selenoprotein GPX4 is essential for mouse development and protects from radiation and oxidative damage insults. *Free Radic. Biol. Med.* **2003**, *34*, 496–502. [CrossRef]
56. Jakupoglu, C.; Przemeck, G.K.; Schneider, M.; Moreno, S.G.; Mayr, N.; Hatzopoulos, A.K.; de Angelis, M.H.; Wurst, W.; Bornkamm, G.W.; Brielmeier, M.; et al. Cytoplasmic thioredoxin reductase is essential for embryogenesis but dispensable for cardiac development. *Mol. Cell. Biol.* **2005**, *25*, 1980–1988. [CrossRef] [PubMed]
57. Ferreiro, A.; Quijano-Roy, S.; Pichereau, C.; Moghadaszadeh, B.; Goemans, N.; Bonnemann, C.; Jungbluth, H.; Straub, V.; Villanova, M.; Leroy, J.P.; et al. Mutations of the selenoprotein N gene, which is implicated in rigid spine muscular dystrophy, cause the classical phenotype of multiminicore disease: Reassessing the nosology of early-onset myopathies. *Am. J. Hum. Genet.* **2002**, *71*, 739–749. [CrossRef] [PubMed]
58. Moghadaszadeh, B.; Petit, N.; Jaillard, C.; Brockington, M.; Quijano Roy, S.; Merlini, L.; Romero, N.; Estournet, B.; Desguerre, I.; Chaigne, D.; et al. Mutations in SEPN1 cause congenital muscular dystrophy with spinal rigidity and restrictive respiratory syndrome. *Nat. Genet.* **2001**, *29*, 17–18. [CrossRef] [PubMed]
59. Jurynec, M.J.; Xia, R.; Mackrill, J.J.; Gunther, D.; Crawford, T.; Flanigan, K.M.; Abramson, J.J.; Howard, M.T.; Grunwald, D.J. Selenoprotein N is required for ryanodine receptor calcium release channel activity in human and zebrafish muscle. *Proc. Natl. Acad. Sci. USA* **2008**, *105*, 12485–12490. [CrossRef] [PubMed]
60. Hornberger, T.A.; McLoughlin, T.J.; Leszczynski, J.K.; Armstrong, D.D.; Jameson, R.R.; Bowen, P.E.; Hwang, E.S.; Hou, H.; Moustafa, M.E.; Carlson, B.A.; et al. Selenoprotein-deficient transgenic mice exhibit enhanced exercise-induced muscle growth. *J. Nutr.* **2003**, *133*, 3091–3097. [CrossRef] [PubMed]
61. Hernandez, A.; St Germain, D.L. Thyroid hormone deiodinases: Physiology and clinical disorders. *Curr. Opin. Pediatr.* **2003**, *15*, 416–420. [CrossRef] [PubMed]
62. Kato, T.; Read, R.; Rozga, J.; Burk, R.F. Evidence for intestinal release of absorbed selenium in a form with high hepatic extraction. *Am. J. Physiol.* **1992**, *262*, G854–G858. [CrossRef] [PubMed]
63. Hill, K.E.; Zhou, J.; McMahan, W.J.; Motley, A.K.; Atkins, J.F.; Gesteland, R.F.; Burk, R.F. Deletion of selenoprotein P alters distribution of selenium in the mouse. *J. Biol. Chem.* **2003**, *278*, 13640–13646. [CrossRef] [PubMed]
64. Schomburg, L.; Schweizer, U.; Holtmann, B.; Flohe, L.; Sendtner, M.; Kohrle, J. Gene disruption discloses role of selenoprotein P in selenium delivery to target tissues. *Biochem. J.* **2003**, *370*, 397–402. [CrossRef] [PubMed]
65. Behne, D.; Hilmert, H.; Scheid, S.; Gessner, H.; Elger, W. Evidence for specific selenium target tissues and new biologically important selenoproteins. *Biochim. Biophys. Acta* **1988**, *966*, 12–21. [CrossRef]
66. Valentine, W.M.; Hill, K.E.; Austin, L.M.; Valentine, H.L.; Goldowitz, D.; Burk, R.F. Brainstem axonal degeneration in mice with deletion of selenoprotein p. *Toxicol. Pathol.* **2005**, *33*, 570–576. [CrossRef] [PubMed]
67. Hill, K.E.; Zhou, J.; McMahan, W.J.; Motley, A.K.; Burk, R.F. Neurological dysfunction occurs in mice with targeted deletion of the selenoprotein P gene. *J. Nutr.* **2004**, *134*, 157–161. [CrossRef] [PubMed]
68. Schweizer, U.; Michaelis, M.; Kohrle, J.; Schomburg, L. Efficient selenium transfer from mother to offspring in selenoprotein-P-deficient mice enables dose-dependent rescue of phenotypes associated with selenium deficiency. *Biochem. J.* **2004**, *378*, 21–26. [CrossRef] [PubMed]
69. Nonn, L.; Williams, R.R.; Erickson, R.P.; Powis, G. The absence of mitochondrial thioredoxin 2 causes massive apoptosis, exencephaly, and early embryonic lethality in homozygous mice. *Mol. Cell. Biol.* **2003**, *23*, 916–922. [CrossRef] [PubMed]
70. Flohe, L.; Gunzler, W.A.; Schock, H.H. Glutathione peroxidase: A selenoenzyme. *FEBS Lett.* **1973**, *32*, 132–134. [CrossRef]
71. Rotruck, J.T.; Pope, A.L.; Ganther, H.E.; Swanson, A.B.; Hafeman, D.G.; Hoekstra, W.G. Selenium: Biochemical role as a component of glutathione peroxidase. *Science* **1973**, *179*, 588–590. [CrossRef] [PubMed]

72. Conrad, M. Transgenic mouse models for the vital selenoenzymes cytosolic thioredoxin reductase, mitochondrial thioredoxin reductase and glutathione peroxidase 4. *Biochim. Biophys. Acta* **2009**, *1790*, 1575–1585. [CrossRef] [PubMed]
73. Schomburg, L.; Schweizer, U. Hierarchical regulation of selenoprotein expression and sex-specific effects of selenium. *Biochim. Biophys. Acta* **2009**, *1790*, 1453–1462. [CrossRef] [PubMed]
74. Burk, R.F.; Hill, K.E.; Awad, J.A.; Morrow, J.D.; Lyons, P.R. Liver and kidney necrosis in selenium-deficient rats depleted of glutathione. *Lab. Investig.* **1995**, *72*, 723–730. [PubMed]
75. Ge, K.; Xue, A.; Bai, J.; Wang, S. Keshan disease-an endemic cardiomyopathy in China. *Virchows Arch. A Pathol. Anat. Histopathol.* **1983**, *401*, 1–15. [CrossRef] [PubMed]
76. Beck, M.A.; Levander, O.A.; Handy, J. Selenium deficiency and viral infection. *J. Nutr.* **2003**, *133*, 1463S–1467S. [CrossRef] [PubMed]
77. Sokoloff, L. Acquired chondronecrosis. *Ann. Rheum. Dis.* **1990**, *49*, 262–264. [CrossRef] [PubMed]
78. Wang, S.J.; Guo, X.; Zuo, H.; Zhang, Y.G.; Xu, P.; Ping, Z.G.; Zhang, Z.; Geng, D. Chondrocyte apoptosis and expression of Bcl-2, Bax, Fas, and iNOS in articular cartilage in patients with Kashin-Beck disease. *J. Rheumatol.* **2006**, *33*, 615–619. [PubMed]
79. Wang, S.J.; Guo, X.; Ren, F.L.; Zhang, Y.G.; Zhang, Z.T.; Zhang, F.J.; Geng, D. Comparison of apoptosis of articular chondrocytes in the pathogenesis of Kashin-beck disease and primary osteoarthritis. *Zhongguo Yi Xue Ke Xue Yuan Xue Bao* **2006**, *28*, 267–270. (In Chinese) [PubMed]
80. Wang, Y.; Guo, X.; Zhang, Z.T.; Wang, M.; Wang, S.J. Expression of Caspase-8 and Bcl-2 in the cartilage loose bodies in patients with Kashin-Beck disease. *Nan Fang Yi Ke Da Xue Xue Bao* **2011**, *31*, 1314–1317. (In Chinese) [PubMed]
81. Yao, Y.; Pei, F.; Kang, P. Selenium, iodine, and the relation with Kashin-Beck disease. *Nutrition* **2011**, *27*, 1095–1100. [CrossRef] [PubMed]
82. Moreno-Reyes, R.; Suetens, C.; Mathieu, F.; Begaux, F.; Zhu, D.; Rivera, M.T.; Boelaert, M.; Neve, J.; Perlmutter, N.; Vanderpas, J. Kashin-Beck osteoarthropathy in rural Tibet in relation to selenium and iodine status. *N. Engl. J. Med.* **1998**, *339*, 1112–1120. [CrossRef] [PubMed]
83. Barrett, C.W.; Reddy, V.K.; Short, S.P.; Motley, A.K.; Lintel, M.K.; Bradley, A.M.; Freeman, T.; Vallance, J.; Ning, W.; Parang, B.; et al. Selenoprotein P influences colitis-induced tumorigenesis by mediating stemness and oxidative damage. *J. Clin. Investig.* **2015**, *125*, 2646–2660. [CrossRef] [PubMed]
84. Hamid, M.; Abdulrahim, Y.; Liu, D.; Qian, G.; Khan, A.; Huang, K. The Hepatoprotective Effect of Selenium-Enriched Yeast and Gum Arabic Combination on Carbon Tetrachloride-Induced Chronic Liver Injury in Rats. *J. Food Sci.* **2018**, *83*, 525–534. [CrossRef] [PubMed]
85. Barrett, C.W.; Short, S.P.; Williams, C.S. Selenoproteins and oxidative stress-induced inflammatory tumorigenesis in the gut. *Cell. Mol. Life Sci.* **2017**, *74*, 607–616. [CrossRef] [PubMed]
86. Nettleford, S.K.; Prabhu, K.S. Selenium and Selenoproteins in Gut Inflammation-A Review. *Antioxidants (Basel)* **2018**, *7*, 36. [CrossRef] [PubMed]
87. Zhang, Z.; Gao, X.; Cao, Y.; Jiang, H.; Wang, T.; Song, X.; Guo, M.; Zhang, N. Selenium Deficiency Facilitates Inflammation Through the Regulation of TLR4 and TLR4-Related Signaling Pathways in the Mice Uterus. *Inflammation* **2015**, *38*, 1347–1356. [CrossRef] [PubMed]
88. Gao, X.; Zhang, Z.; Li, Y.; Shen, P.; Hu, X.; Cao, Y.; Zhang, N. Selenium Deficiency Facilitates Inflammation Following S. aureus Infection by Regulating TLR2-Related Pathways in the Mouse Mammary Gland. *Biol. Trace Elem. Res.* **2016**, *172*, 449–457. [CrossRef] [PubMed]
89. Hoffmann, P.R.; Jourdan-Le Saux, C.; Hoffmann, F.W.; Chang, P.S.; Bollt, O.; He, Q.; Tam, E.K.; Berry, M.J. A role for dietary selenium and selenoproteins in allergic airway inflammation. *J. Immunol.* **2007**, *179*, 3258–3267. [CrossRef] [PubMed]
90. Tsuji, P.A.; Carlson, B.A.; Anderson, C.B.; Seifried, H.E.; Hatfield, D.L.; Howard, M.T. Dietary Selenium Levels Affect Selenoprotein Expression and Support the Interferon-gamma and IL-6 Immune Response Pathways in Mice. *Nutrients* **2015**, *7*, 6529–6549. [CrossRef] [PubMed]
91. Huang, Z.; Rose, A.H.; Hoffmann, P.R. The role of selenium in inflammation and immunity: From molecular mechanisms to therapeutic opportunities. *Antioxid. Redox Signal.* **2012**, *16*, 705–743. [CrossRef] [PubMed]

92. Bentley-Hewitt, K.L.; Chen, R.K.; Lill, R.E.; Hedderley, D.I.; Herath, T.D.; Matich, A.J.; McKenzie, M.J. Consumption of selenium-enriched broccoli increases cytokine production in human peripheral blood mononuclear cells stimulated ex vivo, a preliminary human intervention study. *Mol. Nutr. Food Res.* **2014**, *58*, 2350–2357. [CrossRef] [PubMed]
93. Broome, C.S.; McArdle, F.; Kyle, J.A.; Andrews, F.; Lowe, N.M.; Hart, C.A.; Arthur, J.R.; Jackson, M.J. An increase in selenium intake improves immune function and poliovirus handling in adults with marginal selenium status. *Am. J. Clin. Nutr.* **2004**, *80*, 154–162. [CrossRef] [PubMed]
94. Ivory, K.; Prieto, E.; Spinks, C.; Armah, C.N.; Goldson, A.J.; Dainty, J.R.; Nicoletti, C. Selenium supplementation has beneficial and detrimental effects on immunity to influenza vaccine in older adults. *Clin. Nutr.* **2017**, *36*, 407–415. [CrossRef] [PubMed]
95. Meplan, C.; Johnson, I.T.; Polley, A.C.; Cockell, S.; Bradburn, D.M.; Commane, D.M.; Arasaradnam, R.P.; Mulholland, F.; Zupanic, A.; Mathers, J.C.; et al. Transcriptomics and proteomics show that selenium affects inflammation, cytoskeleton, and cancer pathways in human rectal biopsies. *FASEB J.* **2016**, *30*, 2812–2825. [CrossRef] [PubMed]
96. Mahmoodpoor, A.; Hamishehkar, H.; Shadvar, K.; Ostadi, Z.; Sanaie, S.; Saghaleini, S.H.; Nader, N.D. The Effect of Intravenous Selenium on Oxidative Stress in Critically Ill Patients with Acute Respiratory Distress Syndrome. *Immunol. Investig.* **2018**, 1–13. [CrossRef] [PubMed]
97. Geisberger, R.; Kiermayer, C.; Homig, C.; Conrad, M.; Schmidt, J.; Zimber-Strobl, U.; Brielmeier, M. B- and T-cell-specific inactivation of thioredoxin reductase 2 does not impair lymphocyte development and maintenance. *Biol. Chem.* **2007**, *388*, 1083–1090. [CrossRef] [PubMed]
98. Shrimali, R.K.; Irons, R.D.; Carlson, B.A.; Sano, Y.; Gladyshev, V.N.; Park, J.M.; Hatfield, D.L. Selenoproteins mediate T cell immunity through an antioxidant mechanism. *J. Biol. Chem.* **2008**, *283*, 20181–20185. [CrossRef] [PubMed]
99. Wichman, J.; Winther, K.H.; Bonnema, S.J.; Hegedus, L. Selenium Supplementation Significantly Reduces Thyroid Autoantibody Levels in Patients with Chronic Autoimmune Thyroiditis: A Systematic Review and Meta-Analysis. *Thyroid* **2016**, *26*, 1681–1692. [CrossRef] [PubMed]
100. McLachlan, S.M.; Aliesky, H.; Banuelos, B.; Hee, S.S.Q.; Rapoport, B. Variable Effects of Dietary Selenium in Mice That Spontaneously Develop a Spectrum of Thyroid Autoantibodies. *Endocrinology* **2017**, *158*, 3754–3764. [CrossRef] [PubMed]
101. Hoffmann, F.W.; Hashimoto, A.C.; Shafer, L.A.; Dow, S.; Berry, M.J.; Hoffmann, P.R. Dietary selenium modulates activation and differentiation of CD4+ T cells in mice through a mechanism involving cellular free thiols. *J. Nutr.* **2010**, *140*, 1155–1161. [CrossRef] [PubMed]
102. Mahdavi, M.; Mavandadnejad, F.; Yazdi, M.H.; Faghfuri, E.; Hashemi, H.; Homayouni-Oreh, S.; Farhoudi, R.; Shahverdi, A.R. Oral administration of synthetic selenium nanoparticles induced robust Th1 cytokine pattern after HBs antigen vaccination in mouse model. *J. Infect. Public Health* **2017**, *10*, 102–109. [CrossRef] [PubMed]
103. Roy, M.; Kiremidjian-Schumacher, L.; Wishe, H.I.; Cohen, M.W.; Stotzky, G. Supplementation with selenium restores age-related decline in immune cell function. *Proc. Soc. Exp. Biol. Med.* **1995**, *209*, 369–375. [CrossRef] [PubMed]
104. Hawkes, W.C.; Kelley, D.S.; Taylor, P.C. The effects of dietary selenium on the immune system in healthy men. *Biol. Trace Elem. Res.* **2001**, *81*, 189–213. [CrossRef]
105. Nelson, S.M.; Lei, X.; Prabhu, K.S. Selenium levels affect the IL-4-induced expression of alternative activation markers in murine macrophages. *J. Nutr.* **2011**, *141*, 1754–1761. [CrossRef] [PubMed]
106. Nelson, S.M.; Shay, A.E.; James, J.L.; Carlson, B.A.; Urban, J.F., Jr.; Prabhu, K.S. Selenoprotein Expression in Macrophages Is Critical for Optimal Clearance of Parasitic Helminth Nippostrongylus brasiliensis. *J. Biol. Chem.* **2016**, *291*, 2787–2798. [CrossRef] [PubMed]
107. Carlson, B.A.; Yoo, M.H.; Shrimali, R.K.; Irons, R.; Gladyshev, V.N.; Hatfield, D.L.; Park, J.M. Role of selenium-containing proteins in T-cell and macrophage function. *Proc. Nutr. Soc.* **2010**, *69*, 300–310. [CrossRef] [PubMed]
108. Safir, N.; Wendel, A.; Saile, R.; Chabraoui, L. The effect of selenium on immune functions of J774.1 cells. *Clin. Chem. Lab. Med.* **2003**, *41*, 1005–1011. [CrossRef] [PubMed]
109. Aribi, M.; Meziane, W.; Habi, S.; Boulatika, Y.; Marchandin, H.; Aymeric, J.L. Macrophage Bactericidal Activities against Staphylococcus aureus Are Enhanced In Vivo by Selenium Supplementation in a Dose-Dependent Manner. *PLoS ONE* **2015**, *10*, e0135515. [CrossRef] [PubMed]

110. Bi, C.L.; Wang, H.; Wang, Y.J.; Sun, J.; Dong, J.S.; Meng, X.; Li, J.J. Selenium inhibits Staphylococcus aureus-induced inflammation by suppressing the activation of the NF-kappaB and MAPK signalling pathways in RAW264.7 macrophages. *Eur. J. Pharmacol.* **2016**, *780*, 159–165. [CrossRef] [PubMed]

111. Kose, S.A.; Naziroglu, M. Selenium reduces oxidative stress and calcium entry through TRPV1 channels in the neutrophils of patients with polycystic ovary syndrome. *Biol. Trace Elem. Res.* **2014**, *158*, 136–142. [CrossRef] [PubMed]

112. Ravaglia, G.; Forti, P.; Maioli, F.; Bastagli, L.; Facchini, A.; Mariani, E.; Savarino, L.; Sassi, S.; Cucinotta, D.; Lenaz, G. Effect of micronutrient status on natural killer cell immune function in healthy free-living subjects aged >/=90 y. *Am. J. Clin. Nutr.* **2000**, *71*, 590–598. [CrossRef] [PubMed]

113. Kiremidjian-Schumacher, L.; Roy, M.; Wishe, H.I.; Cohen, M.W.; Stotzky, G. Supplementation with selenium augments the functions of natural killer and lymphokine-activated killer cells. *Biol. Trace Elem. Res.* **1996**, *52*, 227–239. [CrossRef] [PubMed]

114. Enqvist, M.; Nilsonne, G.; Hammarfjord, O.; Wallin, R.P.; Bjorkstrom, N.K.; Bjornstedt, M.; Hjerpe, A.; Ljunggren, H.G.; Dobra, K.; Malmberg, K.J.; et al. Selenite induces posttranscriptional blockade of HLA-E expression and sensitizes tumor cells to CD94/NKG2A-positive NK cells. *J. Immunol.* **2011**, *187*, 3546–3554. [CrossRef] [PubMed]

115. Alvarado, C.; Alvarez, P.; Jimenez, L.; De la Fuente, M. Improvement of leukocyte functions in young prematurely aging mice after a 5-week ingestion of a diet supplemented with biscuits enriched in antioxidants. *Antioxid. Redox Signal.* **2005**, *7*, 1203–1210. [CrossRef] [PubMed]

116. Wang, C.; Wang, H.; Luo, J.; Hu, Y.; Wei, L.; Duan, M.; He, H. Selenium deficiency impairs host innate immune response and induces susceptibility to Listeria monocytogenes infection. *BMC Immunol.* **2009**, *10*, 55. [CrossRef] [PubMed]

117. De Freitas, M.R.B.; da Costa, C.M.B.; Pereira, L.M.; do Prado, J.C.J.; Sala, M.A.; Abrahao, A.A.C. The treatment with selenium increases placental parasitism in pregnant Wistar rats infected with the Y strain of Trypanosoma cruzi. *Immunobiology* **2018**. [CrossRef] [PubMed]

118. Nelson, S.M.; Shay, A.E.; James, J.L.; Carlson, B.A.; Urban, J.F., Jr.; Prabhu, K.S. Selenoprotein Expression in Macrophages Is Critical for Optimal Clearance of Parasitic Helminth Nippostrongylus brasiliensis. *J. Biol. Chem.* **2013**, *291*, 2787–2798. [CrossRef]

119. Smith, A.D.; Cheung, L.; Beshah, E.; Shea-Donohue, T.; Urban, J.F., Jr. Selenium status alters the immune response and expulsion of adult Heligmosomoides bakeri worms in mice. *Infect. Immun.* **2013**, *81*, 2546–2553. [CrossRef] [PubMed]

120. Wiehe, L.; Cremer, M.; Wisniewska, M.; Becker, N.P.; Rijntjes, E.; Martitz, J.; Hybsier, S.; Renko, K.; Buhrer, C.; Schomburg, L. Selenium status in neonates with connatal infection. *Br. J. Nutr.* **2016**, *116*, 504–513. [CrossRef] [PubMed]

121. Liu, Y.; Qiu, C.; Li, W.; Mu, W.; Li, C.; Guo, M. Selenium Plays a Protective Role in Staphylococcus aureus-Induced Endometritis in the Uterine Tissue of Rats. *Biol. Trace Elem. Res.* **2016**, *173*, 345–353. [CrossRef] [PubMed]

122. Varsi, K.; Bolann, B.; Torsvik, I.; Rosvold Eik, T.C.; Hol, P.J.; Bjorke-Monsen, A.L. Impact of Maternal Selenium Status on Infant Outcome during the First 6 Months of Life. *Nutrients* **2017**, *9*, 486. [CrossRef] [PubMed]

123. Yoshizawa, S.; Bock, A. The many levels of control on bacterial selenoprotein synthesis. *Biochim. Biophys. Acta* **2009**, *1790*, 1404–1414. [CrossRef] [PubMed]

124. Grobler, L.; Nagpal, S.; Sudarsanam, T.D.; Sinclair, D. Nutritional supplements for people being treated for active tuberculosis. *Cochrane Database Syst. Rev.* **2016**. [CrossRef] [PubMed]

125. Ramakrishnan, K.; Shenbagarathai, R.; Kavitha, K.; Thirumalaikolundusubramanian, P.; Rathinasabapati, R. Selenium levels in persons with HIV/tuberculosis in India, Madurai City. *Clin. Lab.* **2012**, *58*, 165–168. [PubMed]

126. Eick, F.; Maleta, K.; Govasmark, E.; Duttaroy, A.K.; Bjune, A.G. Food intake of selenium and sulphur amino acids in tuberculosis patients and healthy adults in Malawi. *Int. J. Tuberc. Lung Dis.* **2009**, *13*, 1313–1315. [PubMed]

127. Seyedrezazadeh, E.; Ostadrahimi, A.; Mahboob, S.; Assadi, Y.; Ghaemmagami, J.; Pourmogaddam, M. Effect of vitamin E and selenium supplementation on oxidative stress status in pulmonary tuberculosis patients. *Respirology* **2008**, *13*, 294–298. [CrossRef] [PubMed]

128. Sargazi, A.; Gharebagh, R.A.; Sargazi, A.; Aali, H.; Oskoee, H.O.; Sepehri, Z. Role of essential trace elements in tuberculosis infection: A review article. *Indian J. Tuberc.* **2017**, *64*, 246–251. [CrossRef] [PubMed]
129. Jaquess, P.A.; Smalley, D.L.; Duckworth, J.K. Enhanced growth of Mycobacterium tuberculosis in the presence of selenium. *Am. J. Clin. Pathol.* **1981**, *75*, 209–210. [CrossRef] [PubMed]
130. Steinbrenner, H.; Al-Quraishy, S.; Dkhil, M.A.; Wunderlich, F.; Sies, H. Dietary selenium in adjuvant therapy of viral and bacterial infections. *Adv. Nutr.* **2015**, *6*, 73–82. [CrossRef] [PubMed]
131. Puertollano, M.A.; Puertollano, E.; de Cienfuegos, G.A.; de Pablo, M.A. Dietary antioxidants: Immunity and host defense. *Curr. Top. Med. Chem.* **2011**, *11*, 1752–1766. [CrossRef] [PubMed]
132. Ko, W.S.; Guo, C.H.; Yeh, M.S.; Lin, L.Y.; Hsu, G.S.; Chen, P.C.; Luo, M.C.; Lin, C.Y. Blood micronutrient, oxidative stress, and viral load in patients with chronic hepatitis C. *World J. Gastroenterol.* **2005**, *11*, 4697–4702. [CrossRef] [PubMed]
133. Beck, M.A. Selenium and host defence towards viruses. *Proc. Nutr. Soc.* **1999**, *58*, 707–711. [CrossRef] [PubMed]
134. Jackson, M.J.; Dillon, S.A.; Broome, C.S.; McArdle, A.; Hart, C.A.; McArdle, F. Are there functional consequences of a reduction in selenium intake in UK subjects? *Proc. Nutr. Soc.* **2004**, *63*, 513–517. [CrossRef] [PubMed]
135. Girodon, F.; Galan, P.; Monget, A.L.; Boutron-Ruault, M.C.; Brunet-Lecomte, P.; Preziosi, P.; Arnaud, J.; Manuguerra, J.C.; Herchberg, S. Impact of trace elements and vitamin supplementation on immunity and infections in institutionalized elderly patients: A randomized controlled trial. MIN. VIT. AOX. geriatric network. *Arch. Intern. Med.* **1999**, *159*, 748–754. [CrossRef] [PubMed]
136. Cohen, M.S.; Hellmann, N.; Levy, J.A.; DeCock, K.; Lange, J. The spread, treatment, and prevention of HIV-1: Evolution of a global pandemic. *J. Clin. Investig.* **2008**, *118*, 1244–1254. [CrossRef] [PubMed]
137. Shivakoti, R.; Christian, P.; Yang, W.T.; Gupte, N.; Mwelase, N.; Kanyama, C.; Pillay, S.; Samaneka, W.; Santos, B.; Poongulali, S.; et al. Prevalence and risk factors of micronutrient deficiencies pre- and post-antiretroviral therapy (ART) among a diverse multicountry cohort of HIV-infected adults. *Clin. Nutr.* **2016**, *35*, 183–189. [CrossRef] [PubMed]
138. Anyabolu, H.C.; Adejuyigbe, E.A.; Adeodu, O.O. Serum Micronutrient Status of Haart-Naive, HIV Infected Children in South Western Nigeria: A Case Controlled Study. *AIDS Res. Treat.* **2014**, *2014*, 351043. [CrossRef] [PubMed]
139. Shivakoti, R.; Ewald, E.R.; Gupte, N.; Yang, W.T.; Kanyama, C.; Cardoso, S.W.; Santos, B.; Supparatpinyo, K.; Badal-Faesen, S.; Lama, J.R.; et al. Effect of baseline micronutrient and inflammation status on CD4 recovery post-cART initiation in the multinational PEARLS trial. *Clin. Nutr.* **2018**. [CrossRef] [PubMed]
140. Dworkin, B.M. Selenium deficiency in HIV infection and the acquired immunodeficiency syndrome (AIDS). *Chem. Biol. Interact.* **1994**, *91*, 181–186. [CrossRef]
141. Stone, C.A.; Kawai, K.; Kupka, R.; Fawzi, W.W. Role of selenium in HIV infection. *Nutr. Rev.* **2010**, *68*, 671–681. [CrossRef] [PubMed]
142. Combs, G.F., Jr.; Watts, J.C.; Jackson, M.I.; Johnson, L.K.; Zeng, H.; Scheett, A.J.; Uthus, E.O.; Schomburg, L.; Hoeg, A.; Hoefig, C.S.; et al. Determinants of selenium status in healthy adults. *Nutr. J.* **2011**, *10*, 75. [CrossRef] [PubMed]
143. Irlam, J.H.; Siegfried, N.; Visser, M.E.; Rollins, N.C. Micronutrient supplementation for children with HIV infection. *Cochrane Database Syst. Rev.* **2013**. [CrossRef] [PubMed]
144. Hileman, C.O.; Dirajlal-Fargo, S.; Lam, S.K.; Kumar, J.; Lacher, C.; Combs, G.F., Jr.; McComsey, G.A. Plasma Selenium Concentrations Are Sufficient and Associated with Protease Inhibitor Use in Treated HIV-Infected Adults. *J. Nutr.* **2015**, *145*, 2293–2299. [CrossRef] [PubMed]
145. Akinboro, A.O.; Onayemi, O.; Ayodele, O.E.; Mejiuni, A.D.; Atiba, A.S. The impacts of first line highly active antiretroviral therapy on serum selenium, CD4 count and body mass index: A cross sectional and short prospective study. *Pan. Afr. Med. J.* **2013**, *15*, 97. [CrossRef] [PubMed]
146. Flax, V.L.; Adair, L.S.; Allen, L.H.; Shahab-Ferdows, S.; Hampel, D.; Chasela, C.S.; Tegha, G.; Daza, E.J.; Corbett, A.; Davis, N.L.; et al. Plasma Micronutrient Concentrations Are Altered by Antiretroviral Therapy and Lipid-Based Nutrient Supplements in Lactating HIV-Infected Malawian Women. *J. Nutr.* **2015**, *145*, 1950–1957. [PubMed]
147. Baum, M.K.; Shor-Posner, G. Micronutrient status in relationship to mortality in HIV-1 disease. *Nutr. Rev.* **1998**, *56*, S135–S139. [CrossRef] [PubMed]

148. Kamwesiga, J.; Mutabazi, V.; Kayumba, J.; Tayari, J.C.; Uwimbabazi, J.C.; Batanage, G.; Uwera, G.; Baziruwiha, M.; Ntizimira, C.; Murebwayire, A.; et al. Effect of selenium supplementation on CD4+ T-cell recovery, viral suppression and morbidity of HIV-infected patients in Rwanda: A randomized controlled trial. *AIDS* **2015**, *29*, 1045–1052. [CrossRef] [PubMed]
149. Sappey, C.; Legrand-Poels, S.; Best-Belpomme, M.; Favier, A.; Rentier, B.; Piette, J. Stimulation of glutathione peroxidase activity decreases HIV type 1 activation after oxidative stress. *AIDS Res. Hum. Retroviruses* **1994**, *10*, 1451–1461. [CrossRef] [PubMed]
150. Gupta, S.; Narang, R.; Krishnaswami, K.; Yadav, S. Plasma selenium level in cancer patients. *Indian J. Cancer* **1994**, *31*, 192–197. [PubMed]
151. Duffield-Lillico, A.J.; Reid, M.E.; Turnbull, B.W.; Combs, G.F., Jr.; Slate, E.H.; Fischbach, L.A.; Marshall, J.R.; Clark, L.C. Baseline characteristics and the effect of selenium supplementation on cancer incidence in a randomized clinical trial: A summary report of the Nutritional Prevention of Cancer Trial. *Cancer Epidemiol. Biomarkers Prev.* **2002**, *11*, 630–639. [PubMed]
152. Li, H.; Stampfer, M.J.; Giovannucci, E.L.; Morris, J.S.; Willett, W.C.; Gaziano, J.M.; Ma, J. A prospective study of plasma selenium levels and prostate cancer risk. *J. Natl. Cancer Inst.* **2004**, *96*, 696–703. [CrossRef] [PubMed]
153. Overvad, K.; Wang, D.Y.; Olsen, J.; Allen, D.S.; Thorling, E.B.; Bulbrook, R.D.; Hayward, J.L. Selenium in human mammary carcinogenesis: A case-cohort study. *Eur. J. Cancer* **1991**, *27*, 900–902. [CrossRef]
154. Mannisto, S.; Alfthan, G.; Virtanen, M.; Kataja, V.; Uusitupa, M.; Pietinen, P. Toenail selenium and breast cancer-a case-control study in Finland. *Eur. J. Clin. Nutr.* **2000**, *54*, 98–103. [CrossRef] [PubMed]
155. Hardell, L.; Danell, M.; Angqvist, C.A.; Marklund, S.L.; Fredriksson, M.; Zakari, A.L.; Kjellgren, A. Levels of selenium in plasma and glutathione peroxidase in erythrocytes and the risk of breast cancer. A case-control study. *Biol. Trace Elem. Res.* **1993**, *36*, 99–108. [CrossRef] [PubMed]
156. Hunter, D.J.; Morris, J.S.; Stampfer, M.J.; Colditz, G.A.; Speizer, F.E.; Willett, W.C. A prospective study of selenium status and breast cancer risk. *JAMA* **1990**, *264*, 1128–1131. [CrossRef] [PubMed]
157. Kok, D.E.; Kiemeney, L.A.; Verhaegh, G.W.; Schalken, J.A.; van Lin, E.N.; Sedelaar, J.P.; Witjes, J.A.; Hulsbergen-van de Kaa, C.A.; van 't Veer, P.; Kampman, E.; et al. A short-term intervention with selenium affects expression of genes implicated in the epithelial-to-mesenchymal transition in the prostate. *Oncotarget* **2017**, *8*, 10565–10579. [CrossRef] [PubMed]
158. Radhakrishnan, N.; Dinand, V.; Rao, S.; Gupta, P.; Toteja, G.S.; Kalra, M.; Yadav, S.P.; Sachdeva, A. Antioxidant levels at diagnosis in childhood acute lymphoblastic leukemia. *Indian J. Pediatr.* **2013**, *80*, 292–296. [CrossRef] [PubMed]
159. Masri, D.S. Microquantity for macroquality: Case study on the effect of selenium on chronic neutropenia. *J. Pediatr. Hematol. Oncol.* **2011**, *33*, e361–e362. [CrossRef] [PubMed]
160. Rocha, K.C.; Vieira, M.L.; Beltrame, R.L.; Cartum, J.; Alves, S.I.; Azzalis, L.A.; Junqueira, V.B.; Pereira, E.C.; Fonseca, F.L. Impact of Selenium Supplementation in Neutropenia and Immunoglobulin Production in Childhood Cancer Patients. *J. Med. Food* **2016**, *19*, 560–568. [CrossRef] [PubMed]
161. Rohr-Udilova, N.; Bauer, E.; Timeltthaler, G.; Eferl, R.; Stolze, K.; Pinter, M.; Seif, M.; Hayden, H.; Reiberger, T.; Schulte-Hermann, R.; et al. Impact of glutathione peroxidase 4 on cell proliferation, angiogenesis and cytokine production in hepatocellular carcinoma. *Oncotarget* **2018**, *9*, 10054–10068. [CrossRef] [PubMed]
162. Rohr-Udilova, N.; Sieghart, W.; Eferl, R.; Stoiber, D.; Bjorkhem-Bergman, L.; Eriksson, L.C.; Stolze, K.; Hayden, H.; Keppler, B.; Sagmeister, S.; et al. Antagonistic effects of selenium and lipid peroxides on growth control in early hepatocellular carcinoma. *Hepatology* **2012**, *55*, 1112–1121. [CrossRef] [PubMed]
163. Ren, Y.; Poon, R.T.; Tsui, H.T.; Chen, W.H.; Li, Z.; Lau, C.; Yu, W.C.; Fan, S.T. Interleukin-8 serum levels in patients with hepatocellular carcinoma: Correlations with clinicopathological features and prognosis. *Clin. Cancer Res.* **2003**, *9*, 5996–6001. [PubMed]
164. Gautam, P.K.; Kumar, S.; Tomar, M.S.; Singh, R.K.; Acharya, A.; Kumar, S.; Ram, B. Selenium nanoparticles induce suppressed function of tumor associated macrophages and inhibit Dalton's lymphoma proliferation. *Biochem. Biophys. Rep.* **2017**, *12*, 172–184. [CrossRef] [PubMed]
165. Diwakar, B.T.; Korwar, A.M.; Paulson, R.F.; Prabhu, K.S. The Regulation of Pathways of Inflammation and Resolution in Immune Cells and Cancer Stem Cells by Selenium. *Adv. Cancer Res.* **2017**, *136*, 153–172. [PubMed]

166. Zhang, J.; Basher, F.; Wu, J.D. NKG2D Ligands in Tumor Immunity: Two Sides of a Coin. *Front. Immunol* **2015**, *6*, 97. [CrossRef] [PubMed]
167. Hagemann-Jensen, M.; Uhlenbrock, F.; Kehlet, S.; Andresen, L.; Gabel-Jensen, C.; Ellgaard, L.; Gammelgaard, B.; Skov, S. The selenium metabolite methylselenol regulates the expression of ligands that trigger immune activation through the lymphocyte receptor NKG2D. *J. Biol. Chem.* **2014**, *289*, 31576–31590. [CrossRef] [PubMed]
168. Lennicke, C.; Rahn, J.; Bukur, J.; Hochgrafe, F.; Wessjohann, L.A.; Lichtenfels, R.; Seliger, B. Modulation of MHC class I surface expression in B16F10 melanoma cells by methylseleninic acid. *Oncoimmunology* **2017**, *6*, e1259049. [CrossRef] [PubMed]
169. Rose, A.H.; Bertino, P.; Hoffmann, F.W.; Gaudino, G.; Carbone, M.; Hoffmann, P.R. Increasing dietary selenium elevates reducing capacity and ERK activation associated with accelerated progression of select mesothelioma tumors. *Am. J. Pathol.* **2014**, *184*, 1041–1049. [CrossRef] [PubMed]
170. Faghfuri, E.; Yazdi, M.H.; Mahdavi, M.; Sepehrizadeh, Z.; Faramarzi, M.A.; Mavandadnejad, F.; Shahverdi, A.R. Dose-response relationship study of selenium nanoparticles as an immunostimulatory agent in cancer-bearing mice. *Arch. Med. Res.* **2015**, *46*, 31–37. [CrossRef] [PubMed]
171. Wang, H.; Chan, Y.L.; Li, T.L.; Bauer, B.A.; Hsia, S.; Wang, C.H.; Huang, J.S.; Wang, H.M.; Yeh, K.Y.; Huang, T.H.; et al. Reduction of splenic immunosuppressive cells and enhancement of anti-tumor immunity by synergy of fish oil and selenium yeast. *PLoS ONE* **2013**, *8*, e52912. [CrossRef] [PubMed]
172. Yazdi, M.H.; Mahdavi, M.; Varastehmoradi, B.; Faramarzi, M.A.; Shahverdi, A.R. The immunostimulatory effect of biogenic selenium nanoparticles on the 4T1 breast cancer model: An in vivo study. *Biol. Trace Elem. Res.* **2012**, *149*, 22–28. [CrossRef] [PubMed]
173. Kim, H.Y. The methionine sulfoxide reduction system: Selenium utilization and methionine sulfoxide reductase enzymes and their functions. *Antioxid. Redox Signal.* **2013**, *19*, 958–969. [CrossRef] [PubMed]
174. Lee, B.C.; Peterfi, Z.; Hoffmann, F.W.; Moore, R.E.; Kaya, A.; Avanesov, A.; Tarrago, L.; Zhou, Y.; Weerapana, E.; Fomenko, D.E.; et al. MsrB1 and MICALs regulate actin assembly and macrophage function via reversible stereoselective methionine oxidation. *Mol. Cell.* **2013**, *51*, 397–404. [CrossRef] [PubMed]
175. Saha, S.S.; Hashino, M.; Suzuki, J.; Uda, A.; Watanabe, K.; Shimizu, T.; Watarai, M. Contribution of methionine sulfoxide reductase B (MsrB) to Francisella tularensis infection in mice. *FEMS Microbiol. Lett.* **2017**, *364*. [CrossRef] [PubMed]
176. Fredericks, G.J.; Hoffmann, F.W.; Rose, A.H.; Osterheld, H.J.; Hess, F.M.; Mercier, F.; Hoffmann, P.R. Stable expression and function of the inositol 1,4,5-triphosphate receptor requires palmitoylation by a DHHC6/selenoprotein K complex. *Proc. Natl. Acad. Sci. USA* **2014**, *111*, 16478–16483. [CrossRef] [PubMed]
177. Fredericks, G.J.; Hoffmann, F.W.; Hondal, R.J.; Rozovsky, S.; Urschitz, J.; Hoffmann, P.R. Selenoprotein K Increases Efficiency of DHHC6 Catalyzed Protein Palmitoylation by Stabilizing the Acyl-DHHC6 Intermediate. *Antioxidants (Basel)* **2017**, *7*, 4. [CrossRef] [PubMed]
178. Meiler, S.; Baumer, Y.; Huang, Z.; Hoffmann, F.W.; Fredericks, G.J.; Rose, A.H.; Norton, R.L.; Hoffmann, P.R.; Boisvert, W.A. Selenoprotein K is required for palmitoylation of CD36 in macrophages: Implications in foam cell formation and atherogenesis. *J. Leukoc. Biol.* **2013**, *93*, 771–780. [CrossRef] [PubMed]
179. Norton, R.L.; Fredericks, G.J.; Huang, Z.; Fay, J.D.; Hoffmann, F.W.; Hoffmann, P.R. Selenoprotein K regulation of palmitoylation and calpain cleavage of ASAP2 is required for efficient FcgammaR-mediated phagocytosis. *J. Leukoc. Biol.* **2017**, *101*, 439–448. [CrossRef] [PubMed]

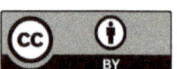

© 2018 by the authors. Licensee MDPI, Basel, Switzerland. This article is an open access article distributed under the terms and conditions of the Creative Commons Attribution (CC BY) license (http://creativecommons.org/licenses/by/4.0/).

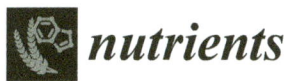

Review

Human Milk Oligosaccharides and Immune System Development

Julio Plaza-Díaz [1,2,3], Luis Fontana [1,2,3] and Angel Gil [1,2,3,4,*]

1. Department of Biochemistry and Molecular Biology II, School of Pharmacy, University of Granada, 18071 Granada, Spain; jrplaza@ugr.es (J.P.-D.); fontana@ugr.es (L.F.)
2. Institute of Nutrition and Food Technology "José Mataix", Biomedical Research Center, Parque Tecnológico Ciencias de la Salud, University of Granada, Armilla, 18100 Granada, Spain
3. Instituto de Investigación Biosanitaria ibs., 18014 Granada, Spain
4. CIBEROBN, Instituto de Salud Carlos III, 28029 Madrid, Spain
* Correspondence: agil@ugr.es; Tel.: +34-9-5824-6139 or +34-9-5824-1000 (ext. 20307)

Received: 19 July 2018; Accepted: 6 August 2018; Published: 8 August 2018

Abstract: Maternal milk contains compounds that may affect newborn immunity. Among these are a group of oligosaccharides that are synthesized in the mammary gland from lactose; these oligosaccharides have been termed human milk oligosaccharides (HMOs). The amount of HMOs present in human milk is greater than the amount of protein. In fact, HMOs are the third-most abundant solid component in maternal milk after lactose and lipids, and are thus considered to be key components. The importance of HMOs may be explained by their inhibitory effects on the adhesion of microorganisms to the intestinal mucosa, the growth of pathogens through the production of bacteriocins and organic acids, and the expression of genes that are involved in inflammation. This review begins with short descriptions of the basic structures of HMOs and the gut immune system, continues with the beneficial effects of HMOs shown in cell and animal studies, and it ends with the observational and randomized controlled trials carried out in humans to date, with particular emphasis on their effect on immune system development. HMOs seem to protect breastfed infants against microbial infections. The protective effect has been found to be exerted through cell signaling and cell-to-cell recognition events, enrichment of the protective gut microbiota, the modulation of microbial adhesion, and the invasion of the infant intestinal mucosa. In addition, infants fed formula supplemented with selected HMOs exhibit a pattern of inflammatory cytokines closer to that of exclusively breastfed infants. Unfortunately, the positive effects found in preclinical studies have not been substantiated in the few randomized, double-blinded, multicenter, controlled trials that are available, perhaps partly because these studies focus on aspects other than the immune response (e.g., growth, tolerance, and stool microbiota).

Keywords: human milk oligosaccharides; intestinal immune system; microbiota

1. Introduction

Breastfeeding has many beneficial effects in newborns. The relative risks of diarrhea incidence, diarrhea mortality, pneumonia incidence, and pneumonia mortality are kept to a minimum in exclusively breastfed infants. These protective effects, although less robust, are also observed in partially breastfed infants when compared with milk formula-fed infants [1]. However, in addition to protecting against infection, human milk has both short-term and long-term effects, such as prevention and protection against allergic reactions; optimal behavioral, cognitive, and gastrointestinal development; and, may protect against chronic diseases, such as diabetes, obesity, hypertension, and autoimmune and cardiovascular diseases [2]. The long-term effects of human milk are related to so-called early programming [3].

Human milk contains many bioactive compounds that may affect immunity (e.g., cytokines, growth factors, hormones, digestive enzymes, transporters, and antimicrobial factors). The latter category of antimicrobial factors includes glycans, among which exists a group of oligosaccharides with different structures that are synthesized from lactose in the mammary gland. These oligosaccharides have been termed human milk oligosaccharides (HMOs). In addition, human milk contains probiotics, which reside in the microbiota of the breast tissue and may also have a role in neonate immunity [4,5].

Although HMOs were originally described and referred to as "gynolactose" by Lespagnol and Polonowski in 1930 [4], they have attracted considerable attention in recent years because of their biological roles. The HMO fraction (5–15 g/L) that is present in human milk is greater than the protein fraction (8 g/L). In fact, HMOs are the third-most abundant solid component in maternal milk after lactose (70 g/L) and lipids (40 g/L), and accordingly, they are considered to be key compounds [4,5].

HMOs have been described to inhibit (i) the adhesion of microorganisms to the intestinal mucosa; (ii) the growth of pathogens through the production of bacteriocins and organic acids; and (iii) the expression of genes involved in inflammation [4–6]. Although many studies regarding the composition of oligosaccharides in human milk have been published, there are few publications about the roles of these compounds in general and in immunity in particular [5,7]. The aim of this review article was to fill this gap by surveying the in vitro and in vivo effects of HMOs, focusing mainly on immunity.

2. Oligosaccharides in Human Milk

More than two hundred different HMOs have been identified to date. HMOs are composed of monosaccharides and monosaccharide derivatives [4]: glucose (Glc), galactose (Gal), N-acetylglucosamine (GlcNAc), fucose (Fuc), and sialic acid (Sia). All of the HMOs contain lactose at their reducing end, which can be elongated by the addition of β1-3- or β1-6-linked lacto-N-biose (Galβ1-3GlcNAc-, type 1 chain) or N-acetyllactosamine (Galβ1-4GlcNAc-, type 2 chain). Elongation with lacto-N-biose appears to terminate the chain, whereas N-acetyllactosamine can be further extended by the addition of either of the two disaccharides. A β1-6 linkage between two disaccharide units introduces chain branching. Branched structures are termed iso-HMOs; linear structures without branches are termed para-HMOs. Lactose or the elongated oligosaccharide chain can be fucosylated with α1-2, α1-3, or α1-4 linkages, and/or sialylated with α2-3 or α2-6 linkages. Some HMOs occur in several isomeric forms, e.g., lacto-N-fucopentaose or sialyllacto-N-tetraose [4]. HMOs with more than 15 disaccharide units have been described; such HMOs form complex structural backbones that can be further modified by the addition of Fuc or/and Sia [8,9]. HMOs are classified into three categories (Figure 1) [8,9]:

(a) Neutral (fucosylated) HMOs are neutral and contain fucose at the terminal position (e.g., 2'-fucosyllactose (2'-FL) and lactodifucopentaose). They represent 35% to 50% of the total HMO content.

(b) Neutral N-containing (nonfucosylated) HMOs are neutral, contain N-acetylglucosamine at the terminal position (e.g., lacto-N-tetraose), and represent 42% to 55% of the total HMO content.

Neutral HMOs account for more than 75% of the total HMOs in human breast milk.

(c) Acid (sialylated) HMOs are acidic and contain sialic acid at the terminal position (e.g., 2'-sialyllactose). They represent 12% to 14% of the total HMO content.

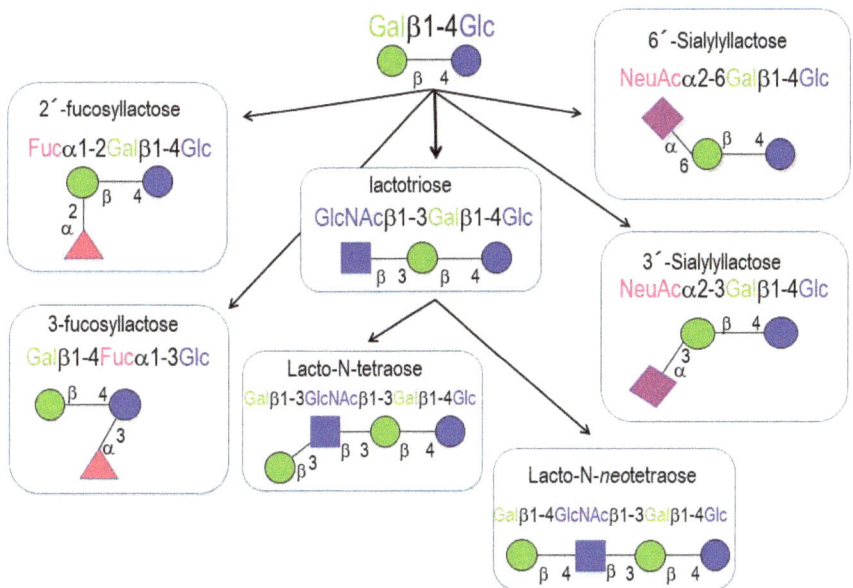

Figure 1. Human milk oligosaccharides (HMO) basic structures.

The amount and composition of HMOs vary among women. The HMO composition is determined genetically and mirrors blood group characteristics, which depend on the expression of certain glycosyltransferases. Four milk groups can be assigned based on the Secretor (Se) and Lewis (Le) blood group system, which is determined by the activity of two gene loci encoding α1-2-fucosyltransferase (FUT2, encoded by the *Se* gene) and α1-3/4-fucosyltransferase (FUT3, encoded by the *Le* gene) [6–17]. Individuals with an active *Se* locus are classified as "secretors". The milk of secretor women is abundant in 2′-FL, lacto-*N*-fucopentaose I (LNFP I), and other α1-2-fucosylated HMOs. In contrast, non-secretor women lack a functional FUT2 enzyme, and their milk does not contain α1-2-fucosylated HMOs. Individuals with an active *Le* locus are classified as *Le*-positive. They express FUT3, which transfers Fuc with a α1-4 linkage to subterminal GlcNAc on type 1 chains. In contrast, the milk of *Le*-negative women lacks these specific α1-4-fucosylated HMOs, e.g., LNFP II [9,10,14]. Therefore, breast milk can be assigned to one of the four groups based on the expression of FUT2 and FUT3: *Le*-positive secretors (*Le+Se+*), *Le*-negative secretors (*Le-Se+*), *Le*-positive nonsecretors (*Le+Se-*), and *Le*-negative nonsecretors (*Le-Se+*) (Table 1) [9,10,14]:

Table 1. Human milk oligosaccharide (HMO) groups.

Genes	Lewis+	Lewis-
Secretor+	Se+Le+ Able to secrete all HMOs	Se+Le- Able to secrete 2′FL, 3FL, LNFP-I, LNFP-III
Secretor-	Se-Le+ Able to secrete 3FL, LNFP-II, LNFP-III	Se-Le- Able to secrete 3FL, LNFP-III, LNFP-V

Abbreviations: FL, fucosyllactose; LNFP, lacto-*N*-fucopentaose. Taken from [18].

This classification, however, is an oversimplification. FUT2 and FUT3 compete for some of the same substrates [19–21], and the levels of enzyme expression and activity translate into different profiles throughout the population. Even the milk of *Le*-negative nonsecretor women who express neither FUT2 nor FUT3 contains fucosylated HMOs, such as 3FL or LNFP III, suggesting that other *Se*-

and *Le*-independent FUTs may be involved [14,22]. In addition, α1-2-fucosylated HMOs have been found in the milk of nonsecretor women near the end of lactation, and Newburg et al. suggested that FUT1 might also participate in HMO fucosylation [22]. In addition, fucosylation in preterm milk is not as well regulated as in term milk, resulting in higher within and between mother variation in women delivering preterm vs term. In fact, of particular clinical interest, the α1,2-linked fucosylated oligosaccharide 2′-fucosyllactose, which is an indicator of secretor status, is not consistently present across the lactation of several mothers that delivered preterm [23].

The amount and composition of HMOs also vary over the course of lactation. Whereas, colostrum contains as much as 20–25 g/L of HMOs, as milk production matures, HMO concentrations decline to 5–20 g/L, which still exceeds the concentration of total milk protein [4]. The milk of mothers delivering preterm infants has higher HMO concentrations than term milk [14], whereas preterm milk contains lower levels of fucosylated HMOs than term milk [24], and no differences in neutral and acidic HMOs are found between preterm and term milk [25].

3. The Intestinal Immune System

The intestinal immune system, also known as gut-associated lymphoid tissue (GALT), is a secondary lymphoid organ that is responsible for the processing of the antigens that interact with the intestinal mucosa and of the dissemination of the immune response [26]. There are two main locations of lymphocytes in the intestine: the inductive sites, that is, where the immune response begins after stimulation by an antigen, of which the Peyer patches are the most typical, and the effector sites, that is, the ones that are responsible for executing and completing the response. There are also two main lymphocyte populations in the gut: the lymphocytes of the lamina propria (LPL), located in the internal part of the villus, and the intraepithelial lymphocytes (IELs), located among the enterocytes along the villus. It is worth mentioning that, in addition to the Peyer patch lymphocytes (PPLs), the peritoneal lymphocytes, particularly the B1 cells, are important precursors of one population of plasmatic cells found in the lamina propria. Therefore, two main inductive populations may be found at the intestinal level: the B2 cells, which reside in the Peyer patches, and the B1 cells, which reside in the peritoneum (Figure 2) [27].

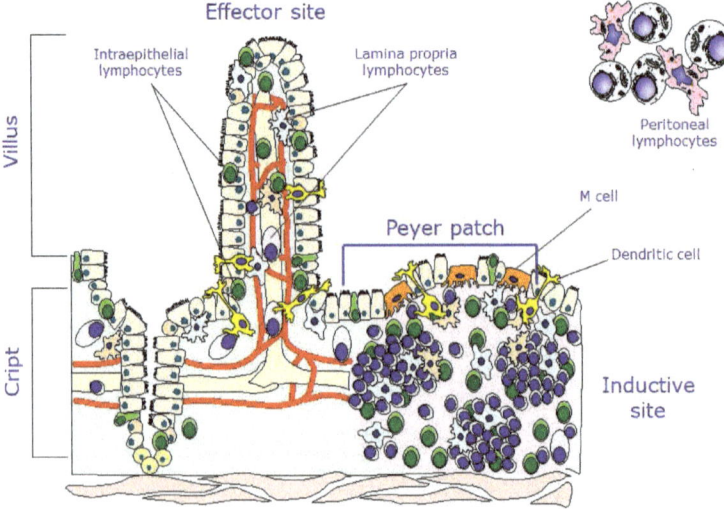

Figure 2. Main lymphocyte populations of the gut-associated lymphoid tissue (GALT). Modified with permission from [26].

The antigens that are present in the intestinal lumen are processed and transported into the Peyer patches via the M cells, which are located among the enterocytes in the epithelium. Once in the Peyer patches, the antigens interact with antigen-presenting cells (APCs), which are responsible for presenting those antigens to immature B and T lymphocytes that are residing in both the germinal centers and interfollicular regions. After their activation by antigens, the immature B and T cells drain down the lymph nodes and migrate through the thoracic duct to the bloodstream. They may circulate for a few days and later differentiate into mature effector cells that migrate to the lamina propria or memory cells, which again travel to the Peyer patches [26,27]. The so-called dendritic cells that are present in the Peyer patches and the lamina propria have been shown to form pseudopods and interact directly with antigens that are present in the intestinal lumen, after which they process the antigens and present them to other underlying cell lineages without the involvement of the M cells [28,29]. Another population of effector cells consisting of IELs may interact with antigens entering the gastrointestinal tract without following the course mentioned above. In recent years, a new type of cells, innate lymphoid cells (ILCs), have been described along with their functions [30]. ILCs are present in the intestine and other mucosae and participate in tissue homeostasis, inflammation, and autoimmunity, although their main function is the development of the gut barrier.

The potential beneficial effects of HMOs might be related to their capacity to interact with a number of receptors that are located in intestinal immune cells [31].

4. Beneficial Effects of HMOs

Humans lack the enzymes (sialidases, fucosidases) that break down HMOs; therefore, these compounds reach the colon intact, where they are digested by bacteria within the intestinal microbiota. In this sense, HMOs are prebiotics and they promote the growth of a favorable microbiota. Moreover, HMOs have been reported to confer additional benefits on the host, among which the three main effects are described below.

4.1. Inhibition of Microorganism Adhesion to the Intestinal Mucosa

The formation of the gut microbiota ecosystem is a complex but continuous process that is affected by endogenous and exogenous determinants of variability. An immediate effect at the time of birth continues for several years during childhood through subsequent stages. *Streptococcus* and *Staphylococcus* species are the most commonly identified bacterial genera in human milk, followed by *Bifidobacterium*, *Lactobacillus*, *Propionibacteria*, *Enterococcus*, and members of the *Enterobacteriaceae* family [32,33].

During early life, several external factors, such as delivery mode, feeding modality, environmental influences, antibiotic exposure, and functional food intake can affect microbiota shaping and composition [34]. The ability of the immune system to coevolve with the microbiota during perinatal life allows for the host and the microbiota to coexist in a mutually beneficial relationship [34]. Metabolic diseases are linked with disruption of both the innate and adaptive immune systems. There is evidence that some cytokines (e.g., TNF-α and IL-1) contribute to insulin resistance, thereby promoting diabetes [35] and leading to metabolic inflammation [36]. Likewise, Gram (−) lipopolysaccharide (LPS) components [37] circulate in the blood transported by LPS-binding proteins and lipoproteins, contributing to inflammation [34].

HMOs might protect breastfed infants against microbial infections due to their structural similarities to cell surface glycoconjugates utilized by microbes [38–40]. Experimental results have shown that oligosaccharides can provide protective effects through cell signaling and cell-to-cell recognition events, the enrichment of protective gut microbiota, and the modulation of microbial adhesion and invasion of the infant intestinal mucosa [41–45]. Most enteric pathogens use cell surface glycans to identify and bind to their target cells, which is the critical first step in pathogenesis.

Fucosylated HMOs have been reported to inhibit (i) the binding of several pathogens, such as *Campylobacter jejuni* [46], Norwald-like virus [47], and *Helicobacter pylori* [48], and (ii) the heat-stable enterotoxin of *Escherichia coli* [49] to intestinal cells.

The addition of HMOs was tested in T84 cell membranes to establish the inhibition of enterotoxin-producing *Escherichia coli*. The administration of HMOs repressed *E. coli* guanylate cyclase activity and cyclic GMP production in these cells [50]. Uropathogenic *E. coli* strains expressing P (Pap) and P-like (Prs) fimbriae are responsible for infections of the urinary tract. The hemagglutination that is mediated by these strains was inhibited by HMOs, especially by the sialylated fraction [51]. Fractions of HMOs were evaluated for their ability to inhibit the adhesion of *E. coli* serotype O119, *Vibrio cholerae*, and *Salmonella fyris* in differentiated Caco-2 cells. The evaluated HMOs inhibited the adhesion of these pathogens to epithelial cells [52]. Oligosaccharides from milk might block the action of PA-IIL, a fucose-binding lectin of the human pathogen *Pseudomonas aeruginosa*, through competition for the receptor and further binding [53]. In particular, a significant reduction in uropathogenic *E. coli* internalization into HMO-pretreated epithelial cells was detected without observing any binding to these cells [54]. HMOs from pooled human milk significantly reduced enteropathogenic *E. coli* strain 2348/69 (serotype O127:H6) attachment to cultured epithelial cells [55]. Likewise, treatment with HMOs reduced the invasion of human premature intestinal epithelial cells by *C. albicans* in a dose-dependent manner [56].

Colonization and invasion require the attachment of trophozoites to the host's mucosa. HMOs reduce *E. histolytica* attachment and cytotoxicity; in fact, pooled HMOs detach *E. histolytica* by more than 80%; moreover, HMOs rescue *E. histolytica*-induced destruction of human intestinal epithelial HT-29 cells in a dose-dependent manner [57].

4.2. Short-Chain Fatty Acid Production by Bifidobacteria

Short-chain fatty acids (SCFAs) are an important source of energy for enterocytes and are key signaling molecules for the maintenance of gut health. HMOs can indirectly increase the production of SCFA, and these augmented levels are mediated by bifidobacteria species. SCFAs can interact with the SCFA receptors GPR41 and GPR43, increasing the intestinal secretion of polypeptide YY (PYY) and glucagon-like peptide 1 (GLP-1), respectively [58,59]. Propionate can increase free-fatty-acid uptake, possibly by affecting the lipoprotein lipase (LPL) inhibitor angiopoietin-like 4 (ANGPTL4). Acetate and propionate might also attenuate intracellular lipolysis by decreasing the phosphorylation of the hormone-sensitive lipase (HSL) through its interaction with the SCFA receptor GPR43. Propionate and butyrate could reduce the secretion of proinflammatory cytokines and chemokines, likely by reducing local macrophage infiltration [58].

Breastfed infants are typically colonized by strains of bacteria that are thought to protect, feed, and communicate with the developing intestine [60]. In 1954, Gyorgy et al. [61] conducted several studies that indicated a unique activity of HMOs as a growth factor for a *Bifidobacterium* that was isolated from the feces of an infant. Ward et al. [62,63] first demonstrated the selective growth of bifidobacteria species on intact HMOs in vitro. A number of studies have characterized the bifidobacterial moieties that specifically bind and catabolize HMOs [64–67].

B. infantis possesses a gene cluster that encodes transport systems and intracellular glycosyl hydrolases [41,68,69]. However, *B. bifidum* employs a different mode of catalytic activity toward HMO consumption: it exports sialidases, fucosidases, and a lacto-N-biosidase to release lacto-N-biose from HMO structures, and lacto-N-biose is then transported and metabolized [70]. Recently, a study revealed a multicomponent transcriptional regulation system that controls the HMO metabolism pathways in *B. breve* UCC2003 [71].

4.3. Inhibition of Inflammatory Genes

Although HMO-mediated changes in the infant microbiota composition or intestinal epithelial cell response may indirectly affect the infant immune system, many in vitro studies suggest that

HMOs also directly modulate immune responses. HMOs may act either locally, on cells of the mucosa-associated lymphoid tissues, or at a systemic level, as 1% of HMOs are absorbed and reach the systemic circulation [4,72–74].

The transcriptional response of colonic epithelial cells that are treated with HMOs was investigated in HT-29 cells. The expression of several cytokines (such as IL-1β, IL-8, colony-stimulating factor 2, IL-17C and platelet factor 4 (PF4)), chemokines (such as CXCL1, CXCL3, CXCL2, CXCL6, CCL5, CCL20, and CX3CL1), and cell surface receptors (interferon γ receptor 1, IFNGR1), intercellular adhesion molecule-1 (ICAM-1), intercellular adhesion molecule-2 (ICAM-2), and IL-10 receptor a (IL10RA) in HT-29 cells was influenced by the administration of HMOs [75]. The aforementioned cytokines, chemokines, and cell surface receptors are implicated in the development and maturation of the intestinal immune response [75].

Using a cellular model with intestinal epithelial cells (T84/HCT8/FHs74) and HeLa cells, He et al. [76] investigated the effects of HMOs from colostrum in fetal human intestinal mucosa cells. These authors identified networks controlling immune cell communication, intestinal mucosal immune system differentiation, and homeostasis. HMOs treatment decreased cytokine protein levels, such as IL-8, IL-6, monocyte chemoattractant protein-1/2 and IL-1β, while increasing the levels of cytokines that are involved in tissue repair and homeostasis [76].

Gram-negative pathogenic bacteria might activate mucosal inflammation through the binding of LPS to intestinal toll-like receptor 4 (TLR4) in epithelial intestinal cells (IECs). Under in vitro conditions, IECs were treated with a strain of enterotoxigenic *E. coli* to evaluate the inhibitory effect of HMO treatment on the secretion of IL-8. Both treatments (a mixture of HMOs and 2′-FL alone) successfully decreased the LPS-dependent stimulation of IL-8 through the attenuation of CD14 induction. CD14 expression mediates the LPS-TLR4 stimulation of portions of the "macrophage migration inhibitory factors" inflammatory pathway via suppressors of cytokine signaling 2/signal transducer and the activator of transcription (STAT) 3/NF-κB [76]. The effects of different oligosaccharide fractions on leukocyte rolling and adhesion were determined. Two active compounds (3′-sialyl-lactose and 3′-sialyl-3-fucosyl-lactose) exhibit an inhibitory effect on leukocyte rolling and adhesion, decreasing the incidence of inflammatory diseases due to their anti-inflammatory activities [77].

The administration of HMOs also demonstrated growth inhibition of *Streptococcus agalactiae* (group B *Streptococcus*). This bacteriostatic activity was mediated through the action of a putative glycosyltransferase that confers resistance to oligosaccharides [78]. The human epithelial cell lines HEp-2 and HT-29 were infected with *C. jejuni* 81-176 and were treated with 2′FL to evaluate the degree of infection and inflammatory response. Treatment with 2′-FL attenuated the majority of *C. jejuni* invasion and decreased the release of IL-8 and IL-1b by 80–90% as well as decreasing the level of the neutrophil chemoattractant macrophage inflammatory protein 2 (MIP-2) [79].

Bacterial strains are not the only pathogens that are inhibited by the action of HMOs. In addition, some evidence suggests that HMOs act against viruses [6]. In particular, 2′-FL and 3-FL can structurally mimic histo-blood group antigens and block the binding of norovirus, which can cause acute gastroenteritis in humans [80]. The effects of 2′FL, 6′-sialyllactose, 3′-sialyllactose and lacto-N-*neo*tetraose on peripheral blood mononuclear cells (PBMCs) following respiratory viral infection were investigated in vitro. The administration of 2′-FL significantly decreased the respiratory syncytial viral load and cytokines that are associated with disease severity (IL-6, IL-8, MIP-1α) and inflammation (TNF-α, MCP-1) in airway epithelial cells. Lacto-N-*neo*tetraose and 6′-sialyllactose treatments decreased the influenza viral load in airway epithelial cells, and only 6′-sialyllactose decreased CXCL10 and TNF-α in respiratory syncytial virus-infected PBMCs [81]. Particularly, HMOs containing more than one unit of fucose may exhibit stronger binding capacities when compared with single fucose HMOs [82].

5. Immunomodulation Mediated by HMOs: Animal Studies

The immunomodulatory effects of HMOs have also been demonstrated in animal studies. The impact of HMOs on mucosal immunity and the response to rotavirus infection has been studied in piglets by Li et al. [83]. The administration of HMOs to these animals decreased the duration of diarrhea and enhanced the expression of IFN-γ and IL-10. HMO treatment failed to prevent the onset of rotavirus infection [83].

Colostrum-deprived newborn pigs were fed HMO formula (2'-FL, lacto-N-neotetraose, 6'-sialyllactose, 3'-sialyllactose, and free sialic acid) or formula containing short-chain galactooligosaccharides and long-chain fructooligosaccharides, and were then inoculated with porcine rotavirus strain OSU at day 10. Pigs that received the HMO treatment had nearly twice as many natural killer cells and five times as many basophils as formula-fed pigs. The authors hypothesized that altered immune cell populations may mediate the effects of dietary HMOs on rotavirus infection susceptibility through the direct stimulation of immune cells, alteration of intestinal bacterial populations, modulation of intestinal barrier function, and the alteration of viral pathogenicity [84].

2'-FL is one of the most prominent short-chain oligosaccharides and it is associated with the anti-infective capacity of human milk. A murine influenza vaccination model was used to determine the effect of 2'-FL on vaccination responsiveness. 2'-FL treatment enhanced the delayed-type hypersensitivity responses and increased the serum levels of immunoglobulin (Ig) G1 and IgG2a and the expression of activation marker CD27 on splenic B cells. Finally, 2'-FL treatment had a direct effect on the maturation status and antigen-presenting capacity of bone marrow-derived dendritic cells [85]. Four-week-old male wild-type C57BL/6 mice were fed antibiotics to reduce their intestinal microbiota and then inoculated with *C. jejuni* 81–176. The effect of treatment with 2'-FL on the resulting acute transient enteric infection and immune response was evaluated. The ingestion of 2'-FL reduced *C. jejuni* colonization and the induction of inflammatory signaling molecules of the acute-phase mucosal immune response by 50–60% [79].

6. Effects of HMOs: Studies in Humans

The positive effects of HMOs found by in vitro and animal studies must be substantiated by findings from clinical studies. The most reliable clinical studies for assessing the benefits of HMOs are randomized, double-blinded, multicenter controlled trials (RCTs). To date, however, the number of RCTs with HMOs is very scarce, and most have focused on aspects other than the immune response.

6.1. Observational Studies

HMOs containing α1,2-fucosyl linkages have been shown to promote the growth of bifidobacteria. *B. longum* subsp. *infantis* and *B. bifidum* possess glycosyl hydrolase family 95 (GH95) fucosidases that act on 2'-fucosylated HMOs [68,86,87]. Mothers with FUT2 (secretor mothers) and nonsecretor mothers (with the nonfunctional enzyme) were recruited to evaluate the effects of maternal secretor status on the developing infant microbiota. Bifidobacteria colonize earlier in infants that are fed by secretor mothers than in infants fed by nonsecretor mothers. In addition, the majority of bifidobacteria were isolated from secretor-fed infants who consumed 2'-FL. Feces with high levels of bifidobacteria contained lower milk oligosaccharide levels and higher lactate levels [86]. The known HMO consumer *Bifidobacterium* were more abundant in the children of secretor mothers than those of nonsecretor mothers. The relative abundance of *Bacteroides plebeius*, a bacterium capable of utilizing sulfated polysaccharides for growth, was decreased in these children [88]. In addition, the FUT2 gene might be related to allergic disease in breastfed infants later in life. At two years of age, but not at five years, a lower incidence of IgE-associated eczema was detected in C-section-born infants who were fed breast milk containing FUT2-dependent oligosaccharides [89]. Additionally, although data suggest that higher lacto-N-fucopentaose III concentrations are associated with the lack of development of cow's milk allergy, they are not required to prevent cow's milk allergy. Therefore, other mechanisms must be in play [90].

HMOs have multiple immunomodulatory functions that influence child´s health [91]. Kuhn et al. evaluated the effects of HMO from breast milk on the survival of uninfected children born to HIV-infected mothers. Higher maternal breast milk concentrations of 2-linked fucosylated HMOs (2'-FL and lacto-N-fucopentaose I, as well as 3FL and lacto-N-fucopentaose II/III) were significantly associated with reduced mortality [91].

Breast milk samples were analyzed to determine the levels of 2-linked fucosyloligosaccharides and their relationship with the incidence of moderate-to-severe diarrhea. The incidence of diarrhea was lower in infants fed milk containing high levels of total 2-linked fucosyloligosaccharides. *Campylobacter*, and calicivirus-induced diarrhea occurred less often in infants whose mother's milk contained high levels of 2'-FL and lacto-N-difucohexaose [92].

6.2. Randomized Controlled Trials

Marriage et al. [93] carried out a prospective, randomized, controlled, multicenter study at 28 sites throughout the United States involving 424 healthy full-term infants enrolled by day five of life to examine infant growth and the tolerance of infant formulas with a caloric density that is closer to that of human milk supplemented with HMOs and to study HMO uptake [93]. Infants were randomly divided into three formula feeding groups: (a) EF1, starter formula (64.3 kcal/100 mL) with galactooligosaccharides (GOS) (2.2 g/L) and 2'-FL at 0.2 g/L (n = 105); (b) EF2, starter formula (64.3 kcal/100 mL) with GOS (1.4 g/L) and 2'-FL at 1 g/L (n = 111); and, CF, control formula (64.3 kcal/100 mL) with only GOS (2.4 g/L) (n = 101). A nonrandomized human milk-fed (HM) group of infants was also enrolled as a reference (n = 107). The study duration was 119 days, and the primary outcome was weight gain per day. Secondary outcomes included measures of tolerance and other anthropometric measures, formula intake, parent responses to questions that are related to satisfaction with the formula and their infant's behavior, concentrations of 2'-FL in human milk in infant plasma and urine, and relative absorption. No significant differences were observed among any groups in growth parameters (weight, length, or head circumference) over the four-month study period. 2'-FL was present in the plasma and urine of infants fed the two formulas containing 2'-FL (EF1, EF2). No significant difference was observed in 2'-FL uptake relative to the concentration fed. All of the formulas were well tolerated and comparable in terms of average stool consistency, number of stools per day, and percentage of feedings associated with spitting up or vomiting. In conclusion, infants fed a lower caloric formula with 2'FL show growth and 2'FL uptake like breast-fed infants [93].

The same authors investigated the effects of feeding formulas supplemented with the HMO 2'-FL on biomarkers of immune function in healthy term infants [94]. For this purpose, they used a subpopulation of the infants that were enrolled in [93]. PBMCs were isolated for cellular phenotyping and stimulated ex vivo with phytohemagglutinin to examine proliferation and cell cycle progression or with respiratory syncytial virus (RSV). Cytokine concentrations were measured in plasma and in ex vivo cultures. Both groups fed EF1 and EF2 exhibited significantly different inflammatory cytokine profiles from those of the group fed the control formula (only GOS) ($p \leq 0.05$) but not different from those of breastfed infants or from each other. The plasma concentrations of the inflammatory cytokines IL-1α, IL-1β, IL-6, and TNF-α, and the anti-inflammatory IL-1 receptor antagonist were significantly higher in the control group (only GOS) than in breastfed infants or the groups fed EF1 and EF2 ($p \leq 0.05$). In ex vivo RSV-stimulated PBMC cultures, breastfed infants were not different from either of the groups fed the experimental formulas (EF1 and EF2), but they had lower concentrations of inflammatory cytokines TNF-α and IFN-Y ($p \leq 0.05$) and tended to have lower IL-1ra, IL-6 and IL-1β than infants fed the control formula. This study suggests that infants fed a formula containing 2'FL have lower inflammatory cytokines, although being similar to those of breastfed infants [94].

Kajzer et al. [95] evaluated the gastrointestinal tolerance of infants fed infant formula supplemented with 2'-FL and short-chain fructo-oligosaccharides (scFOS) in a prospective, randomized, multicenter, double-blinded, controlled study involving 131 full-term infants enrolled between 0 and 8 days of age [95]. Infants were randomly allocated to receive either milk-based infant formula not containing oligosaccharides ($n = 42$) or milk-based infant formula containing 2′-FL (0.2 g/L) and scFOS (2 g/L) ($n = 46$). A group of 43 breastfed infants were also included. The intervention was performed for 35 days. The primary outcome was the average mean rank stool consistency (MRSC) from study day 1 to visit 3, calculated from stool records. From study day 1 to visit 3, no difference in stool consistency was observed. At visit 3, there were no differences between groups in the average volume of study formula intake, the number of study formula feedings per day, anthropometric data, or percentage of feedings with spitting up or vomiting. The conclusion of this study was that the formula containing 2′FL was well tolerated in infants as evidenced by stool consistency, formula intake, anthropometric data and percent feedings with spitup/vomit similar to that of infants fed a formula without oligosaccharides or breast milk [95].

The effects of feeding infant formulas supplemented with two human milk-identical oligosaccharides, 2′FL, and lacto-N-*neo*tetraose (LNnT), on infant growth, tolerability, gut microbiota, and medication use were investigated in a randomized, controlled, multicenter trial in Italy and Belgium [96–98]. One hundred and seventy-five healthy, full-term infants were randomly allocated after birth (between 0–14 days of age) to one of the two formula feeding groups: intact cow's milk-based whey-predominant infant formula with the addition of 2′-FL (1.0 g/L) and LNnT (0.5 g/L) (test group, $n = 88$) or intact cow's milk-based whey-predominant infant formula (control group, $n = 87$). The formulas were given up to six months of age (exclusive formula feeding up to four months). A group of 38 exclusively breastfed infants were enrolled at three months as a reference (breastfed group). The primary endpoint was weight gain through four months of age. The secondary endpoints were anthropometry, stool characteristics, stool microbiota (at 3 and 12 months of age, obtained using 16S rRNA gene sequencing and metagenomics), stool metabolic signature (at 3 and 12 months of age, obtained using proton NMR-based metabolic profiling,), digestive tolerance, and morbidity (reported by parents) through 12 months of age. The weight gain up to four months of age of infants fed formula supplemented with 2′-FL and LNnT was not inferior to the weight gain of infants fed unsupplemented formula. The mean weight, length, head circumference, and BMI up to 12 months of age of infants fed formulas with or without 2′-FL and LNnT were close to the WHO Growth Standards and did not differ between the two groups. Digestive tolerance was similar between the two groups. Infants receiving formula containing 2′-FL and LNnT had significantly fewer parental reports of lower respiratory tract infections (19.3% vs. 34.5%; OR 0.45, 95% CI 0.21–0.95; $p = 0.027$), particularly bronchitis (10.2% vs. 27.6%; OR 0.30, 95% CI 0.11–0.73; $p = 0.004$), up to 12 months of age (42% vs. 60.9%; OR 0.47, 95% CI 0.24–0.89; $p = 0.016$), and lower medication (antibiotics up to 12 months of age, antipyretics (15.9% vs. 29.9%; OR 0.44; 95% CI 0.2–0.98; $p = 0.032$) up to four months of age) than infants fed formula without 2′FL and LNnT [96]. In conclusion, feeding infant formula containing two HMOs (2′FL and LNnT) during the first six months of age are safe, well-tolerated, and supports age-appropriate growth [81]. Also, the observed effects on reduced morbidity and medication use in infants up to 12 months of age, when feeding formula with HMOs, suggest that 2′FL and LNnT may provide immune benefits [81].

In a second work, these authors reported the effects of 2′-FL and LNnT on the infant gut microbiota [97]. The microbiota composition of infants that were fed formula containing 2′-FL and LNnT was significantly different from that of infants fed nonsupplemented formula ($p < 0.001$) at the genus level and closer to that of breastfed infants at three months of age. Three main bacterial genera (*Bifidobacterium*, *Escherichia*, and *Peptostreptococcaceae*) showed significant differences in infants fed formula with or without 2′FL and LNnT at three months of age: greater abundance of beneficial *Bifidobacterium* ($p < 0.01$); and, lower abundance of potentially pathogenic *Escherichia* ($p < 0.01$) as well as of unclassified *Peptostreptococcaceae* ($p < 0.05$) were observed in infants fed formula containing 2′-FL and LNnT as compared to infants fed nonsupplemented formula. These values were closer to the levels that were observed in breastfed infants. The biochemical composition of the stools was explored by the quantitative profiling of major metabolites to gain additional information on the compositional aspects.

The stool contents of some amino acids (phenylalanine, tyrosine, isoleucine), some SCFAs (propionate, butyrate), and some organic acids (lactate) in infants fed formula with 2′-FL and LNnT tended to be closer to those that were observed in breastfed infants than those in infants fed nonsupplemented formula [97]. This study shows that a formula supplemented with 2′FL and LNnT shifts stool microbiota and metabolic signatures of infants born at term closer to that of breastfed infants [97].

Finally, in a third work, the same authors found that, at three months, the microbiota composition in the test group appeared closer to that of the breastfed group than to that of the control group according to alpha (within group) and beta (between groups) diversity analyses of the microbiota and the distribution of microbiota community types (A, B, and C). Supplementation with both HMOs decreased the number of infants with formula-specific C-community (fecal community type/FCT C) and increased those with the breastfed-specific B-community (FCT B). Cumulative antibiotic use up to 12 months was associated with the FCT distribution at three months. Infants with FCT B at 3 months were less likely to be treated with antibiotics (OR 0.4 (95% CI, 0.17–0.93; $p = 0.033$)), while infants with FCT C were more likely to be treated with antibiotics during the first 12 months (OR 3.3 (95% CI, 1.54–7.02; $p = 0.0025$)). The microbiota community type at three months was not associated with other parent-reported infection-related morbidities [98]. This study confirms the microbiota results of the previous one [97] and shows that infants with a breastfed specific microbiota community type (FCT B) are less likely to need antibiotics.

7. Conclusions and Future Perspectives

HMOs have been described to exert immunomodulatory effects. Many in vitro studies suggest that HMOs directly modulate immune responses, acting either locally on cells of the mucosa-associated lymphoid tissues or systemically to inhibit the expression of inflammatory genes, mainly cytokines. Studies in animals have shown that the administration of HMOs decreases the duration of diarrhea and enhances the expression of cytokines. Observational studies in humans have documented that certain HMOs promote the growth of bifidobacteria, which in turn affect the production of lactate and SCFAs that mediate systemic effects, including immunomodulation. Likewise, the intake of 2-linked fucosylated HMOs is associated with a reduced incidence of eczema, as well as reduced mortality in children whose mothers were infected with HIV. Moreover, HMOs play a protective role against bacterial and viral acute diarrhea. HMOs seem to protect breastfed infants against microbial infections due to their structural similarities to pathogen cell surface molecular patterns, and the protective effect has been found to be exerted through cell signaling and cell-to-cell recognition events, enrichment of the protective gut microbiota, and the modulation of microbial adhesion and invasion of the infant intestinal mucosa. Finally, infants fed formula supplemented with selected HMOs exhibit a pattern of inflammatory cytokines that is closer to that of exclusively breastfed infants.

Although new analytical systems that take advantage of the separation of complex carbohydrates by HPLC and identification by mass spectrometry have been developed in recent years, there is a need for a simpler standardized methodology to estimate the HMO patterns and contents in human milk worldwide.

Concerning the potential mechanisms of action of HMOs on immunity, new experimental approaches using human cell intestinal lines and animal models are necessary. In particular, there is a need to know how HMOs, either directly or indirectly though signaling cascade interactions, affect the expression of genes that are involved in antigen tolerance, the development of the GALT, and the response to pathogens, both bacteria and viruses.

A recent development in infant formulas is the incorporation of selected HMOs, mainly neutral, due to new biotechnological processes that are can incorporate human mammary gland glycosyltransferases. However, these formulas lack acidic HMOs, which are known to play relevant biological roles in the inhibition of pathogen and toxin adhesion to the intestine.

The number of RCTs that have evaluated the influence of HMOs on infant health is very scarce, and the number of subjects was calculated to determine the safety and tolerance of the

HMO-supplemented formulas but not to generate actual evidence of the potential preventive effects of HMOs against infectious diseases. Therefore, new RCT studies in infants with the appropriate power should be designed to ascertain the roles of HMOs in the prevention of diarrhea, pneumonia, and other respiratory diseases.

Author Contributions: All three authors participated in the bibliographic search, discussion and writing of the manuscript.

Funding: This research received no external funding.

Acknowledgments: Julio Plaza-Diaz and Angel Gil are part of University of Granada, Plan Propio de Investigación 2016, Excellence actions: Units of Excellence; Unit of Excellence on Exercise and Health (UCEES).

Conflicts of Interest: The authors declare no conflict of interest.

References

1. Black, R.E.; Allen, L.H.; Bhutta, Z.A.; Caulfield, L.E.; de Onis, M.; Ezzati, M.; Mathers, C.; Rivera, J.; Maternal and Child Undernutrition Study Group. Maternal and child undernutrition: Global and regional exposures and health consequences. *Lancet* **2008**, *371*, 243–260. [CrossRef]
2. Dieterich, C.M.; Felice, J.P.; O'Sullivan, E.; Rasmussen, K.M. Breastfeeding and health outcomes for the mother-infant dyad. *Pediatr. Clin. N. Am.* **2013**, *60*, 31–48. [CrossRef] [PubMed]
3. Koletzko, B.; Brands, B.; Grote, V.; Kirchberg, F.F.; Prell, C.; Rzehak, P.; Uhl, O.; Weber, M. Early Nutrition Programming Project. Long-term health impact of early nutrition: The power of programming. *Ann. Nutr. Metab.* **2017**, *70*, 161–169. [CrossRef] [PubMed]
4. Bode, L. Human milk oligosaccharides: Every baby needs a sugar mama. *Glycobiology* **2012**, *22*, 1147–1162. [CrossRef] [PubMed]
5. Musilova, S.; Rada, V.; Vlkova, E.; Bunesova, V. Beneficial effects of human milk oligosaccharides on gut microbiota. *Benef. Microbes* **2014**, *5*, 273–283. [CrossRef] [PubMed]
6. Morozov, V.; Hansman, G.; Hanisch, F.G.; Schroten, H.; Kunz, C. Human milk oligosaccharides as promising antivirals. *Mol. Nutr. Food Res.* **2018**, *62*, e1700679. [CrossRef] [PubMed]
7. Doherty, A.M.; Lodge, C.J.; Dharmage, S.C.; Dai, X.; Bode, L.; Lowe, A.J. Human milk oligosaccharides and associations with immune-mediated disease and infection in childhood: A Systematic Review. *Front. Pediatr.* **2018**, *6*, 91. [CrossRef] [PubMed]
8. Zivkovic, A.M.; German, J.B.; Lebrilla, C.B.; Mills, D.A. Human milk glycobiome and its impact on the infant gastrointestinal microbiota. *Proc. Natl. Acad. Sci. USA* **2011**, *108*, 4653–4658. [CrossRef] [PubMed]
9. Bode, L. The functional biology of human milk oligosaccharides. *Early Hum. Dev.* **2015**, *91*, 619–622. [CrossRef] [PubMed]
10. Smilowitz, J.; Lebrilla, C.; Mills, D.; German, J.; Freeman, S. Breast milk oligosaccharides: Structure-function relationships in the neonate. *Annu. Rev. Nutr.* **2014**, *34*, 143–169. [CrossRef] [PubMed]
11. Kunz, C.; Rudloff, S.; Baier, W.; Klein, N.; Strobel, S. Oligosaccharides in human milk: Structural, functional, and metabolic aspects. *Annu. Rev. Nutr.* **2000**, *20*, 699–722. [CrossRef] [PubMed]
12. Kobata, A. Structures and application of oligosaccharides in human milk. *Proc. Jpn. Acad. Ser. B Phys. Biol. Sci.* **2010**, *86*, 731–747. [CrossRef] [PubMed]
13. Jantscher-Krenn, E.; Bode, L. Human milk oligosaccharides and their potential benefits for the breast-fed neonate. *Minerva Pediatr.* **2012**, *64*, 83–99. [PubMed]
14. Bode, L.; Jantscher-Krenn, E. Structure-function relationships of human milk oligosaccharides. *Adv. Nutr.* **2012**, *3*, 383S–391S. [CrossRef] [PubMed]
15. Goehring, K.C.; Kennedy, A.D.; Prieto, P.A.; Buck, R.H. Direct evidence for the presence of human milk oligosaccharides in the circulation of breastfed infants. *PLoS ONE* **2014**, *9*, e101692. [CrossRef] [PubMed]
16. Blank, D.; Dotz, V.; Geyer, R.; Kunz, C. Human milk oligosaccharides and Lewis blood group: Individual high-throughput sample profiling to enhance conclusions from functional studies. *Adv. Nutr.* **2012**, *3*, 440S–449S. [CrossRef] [PubMed]
17. Austin, S.; De Castro, C.A.; Bénet, T.; Hou, Y.; Sun, H.; Thakkar, S.K.; Vinyes-Pares, G.; Zhang, Y.; Wang, P. Temporal change of the content of 10 oligosaccharides in the milk of chinese urban mothers. *Nutrients* **2016**, *8*, 346. [CrossRef] [PubMed]

18. Kunz, C.; Meyer, C.; Collado, M.C.; Geiger, L.; Garcia-Mantrana, I.; Bertua-Rios, B.; Martinez-Costa, C.; Borsch, C.; Rudloff, S. Influence of gestational age, secretor, and lewis blood group status on the oligosaccharide content of human milk. *J. Pediatr. Gastroenterol. Nutr.* **2017**, *64*, 789–798. [CrossRef] [PubMed]
19. Kumazaki, T.; Yoshida, A. Biochemical evidence that secretor gene, Se, is a structural gene encoding a specific fucosyltransferase. *Proc. Natl. Acad. Sci. USA* **1984**, *81*, 4193–4197. [CrossRef] [PubMed]
20. Johnson, P.H.; Watkins, W.M. Purification of the Lewis blood-group gene associated alpha-3/4-fucosyltransferase from human milk: An enzyme transferring fucose primarily to type 1 and lactose-based oligosaccharide chains. *Glycoconj. J.* **1992**, *9*, 241–249. [CrossRef] [PubMed]
21. Xu, Z.; Vo, L.; Macher, B.A. Structure-function analysis of human α1,3-fucosyltransferase. Amino acids involved in acceptor substrate specificity. *J. Biol. Chem.* **1996**, *271*, 8818–8823. [CrossRef] [PubMed]
22. Newburg, D.S.; Ruiz-Palacios, G.M.; Morrow, A.L. Human milk glycans protect infants against enteric pathogens. *Annu. Rev. Nutr.* **2005**, *25*, 37–58. [CrossRef] [PubMed]
23. De Leoz, M.L.; Gaerlan, S.C.; Strum, J.S.; Dimapasoc, L.M.; Mirmiran, M.; Tancredi, D.J.; Smilowitz, J.T.; Kalanetra, K.M.; Mills, D.A.; German, J.B.; et al. Lacto-N-tetraose, fucosylation, and secretor status are highly variable in human milk oligosaccharides from women delivering preterm. *J. Proteome Res.* **2012**, *11*, 4662–4672. [CrossRef] [PubMed]
24. Davidson, B.; Meinzen-Derr, J.K.; Wagner, C.L.; Newburg, D.S.; Morrow, A.L. Fucosylated oligosaccharides in human milk in relation to gestational age and stage of lactation. *Adv. Exp. Med. Biol.* **2004**, *554*, 427–430. [CrossRef] [PubMed]
25. Dotz, V.; Adam, R.; Lochnit, G.; Schroten, H.; Kunz, C. Neutral oligosaccharides in feces of breastfed and formula-fed infants at different ages. *Glycobiology* **2016**, *26*, 1308–1316. [CrossRef] [PubMed]
26. Rueda-Cabrera, R.; Gil, A. Nutrición en inmunidad en el estado de salud. In *Tratado de Nutrición*; Editorial Médica Panamericana: Madrid, Spain, 2017; Volume 4, ISBN 9788491101932.
27. Rumbo, M.; Schiffrin, E.J. Ontogeny of intestinal epithelium immune functions: Developmental and environmental regulation. *Cell. Mol. Life Sci.* **2005**, *62*, 1288–1296. [CrossRef] [PubMed]
28. Coombes, J.L.; Powrie, F. Dendritic cells in intestinal immune regulation. *Nat. Rev. Immunol.* **2008**, *6*, 411–420. [CrossRef] [PubMed]
29. Gil, A.; Rueda, R. Interaction of early diet and the development of the immune system. *Nutr. Res. Rev.* **2002**, *15*, 263–292. [CrossRef] [PubMed]
30. Klose, C.S.; Artis, D. Innate lymphoid cells as regulators of immunity, inflammation and tissue homeostasis. *Nat. Immunol.* **2016**, *17*, 765–774. [CrossRef] [PubMed]
31. Hardy, H.; Harris, J.; Lyon, E.; Beal, J.; Foey, A.D. Probiotics, prebiotics and immunomodulation of gut mucosal defences: Homeostasis and immunopathology. *Nutrients* **2013**, *5*, 1869–1912. [CrossRef] [PubMed]
32. Pannaraj, P.; Li, F.; Cerini, C.; Bender, J.; Yang, S.; Rollie, A.; Adisetiyo, H.; Zabih, S.; Lincez, P.J.; Bittinger, K.; et al. Association between breast milk bacterial communities and establishment and development of the infant gut microbiome. *JAMA Pediatr.* **2017**, *171*, 647–654. [CrossRef] [PubMed]
33. Fernández, L.; Langa, S.; Martín, V.; Maldonado, A.; Jiménez, E.; Martín, R.; Rodríguez, J.M. The human milk microbiota: Origin and potential roles in health and disease. *Pharmacol. Res.* **2013**, *69*, 1–10. [CrossRef] [PubMed]
34. Putignani, L.; Del Chierico, F.; Petrucca, A.; Vernocchi, P.; Dallapiccola, B. The human gut microbiota: A dynamic interplay with the host from birth to senescence settled during childhood. *Pediatr. Res.* **2014**, *76*, 2–10. [CrossRef] [PubMed]
35. Hotamisligil, G.S.; Peraldi, P.; Budavari, A.; Ellis, R.; White, M.F.; Spiegelman, B.M. IRS-1-mediated inhibition of insulin receptor tyrosine kinase activity in TNF-alpha- and obesity-induced insulin resistance. *Science* **1996**, *271*, 665–668. [CrossRef] [PubMed]
36. Bouloumié, A.; Curat, C.A.; Sengenès, C.; Lolmède, K.; Miranville, A.; Busse, R. Role of macrophage tissue infiltration in metabolic diseases. *Curr. Opin. Clin. Nutr. Metab. Care* **2005**, *8*, 347–354. [CrossRef] [PubMed]
37. Cani, P.D.; Amar, J.; Iglesias, M.A.; Poggi, M.; Knauf, C.; Bastelica, D.; Neyrinck, A.M.; Fava, F.; Tuohy, K.M.; Chabo, C.; et al. Metabolic endotoxemia initiates obesity and insulin resistance. *Diabetes* **2007**, *56*, 1761–1772. [CrossRef] [PubMed]
38. Kunz, C.; Rudloff, S. Biological functions of oligosaccharides in human milk. *Acta Pediatr.* **1993**, *82*, 903–912. [CrossRef]
39. Wold, A.E.; Hanson, L.A. Defence factors in human milk. *Curr. Opin. Gastroenterol.* **1994**, *10*, 652–658. [CrossRef]

40. Zopf, D.; Roth, S. Oligosaccharide anti-infective agents. *Lancet* **1996**, *347*, 1017–1021. [CrossRef]
41. Sela, D.A.; Chapman, J.; Adeuya, A.; Kim, J.; Chen, F.; Whitehead, T.; Lapidus, A.; Rokhsar, D.; Lebrilla, C.; German, J. The genome sequence of *Bifidobacterium longum* subsp. *infantis reveals adaptations for milk utilization within the infant microbiome. Proc. Natl. Acad. Sci. USA* **2008**, *105*, 18964. [CrossRef] [PubMed]
42. Barboza, M.; Pinzon, J.; Wickramasinghe, S.; Froehlich, J.W.; Moeller, I.; Smilowitz, J.T.; Ruhaak, L.R.; Huang, J.; Lonnerdal, B.; German, J.B.; et al. Glycosylation of human milk lactoferrin exhibits dynamic changes during early lactation enhancing its role in pathogenic bacteria-host interactions. *Mol. Cell. Proteomics* **2012**, *11*, M111.015248. [CrossRef] [PubMed]
43. Chichlowski, M.; De Lartigue, G.; German, J.B.; Raybould, H.E.; Mills, D.A. Bifidobacteria isolated from infants and cultured on human milk oligosaccharides affect intestinal epithelial function. *J. Pediatr. Gastroenterol. Nutr.* **2012**, *55*, 321–327. [CrossRef] [PubMed]
44. Newburg, D.S. Do the binding properties of oligosaccharides in milk protect human infants from gastrointestinal bacteria? *J. Nutr.* **1997**, *127*, 980S. [CrossRef] [PubMed]
45. Varki, A. Biological roles of oligosaccharides: All of the theories are correct. *Glycobiology* **1993**, *3*, 97–130. [CrossRef] [PubMed]
46. Ruiz-Palacios, G.M.; Cervantes, L.E.; Ramos, P.; Chavez-Munguia, B.; Newburg, D.S. *Campylobacter jejuni* binds intestinal H(O) antigen (Fuc alpha 1, 2Gal beta 1, 4GlcNAc), and fucosyloligosaccharides of human milk inhibit its binding and infection. *J. Biol Chem.* **2003**, *278*, 14112–14120. [CrossRef] [PubMed]
47. Huang, P.; Farkas, T.; Marionneau, S.; Zhong, W.; Ruvoen-Clouet, N.; Morrow, A.L.; Altaye, M.; Pickering, L.K.; Newburg, D.S.; Le Pendu, J.; et al. Noroviruses bind to human ABO, Lewis, and secretor histo-blood group antigens: Identification of 4 distinct strain-specific patterns. *J. Infect. Dis.* **2003**, *188*, 19–31. [CrossRef] [PubMed]
48. Xu, H.T.; Zhao, Y.F.; Lian, Z.X.; Fan, B.L.; Zhao, Z.H.; Yu, S.Y.; Dai, Y.P.; Wang, L.L.; Niu, H.L.; Li, N.; et al. Effects of fucosylated milk of goat and mouse on *Helicobacter pylori* binding to Lewis b antigen. *World J. Gastroenterol.* **2004**, *10*, 2063–2066. [CrossRef] [PubMed]
49. Newburg, D.S.; Pickering, L.K.; McCluer, R.H.; Cleary, T.G. Fucosylated oligosaccharides of human milk protect suckling mice from heat-stabile enterotoxin of *Escherichia coli*. *J. Infect. Dis.* **1990**, *162*, 1075–1080. [CrossRef] [PubMed]
50. Crane, J.K.; Azar, S.S.; Stam, A.; Newburg, D.S. Oligosaccharides from human milk block binding and activity of the *Escherichia coli* heat-stable enterotoxin (STa) in T84 intestinal cells. *J. Nutr.* **1994**, *124*, 2358–2364. [CrossRef] [PubMed]
51. Martín-Sosa, S.; Martín, M.J.; Hueso, P. The sialylated fraction of milk oligosaccharides is partially responsible for binding to enterotoxigenic and uropathogenic *Escherichia coli* human strains. *J. Nutr.* **2002**, *132*, 3067–3072. [CrossRef] [PubMed]
52. Coppa, G.V.; Zampini, L.; Galeazzi, T.; Facinelli, B.; Ferrante, L.; Capretti, R.; Orazio, G. Human milk oligosaccharides inhibit the adhesion to Caco-2 cells of diarrheal pathogens: *Escherichia coli*, *Vibrio cholerae*, and *Salmonella fyris*. *Pediatr. Res.* **2006**, *59*, 377–382. [CrossRef] [PubMed]
53. Perret, S.; Sabin, C.; Dumon, C.; Pokorná, M.; Gautier, C.; Galanina, O.; Ilia, S.; Bovin, N.; Nicaise, M.; Desmadril, M.; et al. Human milk oligosaccharides shorten rotavirus-induced diarrhea and modulate piglet mucosal immunity and colonic microbiota. *ISME J.* **2014**, *8*, 1609–1620. [CrossRef]
54. Lin, A.E.; Autran, C.A.; Espanola, S.D.; Bode, L.; Nizet, V. Human milk oligosaccharides protect bladder epithelial cells against uropathogenic *Escherichia coli* invasion and cytotoxicity. *J. Infect. Dis.* **2014**, *209*, 389–398. [CrossRef] [PubMed]
55. Manthey, C.F.; Autran, C.A.; Eckmann, L.; Bode, L. Human milk oligosaccharides protect against enteropathogenic *Escherichia coli* attachment in vitro and EPEC colonization in suckling mice. *J. Pediatr. Gastroenterol. Nutr.* **2014**, *58*, 165–168. [CrossRef] [PubMed]
56. Gonia, S.; Tuepker, M.; Heisel, T.; Autran, C.; Bode, L.; Gale, C.A. Human milk oligosaccharides inhibit candida albicans invasion of human premature intestinal epithelial cells. *J. Nutr.* **2015**, *145*, 1992–1998. [CrossRef] [PubMed]
57. Jantscher-Krenn, E.; Lauwaet, T.; Bliss, L.A.; Reed, S.L.; Gillin, F.D.; Bode, L. Human milk oligosaccharides reduce *Entamoeba histolytica* attachment and cytotoxicity in vitro. *Br. J. Nutr.* **2012**, *108*, 1839–1846. [CrossRef] [PubMed]

58. Canfora, E.E.; Jocken, J.W.; Blaak, E.E. Short-chain fatty acids in control of body weight and insulin sensitivity. *Nat. Rev. Endocrinol.* **2015**, *11*, 577–591. [CrossRef] [PubMed]
59. Hur, K.Y.; Lee, M.S. Gut Microbiota and Metabolic Disorders. *Diabetes Metab. J.* **2015**, *39*, 198–203. [CrossRef] [PubMed]
60. Du, X.-L.; Edelstein, D.; Rossetti, L.; Fantus, I.G.; Goldberg, H.; Ziyadeh, F.; Wu, J.; Brownlee, M. Hyperglycemia-induced mitochondrial superoxide overproduction activates the hexosamine pathway and induces plasminogen activator inhibitor-1 expression by increasing Sp1 glycosylation. *Proc. Natl. Acad. Sci. USA* **2000**, *97*, 12222–12226. [CrossRef] [PubMed]
61. Gyorgy, P.; Norris, R.F.; Rose, C.S. *Bifidus* factor. I. A variant of *Lactobacillus bifidus* requiring a special growth factor. *Arch. Biochem. Biophys.* **1954**, *48*, 193–201. [CrossRef]
62. Ward, R.E.; Ninonuevo, M.; Mills, D.A.; Lebrilla, C.B.; German, J.B. In vitro fermentation of breast milk oligosaccharides by *Bifidobacterium infantis* and *Lactobacillus gasseri*. *Appl. Environ. Microbiol.* **2006**, *72*, 4497–4499. [CrossRef] [PubMed]
63. Ward, R.E.; Ninonuevo, M.; Mills, D.A.; Lebrilla, C.B.; German, J.B. In vitro fermentability of human milk oligosaccharides by several strains of bifidobacteria. *Mol. Nutr. Food Res.* **2007**, *51*, 1398–1405. [CrossRef] [PubMed]
64. Garrido, D.; Ruiz-Moyano, S.; Jimenez-Espinoza, R.; Eom, H.J.; Block, D.E.; Mills, D.A. Utilization of galactooligosaccharides by *Bifidobacterium longum* subsp. *infantis* isolates. *Food Microbiol.* **2013**, *33*, 262–270. [CrossRef] [PubMed]
65. LoCascio, R.; Ninonuevo, M.; Freeman, S.; Sela, D.; Grimm, R.; Lebrilla, C.B.; Mills, D.A.; German, J.B. Glycoprofiling of bifidobacterial consumption of human milk oligosaccharides demonstrates strain specific, preferential consumption of small chain glycans secreted in early human lactation. *J. Agric. Food Chem.* **2007**, *55*, 8914–8919. [CrossRef] [PubMed]
66. Marcobal, A.; Barboza, M.; Sonnenburg, E.D.; Pudlo, N.; Martens, E.C.; Desai, P.; Lebrilla, C.B.; Weimer, B.C.; Mills, D.A.; German, J.B.; Sonnenburg, JL. *Bacteroides* in the infant gut consume milk oligosaccharides via mucus-utilization pathways. *Cell Host Microbe* **2011**, *10*, 507–514. [CrossRef] [PubMed]
67. Ruiz-Moyano, S.; Totten, S.M.; Garrido, D.A.; Smilowitz, J.T.; German, J.B.; Lebrilla, C.B.; Mills, D.A. Variation in consumption of human milk oligosaccharides by infant gut-associated strains of *Bifidobacterium breve*. *Appl. Environ. Microbiol.* **2013**, *79*, 6040–6049. [CrossRef] [PubMed]
68. Sela, D.A.; Garrido, D.; Lerno, L.; Wu, S.; Tan, K.; Eom, H.J.; Joachimiak, A.; Lebrilla, C.B.; Mills, D.A. *Bifidobacterium longum* subsp. *infantis* ATCC 15697 α-fucosidases are active on fucosylated human milk oligosaccharides. *Appl. Environ. Microbiol.* **2012**, *78*, 795–803. [CrossRef] [PubMed]
69. Sela, D.A.; Li, Y.; Lerno, L.; Wu, S.; Marcobal, A.M.; German, J.B.; Chen, X.; Lebrilla, C.B.; Mills, D.A. An infant-associated bacterial commensal utilizes breast milk sialyloligosaccharides. *J. Biol. Chem.* **2011**, *286*, 11909–11918. [CrossRef] [PubMed]
70. Kitaoka, M. Bifidobacterial enzymes involved in the metabolism of human milk oligosaccharides. *Adv. Nutr.* **2012**, *3*, 422S–429S. [CrossRef] [PubMed]
71. James, K.; Motherway, M.O.; Penno, C.; O'Brien, R.L.; van Sinderen, D. *Bifidobacterium breve* UCC2003 employs multiple transcriptional regulators to control metabolism of particular human milk oligosaccharides. *Appl. Environ. Microbiol.* **2018**, *10*, 278–279. [CrossRef] [PubMed]
72. Rudloff, S.; Pohlentz, G.; Diekmann, L.; Egge, H.; Kunz, C. Urinary excretion of lactose and oligosaccharides in preterm infants fed human milk or infant formula. *Acta Paediatr.* **1996**, *85*, 598–603. [CrossRef] [PubMed]
73. Rudloff, S.; Pohlentz, G.; Borsch, C.; Lentze, M.J.; Kunz, C. Urinary excretion of in vivo ^{13}C-labelled milk oligosaccharides in breastfed infants. *Br. J. Nutr.* **2012**, *107*, 957–963. [CrossRef] [PubMed]
74. Gnoth, M.J.; Rudloff, S.; Kunz, C.; Kinne, R.K. Investigations of the in vitro transport of human milk oligosaccharides by a Caco-2 monolayer using a novel high performance liquid chromatography-mass spectrometry technique. *J. Biol Chem.* **2001**, *276*, 34363–34370. [CrossRef] [PubMed]
75. Lane, J.A.; O'Callaghan, J.; Carrington, S.D.; Hickey, R.M. Transcriptional response of HT-29 intestinal epithelial cells to human and bovine milk oligosaccharides. *Br. J. Nutr.* **2013**, *110*, 2127–2137. [CrossRef] [PubMed]
76. He, Y.; Liu, S.; Kling, D.E.; Leone, S.; Lawlor, N.T.; Huang, Y.; Feinberg, S.B.; Hill, D.R.; Newburg, D.S. The human milk oligosaccharide 2′-fucosyllactose modulates CD14 expression in human enterocytes, thereby attenuating LPS-induced inflammation. *Gut* **2016**, *65*, 33–46. [CrossRef] [PubMed]

77. Bode, L.; Kunz, C.; Muhly-Reinholz, M.; Mayer, K.; Seeger, W.; Rudloff, S. Inhibition of monocyte, lymphocyte, and neutrophil adhesion to endothelial cells by human milk oligosaccharides. *Thromb. Haemost.* **2004**, *92*, 1402–1410. [CrossRef] [PubMed]
78. Lin, A.E.; Autran, C.A.; Szyszka, A.; Escajadillo, T.; Huang, M.; Godula, K.; Prudden, A.R.; Boons, G.J.; Lewis, A.L.; Doran, K.S.; et al. Human milk oligosaccharides inhibit growth of group B *Streptococcus*. *J. Biol. Chem.* **2017**, *292*, 11243–11249. [CrossRef] [PubMed]
79. Yu, Z.T.; Nanthakumar, N.N.; Newburg, D.S. The human milk oligosaccharide 2′-fucosyllactose quenches *Campylobacter jejuni*-induced inflammation in human epithelial cells HEp-2 and HT-29 and in mouse intestinal mucosa. *J. Nutr.* **2016**, *146*, 1980–1990. [CrossRef] [PubMed]
80. Weichert, S.; Koromyslova, A.; Singh, B.K.; Hansman, S.; Jennewein, S.; Schroten, H.; Hansman, G.S. Structural basis for Norovirus inhibition by human milk oligosaccharides. *J. Virol.* **2016**, *90*, 4843–4848. [CrossRef] [PubMed]
81. Duska-McEwen, G.; Senft, A.P.; Ruetschilling, T.L.; Barrett, E.G.; Buck, R.H. Human milk oligosaccharides enhance innate immunity to respiratory syncytial virus and influenza in vitro. *Food Nutr. Sci.* **2014**, *5*, 1387–1398. [CrossRef]
82. Hanisch, F.G.; Hansman, G.S.; Morozov, V.; Kunz, C.; Schroten, H. Avidity of α-fucose on human milk oligosaccharides and blood group-unrelated oligo/polyfucoses is essential for potent norovirus-binding targets. *J. Biol. Chem.* **2018**, *293*, 11955–11965. [CrossRef] [PubMed]
83. Li, M.; Monaco, M.H.; Wang, M.; Comstock, S.S.; Kuhlenschmidt, T.B.; Fahey, G.C., Jr.; Miller, M.J.; Kuhlenschmidt, M.S.; Donovan, S.M. Human milk oligosaccharides shorten rotavirus-induced diarrhea and modulate piglet mucosal immunity and colonic microbiota. *ISME J.* **2014**, *8*, 1609–1620. [CrossRef] [PubMed]
84. Comstock, S.S.; Li, M.; Wang, M.; Monaco, M.H.; Kuhlenschmidt, T.B.; Kuhlenschmidt, M.S.; Donovan, SM. Dietary human milk oligosaccharides but not prebiotic oligosaccharides increase circulating natural killer cell and mesenteric lymph node memory t cell populations in noninfected and rotavirus-infected neonatal piglets. *J. Nutr.* **2017**, *147*, 1041–1047. [CrossRef] [PubMed]
85. Xiao, L.; Leusink-Muis, T.; Kettelarij, N.; van Ark, I.; Blijenberg, B.; Hesen, N.A.; Stahl, B.; Overbeek, S.A.; Garssen, J.; Folkerts, G.; et al. Human milk oligosaccharide 2′-fucosyllactose improves innate and adaptive immunity in an influenza-specific murine vaccination model. *Front. Immunol.* **2018**, *9*, 452. [CrossRef] [PubMed]
86. Lewis, Z.T.; Totten, S.M.; Smilowitz, J.T.; Popovic, M.; Parker, E.; Lemay, D.G.; Van Tassell, M.L.; Miller, M.J.; Jin, Y.S.; German, J.B.; et al. Maternal fucosyltransferase 2 status affects the gut bifidobacterial communities of breastfed infants. *Microbiome* **2015**, *3*, 13. [CrossRef] [PubMed]
87. Ashida, H.; Miyake, A.; Kiyohara, M.; Wada, J.; Yoshida, E.; Kumagai, H.; Katayama, T.; Yamamoto, K. Two distinct alpha-L-fucosidases from *Bifidobacterium bifidum* are essential for the utilization of fucosylated milk oligosaccharides and glycoconjugates. *Glycobiology* **2009**, *19*, 1010–1017. [CrossRef] [PubMed]
88. Smith-Brown, P.; Morrison, M.; Krause, L.; Davies, P.S. Mothers secretor status affects development of childrens microbiota composition and function: A pilot study. *PLoS ONE* **2016**, *11*, e0161211. [CrossRef] [PubMed]
89. Sprenger, N.; Odenwald, H.; Kukkonen, A.K.; Kuitunen, M.; Savilahti, E.; Kunz, C. FUT2-dependent breast milk oligosaccharides and allergy at 2 and 5 years of age in infants with high hereditary allergy risk. *Eur. J. Nutr.* **2017**, *56*, 1293–1301. [CrossRef] [PubMed]
90. Seppo, A.E.; Autran, C.A.; Bode, L.; Järvinen, K.M. Human milk oligosaccharides and development of cow's milk allergy in infants. *J. Allergy Clin. Immunol.* **2017**, *139*, 708.e5–711.e5. [CrossRef] [PubMed]
91. Kuhn, L.; Kim, H.Y.; Hsiao, L.; Nissan, C.; Kankasa, C.; Mwiya, M.; Thea, D.M.; Aldrovandi, G.M.; Bode, L. Oligosaccharide composition of breast milk influences survival of uninfected children born to HIV-infected mothers in Lusaka, Zambia. *J. Nutr.* **2015**, *145*, 66–72. [CrossRef] [PubMed]
92. Morrow, A.L.; Ruiz-Palacios, G.M.; Altaye, M.; Jiang, X.; Guerrero, M.L.; Meinzen-Derr, J.K.; Farkas, T.; Chaturvedi, P.; Pickering, L.K.; Newburg, D.S. Human milk oligosaccharides are associated with protection against diarrhea in breast-fed infants. *J. Pediatr.* **2004**, *145*, 297–303. [CrossRef] [PubMed]
93. Marriage, B.; Buck, R.; Goehring, K.; Oliver, J.; Williams, J. Infants fed a lower caloric formula with 2′FL show growth and 2′FL uptake like breast-fed infants. *J. Pediatr. Gastroenterol. Nutr.* **2015**, *61*, 649–658. [CrossRef] [PubMed]

94. Goehring, K.; Marriage, B.; Oliver, J.; Wilder, J.; Barrett, E.; Buck, R. Similar to those who are breastfed, infants fed a formula containing 2′-Fucosyllactose have lower inflammatory cytokines in a randomized controlled trial. *J. Nutr.* **2016**, *146*, 2559–2566. [CrossRef] [PubMed]
95. Kajzer, J.; Oliver, J.; Marriage, B.F. Gastrointestinal tolerance of formula supplemented with oligosaccharides. *FASEB J.* **2016**, *30*, 671.
96. Puccio, G.; Alliet, P.; Cajozzo, C.; Janssens, E.; Corsello, G.; Sprenger, N.; Wernimont, S.; Egli, D.; Gosoniu, L.; Steenhout, P.L. Effects of infant formula with human milk oligosaccharides on growth and morbidity: A randomized multicenter trial. *J. Pediatr. Gastroenterol. Nutr.* **2017**, *64*, 624–631. [CrossRef] [PubMed]
97. Steenhout, P.; Sperisen, P.; Martin, F.-P.; Sprenger, N.; Wernimont, S.; Pecquet, S.; Berger, B. Term infant formula supplemented with human milk oligosaccharides (2′-fucosyllactose and lacto-*N*-neotetraose) shifts stool microbiota and metabolic signatures closer to that of breastfed infants. *FASEB J.* **2016**, *30*, 275–277.
98. Berger, B.; Grathwohl, D.; Alliet, P.; Puccio, G.; Steenhout, P.; Sprenger, N. Stool microbiota in term infants fed formula supplemented with human milk oligosaccharides and reduced likelihood of antibiotic use. *J. Pediatr. Gastroenterol. Nutr.* **2016**, *63*, S407.

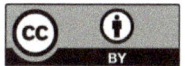

© 2018 by the authors. Licensee MDPI, Basel, Switzerland. This article is an open access article distributed under the terms and conditions of the Creative Commons Attribution (CC BY) license (http://creativecommons.org/licenses/by/4.0/).

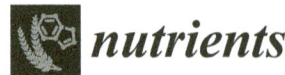

Review

Zinc and Sepsis

Wiebke Alker [1,2] and Hajo Haase [1,2,*]

[1] Department of Food Chemistry and Toxicology, Berlin Institute of Technology, 13355 Berlin, Germany; alker@tu-berlin.de
[2] TraceAge—DFG Research Unit on Interactions of Essential Trace Elements in Healthy and Diseased Elderly, Potsdam-Berlin-Jena, Germany
* Correspondence: Haase@tu-berlin.de; Tel.: +49-30-314-727-01

Received: 25 June 2018; Accepted: 24 July 2018; Published: 27 July 2018

Abstract: Sepsis, defined as a "life-threatening organ dysfunction caused by a dysregulated host-response to infection" is a major health issue worldwide and still lacks a fully elucidated pathobiology and uniform diagnostic tests. The trace element zinc is known to be crucial to ensure an appropriate immune response. During sepsis a redistribution of zinc from serum into the liver has been observed and several studies imply a correlation between zinc and sepsis outcome. Therefore the alterations of zinc concentrations in different tissues might serve as one part of the host's defense mechanism against pathogens during sepsis by diverse mechanisms. It has been suggested that zinc is involved in nutritional immunity, acts as a hepatoprotective agent, or a differentiation signal for innate immune cells, or supports the synthesis of acute phase proteins. Further knowledge about these events could help in the evaluation of how zinc could be optimally applied to improve treatment of septic patients. Moreover, the changes in zinc homeostasis are substantial and correlate with the severity of the disease, suggesting that zinc might also be useful as a diagnostic marker for evaluating the severity and predicting the outcome of sepsis.

Keywords: zinc; sepsis; biomarker; supplementation; homeostasis

1. Introduction

Zinc is of fundamental importance for the immune system and is involved in different pathologies. In recent years, indications have appeared that zinc homeostasis might be an important factor during sepsis. The following review focuses on the alterations of zinc homeostasis during sepsis and possible physiological functions of this process. It further discusses potential risks and benefits of zinc supplementation as well as a possible approach for using serum zinc as a biomarker for sepsis.

1.1. Sepsis

The term "sepsis" in relation to a disease has already been used by Hippocrates, but to this day it remains a challenge to compile a definition comprising its complexity [1]. This results from the fact that sepsis is rather a syndrome than an illness, showing a not yet fully elucidated pathobiology, and with uniform diagnostic tests still lacking [2]. Sepsis is responsible for about 6 million deaths per year, making it a critical illness and one of the major causes of mortality worldwide [3,4]. Its epidemiological burden is assumed to be much higher in low- and middle-income countries and the mortality rate is affected by the global national income [3,5].

There is an urgent need for an easily understandable definition in order to establish public awareness, as well as for improved and uniform diagnostic guidelines for an early recognition of sepsis [2,3]. In the past, different task forces have approached these issues [6,7]. A recent consensus defined sepsis as a "life-threatening organ dysfunction caused by a dysregulated host-response to infection" (Sepsis-3) [2]. To diagnose organ dysfunction in the clinical setting, Singer et al. recommend the Sequential Organ Failure Assessment (SOFA) score. It includes parameters to evaluate the functions of respiration, the liver, the cardiovascular system, the central nervous system, the kidneys, and coagulation. An elevation of the total SOFA score of 2 points or more indicates organ dysfunction [2,8].

Sepsis is initiated by an infection [2]. The pathogen triggers an immune response, comprising pro-inflammatory mechanisms to defeat the pathogen and regenerate the affected tissue, as well as subsequent anti-inflammatory mechanisms to counteract the pro-inflammatory actions in order to limit collateral damage in healthy tissue [9,10]. A dysregulation of this immune response, as it appears during sepsis, leads to an over-reaction of the immune system, which can affect both mechanisms described. Hyper-inflammation in the form of a systemic inflammatory response syndrome (SIRS) can lead to a damage of the host's own tissue. Immune-suppression, also known as compensatory anti-inflammatory response syndrome (CARS), leaves the host more vulnerable to secondary infections [2,11,12]. A wealth of literature is provided about sepsis and its symptoms, diagnostics, and possible medical treatment approaches (e.g., [10,11,13,14]), to which the reader is referred for more detailed information on these aspects of sepsis.

1.2. Zinc

Zinc is an essential trace element [15,16]. In the body it functions, for example, as a co-factor for a high number of enzymes or as a structural element for a variety of proteins [17]. Zinc deficiency can result in growth retardation, dermatitis, and hypogonadism, or symptoms such as delayed wound healing, thymic atrophy or lymphopenia, and high incidence of infection; the latter points are due to its particular importance for the immune system [18–20]. Consequently, zinc deficiency results in multiple immunological changes, including what seems to be a shift toward a predominantly innate immune response when the availability of zinc is limited [21]. One particularly important effect of zinc is a modulation of the production of inflammatory cytokines [22]. Moreover, zinc is crucial for the functioning of virtually all immune cells. For example, the differentiation of immature T-cells depends on zinc, because thymulin, a hormone involved in T-cell differentiation, depends on zinc as a co-factor [23,24]. In addition, the maturation of T-cells is influenced by their zinc status. On the one hand a deficiency results in altered ratios of Th1- and Th2-cells, an increased apoptosis-rate of immature T-cells, and consequently a decrease in T-cells in total [21,25–27]. On the other hand, zinc supplementation has also been shown to promote regulatory T-cell development and to suppress the maturation of Th17-cells, therefore having an inhibitory effect on Th17-mediated autoimmune-diseases [28–30].

On the molecular level, some functions of zinc have been linked to its role as a second messenger in immune cells. It has been shown that alterations in the intracellular free zinc-concentration function as a "zinc signal". Such a change in the intracellular free zinc concentration is induced by the binding of various ligands to their respective receptors, such as lipopolysaccharide (LPS) to Toll-like receptor 4 (TLR-4), or the corresponding antigens to immunoglobulin E when it is present on the high-affinity immunoglobulin E-receptor (FcεRI). Different kinds of immune cells vary in their expression of receptors that utilize zinc; consequently zinc signals mediate diverse events, for example, formation of pro-inflammatory cytokines by monocytes [31], presentation of major histocompatibility complex (MHC) class II molecules at the surface of dendritic cells [32], formation of neutrophil extracellular traps by neutrophil granulocytes [33], or proliferation of T-cells [34].

The essentiality of zinc for the immune system has been known since the 1960s and the corresponding mechanistic knowledge has been expanding ever since. Its importance for the immune system is based on various different mechanisms, each in its own way essential to ensure the functionality of the immune system and the accurate processes of immune response, especially for inflammatory processes. As a complete summary would exceed the scope of this article, the reader is referred to recent review articles on the subject of zinc and immunity for more comprehensive information [35,36] as well as to a recent review on the protective role of zinc during sepsis [37].

2. Zinc Homeostasis during Sepsis

Zinc has not only a crucial role in ensuring a proper immune response. Another observation in the context of zinc and the immune system is an altered zinc homeostasis of the host during an infection, which is discussed below.

2.1. Changes in Zinc Homeostasis

The host's response to an infection or injury is referred to as an acute phase reaction (APR). This process aims to defeat the insult, take actions against ongoing tissue damage, and re-establish homeostasis. One of the characteristics of APR is hypozincemia. To study the time course of hypozincemia and examine possible underlying mechanisms, Gaetke et al. injected LPS to healthy volunteers in order to induce an inflammatory response. Subsequently, an increase in serum tumor necrosis factor α (TNF-α) and interleukin-6 (IL-6) was observed, followed by a decrease in serum zinc concentrations. To explain hypozincemia in their model of infection the authors suggested an internal redistribution of zinc, mediated by cytokines [38]. The analysis of serum from sepsis patients in the intensive care unit (ICU) revealed that serum zinc concentrations were reduced compared to a healthy control group or the normal physiological range [39–41]. Probably these differences were not caused by a zinc-deficient state due to malnutrition, but redistribution of zinc within the patients' bodies. Consistently, a study by Hoeger et al. showed a time-dependent decline of the serum zinc concentrations after induction of sepsis in a porcine model [42]. In order to reveal the mechanisms responsible for the observed hypozincemia, Luizzi et al. used a mouse model and induced inflammation either by turpentine or LPS. Zrt-, Irt-like protein (ZIP)14 mRNA was the transporter transcript that was upregulated the most. This upregulation was liver-specific and an increase of ZIP14 on the plasma membrane of hepatocytes was shown. Further studies indicated a role of the inflammatory cytokines IL-6 and IL-1β in the upregulation of ZIP14. Also, an increase in metallothionein (MT)-1 mRNA in the liver has been observed [43,44]. This observation of enhanced MT expression has been described before in the context of APR [45–47]. As reviewed in detail before, MTs function as intracellular metal-binding proteins and are crucial to maintain the intracellular zinc homeostasis. Their expression is induced by a number of metals, one of them zinc [48]. The increased liver zinc concentrations accompanying hypozincemia lead to an enhanced need for zinc-binding proteins in order to ensure the intracellular zinc homeostasis. The production of MT in the liver seems to be regulated by cytokines as well as zinc [49]. Using a murine model, the already-described decline in serum zinc concentration and an increase in liver zinc level were observed after induction of sepsis. The analysis of the time-course of mRNA expression in the liver first showed a successive upregulation of ZIPs 4, 6, and 10 within the first day, which then returned to near normal levels at 72 h after induction of sepsis. The mRNA expression of ZIP14 increased at 9 h and stayed upregulated for the time of the investigation (72 h), which is in line with the observations described previously and supports a major role for ZIP14 in the redistribution of zinc during sepsis [50]. Taken together, the APR comprises a fundamental change in liver zinc homeostasis and apparent zinc deficiency in the serum [50,51].

The studies mentioned so far aimed, among other things, on understanding the mechanisms responsible for the observed hypozincemia and to track the redistribution of zinc in the body. An alternative approach to broaden the understanding of how certain processes are changed during sepsis is gene expression analysis. The method allows insights into the impact of sepsis at the translational level. The analysis of blood samples from pediatric septic shock patients showed a regulation of genes that are involved in a large number of signaling pathways and gene networks, especially those related to immunity and inflammation. Also, it has been shown that up to 12% of the gene probes that showed a significantly decreased expression compared to the control group are associated with the categories of "zinc, zinc finger, metal-binding and zinc-ion binding" [52]. These results suggest a repression of genes involved in zinc homeostasis, or depending on an intact zinc homeostasis, as a significant feature of pediatric septic shock [52–55]. Further, the question arises as to whether differences in gene expression in pediatric septic shock survivors and non-survivors can be observed. Regarding zinc homeostasis, two isoforms of MT have been identified that showed an increased expression in non-survivors compared to survivors. In addition, non-survivors had a significantly lower serum zinc concentration compared to survivors. Considering the zinc-binding properties of MT, Wong and colleagues interpret these results to indirectly imply that increased MT expression in non survivors might affect zinc homeostasis and thereby serum zinc concentration [53].

Taken together, different approaches imply a contribution of zinc and its altered homeostasis to the pathobiology of sepsis.

2.2. Possible Reasons for the Redistribution of Zinc

With respect to the considerable differences of serum zinc concentrations between sepsis patients and the corresponding control groups, as well as the finely tuned alterations of zinc homeostasis, it can be assumed that these are part of a directed process that aims to benefit the host in defeating the pathogen. This process includes a decrease in serum zinc concentration as well as an increase in liver zinc concentration, whereas both aspects seem to benefit the host's defense against pathogens. Figure 1 gives a brief overview of the processes causing the alterations in zinc concentrations, as well as the possible beneficial effects.

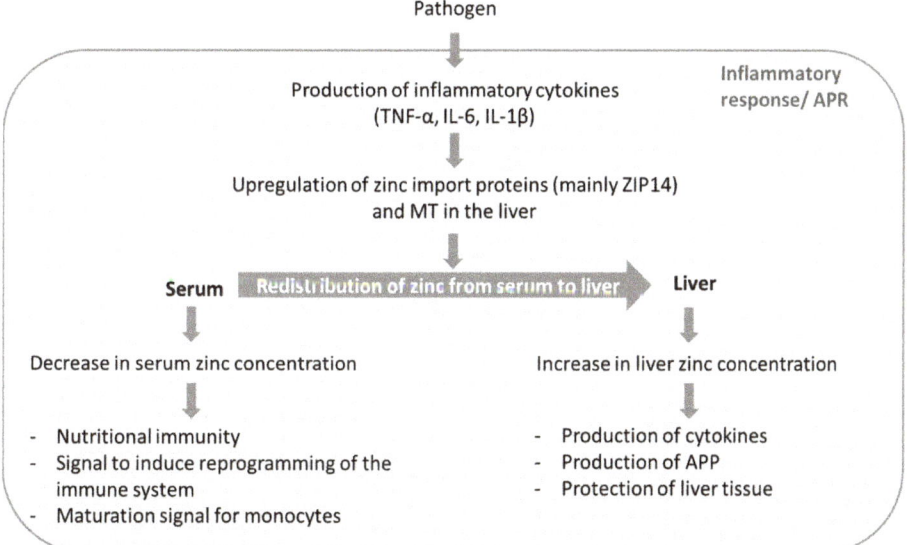

Figure 1. Possible functions of zinc in sepsis. During the APR of sepsis zinc is redistributed from serum to liver. This process results in decreased serum zinc concentration and increased liver zinc. The altered zinc concentrations seem to serve different functions and to be a part of the host's defense against pathogens. APR: acute phase reaction; IL: interleukin; TNF: tumor necrosis factor; MT: metallothionein; APP: acute phase proteins.

Research on zinc homeostasis in the context of sepsis delivered a variety of explanations for the beneficial effects of a redistribution of zinc. The respective studies are discussed below.

One of the main effects of the redistribution of zinc is an accumulation of zinc in the liver. Hence, it seems as is if a higher liver zinc level might benefit the host during infection. Among other things, the APR is not only characterized by the previously mentioned redistribution of zinc, but also by production of acute phase proteins (APP) and the release of cytokines [56,57]. Zinc serves as an important structural element for many proteins and is required by enzymes involved in transcription and translation. Therefore, the higher synthesis rate of APP in the liver could cause an increased requirement for zinc during APR [56–58]. With respect to cytokine production a knockout (k.o.) of ZIP14 in mice, a transporter important for the regulation of zinc homeostasis in hepatocytes, showed lower mRNA expression of TNF-α, IL-6, IL-1β, and IL-10 in the liver compared to wild-type (w.t.) mice after induction of sepsis in a murine model. Simultaneously, plasma levels of TNF-α, IL-6, and IL-10 were significantly higher in k.o. than in w.t. mice. The results indicate a disadvantage of the ZIP14 k.o. mice during sepsis based on increased markers of inflammation and an influence of zinc, transported by ZIP14, on the production of cytokines during APR. However this observation is surprising, because a decrease in mRNA expression would be expected to result in lower cytokine levels. Possible explanations would be elevated cytokine expression elsewhere in the body, or an impact on mechanisms mediating the expression of antagonists of the pro-inflammatory cytokines [50].

Other studies suggest that the altered zinc supply during endotoxemia has a major influence on energy production in the liver. Injection of LPS caused an increase in hepatic zinc and MT in w.t. mice, whereas zinc levels stayed unchanged in MT k.o. mice. At the same time the liver glucose of the former stayed unchanged while the levels in MT k.o. mice decreased significantly. These results imply a lack of hepatic gluconeogenesis in the MT KO mice and a role for MT, and most likely also for zinc, in maintaining glycaemia after induction of an infection [59].

A protective role of zinc for the liver has also been suggested. Using murine models it was shown that after injection of endotoxin, zinc-deficient nutrition resulted in enhanced lipid peroxidation in the liver compared to the zinc adequate group [60]. Another study showed that zinc pre-treatment of mice resulted in an increased intracellular availability of zinc in liver cells and was accompanied by decreased accumulation of superoxide and necrotic cell death in the liver after injection of LPS [61]. Both experimental observations support a protective role of zinc in the liver during infection. Interestingly, after injection of endotoxin, Sakagouchi et al. saw an increase in MT only in the zinc adequate group, but not in zinc-deficient animals, and therefore suggested a relation between zinc concentration, endotoxin-induced MT and lipid peroxidation [60]. In contrast, Zhou et al. observed the protective effects of zinc pre-treatment on liver cells in w.t. mice as well as MT k.o. mice, leading them to propose an effect of zinc independent of MT [61]. These results are not necessarily contradictory, but could imply that the protective effect of zinc on the liver could work in more than one way. Further studies on this topic would be useful, since organ dysfunction is one of the hallmarks of sepsis and a better understanding of its mechanisms is the basis of a possible prevention. In summary, studies show multiple and diverse functions of zinc in the liver during the onset of sepsis, suggesting a physiological basis for the accumulation of zinc.

The redistribution of zinc and accumulation in the liver is accompanied by a decrease in serum zinc concentration. With regard to the host's defense against pathogens, this effect might have some benefits as well. One protective mechanism of the host is referred to as nutritional immunity. Pathogens, just like all living organisms, require transition metals for their survival. The host's strategy is to restrict the pathogens' access to essential transition metals, for example by lowering their concentrations in the serum or secretion of metal ion binding proteins. This process is not limited to zinc but has been described for other micronutrients, such as iron or manganese [62].

A decrease in the serum zinc concentration has also been shown to influence the respective number and maturation of immune cells. Therefore, the alteration of serum zinc during the APR might function as a signal. Using a murine model of zinc deficiency, a downregulation of lymphopoiesis and upregulation of myelopoiesis was found [19,21,27,63]. In line with this observation, a decrease of intracellular zinc occurred as a result of homeostatic changes during monocytic differentiation of HL60 cells. Moreover, experiments simulating zinc deficiency showed that lower zinc levels promoted the development of HL-60 cells along the myeloid lineage into functionally mature macrophages [64].

The immune cells that benefit from a decline of serum zinc are part of the innate immune system. They represent the first line of host defense and provide a faster response than the cells of the adaptive immune system. Fraker and King proposed the hypothesis of a "reprogramming of the immune system" during zinc deficiency in the form of a shift from adaptive immunity to predominantly innate immunity [65]. Here, limited resources would be directed toward an immediate defense on the expense of long-term protection. In the context of sepsis, the reduction of serum zinc as a promoting signal for the innate immune system might be an attempt to focus the defense mechanisms toward a fast innate immune reaction in the face of a potentially overwhelming infection.

The various aspects by which zinc homeostasis seems to be involved in the body's defense against pathogens suggest that the redistribution of zinc in the course of sepsis could serve multiple physiological purposes. However, further research will be required to evaluate the physiological significance of the different processes, thereby widening our understanding of the zinc-dependent endogenous defense mechanisms. This knowledge is required to develop medical approaches in order to support the host's body and its defense during sepsis.

2.3. Possible Adverse Effects of Zinc-Redistribution

Despite the potential physiological roles of the redistribution of zinc, this process might also cause some adverse effects, especially the decrease in serum zinc concentration. Possible symptoms of a low serum zinc concentration due to zinc deficiency caused by malnutrition are higher levels of pro-inflammatory cytokines, higher markers of oxidative stress, and oxidative damage to proteins, lipids, and DNA [66–70]. Notably, zinc deficiency and sepsis show several parallels in addition to low serum zinc concentrations. The severe effects of zinc deficiency on the functionality of the immune system have already been described in the introduction, including a decrease in T-cell numbers and function [20]. Dysfunction and apoptosis of T-cells have also been observed in the context of sepsis [71–73]. Other symptoms of zinc deficiency have been found during sepsis as well, for example the overproduction of pro-inflammatory cytokines and SIRS, which is a hallmark of sepsis and a major factor in the host's dysregulation to an infection during sepsis [11]. Furthermore, effects such as lipid peroxidation and oxidative damage of DNA, proteins, and mitochondria have been observed [74–76]. In light of the parallels between symptoms of zinc deficiency and sepsis, further research should elucidate the question whether the body's reaction to an infection might cause a decrease in bioavailable zinc severe enough to contribute to, or maybe even cause, these common symptoms during sepsis.

In this context it is of interest to mention that several studies have shown a correlation between a patient's serum zinc concentration and the severity of the inflammatory response or sepsis. In critically ill patients, those with a high SOFA score showed a significantly lower serum zinc concentration than patients with a low SOFA score, whereby a higher SOFA score was associated with higher mortality [2,58]. In line with these results serum zinc concentrations were found to be inversely correlated with the SOFA score in other studies, as well [39,77]. Yet another study revealed a significantly lower serum zinc concentration in sepsis patients who developed a recurrent sepsis compared to those that did not. Additionally, sepsis non-survivors had a significantly lower serum zinc concentration than survivors [41]. Because zinc fulfils a great number of crucial functions in the body, and especially the immune system, it seems reasonable that a decrease of bioavailable zinc in the serum could contribute to some adverse effects, thereby aggravating sepsis.

3. Zinc Supplementation

The correlation between low serum zinc concentrations and a higher mortality rate or chance of recurrence raises the question, if supplementation of zinc might be a treatment option to improve the outcomes of sepsis. Table 1 gives an overview of zinc supplementation studies in the context of sepsis in humans. In these studies zinc supplementation took place after the onset of sepsis. Some of them show a beneficial effect of zinc in form of a lower mortality rate and a better neurological development of neonates [78–80]. However, it was also observed that supplementation did not result in any significant differences between the zinc group and the control group [81] or even showed a harmful effect [82].

The published animal studies mostly examined the effects of prophylactic zinc supplementation (Table 2). In several of them the supplementation of zinc prior to induction of sepsis showed beneficial effects, such as improved survival, lower serum concentrations of pro-inflammatory cytokines, lower bacterial burden or improved pulmonary function compared to the control-group [50,83–85]. However, for the animal studies the results are also not consistent and a missing effect of zinc supplementation is reported [86] as well as a harmful outcome in a case where zinc was applied during the acute phase [87]. The negative results of zinc supplementation may be explained by the fact that the reduction of zinc levels during sepsis may occur for a reason, such as the above-mentioned physiological functions. High doses of zinc were shown to have a pro-inflammatory effect [88] and might therefore aggravate inflammation, or zinc supplementation could potentially interfere with nutritional immunity, one of the endogenous defense mechanisms based on a shortage of zinc in the serum [62].

Another important factor is the bioavailability of serum zinc. Albumin is the major zinc-buffering protein [89] as well as a negative APP [56,90]. Its concentration decreases during sepsis, leading to a decreased zinc-binding capacity of the serum [42]. As a consequence, supplementing sepsis patients until the "normal" total serum zinc concentration is restored would result in a supraphysiological concentration of free, and thereby bioavailable, zinc in these patients.

Correcting zinc deficiency prior to sepsis is certainly beneficial, but difficult to realize, as in most cases sepsis cannot be predicted. Moderate supplementation during sepsis might, in some cases, turn out to be helpful, as well. This may be particularly so in patients with pre-existing zinc deficiency that is so pronounced that the liver cannot accumulate sufficient amounts to exert the abovementioned protective effects of zinc. However, as the reduction of serum zinc seems to be a necessary physiological process, in these cases extreme care needs to be taken in order not to exceed the zinc-binding capacity of the serum to avoid negative effects, such as counteracting nutritional immunity or aggravating inflammation.

The endogenous processes, which are supposed to be affected by the supplementation of zinc, are quite complex and fine-tuned. As illustrated by the divergence of the study results, effective zinc supplementation has to be just as elaborate with regard to timing as well as dosage in order to achieve optimal results.

Table 1. Zinc supplementation studies in septic patients.

Study Population	Intervention/Zn-Supply	Observation Time Points	Results (Zinc Group vs. Control Group)	Reference
Neonates with clinical signs suggestive of sepsis and at least two screening tests positive	Zinc group *: Antibiotic treatment, dose of 3 mg/kg bodyweight (BW) zinc sulfate monohydrate twice a day for 10 days (corresponding to 2.1 mg/kg BW Zn^{2+} per day) Control group: Antibiotic treatment	Measurement of blood samples from base line (BL) and after 10 days	• Significant increase in serum zinc concentrations compared to BL • Significant decrease in TNF-α compared to BL • Lower mortality rate, but not reaching significance (7.4% compared to 16.4%) • Similar duration of hospitalization	[78]
Neonates with clinical features of sepsis and positive blood culture or positive sepsis screening tests	Zinc group *: Antibiotic treatment, dose of 3 mg/kg BW zinc sulfate monohydrate twice a day for 10 days (corresponding to 2.1 mg/kg BW Zn^{2+} per day) Control group: Antibiotic treatment	Measurement of blood samples from BL and after 10 days	• Increase in serum zinc concentrations compared to BL, but not reaching significance • Lower mortality rate, but not reaching significance (4.5% compared to 13.6%) • Better neurological status (chance of having abnormalities is 70% less) at one month of age • Similar duration of hospitalization	[79]
Neonates with clinical manifestations of sepsis who exhibited two positive screening tests	Zinc group *: Antibiotic treatment, dose of 3 mg/kg BW zinc sulfate monohydrate twice a day for 10 days (corresponding to 2.1 mg/kg BW Zn^{2+} per day) Control group: Antibiotic treatment	Measurement of blood samples from BL and after 10 days	• Significant increase in serum zinc concentrations • Significantly lower mortality rate (6.6% compared to 17.3%) • Better neurodevelopment (significantly better Mental Development Quotient) at 12 month of age	[80]

Table 1. *Cont.*

Study Population	Intervention/Zn-Supply	Observation Time Points	Results (Zinc Group vs. Control Group)	Reference
Neonates with probable sepsis	Zinc group *: Antibiotic treatment, dose of 1 mg/kg BW zinc sulfate per day until the final outcome (discharge/death) (corresponding to 0.4 mg/kg BW Zn^{2+} per day) Control group: Antibiotic treatment, dose of placebo until the final outcome (discharge/death)	Final outcome at discharge/death	• No significant differences in mortality rate • No significant differences in duration of hospital stay • No significant differences in requirement of antibiotic treatment	[81]
Patients with pancreatitis or catheter sepsis	Zinc group *: Total parenteral nutrition, 30 mg zinc sulfate per day for 3 days (corresponding to 12.1 mg Zn^{2+} per day) Control group: Total parenteral nutrition, 0 mg zinc sulfate for 3 days	Measurement of blood samples from BL, day 1, 2, 3; highest temperatures from patients' bedside charts from day 1, 2, 3	• Higher temperatures, reaching significance on day 3 • No difference in serum IL-6 and ceruloplasmin	[82]

* In all studies, zinc supplementation was started after the onset of sepsis.

Table 2. Zinc supplementation studies in animal models of sepsis. LPS: lipopolysaccharide.

Animals	Sepsis Model	Intervention/Zn-Supply	Results (Zinc Group vs. Control Group)	Reference
Male mice (C57BL/6)	Intraperitoneal (i. p.) fecal slurry injection; sacrifice of mice at 24 h to conduct assays or observed 72 h for survival study	Zinc group: Injection of 10 mg/kg BW zinc gluconate every 24 h for 3 days prior to induction of sepsis, injection continued every 24 h after induction of peritonitis (corresponding to 1.4 mg/kg BW Zn^{2+} per day) Control group: Injection of equal volume of saline at the same time points as for the zinc group	• Significantly improved survival following sepsis at 72 h after induction • Significantly lower myeloperoxidase activity in lung tissue (at 24 h) • Significantly lower bacterial burden in blood and spleen (at 24 h) • Significantly lower serum keratinocyte chemoattractant concentration (at 24 h) • No significant difference between serum concentration of IL6, IL-1β, IL-10	[84]
Male and female mice (C57BL/6)	Cecal ligation and puncture; sacrifice of mice at 24 h	Zinc group: High-zinc diet (180 mg/kg) for 7 days prior to induction of sepsis Control group: Zinc-adequate diet (30 mg/kg) for 7 days prior to induction of sepsis	• Significantly lower IL-6 mRNA expression in hepatocytes • Significantly lower TNF-α mRNA expression in hepatic leukocytes • Significantly lower S100A9 mRNA expression in white blood cells • Significantly lower serum concentrations of TNF-α, S100A8 and S100A9 • Significantly lower serum concentration of plasma alanine aminotransferase • Significantly lower bacterial burden in blood and spleen	[50]
Male and female juvenile mice (C57BL/6)	I. p. cecal-slurry injection and measurement of blood samples at 6 and 12 h; mice were sacrificed at 6 h or 12 h or observed for 72 h for survival study	Zinc group: Injection of 10 mg/kg BW zinc gluconate once a day for 3 days prior to induction of sepsis (corresponding to 1.4 mg/kg BW Zn^{2+} per day) Control group: Injection of equal volume of saline for 3 days prior to induction of sepsis	• Significantly improved survival of following sepsis at 72 h after induction • Significantly lower myeloperoxidase activity in lung tissue (at 12 h) • Significantly lower bacterial burden in peritoneal fluid (at 12 h) • Significantly lower serum concentrations of IL-2 (at 6 h, 12 h), IL-6 (at 6 h, 12 h), IL-1β (at 6 h), and keratinocyte-derived chemokines (at 12 h)	[83]

Table 2. Cont.

Animals	Sepsis Model	Intervention/Zn-Supply	Results (Zinc Group vs. Control Group)	Reference
Female farm pigs (Deutsche Landrasse)	Intravenous infusion of LPS and measurement of the parameters for a duration of 300 min after infusion of LPS; pigs were sacrificed at 500 min of total registration time	Zinc group: Infusion of 25 mg/kg BW zinc-bis-(DL-hydrogenaspartate) 24 h prior to infusion of LPS (corresponding to 5 mg/kg BW Zn^{2+} per day) Control group: Infusion of saline 24 h prior to infusion of LPS	• Increased arterial and venous oxygen pressure (reaching significance at 45 min or 210 min) • Increased arterial and venous oxygen saturation (reaching significance at 210 min) • Stable intrapulmonary shunt (instead of an increase in the control group) • Stable extravascular lung water (EVLW) (instead of an increase in the control group)	[85]
Female farm pigs (Deutsche Landrasse)	Intravenous infusion of LPS and measurement of parameters for a duration of 60 min after infusion of LPS; pigs were sacrificed at 60 min and organs removed for analysis	Zinc group: Infusion of 25 mg/kg BW zinc-bis-(DL-hydrogenaspartate) 2 h prior to infusion of LPS (corresponding to 5 mg/kg BW Zn^{2+} per day) Control group: Infusion of saline 2 h prior to infusion of LPS	• Decrease in arterial and venous oxygen pressure (reaching significance at 30 min) • Decrease in arterial and venous oxygen saturation (reaching significance at 30 min or 15 min) • Increase in intrapulmonary shunt (reaching significance at 30 min) • Increase in EVLW (reaching significance at 45 min) • Increase in mean hemoglobin (reaching significance at 30 min) • Increase in IL-6 and TNF-α plasma concentrations (reaching significance at 0 min or 45 min) • Significant higher weights of lungs, width of alveolar septae and rate of paracentral liver necrosis	[87]
Female farm pigs (Deutsche Landrasse)	Intravenous infusion of LPS and measurement of parameters for a duration of 1020 min, with infusion of zinc from 600 to 720 min; pigs were sacrificed at the end of the study period and a necropsy carried out	Zinc group: Infusion of LPS at 0 h, 5 h and 12 h, infusion of 25 mg/kg BW zinc-bis-(DL-hydrogenaspartate) (corresponding to 5 mg/kg BW Zn^{2+} per day) at 10 h during sepsis Control group: Infusion of LPS at 0 h, 5 h and 12 h, infusion of saline at 10 h during sepsis	• Trend to higher arterial and venous oxygen pressure • Trend to higher arterial and venous oxygen saturation • No significant differences in intrapulmonary shunt • No significant differences in EVLW • Different courses in IL-6 and TNF-α plasma concentrations, at the end almost similar levels	[86]

4. Serum Zinc Concentration as a Possible Biomarker for Sepsis

In addition to a potential therapeutic value of zinc supplementation, the altered zinc homeostasis could have potential to be utilized for establishing a biomarker based on the serum zinc level of a patient. In a porcine model of sepsis, the decline of the serum zinc concentration was the first marker of inflammation, already statistically significant one hour after induction of sepsis. Thereby, it was an earlier indicator for inflammation than the increase of the pro-inflammatory cytokines IL-6 and TNF-α, which reached statistical significance two hours after induction of sepsis [42]. However, hypozincemia is activated in non-infectious as well as infectious inflammation. The ability to discriminate between the different causes for hypozincemia would be relevant for a use of zinc as a biomarker for sepsis. So far the studies vary in their results as to whether there is a significant difference in the serum zinc concentration of sepsis patients and a critically ill control group, surgical control group, or trauma patients [39,41,91]. Further studies would be required to evaluate the potential of serum zinc concentration as a biomarker for sepsis, including large clinical studies and the evaluation of clinical data sets to proof its validity and prospective value.

According to Singer et al., a diagnostic marker for sepsis should be easily to obtain and available promptly at reasonable cost [2]. Provided the evaluation studies on serum zinc concentration as a biomarker for sepsis turn out to be positive, this marker would fulfil Singer et al.'s demands [2]: It would allow for early recognition, which is crucial to improve the patient's outcome and decrease the sepsis-related mortality rate. Also, patient serum is easily to obtain and the parameter could be monitored closely once the patient is under medical supervision. If the required infrastructure is available, an analysis of the serum zinc concentration delivers fast results at reasonable cost.

One hindrance for the use of zinc as a marker in sepsis might be the necessary infrastructure. Presently, atomic absorption spectrometry or inductively-coupled plasma mass spectrometry are being used to quantify zinc. Even with the required instruments available the quality of the results strongly depends on the analytical abilities of the performing personnel or laboratory [92]. If this sophisticated equipment is not available, e.g., in rural areas or countries with a less developed infrastructure, sending the samples to external labs might cause significant delay in obtaining these time-sensitive results, nullifying the advantage of an early diagnostic marker. Some basic work on easier point-of-care devices to measure the serum zinc concentrations has been reported, but these still have to reach clinical applications [93,94].

Other tools widely used to detect zinc in biological samples are fluorescent probes [95]. However, they have only sparsely been used in the context of sepsis thus far. One example is the application of Zinpyr-1 by Hoeger et al. in serum samples from a porcine model of sepsis [42]. It should be noted that these probes do not measure total zinc, but determine the amount of free zinc in the sample. Still, this parameter might be interesting to look at in the context of sepsis, because it represents the amount of bioavailable zinc and has been suggested as an alternative biomarker for a person's zinc status [96].

Some aspects regarding the mechanism mediating the redistribution of zinc have not been fully revealed yet. Once understood, they might contribute to an even better use of zinc homeostasis as a diagnostic parameter in sepsis. Hoeger et al. observed a continuous decline of serum zinc concentration from one hour after induction of sepsis in vivo. However, for up to two hours no induction of mRNA expression of MT-1, MT-2, and ZIP14 was observed in an in vitro model of hepatoma cells after incubation with IL-1β, IL-6, or LPS [42]. Wessels et al. reported the lowest serum zinc concentration in their sepsis model at 9 h after induction whereas the upregulation of ZIP14 in the liver and the increase in liver zinc have been observed from hour 9 on after induction [50]. These studies raise further questions, mainly as to how the decline of serum zinc concentration is mediated in the initial phase, and if zinc may be located in some other part of the body in the period from its disappearance from the serum until it is finally detected in the liver.

5. Conclusions

Zinc is an essential trace element and has been shown to be crucial for ensuring an adequate immune response. In the context of sepsis the host's zinc homeostasis is altered. Various study results imply some of the alterations to be part of the host's defense mechanism against pathogens (Figure 1). There are indications that a patient's zinc supply and serum zinc concentration is associated with severity, outcome, and recurrence of sepsis. Zinc seems to have potential to be used as a biomarker or even as a starting point for a therapeutic approach. Further research is required to broaden the understanding of zinc homeostasis during sepsis and the underlying mechanisms as well as to evaluate the possible clinical applicability of this knowledge.

Funding: This work was funded by a grant from Deutsche Forschungsgemeinschaft (HA 4318/4-1) within the TraceAge—DFG Research Unit on Interactions of essential trace elements in healthy and diseased elderly, Potsdam-Berlin-Jena, FOR 2558/1.

Conflicts of Interest: The authors declare no conflict of interest.

References

1. Funk, D.J.; Parrillo, J.E.; Kumar, A. Sepsis and septic shock: A history. *Crit. Care Clin.* **2009**, *25*, 83–101. [CrossRef] [PubMed]
2. Singer, M.; Deutschman, C.S.; Seymour, C.W.; Shankar-Hari, M.; Annane, D.; Bauer, M.; Bellomo, R.; Bernard, G.R.; Chiche, J.-D.; Coopersmith, C.M.; et al. The third international consensus definitions for sepsis and septic shock (Sepsis-3). *JAMA* **2016**, *315*, 801–810. [CrossRef] [PubMed]
3. WHO (The World Health Organization). *WHA Resolution A70/13—Improving the Prevention, Diagnosis and Clinical Management of Sepsis*; WHO: Geneva, Switzerland, 2017.
4. WHO (The World Health Organization). *WHO Secretariat Report A70/13—Improving the Prevention, Diagnosis and Clinical Management of Sepsis*; WHO: Geneva, Switzerland, 2017.
5. Vincent, J.-L.; Marshall, J.C.; Ñamendys-Silva, S.A.; François, B.; Martin-Loeches, I.; Lipman, J.; Reinhart, K.; Antonelli, M.; Pickkers, P.; Njimi, H.; et al. Assessment of the worldwide burden of critical illness: The Intensive Care Over Nations (ICON) audit. *Lancet Respir. Med.* **2014**, *2*, 380–386. [CrossRef]
6. Bone, R.C.; Balk, R.A.; Cerra, F.B.; Dellinger, R.P.; Fein, A.M.; Knaus, W.A.; Schein, R.M.H.; Sibbald, W.J. Definitions for Sepsis and Organ Failure and Guidelines for the Use of Innovative Therapies in Sepsis. *Chest* **1992**, *101*, 1644–1655. [CrossRef] [PubMed]
7. Levy, M.M.; Fink, M.P.; Marshall, J.C.; Abraham, E.; Angus, D.; Cook, D.; Cohen, J.; Opal, S.M.; Vincent, J.; Ramsay, G. 2001 SCCM/ESICM/ACCP/ATS/SIS international sepsis definitions conference. *Crit. Care Med.* **2003**, *31*, 1250–1256. [CrossRef] [PubMed]
8. Vincent, J.-L.; Moreno, R.; Takala, J.; Willatts, S.; Mendonça, A.D.; Bruining, H.; Reinhart, C.K.; Suter, P.M.; Thijs, L.G. The SOFA (Sepsis-related Organ Failure Assessment) score to describe organ dysfunction/failure. *Intensive Care Med.* **1996**, *22*, 707–710. [CrossRef] [PubMed]
9. Takeuchi, O.; Akira, S. Pattern recognition receptors and inflammation. *Cell* **2010**, *140*, 805–820. [CrossRef] [PubMed]
10. Van der Poll, T.; Opal, S.M. Host–pathogen interactions in sepsis. *Lancet Infect. Dis.* **2008**, *8*, 32–43. [CrossRef]
11. Angus, D.C.; van der Poll, T. Severe sepsis and septic shock. *N. Engl. J. Med.* **2013**, *369*, 840–851. [CrossRef] [PubMed]
12. Bone, R.C.; Grodzin, C.J.; Balk, R.A. Sepsis: A New hypothesis for pathogenesis of the disease process. *CHEST* **1997**, *112*, 235–243. [CrossRef] [PubMed]
13. Chong, J.; Dumont, T.; Francis-frank, L.; Balaan, M. Sepsis and septic shock: A review. *Crit. Care Nurs. Q.* **2015**, *38*, 111–120. [CrossRef] [PubMed]
14. Ward, N.S.; Casserly, B.; Ayala, A. The Compensatory Anti-inflammatory Response syndrome (CARS) in critically ill patients. *Clin. Chest Med.* **2008**, *29*, 617–625. [CrossRef] [PubMed]
15. Prasad, A.S.; Halsted, J.A.; Nadimi, M. Syndrome of iron deficiency anemia, hepatosplenomegaly, hypogonadism, dwarfism and geophagia. *Am. J. Med.* **1961**, *31*, 532–546. [CrossRef]
16. Prasad, A.S. Importance of zinc in human nutrition. *Am. J. Clin. Nutr.* **1967**, *20*, 648–652. [CrossRef] [PubMed]

17. Coleman, J.E. Zinc proteins: Enzymes, storage proteins, transcription factors, and replication proteins. *Annu. Rev. Biochem.* **1992**, *61*, 897–946. [CrossRef] [PubMed]
18. Evans, G.W. Zinc and its deficiency diseases. *Clin. Physiol. Biochem.* **1986**, *4*, 94–98. [PubMed]
19. King, L.E.; Frentzel, J.W.; Mann, J.J.; Fraker, P.J. Chronic zinc deficiency in mice disrupted T cell lymphopoiesis and erythropoiesis while B cell lymphopoiesis and myelopoiesis were maintained. *J. Am. Coll. Nutr.* **2005**, *24*, 494–502. [CrossRef] [PubMed]
20. Prasad, A.S.; Meftah, S.; Abdallah, J.; Kaplan, J.; Brewer, G.J.; Bach, J.F.; Dardenne, M. Serum thymulin in human zinc deficiency. *J. Clin. Investig.* **1988**, *82*, 1202–1210. [CrossRef] [PubMed]
21. Fraker, P.J.; King, L.E. A distinct role for apoptosis in the changes in lymphopoiesis and myelopoiesis created by deficiencies in zinc. *FASEB J.* **2001**, *15*, 2572–2578. [CrossRef] [PubMed]
22. Mayer, L.S.; Uciechowski, P.; Meyer, S.; Schwerdtle, T.; Rink, L.; Haase, H. Differential impact of zinc deficiency on phagocytosis, oxidative burst, and production of pro-inflammatory cytokines by human monocytes. *Metallomics* **2014**, *6*, 1288–1295. [CrossRef] [PubMed]
23. Dardenne, M.; Pléau, J.M.; Nabarra, B.; Lefrancier, P.; Derrien, M.; Choay, J.; Bach, J.F. Contribution of zinc and other metals to the biological activity of the serum thymic factor. *Proc. Natl. Acad. Sci. USA* **1982**, *79*, 5370–5373. [CrossRef] [PubMed]
24. Incefy, G.S.; Mertelsmann, R.; Yata, K.; Dardenne, M.; Bach, J.F.; Good, R.A. Induction of differentiation in human marrow T cell precursors by the synthetic serum thymic factor, FTS. *Clin. Exp. Immunol.* **1980**, *40*, 396–406. [PubMed]
25. Prasad, A.S. Effects of zinc deficiency on Th1 and Th2 cytokine shifts. *J. Infect. Dis.* **2000**, *182*, S62–S68. [CrossRef] [PubMed]
26. Beck, F.W.; Prasad, A.S.; Kaplan, J.; Fitzgerald, J.T.; Brewer, G.J. Changes in cytokine production and T cell subpopulations in experimentally induced zinc-deficient humans. *Am. J. Physiol. Endocrinol. Metab.* **1997**, *272*, E1002–E1007. [CrossRef] [PubMed]
27. King, L.E.; Osati-Ashtiani, F.; Fraker, P.J. Apoptosis plays a distinct role in the loss of precursor lymphocytes during zinc deficiency in mice. *J. Nutr.* **2002**, *132*, 974–979. [CrossRef] [PubMed]
28. Rosenkranz, E.; Maywald, M.; Hilgers, R.-D.; Brieger, A.; Clarner, T.; Kipp, M.; Plümakers, B.; Meyer, S.; Schwerdtle, T.; Rink, L. Induction of regulatory T cells in Th1-/Th17-driven experimental autoimmune encephalomyelitis by zinc administration. *J. Nutr. Biochem.* **2016**, *29*, 116–123. [CrossRef] [PubMed]
29. Lee, H.; Kim, B.; Choi, Y.H.; Hwang, Y.; Kim, D.H.; Cho, S.; Hong, S.J.; Lee, W. Inhibition of interleukin-1β-mediated interleukin-1 receptor-associated kinase 4 phosphorylation by zinc leads to repression of memory T helper type 17 response in humans. *Immunology* **2015**, *146*, 645–656. [CrossRef] [PubMed]
30. Kitabayashi, C.; Fukada, T.; Kanamoto, M.; Ohashi, W.; Hojyo, S.; Atsumi, T.; Ueda, N.; Azuma, I.; Hirota, H.; Murakami, M.; et al. Zinc suppresses Th17 development via inhibition of STAT3 activation. *Int. Immunol.* **2010**, *22*, 375–386. [CrossRef] [PubMed]
31. Haase, H.; Ober-Blöbaum, J.L.; Engelhardt, G.; Hebel, S.; Heit, A.; Heine, H.; Rink, L. Zinc signals are essential for lipopolysaccharide-induced signal transduction in monocytes. *J. Immunol.* **2008**, *181*, 6491–6502. [CrossRef] [PubMed]
32. Kitamura, H.; Morikawa, H.; Kamon, H.; Iguchi, M.; Hojyo, S.; Fukada, T.; Yamashita, S.; Kaisho, T.; Akira, S.; Murakami, M.; et al. Toll-like receptor–mediated regulation of zinc homeostasis influences dendritic cell function. *Nat. Immunol.* **2006**, *7*, 971. [CrossRef] [PubMed]
33. Hasan, R.; Rink, L.; Haase, H. Zinc signals in neutrophil granulocytes are required for the formation of neutrophil extracellular traps. *Innate Immun.* **2013**, *19*, 253–264. [CrossRef] [PubMed]
34. Kaltenberg, J.; Plum, L.M.; Ober-Blöbaum, J.L.; Hönscheid, A.; Rink, L.; Haase, H. Zinc signals promote IL-2-dependent proliferation of T cells. *Eur. J. Immunol.* **2010**, *40*, 1496–1503. [CrossRef] [PubMed]
35. Maares, M.; Haase, H. Zinc and immunity: An essential interrelation. *Arch. Biochem. Biophys.* **2016**, *611*, 58–65. [CrossRef] [PubMed]
36. Wessels, I.; Maywald, M.; Rink, L. Zinc as a Gatekeeper of Immune Function. *Nutrients* **2017**, *9*, 1286. [CrossRef] [PubMed]
37. Souffriau, J.; Libert, C. Mechanistic insights into the protective impact of zinc on sepsis. *Cytokine Growth Factor Rev.* **2017**. [CrossRef] [PubMed]

38. Gaetke, L.M.; McClain, C.J.; Talwalkar, R.T.; Shedlofsky, S.I. Effects of endotoxin on zinc metabolism in human volunteers. *Am. J. Physiol. Endocrinol. Metab.* **1997**, *272*, E952–E956. [CrossRef] [PubMed]
39. Besecker, B.Y.; Exline, M.C.; Hollyfield, J.; Phillips, G.; DiSilvestro, R.A.; Wewers, M.D.; Knoell, D.L. A comparison of zinc metabolism, inflammation, and disease severity in critically ill infected and noninfected adults early after intensive care unit admission123. *Am. J. Clin. Nutr.* **2011**, *93*, 1356–1364. [CrossRef] [PubMed]
40. Mertens, K.; Lowes, D.A.; Webster, N.R.; Talib, J.; Hall, L.; Davies, M.J.; Beattie, J.H.; Galley, H.F. Low zinc and selenium concentrations in sepsis are associated with oxidative damage and inflammation. *Br. J. Anaesth.* **2015**, *114*, 990–999. [CrossRef] [PubMed]
41. Hoeger, J.; Simon, T.-P.; Beeker, T.; Marx, G.; Haase, H.; Schuerholz, T. Persistent low serum zinc is associated with recurrent sepsis in critically ill patients—A pilot study. *PLoS ONE* **2017**, *12*, e0176069. [CrossRef] [PubMed]
42. Hoeger, J.; Simon, T.-P.; Doemming, S.; Thiele, C.; Marx, G.; Schuerholz, T.; Haase, H. Alterations in zinc binding capacity, free zinc levels and total serum zinc in a porcine model of sepsis. *BioMetals* **2015**, *28*, 693–700. [CrossRef] [PubMed]
43. Liuzzi, J.P.; Lichten, L.A.; Rivera, S.; Blanchard, R.K.; Aydemir, T.B.; Knutson, M.D.; Ganz, T.; Cousins, R.J. Interleukin-6 regulates the zinc transporter Zip14 in liver and contributes to the hypozincemia of the acute-phase response. *Proc. Natl. Acad. Sci. USA* **2005**, *102*, 6843–6848. [CrossRef] [PubMed]
44. Lichten, L.A.; Liuzzi, J.P.; Cousins, R.J. Interleukin-1β contributes via nitric oxide to the upregulation and functional activity of the zinc transporter Zip14 (Slc39a14) in murine hepatocytes. *Am. J. Physiol. Gastrointest. Liver Physiol.* **2009**, *296*, G860–G867. [CrossRef] [PubMed]
45. Sobocinski, P.Z.; Canterbury, W.J.; Mapes, C.A.; Dinterman, R.E. Involvement of hepatic metallothioneins in hypozincemia associated with bacterial infection. *Am. J. Physiol. Endocrinol. Metab.* **1978**, *234*, E399. [CrossRef] [PubMed]
46. Sobocinski, P.Z.; Canterbury, W.J. Hepatic metallothionein induction in inflammation. *Ann. N. Y. Acad. Sci.* **1982**, *389*, 354–367. [CrossRef]
47. Cousins, R.J.; Leinart, A.S. Tissue-specific regulation of zinc metabolism and metallothionein genes by interleukin 1. *FASEB J. Off. Publ. Fed. Am. Soc. Exp. Biol.* **1988**, *2*, 2884–2890. [CrossRef]
48. Coyle, P.; Philcox, J.C.; Carey, L.C.; Rofe, A.M. Metallothionein: The multipurpose protein. *Cell. Mol. Life Sci. CMLS* **2002**, *59*, 627–647. [CrossRef] [PubMed]
49. Huber, K.L.; Cousins, R.J. Metallothionein expression in rat bone marrow is dependent on dietary zinc but not dependent on interleukin-1 or interleukin-6. *J. Nutr.* **1993**, *123*, 642–648. [CrossRef] [PubMed]
50. Wessels, I.; Cousins, R.J. Zinc dyshomeostasis during polymicrobial sepsis in mice involves zinc transporter Zip14 and can be overcome by zinc supplementation. *Am. J. Physiol. Gastrointest. Liver Physiol.* **2015**, *309*, G768–G778. [CrossRef] [PubMed]
51. Rech, M.; To, L.; Tovbin, A.; Smoot, T.; Mlynarek, M. Heavy metal in the intensive care unit: A review of current literature on trace element supplementation in critically ill patients. *Nutr. Clin. Pract.* **2014**, *29*, 78–89. [CrossRef] [PubMed]
52. Wong, H.R. Pediatric septic shock treatment: New clues from genomic profiling. *Pharmacogenomics* **2007**, *8*, 1287–1290. [CrossRef] [PubMed]
53. Wong, H.R.; Shanley, T.P.; Sakthivel, B.; Cvijanovich, N.; Lin, R.; Allen, G.L.; Thomas, N.J.; Doctor, A.; Kalyanaraman, M.; Tofil, N.M.; et al. Genome-level expression profiles in pediatric septic shock indicate a role for altered zinc homeostasis in poor outcome. *Physiol. Genom.* **2007**, *30*, 146–155. [CrossRef] [PubMed]
54. Shanley, T.P.; Wong, H.R. Molecular genetics in the pediatric intensive care unit. *Crit. Care Clin.* **2003**, *19*, 577–594. [CrossRef]
55. Cvijanovich, N.; Shanley, T.P.; Lin, R.; Allen, G.L.; Thomas, N.J.; Checchia, P.; Anas, N.; Freishtat, R.J.; Monaco, M.; Odoms, K.; et al. Validating the genomic signature of pediatric septic shock. *Physiol. Genom.* **2008**, *34*, 127–134. [CrossRef] [PubMed]
56. Moshage, H. Cytokines and the hepatic acute phase response. *J. Pathol.* **1997**, *181*, 257–266. [CrossRef]
57. Baumann, H.; Gauldie, J. The acute phase response. *Immunol. Today* **1994**, *15*, 74–80. [CrossRef]
58. Florea, D.; Molina-López, J.; Hogstrand, C.; Lengyel, I.; de la Cruz, A.P.; Rodríguez-Elvira, M.; Planells, E. Changes in zinc status and zinc transporters expression in whole blood of patients with Systemic Inflammatory Response Syndrome (SIRS). *J. Trace Elem. Med. Biol.* **2017**. [CrossRef] [PubMed]

59. Rofe, A.M.; Philcox, J.C.; Coyle, P. Trace metal, acute phase and metabolic response to endotoxin in metallothionein-null mice. *Biochem. J.* **1996**, *314*, 793–797. [CrossRef] [PubMed]
60. Sakaguchi, S.; Iizuka, Y.; Furusawa, S.; Ishikawa, M.; Satoh, S.; Takayanagi, M. Role of Zn^{2+} in oxidative stress caused by endotoxin challenge. *Eur. J. Pharmacol.* **2002**, *451*, 309–316. [CrossRef]
61. Zhou, Z.; Wang, L.; Song, Z.; Saari, J.T.; McClain, C.J.; Kang, Y.J. Abrogation of nuclear factor-κB activation is involved in zinc inhibition of lipopolysaccharide-induced tumor necrosis factor-α production and liver injury. *Am. J. Pathol.* **2004**, *164*, 1547–1556. [CrossRef]
62. Hood, M.I.; Skaar, E.P. Nutritional immunity: Transition metals at the pathogen-host interface. *Nat. Rev. Microbiol.* **2012**, *10*. [CrossRef] [PubMed]
63. King, L.E.; Osati-Ashtiani, F.; Fraker, P.J. Depletion of cells of the B lineage in the bone marrow of zinc-deficient mice. *Immunology* **1995**, *85*, 69–73. [PubMed]
64. Dubben, S.; Hönscheid, A.; Winkler, K.; Rink, L.; Haase, H. Cellular zinc homeostasis is a regulator in monocyte differentiation of HL-60 cells by 1α,25-dihydroxyvitamin D3. *J. Leukoc. Biol.* **2010**, *87*, 833–844. [CrossRef] [PubMed]
65. Fraker, P.J.; King, L.E. Reprogramming of the immune system during zinc deficiency. *Annu. Rev. Nutr.* **2004**, *24*, 277–298. [CrossRef] [PubMed]
66. Prasad, A.S.; Beck, F.W.; Bao, B.; Fitzgerald, J.T.; Snell, D.C.; Steinberg, J.D.; Cardozo, L.J. Zinc supplementation decreases incidence of infections in the elderly: Effect of zinc on generation of cytokines and oxidative stress. *Am. J. Clin. Nutr.* **2007**, *85*, 837–844. [CrossRef] [PubMed]
67. Wessels, I.; Haase, H.; Engelhardt, G.; Rink, L.; Uciechowski, P. Zinc deficiency induces production of the proinflammatory cytokines IL-1β and TNFα in promyeloid cells via epigenetic and redox-dependent mechanisms. *J. Nutr. Biochem.* **2013**, *24*, 289–297. [CrossRef] [PubMed]
68. Oteiza, P.I.; Clegg, M.S.; Zago, M.P.; Keen, C.L. Zinc deficiency induces oxidative stress and AP-1 activation in 3T3 cells. *Free Radic. Biol. Med.* **2000**, *28*, 1091–1099. [CrossRef]
69. Oteiza, P.I.; Olin, K.L.; Fraga, C.G.; Keen, C.L. Zinc deficiency causes oxidative damage to proteins, lipids and DNA in rat testes. *J. Nutr.* **1995**, *125*, 823–829. [CrossRef] [PubMed]
70. Song, Y.; Chung, C.S.; Bruno, R.S.; Traber, M.G.; Brown, K.H.; King, J.C.; Ho, E. Dietary zinc restriction and repletion affects DNA integrity in healthy men. *Am. J. Clin. Nutr.* **2009**, *90*, 321–328. [CrossRef] [PubMed]
71. Hotchkiss, R.S.; Osmon, S.B.; Chang, K.C.; Wagner, T.H.; Coopersmith, C.M.; Karl, I.E. Accelerated lymphocyte death in sepsis occurs by both the death receptor and mitochondrial pathways. *J. Immunol.* **2005**, *174*, 5110–5118. [CrossRef] [PubMed]
72. Hotchkiss, R.S.; Swanson, P.E.; Freeman, B.D.; Tinsley, K.W.; Cobb, J.P.; Matuschak, G.M.; Buchman, T.G.; Karl, I.E. Apoptotic cell death in patients with sepsis, shock, and multiple organ dysfunction. *Crit. Care Med.* **1999**, *27*, 1230. [CrossRef] [PubMed]
73. Heidecke, C.-D.; Hensler, T.; Weighardt, H.; Zantl, N.; Wagner, H.; Siewert, J.-R.; Holzmann, B. Selective defects of T lymphocyte function in patients with lethal intraabdominal infection. *Am. J. Surg.* **1999**, *178*, 288–292. [CrossRef]
74. Andresen, M.; Regueira, T.; Bruhn, A.; Perez, D.; Strobel, P.; Dougnac, A.; Marshall, G.; Leighton, F. Lipoperoxidation and protein oxidative damage exhibit different kinetics during septic shock. *Mediat. Inflamm.* **2008**, *2008*. [CrossRef] [PubMed]
75. Kaymak, C.; Kadioglu, E.; Ozcagli, E.; Osmanoglu, G.; Izdes, S.; Agalar, C.; Basar, H.; Sardas, S. Oxidative DNA damage and total antioxidant status in rats during experimental gram-negative sepsis. *Hum. Exp. Toxicol.* **2008**, *27*, 485–491. [CrossRef] [PubMed]
76. Galley, H.F. Oxidative stress and mitochondrial dysfunction in sepsis. *Br. J. Anaesth.* **2011**, *107*, 57–64. [CrossRef] [PubMed]
77. Cander, B.; Dundar, Z.D.; Gul, M.; Girisgin, S. Prognostic value of serum zinc levels in critically ill patients. *J. Crit. Care* **2011**, *26*, 42–46. [CrossRef] [PubMed]
78. Newton, B.; Ballambattu, V.B.; Bosco, D.B.; Gopalakrishna, S.M.; Subash, C.P. Efficacy of zinc supplementation on serum calprotectin, inflammatory cytokines and outcome in neonatal sepsis—A randomized controlled trial. *J. Matern. Fetal Neonatal Med.* **2017**, *30*, 1627–1631. [CrossRef]
79. Newton, B.; Bhat, B.V.; Bosco Dhas, B.; Mondal, N.; Gopalakrishna, S.M. Effect of zinc supplementation on early outcome of neonatal sepsis—A randomized controlled trial. *Indian J. Pediatr.* **2016**, *83*, 289–293. [CrossRef] [PubMed]

80. Newton, B.; Bhat, B.V.; Bosco Dhas, B.; Christina, C.; Gopalakrishna, S.M.; Subhash Chandra, P. Short term oral zinc supplementation among babies with neonatal sepsis for reducing mortality and improving outcome—A double-blind randomized controlled trial. *Indian J. Pediatr.* **2018**, *85*, 5–9. [CrossRef]
81. Mehta, K.; Bhatta, N.K.; Majhi, S.; Shrivastava, M.K.; Singh, R.R. Oral zinc supplementation for reducing mortality in probable neonatal sepsis: A double blind randomized placebo controlled trial. *Indian Pediatr.* **2013**, *50*, 390–393. [CrossRef] [PubMed]
82. Braunschweig, C.L.; Sowers, M.; Kovacevich, D.S.; Hill, G.M.; August, D.A. Parenteral zinc supplementation in adult humans during the acute phase response increases the febrile response. *J. Nutr.* **1997**, *127*, 70–74. [CrossRef] [PubMed]
83. Ganatra, H.A.; Varisco, B.M.; Harmon, K.; Lahni, P.; Opoka, A.; Wong, H.R. Zinc supplementation leads to immune modulation and improved survival in a juvenile model of murine sepsis. *Innate Immun.* **2017**, *23*, 67–76. [CrossRef] [PubMed]
84. Nowak, J.E.; Harmon, K.; Caldwell, C.C.; Wong, H.R. Prophylactic zinc supplementation reduces bacterial load and improves survival in a murine model of sepsis. *Pediatr. Crit. Care Med. J. Soc. Crit. Care Med. World Fed. Pediatr. Intensive Crit. Care Soc.* **2012**, *13*, e323–e329. [CrossRef] [PubMed]
85. Krones, C.J.; Klosterhalfen, B.; Butz, N.; Hoelzl, F.; Junge, K.; Stumpf, M.; Peiper, C.; Klinge, U.; Schumpelick, V. Effect of zinc pretreatment on pulmonary endothelial cells in vitro and pulmonary function in a porcine model of endotoxemia. *J. Surg. Res.* **2005**, *123*, 251–256. [CrossRef] [PubMed]
86. Krones, C.J.; Klosterhalfen, B.; Anurov, M.; Stumpf, M.; Klinge, U.; Oettinger, A.P.; Schumpelick, V. Missing effects of zinc in a porcine model of recurrent endotoxemia. *BMC Surg.* **2005**, *5*, 22. [CrossRef] [PubMed]
87. Krones, C.J.; Klosterhalfen, B.; Fackeldey, V.; Junge, K.; Rosch, R.; Schwab, R.; Stumpf, M.; Klinge, U.; Schumpelick, V. Deleterious effect of zinc in a pig model of acute endotoxemia. *J. Investig. Surg.* **2004**, *17*, 249–256. [CrossRef] [PubMed]
88. Driessen, C.; Hirv, K.; Rink, L.; Kirchner, H. Induction of cytokines by zinc ions in human peripheral blood mononuclear cells and separated monocytes. *Lymphokine Cytokine Res.* **1994**, *13*, 15–20. [PubMed]
89. Foote, J.W.; Delves, H.T. Albumin bound and alpha 2-macroglobulin bound zinc concentrations in the sera of healthy adults. *J. Clin. Pathol.* **1984**, *37*, 1050–1054. [CrossRef] [PubMed]
90. Castell, J.V.; Gómez-Lechón, M.J.; David, M.; Andus, T.; Geiger, T.; Trullenque, R.; Fabra, R.; Heinrich, P.C. Interleukin-6 is the major regulator of acute phase protein synthesis in adult human hepatocytes. *FEBS Lett.* **1989**, *242*, 237–239. [CrossRef]
91. Jang, J.Y.; Shim, H.; Lee, S.H.; Lee, J.G. Serum selenium and zinc levels in critically ill surgical patients. *J. Crit. Care* **2014**, *29*, 317.e5–317.e8. [CrossRef] [PubMed]
92. Trame, S.; Wessels, I.; Haase, H.; Rink, L. A short 18 items food frequency questionnaire biochemically validated to estimate zinc status in humans. *J. Trace Elem. Med. Biol.* **2018**, *49*, 285–295. [CrossRef] [PubMed]
93. Sukhavasi, S.; Jothimuthu, P.; Papautsky, I.; Beyette, F.R. Development of a Point-of-Care device to quantify serum zinc to aid the diagnosis and follow-up of pediatric septic shock. In Proceedings of the 2011 Annual International Conference of the IEEE Engineering in Medicine and Biology Society, Boston, MA, USA, 30 August–3 September 2011; pp. 3676–3679. [CrossRef]
94. Zerhusen, B.; de Silva, G.; Pei, X.; Papautsky, I.; Beyette, F.R. Rapid quantification system for zinc in blood serum. In Proceedings of the 2013 IEEE 56th International Midwest Symposium on Circuits and Systems (MWSCAS), Columbus, OH, USA, 4–7 August 2013; pp. 400–403.
95. Maret, W. Analyzing free zinc(II) ion concentrations in cell biology with fluorescent chelating molecules. *Metallomics* **2015**, *7*, 202–211. [CrossRef] [PubMed]
96. Bornhorst, J.; Kipp, A.P.; Haase, H.; Meyer, S.; Schwerdtle, T. The crux of inept biomarkers for risks and benefits of trace elements. *TrAC Trends Anal. Chem.* **2017**. [CrossRef]

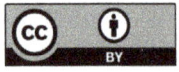

© 2018 by the authors. Licensee MDPI, Basel, Switzerland. This article is an open access article distributed under the terms and conditions of the Creative Commons Attribution (CC BY) license (http://creativecommons.org/licenses/by/4.0/).

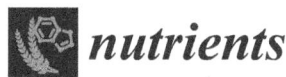

Review

Immunomodulatory Protein Hydrolysates and Their Application

Mensiena B. G. Kiewiet *, Marijke M. Faas and Paul de Vos

Immunoendocrinology, Division of Medical Biology, Department of Pathology and Medical Biology, University Medical Center Groningen, University of Groningen, Hanzeplein 1, 9700 RB Groningen, The Netherlands; m.m.faas@umcg.nl (M.M.F.); p.de.vos@umcg.nl (P.d.V.)
* Correspondence: m.b.g.kiewiet@umcg.nl; Tel.: +31-50-361-0109

Received: 21 June 2018; Accepted: 12 July 2018; Published: 14 July 2018

Abstract: Immunomodulatory protein hydrolysate consumption may delay or prevent western immune-related diseases. In order to purposively develop protein hydrolysates with an optimal and reproducible immunomodulatory effect, knowledge is needed on which components in protein hydrolysates are responsible for the immune effects. Important advances have been made on this aspect. Also, knowledge on mechanisms underlying the immune modulating effects is indispensable. In this review, we discuss the most promising application possibilities for immunomodulatory protein hydrolysates. In order to do so, an overview is provided on reported in vivo immune effects of protein hydrolysates in both local intestinal and systemic organs, and the current insights in the underlying mechanisms of these effects. Furthermore, we discuss current knowledge and physicochemical approaches to identify the immune active protein sequence(s). We conclude that multiple hydrolysate compositions show specific immune effects. This knowledge can improve the efficacy of existing hydrolysate-containing products such as sports nutrition, clinical nutrition, and infant formula. We also provide arguments for why immunomodulatory protein hydrolysates could be applied to manage the immune response in the increasing number of individuals with a higher risk of immune dysfunction due to, for example, increasing age or stress.

Keywords: protein hydrolysate; bioactive peptide; immunomodulation; Toll-like receptor; functional foods

1. Introduction

Protein hydrolysates are commonly used as an alternative protein source in commercial products. They consist of a mixture of different proteins and peptides which is formed by the hydrolysis of intact proteins. During this process, peptide bonds of intact proteins are broken (Figure 1A), which results in the formation of a range of peptides of different sizes. Depending on their properties, protein hydrolysates are applied in different products. Mildly hydrolyzed proteins are, for example, used in clinical and sport nutrition to support digestibility, while extensively hydrolyzed proteins are used in infant formulas as a hypo-allergenic alternative for intact cow's milk proteins (Figure 1B).

Furthermore, protein hydrolysates are recognized as a potent source of bioactive peptides. Different peptides with, for example, anti-thrombotic, anti-hypertensive, anti-microbial, anti-cancer, anti-oxidative, and many immunomodulatory effects have been identified [1]. Consuming protein hydrolysates containing these peptides might be helpful in the management of many western diseases [2,3]. Since many of these diseases are immune-related, immunomodulatory products have gained special attention from both academical and industrial researchers for the management and amelioration of, for example, inflammatory bowel diseases, allergies, and diabetes [4,5].

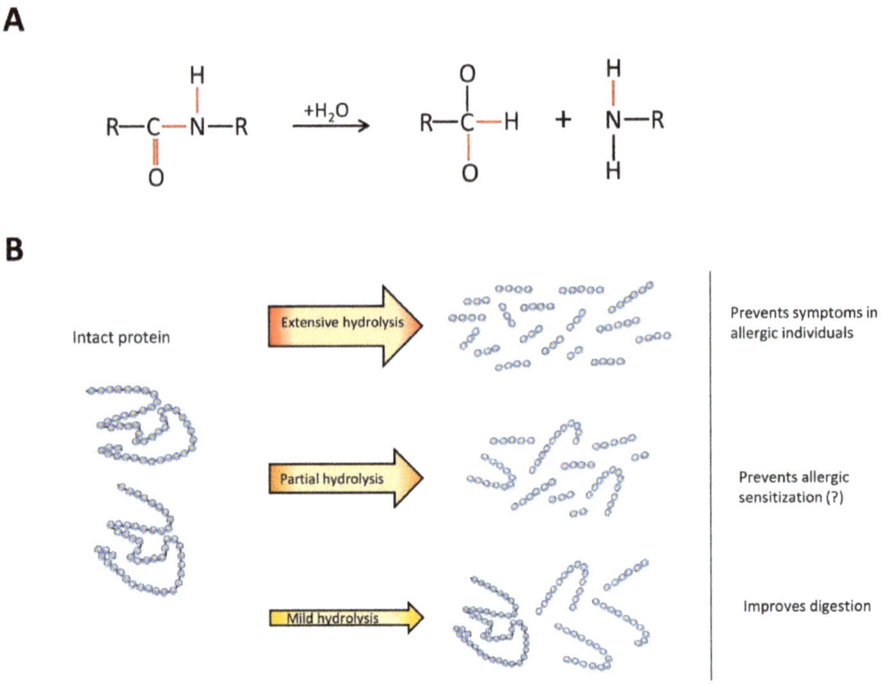

Figure 1. The process of protein hydrolysis and its products. (**A**) chemical reaction of protein hydrolysis; (**B**) different hydrolysates serve different purposes.

Purposively deploying the immunomodulating effects of protein hydrolysates in existing or new dietary products is an attractive opportunity to manage immune-related diseases. In order to achieve this, the identification of specific peptides and a better understanding of their working mechanisms is required. This review aims to provide an overview of studies on reported in vivo immune effects of hydrolysates in both local intestinal and systemic organs. The current insights in underlying mechanisms are also discussed. As the design of effective protein hydrolysates may benefit from the identification of specific bioactive peptides, we review current knowledge and physicochemical approaches to identify the protein sequence(s). Based on the discussed topics, we provide our view on the possible application of immunomodulatory protein hydrolysates or peptides in specific target groups.

2. Immune Effects of Hydrolysates

In 1984, immune effects were detected for the first time in a fraction of a casein hydrolysate [6]. The studied protein fraction was found to both increase the production of hemolytic antibodies in mice splenocytes, and to enhance the phagocytic capacity of murine macrophages against sheep red blood cells in vitro. In vivo, the protein fraction protected mice against a lethal infection with *Klebsiella pneumoniae*. Since then, measuring lymphocyte proliferation and macrophage phagocytosis capacity have been the main in vitro assays used to study the immune effects of protein hydrolysates.

An increase in lymphocyte proliferation was observed after stimulation with other protein hydrolysates which were derived from soy, wheat, whey, casein, and mollusk [7–13]. Not all protein hydrolysates were found to stimulate proliferation. Hydrolysates derived from egg white were shown to decrease instead of enhance lymphocyte proliferation [14]. Different hydrolysates from casein were found to possess either proliferation increasing [10] or inhibiting effects [15], showing that individual protein hydrolysates from the same protein source also have remarkably different immunomodulating properties. Phagocytosis modulation was source dependent as well. Most protein hydrolysates were found to increase macrophage phagocytosis capacity in vitro, for example, soy, egg, wheat, and casein hydrolysates had such an effect [9,12,16,17]. However, a rice protein hydrolysate was found to inhibit the phagocytic activity of RAW264.7 macrophages [18].

These early in vitro experiments investigating the immune effects of protein hydrolysates have led to many more in vitro and in vivo studies on the effects of protein hydrolysates on immunity. In the sections below, these in vivo studies are reviewed (an overview of the studies is given in Table 1). In this part, a distinction was made between local intestinal immune effects and systemic effects. All effects discussed below are also visualized in Figure 2. To start with, protein hydrolysates have an effect on the epithelial cells aligning the gut and by that induce crosstalk between the epithelial cells and immune cells [5].

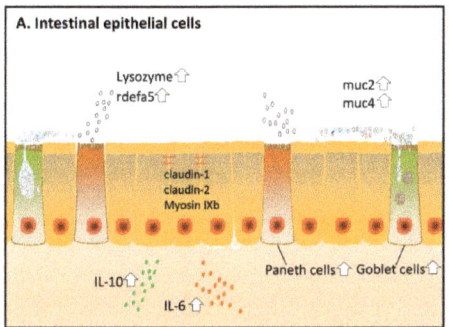
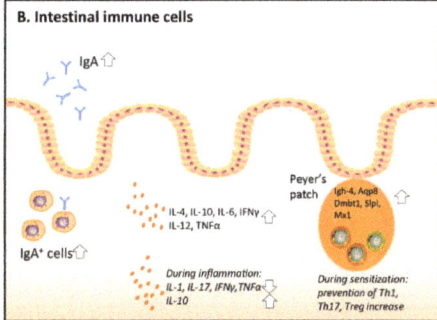
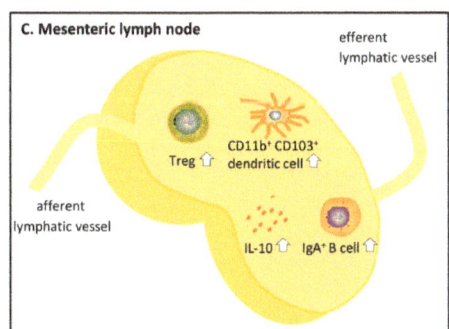
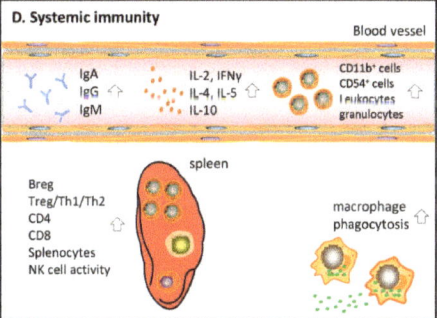

Figure 2. Overview of immune effects induced by protein hydrolysates on the (**A**) intestinal epithelial cells; (**B**) intestinal immune cells; (**C**) mesenteric lymph nodes; (**D**) systemic immune system.

Table 1. Overview of hydrolysates and their immune effects.

Hydrolysate/Peptide	Enzyme/Treatment	Immune Effects	Species	Reference
Casein hydrolysate diet (200 g/kg casein, TD99482, Harlan-Teklad Custom Research, Madison, WI, USA	Not applicable (NA)	Reduction of autoimmune diabetes by 50%, decreased lactulose/mannitol ratio, decreased serum zonulin levels, increased ileal TEER, altered ileal mRNA expression of Myo9b, claudin-1, and claudin-2.	Diabetes prone BB rat	[19]
Casein hydrolysate (20% of diet Pancase S™ (Sensient Flavours, Strassbourg, France) or Nutramigen™ (Mead Johnson Nutrition, Zeeland, MI, USA))	NA	Reduction of autoimmune diabetes, decreased lactulose/mannitol ratio, increased ileal IL-10 levels, beneficial gut microbiota changes (increased $Lactobacilli$ and reduced $Bacteroides$ spp. levels)	Diabetes prone BB rat	[20]
β-CN(94-123) from commercial yoghurt	NA	Enhanced numbers of goblet and Paneth cells in the small intestine, increased expression of Muc2, Muc4, lysozyme, and rdefa5.	rat	[21]
Yoghurt or Milk Fermented by $Lactobacillus\ casei$ DN-114 001	$Lactobacillus\ casei$ DN-114 001	Increased cell proliferation and villous area in the proximal intestine, hypertrophy and hyperplasia of Paneth and goblet cells.	mouse	[22]
Milk fermentation products of $L.\ Helveticus$ R389	$L.\ Helveticus$ R389	Enhanced expression of calcineurin in the small intestine, upregulated IL-2 and TNF production, increased number of mucosal mast cells and goblet cells	mouse	[23]
Egg yolk digests	Pepsin	Increase of the IL-6 secretion by small intestinal epithelial cells, increase in IgA$^+$ cells, orchestrating the Th1/Th2 response.	mouse	[24]
Common carp egg hydrolysate	Pepsin, alcalase	Increase of secretory immunoglobulin A in the gut. Pepsin hydrolysate increased the splenic NK cell cytotoxicity, macrophage phagocytosis and level of serum immunoglobulin A (IgA). S-IgA in the gut was significantly enhanced by pepsin and alcalase hydrolysates. Trypsin hydrolysate increased the percentages of CD4$^+$ and CD8$^+$ cells in the spleen.	mouse	[25]
Yellow field pea hydrolysate	Thermolysin	Increased number of IgA$^+$ cells in the small intestine lamina propria, accompanied by an increase in the number of IL-4$^+$, IL-10$^+$, and IFNγ$^+$ cells.	mouse	[26]
Fermented pacific whiting protein	Yeast	Enhanced phagocytic activity of peritoneal macrophages, increased number of IgA$^+$ cells, and increased IL-4, IL-6, IL-10, IFNγ, and TNFα levels in the small intestine lamina propria	mouse	[27]
Shark protein hydrolysate Peptibal™ (innoVactiv Inc)	Trypsin and chymotrypsin	Increase of small intestinal immunoglobulin A-producing cells and intestinal IL-6, TNFα, TGFβ, and IL-10	mouse	[28]

Table 1. *Cont.*

Hydrolysate/Peptide	Enzyme/Treatment	Immune Effects	Species	Reference
Peptide fraction from *Lactobacillus helveticus*-Fermented Milk	Lactobacillus Helveticus	Increased intestinal and serum IgA levels, increase in the number of IgA-secreting B lymphocytes in the intestinal lamina propria, stimulation of Th2 response (IL-4 vs. IFNγ)	mouse	[29]
κ-casein–derived glycomacropeptide	NA	Decreased body weight loss, decreased anorexia, colonic damage, a reduction in colonic alkaline phosphatase activity, IL-1, trefoil factor 3, and iNOS mRNA levels.	Rat (TNBS induced colitis)	[30]
β-Casein hydrolysate	Cell envelope-associated proteinase of Lactobacillus delbrueckii ssp. lactis CRL 581	Decreased mortality rates, faster recovery of initial body weight loss, less microbial translocation to the liver, decreased β-glucuronidase and myeloperoxidase activities in the gut, decreased colonic macroscopic and microscopic damage, increased IL-10 and decreased IFNγ.	Mouse (TNBS induced colitis)	[31]
κ-casein–derived glycomacropeptide	NA	$Rag1^{-/-}$: increased body-weight gain, decreased colonic damage score and myeloperoxidase (MPO) activity, reduced percentage of $CD4^+$ interferon $IFNγ^+$ cells and increased IL-6 in MLN. Increased colonic expression of TNFα and IFNγ and increased IL-10 in MLN, by MLN. DSS: decreased MPO activity, increased IL-10 production in MLN.	Mouse (DSS induced colitis and $Rag1^{-/-}$)	[32]
bovine glycomacropeptide	NA	Decrease of inflammatory injury, as assessed by lower extension of necrosis and damage score, myeloperoxidase, alkaline phosphatase, inducible nitric oxide synthase, IL-1β, TNFα, and IL-17.	Rat (TNBS induced colitis)	[33]
Egg white hydrolysate	Aminopeptidase	Attenuated DSS-induced clinical symptoms, including weight loss, mucosal and submucosal inflammation, crypt distortion, and colon muscle thickening, and decreased intestinal permeability and increased mucin gene expression, reduced intestinal expression of pro-inflammatory cytokines TNFα, IL-6, IL-1β, IFNγ, IL-8, and IL-17.	Pig (DSS induced colitis)	[34]
Soybean protein hydrolysate	*Rhizopus oryzae* neutral protease preparation	Increased number of $IL-12^+ CD11b^+$ in spleens, increased cytotoxic activity of spleen cells, increased *Igh-4*, *Aqp8*, *Umbt1*, *Slpi*, and *Mx1* in Peyer's patch cells.	Mouse	[35]
Partially hydrolyzed whey protein	NA	Increased Breg and Treg in the spleen, increased IgA^+ B-cells in the MLN, increased Th1, activated Treg and activated Th17 cells in the Peyer's patches	Mouse	[36]

Table 1. Cont.

Hydrolysate/Peptide	Enzyme/Treatment	Immune Effects	Species	Reference
LLDAQSAPLRVYVEELKP (from whey)	NA	Reduced acute allergic skin response, decreased whey-specific antibody levels, increased the percentages of CD11b$^+$CD103$^+$ dendritic cells and CD25$^+$Foxp3$^+$ T cells in the MLN.	Mouse	[37]
Partial whey hydrolysate	NA	Reduced acute allergic skin response and mast cell degranulation after whey challenge, increased Foxp3$^+$ regulatory T-cell numbers in the MLN.	Mouse	[38]
oyster peptide-based enteral nutrition formula	Bromelain, pepsin, trypsin	Enhanced spleen lymphocyte proliferation of and of NK cell activity	Mouse	[39]
Casein hydrolysate	Trypsin	Phagocytosing capacity of phagocytic cells was increased	Mouse	[17]
Milk protein hydrolysate	Complex protease	Improved the level of hemolysin in serum, and enhanced phagocytosis of macrophages. In ovalbumin-sensitized mice, the milk protein hydrolysates reduced IgE levels, reduced IL-4 in serum, reduced the release of histamine and bicarbonate in peritoneal mast cells, and enhanced TGFβ levels.	ICR mouse	[40]
Chum salmon oligopeptide preparation	Complex protease	Enhanced lymphocyte proliferation capacity increased number of plaque-forming cells, increased NK cell activity, increased percentage of CD4$^+$ T helper (Th) cells in spleen and secretion of Th1 (IL-2, IFNγ) and Th2 (IL-5, IL-6) type cell cytokines.	ICR mouse	[41]
Tuna cooking drip hydrolysate	Enzyme A and B	Increased weight of the spleen and thymus and enhanced the proliferation of splenocytes. Increased production of IL-10 and IL-2. Increased serum IgG1 and IgG2a levels.	Mouse	[42]
Soy protein hydrolysate	Pepsin	Increased serum IgA and IgG levels	Rat	[7]
Soy protein hydrolysate	Theroase, bioprase, Sumizyme FP	Total lymphocyte and granulocyte numbers were altered, and the numbers of CD11b$^+$ cells and CD56$^+$ cells increased.	Human	[43]
Wheat gluten hydrolysate	NA	NK cell activity increased significantly	Human	[44]
Fish protein hydrolysate (Amizate)	NA	No effects observed	Human	[45]

3. Effects of Protein Hydrolysates on the Gut Barrier

Epithelial cells form a first layer of defense against harmful pathogens and molecules in the intestinal lumen. These cells are covered by a layer of mucus. Together, this forms a physical barrier between the luminal content and the human body [46]. Protein hydrolysates and bioactive peptides in the lumen of the intestine were found to affect barrier function in multiple ways (Figure 2A). First, protein hydrolysates are able to strengthen the epithelial barrier. Second, they enhance the production of mucus and so-called anti-microbial proteins that delete pathogens.

Barrier enhancing effects by protein hydrolysates were shown by Visser et al., [19,20], who fed diabetes prone rats casein hydrolysates for up to 150 days and measured the barrier function by determining the lactulose-mannitol ratio in urine. They showed that casein hydrolysate intake decreased the epithelial permeability compared to a diet with sole amino acids. In the ileum of diabetic rats on the casein hydrolysates, a normalization of the tight junction mRNA expression, including myosin IXb, claudin-1, and claudin-2, was observed, together with an upregulation of the regulatory cytokine Interleukin (IL)-10. Multiple other dairy derived peptides have been found to increase the amount of goblet and Paneth cells in the intestine [21–23], which are specialized epithelial cells regulating the production of mucus and anti-bacterial peptides. The consumption of yoghurt peptides did not only increase the amount of these cell types, but also increased the expression of Muc2 and 4, as well as the anti-bacterial factors lysozyme and rdefa5 [21].

Another function of epithelial cells is sampling the lumen and skewing the differentiation of immune cells in the lamina propria accordingly, mainly by basolateral cytokine secretion [47]. In a healthy situation, egg yolk peptide digest consumption in mice was able to increase IL-6 production in epithelial cells ex vivo [24]. IL-6 has been described to affect both innate and adaptive immune responses [48,49], meaning that protein hydrolysates might influence the immune system via epithelial cells in this way. However, due to the pleiotropic nature of this cytokine [50], its impact is different in different cell types and conditions, and the overall effect of increased IL-6 is difficult to predict.

4. Effects of Protein Hydrolysates on the Intestinal Immune System

One of the most studied immune effects in the intestine after hydrolysate administration in vivo is the level of IgA (Figure 2B). This typical intestinal immunoglobulin can easily be measured in the faeces and is instrumental in the clearance of toxins, pathogens, and other harmful molecules [51]. Hydrolysate intake can cause an increase in IgA, as shown for a common carp egg hydrolysate [25]. Corresponding to this, studies investigating intestinal immunity after pacific whiting, shark hydrolysate, and yellow field pea hydrolysate consumption in mice detected an increased amount of IgA$^+$ B cells [26–28]. Leblanc et al. studied IgA secretion in an infection mouse model fed *Lactobacillus helveticus*-fermented milk, and found an increase of IgA both in the intestinal fluid and blood, together with an increased amount of IgA$^+$ cells in the lamina propria [29]. Increased IgA levels seem to be a general effect of hydrolysate intake and seem to be independent of the hydrolysate protein source.

Besides enhancing IgA production, protein hydrolysates have more effects on the immune system which might lead to a more matured and developed immune response. Levels of multiple cytokines, including IL-4, IL-10, IL-6, IFNγ, IL-12, and TNFα, have been found to be elevated in healthy mice after consuming egg yolk, fish, and yellow pea hydrolysate [24,26,27]. For the shark hydrolysate, these increased cytokine levels were associated with a better response of the mice against *E. Coli* infection [28]. The enhancement of IL-4, IL-10, IFNγ, and IL-12 suggests that T cells in the intestine are activated by the hydrolysate. To understand what the administration of protein hydrolysates could mean in situations such as pathogenic infections or inflammatory bowel disease, it would be helpful to know which types of T cells are stimulated. To this end, Leblanc et al., compared the amount of IL-4 (Th2) and IFNγ (T helper (Th)1) in the intestine of a mouse model fed *Lactobacillus helveticus*-fermented milk, and found a predominant Th2 response after feeding the milk peptides [29].

Anti-inflammatory properties are another often observed feature of protein hydrolysates. This is a characteristic mainly attributed to the hydrolysates of bovine milk. To study these effects, experimental models with colitis and ileitis have been used. In all cases, oral pretreatment of the animals with casein hydrolysate or a casein glycomacropeptide reduced damage to the intestine, leading to a decrease in weight loss [30–33]. They also observed a decrease in the pro-inflammatory cytokines IL-1β, IL-17, TNFα, and IFNγ, while in one study, an increase of the regulatory cytokine IL-10 was observed [31]. Similar outcomes were observed when egg white peptides were administered to pigs with dextran sodium sulphate (DSS) induced colitis [34].

The effects of protein hydrolysates in the Peyer's patches (PP), which are part of the gut-associated lymphoid tissue, have been studied to a lesser extent but are essential as this tissue is the central immune sampling and signaling site in the gut. Egusa et al. studied the effects of a specific soybean protein digest in the PP [35]. After five weeks of feeding mice a soybean hydrolysate enriched diet, the genome wide gene expression of PP derived cells was examined. They found that several genes related to innate immunity and host defense were upregulated. They observed the upregulation of *Igh-4* and *Aqp8*, which enhance phagocytosis, and of Dmbt1, *Slpi*, and *Mx1*, which are anti-bacterial and anti-viral components [52–54]. When looking at adaptive responses in the PP, we found in our own study that sensitization with a partially hydrolyzed whey protein prevented the increase of Th1, Th17, and regulatory T cells (Treg) in the PP after a challenge with intact whey [36].

5. Effects of Protein Hydrolysates on the Mesenteric Lymph Nodes (MLN)

Tolerance induction and other antigen presenting dependent processes occur predominantly in the MLN [55]. Antigen loaded dendritic cells from the PP and lamina propria in the intestine migrate to the MLN and subsequently activate T and B cells. Depending on the nature of the antigen, either an immune response is evoked or tolerance is induced via the formation of Treg. A number of studies investigating the effects of bovine milk hydrolysates or peptides in murine sensitization models assessed which cell types were present in the MLN of the mice after hydrolysate consumption (Figure 2C). When mice were fed milk peptides, either alone or in combination with indigestible oligosaccharides, before the start of the sensitization against intact whey, the number of Treg in the MLN increased [37,38]. One study showed that the number of dendritic cells responsible for the transport of antigens from the lamina propria to the MLNs, i.e., the CD11b$^+$ and CD103$^+$ dendritic cells, was increased [37]. Casein derived glycomacropeptide consumption increased ex vivo tolerogenic IL-10 production in MLN cells of a DSS induced colitis mouse model [32], which also suggests an increase in Treg here. However, in a rat model for ileitis, the glycomacropeptide did not influence MLN cytokine levels [33]. This might be explained by differences in species, inflammation models, or glycomacropeptide dosing.

Not only T cell responses are induced in the MLN, but also B cells can be activated, after which they expand in specialized follicles. It was found that sensitization with a partially hydrolyzed whey protein increased the number of IgA$^+$ B cells [36]. However, since the role of the MLN in intestinal IgA production is still under debate, more research is needed to evaluate the contribution of this observed phenomenon to intestinal and systemic IgA levels [56].

6. Effects of Protein Hydrolysates on Systemic Immunity

Protein hydrolysates do not only affect the immune response locally in the intestine, but also have effects on the systemic immunity, mostly measured in splenic and peritoneal cells, and in the blood (Figure 2D). Small peptides are probably able to pass through the gut barrier and have been detected in the blood of volunteers who consumed dairy and soy products, [57,58] allowing a direct impact on immune cells in the systemic circulation. Administration of many protein hydrolysates made from casein and other milk products, oyster, salmon, and fish [17,27,39–41] increased the ex vivo phagocytotic capacity of macrophages isolated from the peritoneal cavity of mice. Oyster, salmon, and common carp egg were furthermore found to increase NK cell activity in the spleen [25,39,41].

Similar to results after direct in vitro stimulation of splenocytes, oral administration of protein hydrolysate derived from oyster, tuna cooking drip, salmon, and multiple common carp egg hydrolysates increased ex vivo splenocyte proliferation [25,39,41,42]. Some of these studies looked into the cell types present in the spleens of these animals in more detail. Alcalase common carp egg hydrolysate was found to increase $CD4^+$ and $CD8^+$ cells in the spleen [25], while salmon hydrolysate only increased $CD4^+$ [41]. These cells were expected to be both Th1 and Th2 cells, since both Th1 (IL-2, IFNγ) and Th2 (IL-4, IL-5) cytokines were detected in the blood of these animals. These effects might differ between protein hydrolysates, since a tuna cooking drip hydrolysate was found to increase IL-2 and IL-10 [42], and sensitization with a partial whey hydrolysate increased Treg in the spleen [36].

Together with an increase in Treg, an increase in regulatory B cells (Breg) was observed in the spleen after whey hydrolysate administration [36]. Breg are increasingly recognized to be important in regulatory immune responses and induce the differentiation of T cells into Treg [59]. Another study also found an increase in IL-10 producing Breg when inducing oral tolerance using intact casein in casein-allergic mice [60]. Here, casein might be digested in the intestine of the mice, after which the newly formed bioactive peptide(s) derived from casein increased Breg. An adoptive transfer of these Breg could even prevent the onset of allergy in recipients [60], demonstrating the importance of this cell type in tolerance induction.

Other evidence that hydrolysate consumption affects B cell responses is the observation of increased antibody levels observed in the blood. A soy protein hydrolysate was found to induce IgG and IgA in the blood of rats [7], while the common carp egg hydrolysate increased IgA in mice [25]. Therefore, it is likely that protein hydrolysates not only affect B cell differentiation, but also induce class-switching and antibody production.

Only a few studies investigated the effects of protein hydrolysates on immune parameters in the blood of humans. The effect of a single dose of soybean hydrolysate was studied in a small group of volunteers, and it was found to change leukocyte numbers and increase granulocytes. More specifically, it significantly increased $CD11b^+$ (macrophages and/or dendritic cells) and $CD56^+$ cells (NK cells) in blood [43]. When nine subjects were fed a wheat hydrolysate for six days, an increase in NK cell activity was observed [44]. A larger group of undernourished Indian children was given a fish hydrolysate for 120 days. After this period, the CD4/CD8 ratio and antibody levels were measured, but no significant differences were detected [45]. These studies show that protein hydrolysates have immunomodulatory effects in humans, which are similar to some of the previously mentioned in vitro and in vivo effects, although the protein hydrolysates used are different. However, in these studies, only a few immunological parameters were measured, and/or only included a small group of volunteers, which makes it difficult to draw firm conclusions. Well-designed, extensive human studies are lacking at the moment, but are needed to better understand the effects of protein hydrolysates in humans.

7. Understanding Hydrolysate Compositions

A mandatory assignment for the coming years for researchers in the field is to identify the exact peptide sequence(s) responsible for the reported effects described above. This will make the design of formulations possible for specific health effects. Currently, protein hydrolysates are mainly characterized by determining their degree of hydrolysis (DH). The DH is a measure for how extensively a protein has been hydrolyzed, and therefore gives an indication of the size of the peptides present in the hydrolysate. The DH is calculated by determining the amount of cleaved peptide bonds [61]. Different methods have been developed to obtain the DH, including the pH-stat, trinitrobenzenesulfonic acid (TNBS), o-phthaldialdehyde (OPA), trichloroacetic acid soluble nitrogen (SN-TCA), and formol titration methods [62].

However, the DH does not give any indication of the presence or absence of specific bioactive peptides. Protein hydrolysates with a similar DH can still have a different peptide composition. Therefore, protein hydrolysates are often further characterized by using techniques to separate the peptides in the hydrolysate based on their physicochemical properties, mainly size, hydrophobicity, or a combination thereof. Techniques which are often used to characterize peptide composition are, for example sodium, dodecyl sulfate polyacrylamide gel electrophoresis (SDS-PAGE), size exclusion chromatography, and High Performance Liquid Chromatography (HPLC) [63]. All these techniques are used to obtain a molecular weight distribution, which gives an overall indication of the hydrolysate composition based on size. One can focus on a specific fraction of the protein hydrolysates by choosing the most appropriate technique and optimizing the settings used.

HPLC, especially Reverse Phase-HPLC, has, for a long time, been found to be useful in separating peptides from protein hydrolysates based on their size and hydrophobicity [64]. When this method is coupled to a mass spectrometer (MS), it is also possible to determine the amino acid sequence of the detected peptides [65]. In this way, a very detailed characterization of the hydrolysate can be obtained, which can be used to identify structure-effector relationships between, for example, immune effects and specific peptides in a hydrolysate. However, protein hydrolysates consist of thousands of different peptides, which will all be detected by HPLC-MS when a complete hydrolysate is analyzed. Therefore, studies aiming for the identification of bioactive peptides often compare the bioactivity of size-based fractions of the hydrolysate first [66,67], after which the bioactive fraction alone can be further analyzed using HPLC-MS. Ultimately, the peptides present in the bioactive fraction should be tested individually for bioactivity in order to obtain the peptide responsible for the observed effect [65].

Using this and similar methods has led to the discovery of a range of bioactive peptides from protein mixtures, as reviewed by Sanchez et al., and Lafarga et al., [1,68]. However, most of the identified bioactive peptides possess anti-hypertensive, anti-microbial, or anti-oxidative effects, but peptides with immunomodulatory properties have not widely been identified yet. Comparing the characteristics of the immunomodulatory peptides that have been identified generated new knowledge about which peptide properties are associated with immune effects. It is known that immunomodulatory peptides are mostly two to 20 amino acids long and hydrophobic [61]. Chalamaiah et al., concluded by listing known peptides with immunomodulatory effects that glycine (Gly), valine (Val), leucine (Leu), proline (Pro), phenylalanine (Phe), negatively charged amino acid glutamic acid (Glu), and aromatic amino acid tyrosine (Tyr) were most frequently present in peptides with immune effects [69].

Recently, we also found that larger fractions in whey and soy protein hydrolysates can have immunomodulatory effects. These fractions have a size of over 1000 kDa and were composed of aggregates which are formed during the hydrolysis process [66]. In this process, the proteins are heated, which is a known cause of protein denaturation and aggregation [70]. By performing PAGE under different conditions, it was found that these aggregates were formed due to electrostatic forces and disulfide bridges between single proteins and induce responses in human dendritic cells. The fact that these aggregates were found in both a whey and soy hydrolysate suggests that aggregate formation is not protein source specific and might be present in a wide range of different protein hydrolysates.

8. Underlying Mechanisms of Immunomodulatory Effects

In order to understand the immune effects that can be induced by protein hydrolysates and to ultimately apply protein hydrolysates in specific conditions, it is of crucial importance to understand exactly how the observed immune effects come about. Up to now, only a few studies have focused on elucidation of the underlying mechanisms of immunomodulatory effects by protein hydrolysates and are reviewed below. Recent research suggests that hydrolysate peptides bind to specific immune-receptors and that multiple receptors might be involved (Figure 3A).

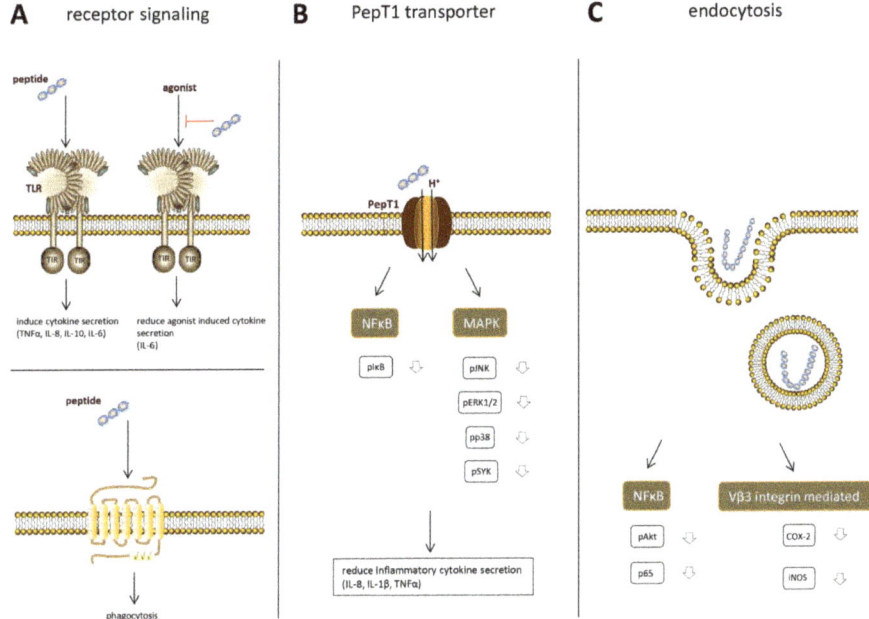

Figure 3. Overview of mechanisms described in the literature via which peptides can exert immunomodulatory effects in the cell. Peptides can (**A**) directly stimulate receptors; (**B**) be taken up in the cell via a peptide transporter and interfere with inflammatory signaling pathways; or (**C**) be taken up into the cell via endocytosis and inhibit inflammatory signaling pathways.

9. Receptor Binding

One of the most studied receptor types in immune signaling is Toll-like receptors (TLRs). This is a family of pathogen recognition receptors. They are not only expressed by most immune cells [71,72], but also by epithelial cells [73]. Multiple protein hydrolysates were found to affect TLRs, but the effects were very hydrolysate dependent. By studying a range of cow's milk hydrolysates in a TLR reporter cell platform, we previously found that especially mildly hydrolyzed whey hydrolysates were able to activate multiple TLRs, including TLR2, 3, 4, 5, 7, 8, and 9 [74]. This activation does lead to the production of TNFα, IL-10, and IL-8 in human peripheral blood mononuclear cells (PBMCs). The protein source of the hydrolysates was crucial for its final effects, as it was observed that casein hydrolysates only inhibited TLR activation. Which TLRs were inhibited also differed per hydrolysate, but TLR5 and 9 were the most profoundly inhibited. Other studies focused mainly on TLR2 and 4. Tobita et al., described that a casein phosphopeptide was able to induce proliferation and IL-6 production in CD19+ cells from mice after stimulation in vitro. This effect was gone after the administration of an anti-TLR4 antibody, suggesting that the effects were induced via TLR4 [75]. A primary culture of murine intestinal epithelial cells was also thought to secrete IL-6 via the stimulation of both TLR2 and TLR4 when the mice were fed with yellow pea hydrolysate [26] and shark protein hydrolysate [28]. A pressurized whey hydrolysate was able to suppress lipopolysaccharide (LPS) induced IL-8 production in respiratory epithelial cell lines, likely via binding to TLR4 [76].

There is evidence that other transmembrane receptors are also involved in immune effects by protein hydrolysates. Tsuruki et al., described that a peptide derived from the soybean β-conglycinin A' subunit, which stimulated phagocytosis in human neutrophils, showed a low affinity for the N-formyl-methionyl-leucyl-phenylalanine (fMLP) receptor [77]. The phagocytosis stimulating effect disappeared when this receptor was blocked. The authors discuss that its low affinity for the fMLP receptor allows it to stimulate the immune response in a safe way, without causing inflammation.

Peptides derived from many different food protein sources are known to bind opioid receptors [78]. Although endogenous opioid peptides have a main function as neurotransmitters, they are also known to modulate innate and acquired immune responses [79]. Opioid receptor signaling can, for example, skew T cell differentiation, increase antibody production in B cells, and affect phagocytosis in macrophages [80–82]. These effects have also been described in immune cells after hydrolysate administration. Therefore, it cannot be excluded that protein hydrolysates also modulate the immune system via opioid receptors.

10. PepT1 Dependent Intracellular Effects

Multiple bioactive tri- and tetrapeptides derived from soy and whey have been found to induce anti-inflammatory effects after being taken up into the cell [83–85]. This cellular uptake, and therefore the anti-inflammatory effects of the peptides, depends on the peptide transporter PepT1 (Figure 3B). PepT1 is an H^+ coupled oligopeptide transporter, mediating the uptake of a broad range of di-and tripeptides in intestinal epithelial cells in order to transport the peptides into the bloodstream. Normally, it is expressed in the small intestine, but during inflammation, it is also upregulated in the colon [86]. Treatment with the soy peptides KVP and VPY and the whey peptide IPAV all showed a decrease in the production of the pro-inflammatory cytokines IL-6, IL-8, and TNFα in Caco2 cells. This effect disappeared when PepT1-activity was inhibited, indicating that transport via PepT1 is necessary for the anti-inflammatory effects. Once taken up in the cytosol, the peptides were shown to inhibit the main inflammatory signaling pathways in order to decrease the pro-inflammatory cytokine secretion. A decrease in phosphorylated nuclear factor kappa-light-chain-enhancer of activated B cells (NFκB), mitogen-activated protein kinase (MAPK), extracellular signal-regulated kinase (ERK)1/2, c-Jun N-terminal kinase (JNK)1/2, p38, and spleen tyrosine kinase (SYK) was observed after pretreatment with the bioactive peptides.

As described above, gut epithelial cells can influence the immune response in the intestine [47]. Therefore, an anti-inflammatory status of the epithelial cells is expected to also regulate the underlying immune cells [87]. Furthermore, the soy and whey proteins can be transported over the epithelial barrier and interact directly with immune cells. The soy peptide VPY was also found to induce anti-inflammatory effects in THP-1 human monocytes [84], while the soy peptide KVP showed anti-inflammatory effects in T cells [83]. Interestingly, both monocytes and T cells express the PepT1 transporter [88], suggesting that the bioactive peptides might induce anti-inflammatory effects in innate and adaptive immune cells via a similar mechanism as described for epithelial cells.

The relevance of these effects in vivo was shown by treating mice with DSS and TNBS induced colitis with the bioactive soy peptides [83,84]. In these models, KVP and VPY were shown to reduce colitis symptoms, reduce body weight loss, and decrease pro-inflammatory cytokines in the intestine.

11. Endocytosis

Once immunomodulatory peptides are taken up in epithelial or immune cells, they can exert their effects by interfering with signaling pathways. However, not all peptides and protein can be internalized via the PepT1 transporter, since this transporter is specific for di- and tripeptides. Larger food derived peptides, which are too large for the PepT1 transporter, can also be taken up into the cell by fluid phase endocytosis (Figure 3C), which is a non-specific form of vesicle mediated internalization. In this type of endocytosis, hydrophobic interactions between the peptide and the cell membrane are involved in the internalization of the peptide [89]. Differences in physicochemical properties of peptides, including size, hydrophobicity, and charge determine the kinetics of uptake of individual peptides.

The involvement of this type of peptide uptake in immunomodulation by peptides was confirmed by Regazzo et al., [90]. They showed that a relatively large, hydrophobic casein peptide which showed multiple stimulating effects in immune cells, could be taken up in a layer of Caco2 cells via endocytosis. They did not see a difference in casein peptide uptake when they used an inhibitor for the PepT1 transporter or cytochalasin D to open the tight junctions (and increase the paracellular route), but found a significant inhibitory effect on peptide uptake after treatment with wortmannin, which inhibits endocytosis [90]. When the peptide is translocated over the epithelial cells via this mechanism, it may affect immune cell functioning in the lamina propria or in the blood.

A study investigating the well-characterized soy peptide lunasin showed that endocytosis is also used by immune cells to take up immunomodulatory peptides [91]. Lunasin is a 43-amino acid peptide which was shown to interact with the $\alpha V\beta 3$ integrin, which led to inhibiting $\alpha V\beta 3$ integrin-mediated pro-inflammatory markers and to downregulation of the Akt-mediated NF-κB pathway. By using different inhibitors, it was found that lunasin was mainly taken up by endocytic mechanisms that involve integrin signaling, clathrin-coated structures, and macropinosomes [91]. Interestingly, this lunasin uptake was increased under inflammatory conditions.

12. Possibilities for Hydrolysate Application

Since immune effects were found to be hydrolysate specific, many immune-related conditions could potentially benefit from hydrolysate administration by selecting specific protein hydrolysates. However, up to now, research has mainly focused on the discovery of immune effects in vitro and animal studies, while follow up studies in humans are rare. To develop an immunomodulatory product containing a hydrolysate, these studies are indispensable in order to investigate the safety, bioavailability, and inducible immune effects in the human body. Protein hydrolysates with the most promising effects should be chosen for further research. Based on the knowledge on immune effects and the underlying mechanisms involved, of which an overview was given above, protein hydrolysates can be selected for application in specific products.

13. Existing Products

Existing hydrolysate containing products can benefit from applying a different protein hydrolysate with the same nutritional value as the currently used protein hydrolysates, but with an additional immune modulating effect (Figure 4). Hypo-allergenic infant formulas are the main market for protein hydrolysates nowadays. By hydrolyzing proteins, epitopes which are recognized by the immune system of allergic infants are destroyed. Therefore, infant formulas containing extensively hydrolyzed proteins can be tolerated by allergic infants [92]. However, allergic reactions may also be reduced by modulating the immune system [5]. When the allergic reaction develops, the intestinal immune system induces an inappropriate immune response against a harmless food molecule [93], which is characterized by an increased Th2 response [94] (Figure 5). Since multiple cow's milk hydrolysates have been described to induce Treg cell differentiation in the MLN and spleen [36,38] which reduces the Th2 response [95], these protein hydrolysates might help to reduce allergic symptoms.

T cell differentiation can be regulated via TLRs [96,97]. Therefore, protein hydrolysates might affect the T cell response via TLRs, as they have been found to modulate TLR signaling [74]. This knowledge could help in selecting allergy reducing protein hydrolysates, since TLR signaling of protein hydrolysates can be measured in reporter cell platforms [74]. Furthermore, protein hydrolysates have also been found to reduce the permeability of the intestinal epithelial barrier [19]. This might provide an alternative mechanism for reducing the allergic reaction, since it reduces the uptake of antigens and prevents the interaction of lamina propria immune cells with antigens.

Another product in which protein hydrolysates are already used is clinical nutrition. In general, a high protein intake was found to decrease mortality in hospitalized patients [98]. Protein hydrolysates are used instead of intact proteins because of their ease of digestion. Anti-inflammatory protein hydrolysates might have an additional benefit in patients consuming clinical nutrition because of intestinal inflammation, because many studies have found beneficial effects of anti-inflammatory protein hydrolysates in multiple colitis mouse models [30–33]. Therefore, anti-inflammatory protein hydrolysates may be expected to reduce symptoms of, for example, inflammatory bowel disease and irritable bowel syndrome in patients.

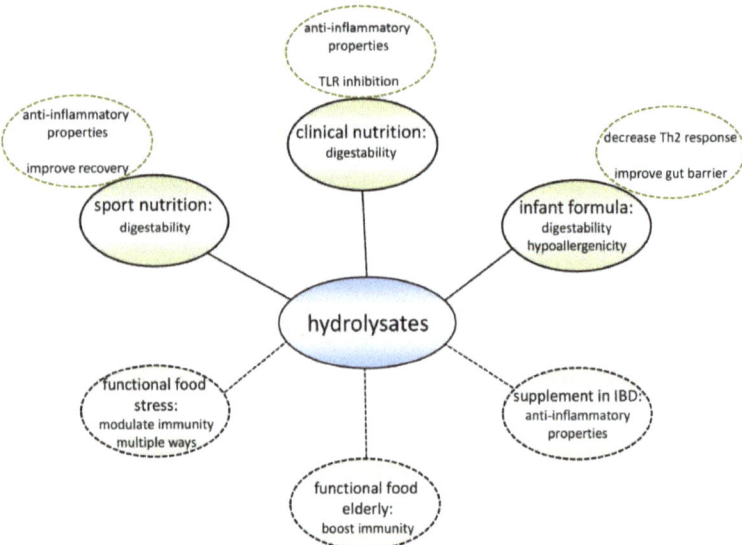

Figure 4. Summary of the application possibilities of protein hydrolysates. These hydrolysates are currently being used in sport nutrition, clinical nutrition, and infant formula, mainly because of their good digestibility and hypoallergenicity. Recent research indicates that specific protein hydrolysates could optimize the current products in multiple ways. Also, there is evidence that new protein hydrolysate products could be beneficial for specific target groups.

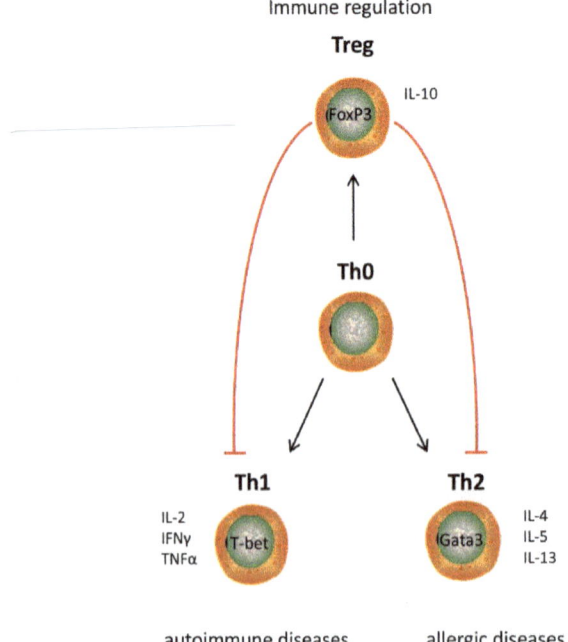

Figure 5. Overview of T helper cell subsets and their interactions and their relation to specific diseases.

Intestinal inflammation is also a common side-effect of chemotherapy [99]. Therefore, individuals undergoing chemotherapy could be another target group for anti-inflammatory protein hydrolysates. Interestingly, some chemotherapeutic agents induce inflammation via specific TLRs [100,101]. During chemotherapy, intestinal epithelial cells are damaged, which leads to the release of Damage associated molecular patterns (DAMPs). DAMPs are able to activate TLR activation, which initiates an inflammatory response [102,103]. Therefore, inhibiting TLR signaling protects against chemotherapy induced inflammation. It was indeed found that the intake of food molecules could reduce the inflammation caused by the chemotherapeutic agent doxorubicin, by the inhibition of TLR2 [104]. Since protein hydrolysates can also inhibit TLRs [74], they might elicit similar effects.

Protein hydrolysates are also applied in sport nutrition. Proteins are known to be essential in the recovery after exercise [105], and peptides are more rapidly taken up compared to intact protein [106]. Reducing inflammatory responses was found to reduce muscle pain and aid in the recovery after exercise. This can be done by taking anti-inflammatory food products, for example, tart cherry juice, which decreased pain and increased muscle recovery after running long distances when ingested prior to the exercise [107,108]. Protein hydrolysates with an anti-inflammatory effect could therefore simultaneously provide a protein source needed for muscle anabolism, and aid in the recovery due to anti-inflammatory effects. Some studies indeed suggest that the administration of whey protein hydrolysate or wheat gluten hydrolysate prior or after exercise decreased muscle damage, improved muscle repair, and improved the performance [109–111]. Furthermore, excessive exercise may result in impaired immunity [112]. Immune modulating protein hydrolysates could also be beneficial for athletes in this respect.

14. Target Groups for New Products

Protein hydrolysates could also be used to develop completely new products with immunomodulatory effects (Figure 5). Many studies showing a new immunomodulating effect of a hydrolysate suggest that the hydrolysate could be used as a nutraceutical or functional food. Both terms are used for food products with an additional health effect besides their nutritional value. As outlined in the introduction, we and others feel that immunomodulating products will be particularly useful in modern Western society, since the occurrence of immune-related diseases is currently increasing [113].

As mentioned before, protein hydrolysates have a good chance of ameliorating symptoms in local intestinal diseases like inflammatory bowel disease and irritable bowel syndrome. In addition, patients suffering from systemic immune diseases are likely to benefit from hydrolysate consumption. Type 1 diabetes is an example of an autoimmune disease with a rapidly increasing prevalence [114]. Animals studies suggest that casein hydrolysate can prevent autoimmune diabetes by modulating multiple immune responses in the intestine [19,20]. Management of autoimmunity to delay or prevent disease may therefore be another promising field of application for specific protein hydrolysates.

In our view, some specific target groups might also specifically benefit from specific immunomodulatory protein hydrolysates in order to delay or prevent disease. The number of elderly in the population is increasing. With increasing age, the immune system deteriorates and becomes more proinflammatory. This leads, for example, to more infections, and therefore a higher mortality rate [115]. The innate immune response is affected in multiple ways during immunoscenesence. An altered cytokine production by monocytes and macrophages has been found, together with a decreased phagocytotic capacity and a reduced TLR expression [116,117]. Since it was found that specific protein hydrolysates are able to modulate these immune aspects [27,74], protein hydrolysates might be beneficial in keeping the elderly healthy for a longer period of time. This improves quality of life and reduces health care costs.

Stress is another common cause of immune dysfunction [118]. Currently, an increasing number of people experience significant levels of stress, leading to more immune-related diseases [119,120]. Both acute and chronic stress has been found to induce immune dysfunction, resulting in inflammatory, autoimmune, and allergic diseases [121,122]. Effects associated with the development of immune diseases due to stress are increased pro-inflammatory cytokines, more Th2-related cytokines, and changes in leukocyte number and distribution [123–126]. As described above, specific protein hydrolysates are able to counteract these effects. Therefore, functional food containing protein hydrolysates may contribute to healthy immunity in people experiencing significant stress levels.

15. Conclusions

A wide range of protein hydrolysates have immunomodulatory capacities. However, before protein hydrolysates can serve as functional foods, physicochemical approaches to identify the protein sequence(s) are needed to be able to design effective protein hydrolysates. Also, specific target groups have to be identified. In this way, specific protein hydrolysates can be designed to ameliorate, delay, or prevent the onset of a wide variety of Western immune-related conditions.

Author Contributions: Writing-Original Draft Preparation, M.B.G.K.; Writing-Review & Editing, M.M.F. and P.d.V.

Conflicts of Interest: The authors declare no conflict of interest.

References

1. Sánchez, A.; Vázquez, A. Bioactive peptides: A review. *Food Qual. Saf.* **2017**, *1*, 29–46. [CrossRef]
2. Li-Chan, E.C.Y. Bioactive peptides and protein hydrolysates: Research trends and challenges for application as nutraceuticals and functional food ingredients. *Curr. Opin. Food Sci.* **2015**, *1*, 28–37. [CrossRef]
3. Dhaval, A.; Yadav, N.; Purwar, S. Potential Applications of Food Derived Bioactive Peptides in Management of Health. *Int. J. Pept. Res. Ther.* **2016**, *22*, 377–398. [CrossRef]
4. Bouglé, D.; Bouhallab, S. Dietary bioactive peptides: Human studies. *Crit. Rev. Food Sci. Nutr.* **2015**, *57*, 335–343. [CrossRef] [PubMed]
5. Kiewiet, M.B.G.; Gros, M.; van Neerven, R.J.J.; Faas, M.M.; de Vos, P. Immunomodulating properties of protein hydrolysates for application in cow's milk allergy. *Pediatr. Allergy Immunol.* **2015**, *26*, 206–217. [CrossRef] [PubMed]
6. Parker, F.; Migliore-Samour, D.; Floch, F.; Zerial, A.; Werner, G.H.; Jollès, J.; Casaretto, M.; Zahn, H.; Jollès, P. Immunostimulating hexapeptide from human casein: Amino acid sequence, synthesis and biological properties. *Eur. J. Biochem.* **1984**, *145*, 677–682. [CrossRef] [PubMed]
7. Ashaolu, T.J.; Yanyiam, N.; Yupanqui, C.T. Immunomodulatory effects of pepsin-educed soy protein hydrolysate in rats and murine cells. *Funct. Foods Health Dis.* **2017**, *7*, 889–900.
8. Caron, S.; Samanez, C.H.; Dehondt, H.; Ploton, M.; Briand, O.; Lien, F.; Dorchies, E.; Dumont, J.; Postic, C.; Cariou, B.; et al. Farnesoid X receptor inhibits the transcriptional activity of carbohydrate response element binding protein in human hepatocytes. *Mol. Cell. Biol.* **2013**, *33*, 2202–2211. [CrossRef] [PubMed]
9. Kong, X.; Guo, M.; Hua, Y.; Cao, D.; Zhang, C. Enzymatic preparation of immunomodulating hydrolysates from soy proteins. *Bioresour. Technol.* **2008**, *99*, 8873–8879. [CrossRef] [PubMed]
10. Mao, X.Y.; Yang, H.Y.; Song, J.P.; Li, Y.H.; Ren, F.Z. Effect of yak milk casein hydrolysate on Th1/Th2 cytokines production by murine spleen lymphocytes in vitro. *J. Agric. Food Chem.* **2007**, *55*, 638–642. [CrossRef] [PubMed]
11. Rodríguez-Carrio, J.; Fernández, A.; Riera, F.A.; Suárez, A. Immunomodulatory activities of whey β-lactoglobulin tryptic-digested fractions. *Int. Dairy J.* **2014**, *34*, 65–73. [CrossRef]
12. Wu, W.; Zhang, M.; Sun, C.; Brennan, M.; Li, H.; Wang, G.; Lai, F.; Wu, H. Enzymatic preparation of immunomodulatory hydrolysates from defatted wheat germ (Triticum Vulgare) globulin. *Int. J. Food Sci. Technol.* **2016**, *51*, 2556–2566. [CrossRef]
13. He, X.Q.; Cao, W.H.; Pan, G.K.; Yang, L.; Zhang, C.H. Enzymatic hydrolysis optimization of Paphia undulata and lymphocyte proliferation activity of the isolated peptide fractions. *J. Sci. Food Agric.* **2015**, *95*, 1544–1553. [CrossRef] [PubMed]
14. Lozano-Ojalvo, D.; Molina, E.; López-Fandiño, R. Hydrolysates of egg white proteins modulate T- and B-cell responses in mitogen-stimulated murine cells. *Food Funct.* **2016**, *7*, 1048–1056. [CrossRef] [PubMed]

15. Sutas, Y.; Soppi, E.; Korhonen, H.; Syvaoja, E.L.; Saxelin, M.; Rokka, T.; Isolauri, E. Suppression of lymphocyte proliferation in vitro by bovine caseins hydrolyzed with Lactobacillus casei GG-derived enzymes. *J. Allergy Clin. Immunol.* **1996**, *98*, 216–224. [CrossRef]
16. Meram, C.; Wu, J. Anti-inflammatory effects of egg yolk livetins (α, β, and γ-livetin) fraction and its enzymatic hydrolysates in lipopolysaccharide-induced RAW 264.7 macrophages. *Food Res. Int.* **2017**, *100*, 449–459. [CrossRef] [PubMed]
17. Kazlauskaite, J.; Biziulevicius, G.A.; Zukaite, V.; Biziuleviciene, G.; Miliukiene, V.; Siaurys, A. Oral tryptic casein hydrolysate enhances phagocytosis by mouse peritoneal and blood phagocytic cells but fails to prevent induced inflammation. *Int. Immunopharmacol.* **2005**, *5*, 1936–1944. [CrossRef] [PubMed]
18. Wen, L.; Chen, Y.; Zhang, L.; Yu, H.; Xu, Z.; You, H.; Cheng, Y. Rice protein hydrolysates (RPHs) inhibit the LPS-stimulated inflammatory response and phagocytosis in RAW264.7 macrophages by regulating the NF-κB signaling pathway. *RSC Adv.* **2016**, *6*, 71295–71304. [CrossRef]
19. Visser, J.; Lammers, K.; Hoogendijk, A.; Boer, M.; Brugman, S.; Beijer-Liefers, S.; Zandvoort, A.; Harmsen, H.; Welling, G.; Stellaard, F.; et al. Restoration of impaired intestinal barrier function by the hydrolysed casein diet contributes to the prevention of type 1 diabetes in the diabetes-prone BioBreeding rat. *Diabetologia* **2010**, *53*, 2621–2628. [CrossRef] [PubMed]
20. Visser, J.; Bos, N.; Harthoorn, L.; Stellaard, F.; Beijer-Liefers, S.; Rozing, J.; van Tol, E.A.F. Potential mechanisms explaining why hydrolyzed casein-based diets outclass single amino acid-based diets in the prevention of autoimmune diabetes in diabetes-prone BB rats. *Diabete Metab. Res. Rev.* **2012**, *28*, 505–513. [CrossRef] [PubMed]
21. Plaisancié, P.; Claustre, J.; Estienne, M.; Henry, G.; Boutrou, R.; Paquet, A.; Léonil, J. A novel bioactive peptide from yoghurts modulates expression of the gel-forming MUC2 mucin as well as population of goblet cells and Paneth cells along the small intestine. *J. Nutr. Biochem.* **2013**, *24*, 213–221. [CrossRef] [PubMed]
22. Thoreux, K.; Balas, D.; Bouley, C.; Senegas-Balas, F. Diet Supplemented with Yoghurt or Milk Fermented by Lactobacillus casei DN-114 001 Stimulates Growth and Brush-Border Enzyme Activities in Mouse Small Intestine. *Digestion* **1998**, *59*, 349–359. [CrossRef] [PubMed]
23. Vinderola, G.; Matar, C.; Perdigón, G. Milk fermentation products of L. helveticus R389 activate calcineurin as a signal to promote gut mucosal immunity. *BMC Immunol.* **2007**, *8*, 19. [CrossRef] [PubMed]
24. Nelson, R.; Katayama, S.; Mine, Y.; Duarte, J.; Matar, C. Immunomodulating effects of egg yolk low lipid peptic digests in a murine model. *Food Agric. Immunol.* **2007**, *18*, 1–15. [CrossRef]
25. Chalamaiah, M.; Hemalatha, R.; Jyothirmayi, T.; Diwan, P.V.; Bhaskarachary, K.; Vajreswari, A.; Ramesh Kumar, R.; Dinesh Kumar, B. Chemical composition and immunomodulatory effects of enzymatic protein hydrolysates from common carp (Cyprinus carpio) egg. *Nutrition* **2015**, *31*, 388–398. [CrossRef] [PubMed]
26. Ndiaye, F.; Vuong, T.; Duarte, J.; Aluko, R.E.; Matar, C. Anti-oxidant, anti-inflammatory and immunomodulating properties of an enzymatic protein hydrolysate from yellow field pea seeds. *Eur. J. Nutr.* **2012**, *51*, 29–37. [CrossRef] [PubMed]
27. Duarte, J.; Vinderola, G.; Ritz, B.; Perdigón, G.; Matar, C. Immunomodulating capacity of commercial fish protein hydrolysate for diet supplementation. *Immunobiology* **2006**, *211*, 341–350. [CrossRef] [PubMed]
28. Mallet, J.F.; Duarte, J.; Vinderola, G.; Anguenot, R.; Beaulieu, M.; Matar, C. The immunopotentiating effects of shark-derived protein hydrolysate. *Nutrition* **2014**, *30*, 706–712. [CrossRef] [PubMed]
29. LeBlanc, J.; Fliss, I.; Matar, C. Induction of a Humoral Immune Response following an Escherichia coli O157:H7 Infection with an Immunomodulatory Peptidic Fraction Derived from Lactobacillus helveticus-Fermented Milk. *Clin. Diagn. Lab. Immunol.* **2004**, *11*, 1171–1181. [CrossRef] [PubMed]
30. Daddaoua, A.; Puerta, V.; Zarzuelo, A.; Suárez, M.D.; Sánchez de Medina, F.; Martínez-Augustin, O. Bovine Glycomacropeptide Is Anti-Inflammatory in Rats with Hapten-Induced Colitis. *J. Nutr.* **2005**, *135*, 1164–1170. [CrossRef] [PubMed]
31. Espeche Turbay, M.B.; De Leblanc, A.D.M.; Perdigón, G.; Savoy de Giori, G.; Hebert, E.M. β-Casein hydrolysate generated by the cell envelope-associated proteinase of Lactobacillus delbrueckii ssp. lactis CRL 581 protects against trinitrobenzene sulfonic acid-induced colitis in mice. *J. Dairy Sci.* **2012**, *95*, 1108–1118. [CrossRef] [PubMed]

32. Ortega-Gonzalez, M.; Capitan-Canadas, F.; Requena, P.; Ocon, B.; Romero-Calvo, I.; Aranda, C.; Suarez, M.D.; Zarzuelo, A.; de Medina, F.S.; Martinez-Augustin, O. Validation of bovine glycomacropeptide as an intestinal anti-inflammatory nutraceutical in the lymphocyte-transfer model of colitis. *Br. J. Nutr.* **2014**, *111*, 1202–1212. [CrossRef] [PubMed]
33. Requena, P.; Daddaoua, A.; Martínez-Plata, E.; González, M.; Zarzuelo, A.; Suárez, M.D.; Sánchez de Medina, F.; Martínez-Augustin, O. Bovine glycomacropeptide ameliorates experimental rat ileitis by mechanisms involving downregulation of interleukin 17. *Br. J. Pharmacol.* **2009**, *154*, 825–832. [CrossRef] [PubMed]
34. Lee, M.; Kovacs-Nolan, J.; Archbold, T.; Fan, M.Z.; Juneja, L.R.; Okubo, T.; Mine, Y. Therapeutic potential of hen egg white peptides for the treatment of intestinal inflammation. *J. Funct. Foods* **2009**, *1*, 161–169. [CrossRef]
35. Egusa, S.; Otani, H. Soybean protein fraction digested with neutral protease preparation, "Peptidase R", produced by Rhizopus oryzae, stimulates innate cellular immune system in mouse. *Int. Immunopharmacol.* **2009**, *9*, 931–936. [CrossRef] [PubMed]
36. Kiewiet, M.; van Esch, B.; Garssen, J.; Faas, M.; de Vos, P. Partially hydrolyzed whey proteins prevent clinical symptoms in a cow's milk allergy mouse model and enhance regulatory T and B cell frequencies. *Mol. Nutr. Food Res.* **2017**, *61*. [CrossRef] [PubMed]
37. Meulenbroek, L.A.P.M.; van Esch, B.C.A.M.; Hofman, G.A.; den Hartog Jager, C.F.; Nauta, A.J.; Willemsen, L.E.M.; Bruijnzeel-Koomen, C.A.F.M.; Garssen, J.; van Hoffen, E.; Knippels, L.M.J. Oral treatment with beta-lactoglobulin peptides prevents clinical symptoms in a mouse model for cow's milk allergy. *Pediatr. Allergy Immunol.* **2013**, *24*, 656–664. [CrossRef] [PubMed]
38. Van Esch, B.C.A.M.; Schouten, B.; de Kivit, S.; Hofman, G.A.; Knippels, L.M.J.; Willemsen, L.E.M.; Garssen, J. Oral tolerance induction by partially hydrolyzed whey protein in mice is associated with enhanced numbers of Foxp3(+) regulatory T-cells in the mesenteric lymph nodes. *Pediatr. Allergy Immunol.* **2011**, *22*, 820–826. [CrossRef] [PubMed]
39. Cai, B.; Pan, J.; Wu, Y.; Wan, P.; Sun, H. Immune functional impacts of oyster peptide-based enteral nutrition formula (OPENF) on mice: A pilot study. *Chin. J. Oceanol. Limnol.* **2013**, *31*, 813–820. [CrossRef]
40. Pan, D.D.; Wu, Z.; Liu, J.; Cao, X.Y.; Zeng, X.Q. Immunomodulatory and hypoallergenic properties of milk protein hydrolysates in ICR mice. *J. Dairy Sci.* **2013**, *96*, 4958–4964. [CrossRef] [PubMed]
41. Yang, R.; Zhang, Z.; Pei, X.; Han, X.; Wang, J.; Wang, L.; Long, Z.; Shen, X.; Li, Y. Immunomodulatory effects of marine oligopeptide preparation from Chum Salmon (Oncorhynchus keta) in mice. *Food Chem.* **2009**, *113*, 464–470. [CrossRef]
42. Kim, M.J.; Kim, K.B.W.R.; Sung, N.Y.; Byun, E.H.; Nam, H.S.; Ahn, D.H. Immune-enhancement effects of tuna cooking drip and its enzymatic hydrolysate in Balb/c mice. *Food Sci. Biotechnol.* **2018**, *27*, 131–137. [CrossRef]
43. Yimit, D.; Hoxur, P.; Amat, N.; Uchikawa, K.; Yamaguchi, N. Effects of soybean peptide on immune function, brain function, and neurochemistry in healthy volunteers. *Nutrition* **2012**, *28*, 154–159. [CrossRef] [PubMed]
44. Horiguchi, N.; Horiguchi, H.; Suzuki, Y. Effect of wheat gluten hydrolysate on the immune system in healthy human subjects. *Biosci. Biotechnol. Biochem.* **2005**, *69*, 2445–2449. [CrossRef] [PubMed]
45. Nesse, K.O.; Nagalakshmi, A.P.; Marimuthu, P.; Singh, M. Efficacy of a Fish Protein Hydrolysate in Malnourished Children. *Indian J. Clin. Biochem.* **2011**, *26*, 360–365. [CrossRef] [PubMed]
46. Farhadi, A.; Banan, A.; Fields, J.; Keshavarzian, A. Intestinal barrier: An interface between health and disease. *J. Gastroenterol. Hepatol.* **2003**, *18*, 479–497. [CrossRef] [PubMed]
47. Peterson, L.W.; Artis, D. Intestinal epithelial cells: Regulators of barrier function and immune homeostasis. *Nat. Rev. Immunol.* **2014**, *14*, 141–153. [CrossRef] [PubMed]
48. Liu, F.; Poursine-Laurent, J.; Wu, H.; Link, D.C. Interleukin-6 and the granulocyte colony-stimulating factor receptor are major independent regulators of granulopoiesis in vivo but are not required for lineage commitment or terminal differentiation. *Blood* **1997**, *90*, 2583–2590. [PubMed]
49. Smith, K.A.; Maizels, R.M. IL-6 controls susceptibility to helminth infection by impeding Th2 responsiveness and altering the Treg phenotype in vivo. *Eur. J. Immunol.* **2014**, *44*, 150–161. [CrossRef] [PubMed]
50. Hunter, C.A.; Jones, S.A. IL-6 as a keystone cytokine in health and disease. *Nat. Immunol.* **2015**, *16*, 448–457. [CrossRef] [PubMed]
51. Pabst, O. New concepts in the generation and functions of IgA. *Nat. Rev. Immunol.* **2012**, *12*, 821–832. [CrossRef] [PubMed]

52. Ligtenberg, A.; Veerman, E.; Nieuw Amerongen, A.; Mollenhauer, J. Salivary agglutinin/glycoprotein-340/DMBT1: A single molecule with variable composition and with different functions in infection, inflammation and cancer. *Biol. Chem.* **2007**, *388*, 1275–1289. [CrossRef] [PubMed]
53. Fernie-King, B.; Seilly, D.; Binks, M.; Sriprakash, K.; Lachmann, P. Streptococcal DRS (distantly related to SIC) and SIC inhibit antimicrobial peptides, components of mucosal innate immunity: A comparison of their activities. *Microbes Infect.* **2007**, *9*, 300–307. [CrossRef] [PubMed]
54. Samuel, C.E. Antiviral actions of interferons. *Clin. Microbiol. Rev.* **2001**, *14*, 778–809. [CrossRef] [PubMed]
55. Macpherson, A.J.; Smith, K. Mesenteric lymph nodes at the center of immune anatomy. *J. Exp. Med.* **2006**, *203*, 497–500. [CrossRef] [PubMed]
56. Santiago, A.F.; Fernandes, R.M.; Santos, B.P.; Assis, F.A.; Oliveira, R.P.; Carvalho, C.R.; Faria, A.M.C. Role of mesenteric lymph nodes and aging in secretory IgA production in mice. *Cell. Immunol.* **2008**, *253*, 5–10. [CrossRef] [PubMed]
57. Chabance, B.; Marteau, P.; Rambaud, J.C.; Migliore-Samour, D.; Boynard, M.; Perrotin, P.; Guillet, R.; Jolles, P.; Fiat, A.M. Casein peptide release and passage to the blood in humans during digestion of milk or yogurt. *Biochimie* **1998**, *80*, 155–165. [CrossRef]
58. Dia, V.P.; Torres, S.; De Lumen, B.O.; Erdman, J.W.; Gonzalez De Mejia, E. Presence of lunasin in plasma of men after soy protein consumption. *J. Agric. Food Chem.* **2009**, *57*, 1260–1266. [CrossRef] [PubMed]
59. Rosser, E.C.; Mauri, C. Regulatory B Cells: Origin, Phenotype, and Function. *Immunity* **2015**, *42*, 607–612. [CrossRef] [PubMed]
60. Kim, A.R.; Kim, H.S.W.H.S.; Kim, D.K.; Nam, S.T.; Kim, H.S.W.H.S.; Park, Y.H.; Lee, D.; Lee, M.B.; Lee, J.H.; Kim, B.; et al. Mesenteric IL-10-producing CD5(+) regulatory B cells suppress cow's milk casein-induced allergic responses in mice. *Sci. Rep.* **2016**, *6*, 19685. [CrossRef] [PubMed]
61. Agyei, D.; Ongkudon, C.M.; Wei, C.Y.; Chan, A.S.; Danquah, M.K. Bioprocess challenges to the isolation and purification of bioactive peptides. *Food Bioprod. Process.* **2016**, *98*, 244–256. [CrossRef]
62. Rutherfurd, S.M. Methodology for determining degree of hydrolysis of proteins in Hydrolysates: A review. *J. AOAC Int.* **2010**, *93*, 1515–1522. [PubMed]
63. Silvestre, M.P.C. Review of methods for the analysis of protein hydrolysates. *Food Chem.* **1997**, *60*, 263–271. [CrossRef]
64. Lemieux, L.; Piot, J.-M.; Guillochon, D.; Amiot, J. Study of the efficiency of a mobile phase used in size-exclusion HPLC for the separation of peptides from a casein hydrolysate according to their hydrodynamic volume. *Chromatographia* **1991**, *32*, 499–504. [CrossRef]
65. Chen, H.-M.; Muramoto, K.; Yamauchi, F. Structural Analysis of Antioxidative Peptides from Soybean .beta.-Conglycinin. *J. Agric. Food Chem.* **1995**, *43*, 574–578. [CrossRef]
66. Kiewiet, M.B.G.; Dekkers, R.; Ulfman, L.H.; Groeneveld, A.; de Vos, P.; Faas, M.M. Immunomodulating protein aggregates in soy and whey hydrolysates and their resistance to digestion in an in vitro infant gastrointestinal model: New insights in the mechanism of immunomodulatory hydrolysates. *Food Funct.* **2018**, *9*, 604–613. [CrossRef] [PubMed]
67. Mukhopadhya, A.; Noronha, N.; Bahar, B.; Ryan, M.T.; Murray, B.A.; Kelly, P.M.; O'Loughlin, I.B.; O'Doherty, J.V.; Sweeney, T. The anti-inflammatory potential of a moderately hydrolysed casein and its 5 kDa fraction in in vitro and ex vivo models of the gastrointestinal tract. *Food Funct.* **2015**, *6*, 612–621. [CrossRef] [PubMed]
68. Lafarga, T.; Hayes, M. Bioactive protein hydrolysates in the functional food ingredient industry: Overcoming current challenges. *Food Rev. Int.* **2017**, *33*, 217–246. [CrossRef]
69. Chalamaiah, M.; Yu, W.; Wu, J. Immunomodulatory and anticancer protein hydrolysates (peptides) from food proteins: A review. *Food Chem.* **2018**, *245*, 205–222. [CrossRef] [PubMed]
70. Monahan, F.J.; German, J.B.; Kinsella, J.E. Effect of Ph and Temperature on Protein Unfolding and Thiol-Disulfide Interchange Reactions during Heat-Induced Gelation of Whey Proteins. *J. Agric. Food Chem.* **1995**, *43*, 46–52. [CrossRef]
71. Gordon, S. Pattern recognition receptors: Doubling up for the innate immune response. *Cell* **2002**, *111*, 927–930. [CrossRef]
72. Michallet, M.-C.; Rota, G.; Maslowski, K.; Guarda, G. Innate receptors for adaptive immunity. *Curr. Opin. Microbiol.* **2013**, *16*, 296–302. [CrossRef] [PubMed]

73. Abreu, M.T. Toll-like receptor signalling in the intestinal epithelium: How bacterial recognition shapes intestinal function. *Nat. Rev. Immunol.* **2010**, *10*, 131–143. [CrossRef] [PubMed]
74. Kiewiet, M.B.G.; Dekkers, R.; Gros, M.; van Neerven, R.J.J.; Groeneveld, A.; de Vos, P.; Faas, M.M. Toll-like receptor mediated activation is possibly involved in immunoregulating properties of cow's milk hydrolysates. *PLoS ONE* **2017**, *12*, e0178191. [CrossRef] [PubMed]
75. Tobita, K.; Kawahara, T.; Otani, H. Bovine beta-casein (1-28), a casein phosphopeptide, enhances proliferation and IL-6 expression of mouse CD19(+) cells via toll-like receptor 4. *J. Agric. Food Chem.* **2006**, *54*, 8013–8017. [CrossRef] [PubMed]
76. Iskandar, M.M.; Lands, L.C.; Sabally, K.; Azadi, B.; Meehan, B.; Mawji, N.; Skinner, C.D.; Kubow, S. High Hydrostatic Pressure Pretreatment of Whey Protein Isolates Improves Their Digestibility and Antioxidant Capacity. *Foods* **2015**, *4*, 184–207. [CrossRef] [PubMed]
77. Tsuruki, T.; Kishi, K.; Takahashi, M.; Tanaka, M.; Matsukawa, T.; Yoshikawa, M. Soymetide, an immunostimulating peptide derived from soybean beta-conglycinin, is an fMLP agonist. *FEBS Lett.* **2003**, *540*, 206–210. [CrossRef]
78. Stefanucci, A.; Mollica, A.; Macedonio, G.; Zengin, G.; Ahmed, A.A.; Novellino, E. Exogenous opioid peptides derived from food proteins and their possible uses as dietary supplements: A critical review. *Food Rev. Int.* **2018**, *34*, 70–86. [CrossRef]
79. Liang, X.; Liu, R.; Chen, C.; Ji, F.; Li, T. Opioid System Modulates the Immune Function: A Review. *Transl. Perioper. Pain Med.* **2016**, *1*, 5–13. [CrossRef] [PubMed]
80. Börner, C.; Lanciotti, S.; Koch, T.; Höllt, V.; Kraus, J. μ opioid receptor agonist-selective regulation of interleukin-4 in T lymphocytes. *J. Neuroimmunol.* **2013**, *263*, 35–42. [CrossRef] [PubMed]
81. Cheido, M.A.; Gevorgyan, M.M.; Zhukova, E.N. Comparative Evaluation of Opioid-Induced Changes in Immune Reactivity of CBA Mice. *Bull. Exp. Biol. Med.* **2014**, *156*, 363–365. [CrossRef] [PubMed]
82. Tomassini, N.; Renaud, F.; Roy, S.; Loh, H.H. Morphine inhibits Fc-mediated phagocytosis through mu and delta opioid receptors. *J. Neuroimmunol.* **2004**, *147*, 131–133. [CrossRef] [PubMed]
83. Dalmasso, G.; Charrier-Hisamuddin, L.; Thu Nguyen, H.T.; Yan, Y.; Sitaraman, S.; Merlin, D. PepT1-Mediated Tripeptide KPV Uptake Reduces Intestinal Inflammation. *Gastroenterology* **2008**, *134*, 166–178. [CrossRef] [PubMed]
84. Kovacs-Nolan, J.; Zhang, H.; Ibuki, M.; Nakamori, T.; Yoshiura, K.; Turner, P.V.; Matsui, T.; Mine, Y. The PepT1-transportable soy tripeptide VPY reduces intestinal inflammation. *Biochim. Biophys. Acta Gen. Subj.* **2012**, *1820*, 1753–1763. [CrossRef] [PubMed]
85. Oyama, M.; Van Hung, T.; Yoda, K.; He, F.; Suzuki, T. A novel whey tetrapeptide IPAV reduces interleukin-8 production induced by TNF-α in human intestinal Caco-2 cells. *J. Funct. Foods* **2017**, *35*, 376–383. [CrossRef]
86. Adibi, S.A. Regulation of expression of the intestinal oligopeptide transporter (Pept-1) in health and disease. *Am. J. Physiol. Liver Physiol.* **2003**, *285*, G779–G788. [CrossRef] [PubMed]
87. Bermudez-Brito, M.; Sahasrabudhe, N.M.; Rösch, C.; Schols, H.A.; Faas, M.M.; de Vos, P. The impact of dietary fibers on dendritic cell responses in vitro is dependent on the differential effects of the fibers on intestinal epithelial cells. *Mol. Nutr. Food Res.* **2015**, *59*, 698–710. [CrossRef] [PubMed]
88. Charrier, L.; Driss, A.; Yan, Y.; Nduati, V.; Klapproth, J.-M.; Sitaraman, S.V.; Merlin, D. hPepT1 mediates bacterial tripeptide fMLP uptake in human monocytes. *Lab. Investig.* **2006**, *86*, 490–503. [CrossRef] [PubMed]
89. Knipp, G.T.; Vander Velde, D.G.; Siahaan, T.J.; Borchardt, R.T. The effect of beta-turn structure on the passive diffusion of peptides across Caco-2 cell monolayers. *Pharm. Res.* **1997**, *14*, 1332–1340. [CrossRef] [PubMed]
90. Regazzo, D.; Molle, D.; Gabai, G.; Tome, D.; Dupont, D.; Leonil, J.; Boutrou, R. The (193-209) 17-residues peptide of bovine beta-casein is transported through Caco-2 monolayer. *Mol. Nutr. Food Res.* **2010**, *54*, 1428–1435. [CrossRef] [PubMed]
91. Cam, A.; Sivaguru, M.; Gonzalez de Mejia, E. Endocytic Mechanism of Internalization of Dietary Peptide Lunasin into Macrophages in Inflammatory Condition Associated with Cardiovascular Disease. *PLoS ONE* **2013**, *8*, e72115. [CrossRef] [PubMed]
92. Kneepkens, C.M.F.; Meijer, Y. Clinical practice. Diagnosis and treatment of cow's milk allergy. *Eur. J. Pediatr.* **2009**, *168*, 891–896. [CrossRef] [PubMed]
93. Turcanu, V.; Brough, H.A.; Du Toit, G.; Foong, R.-X.; Marrs, T.; Santos, A.F.; Lack, G. Immune mechanisms of food allergy and its prevention by early intervention. *Curr. Opin. Immunol.* **2017**, *48*, 92–98. [CrossRef] [PubMed]

94. Berin, M.C.; Sampson, H.A. Review Mucosal Immunology of Food Allergy. *Curr. Biol.* **2013**, *23*, R389–R400. [CrossRef] [PubMed]
95. Curotto de Lafaille, M.A.; Kutchukhidze, N.; Shen, S.; Ding, Y.; Yee, H.; Lafaille, J.J. Adaptive Foxp3+ Regulatory T Cell-Dependent and -Independent Control of Allergic Inflammation. *Immunity* **2008**, *29*, 114–126. [CrossRef] [PubMed]
96. Morgan, M.E.; Koelink, P.J.; Zheng, B.; den Brok, M.H.M.G.M.; van de Kant, H.J.; Verspaget, H.W.; Folkerts, G.; Adema, G.J.; Kraneveld, A.D. Toll-like receptor 6 stimulation promotes T-helper 1 and 17 responses in gastrointestinal-associated lymphoid tissue and modulates murine experimental colitis. *Mucosal Immunol.* **2014**, *7*, 1266–1277. [CrossRef] [PubMed]
97. Dolina, J.S.; Schoenberger, S.P. Toll-like receptor 9 is required for the maintenance of $CD25^+FoxP3^+CD4^+$ Treg cells during *Listeria monocytogenes* infection. *J. Immunol.* **2017**, *198* (Suppl. 1), 151.9.
98. Deutz, N.E.; Matheson, E.M.; Matarese, L.E.; Luo, M.; Baggs, G.E.; Nelson, J.L.; Hegazi, R.A.; Tappenden, K.A.; Ziegler, T.R.; Grp, N.S. Readmission and mortality in malnourished, older, hospitalized adults treated with a specialized oral nutritional supplement: A randomized clinical trial. *Clin. Nutr.* **2016**, *35*, 18–26. [CrossRef] [PubMed]
99. Elting, L.S.; Cooksley, C.; Chambers, M.; Cantor, S.B. The burdens of cancer therapy—Clinical and economic outcomes of chemotherapy-induced mucositis. *Cancer* **2003**, *98*, 1531–1539. [CrossRef] [PubMed]
100. Kaczmarek, A.; Brinkman, B.M.; Heyndrickx, L.; Vandenabeele, P.; Krysko, D.V. Severity of doxorubicin-induced small intestinal mucositis is regulated by the TLR-2 and TLR-9 pathways. *J. Pathol.* **2012**, *226*, 598–608. [CrossRef] [PubMed]
101. De Koning, B.A.E.; van Dieren, J.M.; Lindenbergh-Kortleve, D.J.; van der Sluis, M.; Matsumoto, T.; Yamaguchi, K.; Einerhand, A.W.; Samsom, J.N.; Pieters, R.; Nieuwenhuis, E.E.S. Contributions of mucosal immune cells to methotrexate-induced mucositis. *Int. Immunol.* **2006**, *18*, 941–949. [CrossRef] [PubMed]
102. Cario, E. Toll-like receptors in the pathogenesis of chemotherapy-induced gastrointestinal toxicity. *Curr. Opin. Support. Palliat. Care* **2016**, *10*, 157–164. [CrossRef] [PubMed]
103. Villa, A.; Sonis, S.T. Mucositis: Pathobiology and management. *Curr. Opin. Oncol.* **2015**, *27*, 159–164. [CrossRef] [PubMed]
104. Sahasrabudhe, N.M.; Beukema, M.; Tian, L.; Troost, B.; Scholte, J.; Bruininx, E.; Bruggeman, G.; van den Berg, M.; Scheurink, A.; Schols, H.A.; et al. Dietary Fiber Pectin Directly Blocks Toll-Like Receptor 2–1 and Prevents Doxorubicin Induced Ileitis. *Front. Immunol.* **2018**, *9*, 383. [CrossRef] [PubMed]
105. Crittenden, R.; Buckley, J.; Cameron-Smith, D.; Brown, A.; Thomas, K.; Davey, S.; Hobman, P. Functional dairy protein supplements for elite athletes. *Aust. J. Dairy Technol.* **2009**, *64*, 133–138.
106. Foltz, M.; Ansems, P.; Schwarz, J.; Tasker, M.C.; Lourbakos, A.; Gerhardt, C.C. Protein hydrolysates induce CCK release from enteroendocrine cells and act as partial agonists of the CCK1receptor. *J. Agric. Food Chem.* **2008**, *56*, 837–843. [CrossRef] [PubMed]
107. Kuehl, K.S.; Perrier, E.T.; Elliot, D.L.; Chesnutt, J.C. Efficacy of tart cherry juice in reducing muscle pain during running: A randomized controlled trial. *J. Int. Soc. Sports Nutr.* **2010**, *7*, 1–6. [CrossRef] [PubMed]
108. Howatson, G.; McHugh, M.P.; Hill, J.A.; Brouner, J.; Jewell, A.P.; Van Someren, K.A.; Shave, R.E.; Howatson, S.A. Influence of tart cherry juice on indices of recovery following marathon running. *Scand. J. Med. Sci. Sport.* **2010**, *20*, 843–852. [CrossRef] [PubMed]
109. Koikawa, N.; Nakamura, A.; Ngaoka, I.; Aoki, K.; Sawaki, K.; Suzuki, Y. Delayed-onset muscle injury and its modification by wheat gluten hydrolysate. *Nutrition* **2009**, *25*, 493–498. [CrossRef] [PubMed]
110. Hansen, M.; Bangsbo, J.; Bibby, B.M.; Madsen, K. Effect of whey protein hydrolysate on performance and recovery of top-clas orienteering runners. *Int. J. Sport Nutr. Exerc. Metab.* **2014**, *25*, 97–109. [CrossRef] [PubMed]
111. Buckley, J.D.; Thomson, R.L.; Coates, A.M.; Howe, P.R.C.; DeNichilo, M.O.; Rowney, M.K. Supplementation with a whey protein hydrolysate enhances recovery of muscle force-generating capacity following eccentric exercise. *J. Sci. Med. Sport* **2010**, *13*, 178–181. [CrossRef] [PubMed]
112. Cruzat, V.F.; Krause, M.; Newsholme, P. Amino acid supplementation and impact on immune function in the context of exercise. *J. Int. Soc. Sports Nutr.* **2014**, *11*, 1–13. [CrossRef] [PubMed]
113. Okada, H.; Kuhn, C.; Feillet, H.; Bach, J.-F. The "hygiene hypothesis" for autoimmune and allergic diseases: An update. *Clin. Exp. Immunol.* **2010**, *160*, 1–9. [CrossRef] [PubMed]

114. Dabelea, D.; Mayer-Davis, E.J.; Saydah, S.; Imperatore, G.; Linder, B.; Divers, J.; Bell, R.; Badaru, A.; Talton, J.W.; Crume, T.; et al. Prevalence of Type 1 and Type 2 Diabetes Among Children and Adolescents From 2001 to 2009. *JAMA* **2014**, *311*, 1778. [CrossRef] [PubMed]
115. Aw, D.; Silva, A.B.; Palmer, D.B. Immunosenescence: Emerging challenges for an ageing population. *Immunology* **2007**, *120*, 435–446. [CrossRef] [PubMed]
116. Plowden, J.; Renshaw-Hoelscher, M.; Engleman, C.; Katz, J.; Sambhara, S. Innate immunity in aging: Impact on macrophage function. *Aging Cell* **2004**, *3*, 161–167. [CrossRef] [PubMed]
117. Lloberas, J.; Celada, A. Effect of aging on macrophage function. *Exp. Gerontol.* **2002**, *37*, 1325–1331. [CrossRef]
118. Morey, J.N.; Boggero, I.A.; Scott, A.B.; Segerstrom, S.C. Current directions in stress and human immune function. *Curr. Opin. Psychol.* **2015**, *5*, 13–17. [CrossRef] [PubMed]
119. Organization, W.H. Mental health: Facing the challenges, building solutions. In Proceedings of the First WHO European Ministerial Conference on Mental Health, Helsinki, Finland, 12–15 January 2005.
120. Corazon, S.; Nyed, P.; Sidenius, U.; Poulsen, D.; Stigsdotter, U. A Long-Term Follow-Up of the Efficacy of Nature-Based Therapy for Adults Suffering from Stress-Related Illnesses on Levels of Healthcare Consumption and Sick-Leave Absence: A Randomized Controlled Trial. *Int. J. Environ. Res. Public Health* **2018**, *15*, 137. [CrossRef] [PubMed]
121. Dhabhar, F.S. Effects of stress on immune function: The good, the bad, and the beautiful. *Immunol. Res.* **2014**, *58*, 193–210. [CrossRef] [PubMed]
122. Godbout, J.P.; Glaser, R. Stress-induced immune dysregulation: Implications for wound healing, infectious disease and cancer. *J. Neuroimmune Pharmacol.* **2006**, *1*, 421–427. [CrossRef] [PubMed]
123. Steptoe, A.; Hamer, M.; Chida, Y. The effects of acute psychological stress on circulating inflammatory factors in humans: A review and meta-analysis. *Brain Behav. Immun.* **2007**, *21*, 901–912. [CrossRef] [PubMed]
124. Glaser, R.; MacCallum, R.C.; Laskowski, B.F.; Malarkey, W.B.; Sheridan, J.F.; Kiecolt-Glaser, J.K. Evidence for a shift in the Th-1 to Th-2 cytokine response associated with chronic stress and aging. *J. Gerontol. A. Biol. Sci. Med. Sci.* **2001**, *56*, M477–M482. [CrossRef] [PubMed]
125. Veru, F.; Dancause, K.; Laplante, D.P.; King, S.; Luheshi, G. Prenatal maternal stress predicts reductions in CD4+ lymphocytes, increases in innate-derived cytokines, and a Th2 shift in adolescents: Project Ice Storm. *Physiol. Behav.* **2015**, *144*, 137–145. [CrossRef] [PubMed]
126. Dhabhar, F.S.; Malarkey, W.B.; Neri, E.; McEwen, B.S. Stress-induced redistribution of immune cells—From barracks to boulevards to battlefields: A tale of three hormones—Curt Richter Award Winner. *Psychoneuroendocrinology* **2012**, *37*, 1345–1368. [CrossRef] [PubMed]

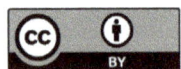

© 2018 by the authors. Licensee MDPI, Basel, Switzerland. This article is an open access article distributed under the terms and conditions of the Creative Commons Attribution (CC BY) license (http://creativecommons.org/licenses/by/4.0/).

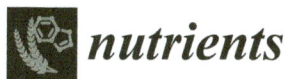

Review

Obesity, Inflammation, Toll-Like Receptor 4 and Fatty Acids

Marcelo Macedo Rogero [1,2,*] and Philip C. Calder [3,4]

1. Nutritional Genomics and Inflammation Laboratory, Department of Nutrition, School of Public Health, University of São Paulo, 01246-904 São Paulo, Brazil
2. Food Research Center (FoRC), CEPID-FAPESP, Research Innovation and Dissemination Centers São Paulo Research Foundation, São Paulo 05468-140, Brazil
3. Human Development and Health Academic Unit, Faculty of Medicine, University of Southampton, Southampton SO16 6YD, UK; P.C.Calder@soton.ac.uk
4. National Institute for Health Research Southampton Biomedical Research Centre, University Hospital Southampton National Health Service Foundation Trust and University of Southampton, Southampton SO16 6YD, UK
* Correspondence: mmrogero@usp.br; Tel.: +55-11-3061-7850

Received: 28 February 2018; Accepted: 28 March 2018; Published: 30 March 2018

Abstract: Obesity leads to an inflammatory condition that is directly involved in the etiology of cardiovascular diseases, type 2 diabetes mellitus, and certain types of cancer. The classic inflammatory response is an acute reaction to infections or to tissue injuries, and it tends to move towards resolution and homeostasis. However, the inflammatory process that was observed in individuals affected by obesity and metabolic syndrome differs from the classical inflammatory response in certain respects. This inflammatory process manifests itself systemically and it is characterized by a chronic low-intensity reaction. The toll-like receptor 4 (TLR4) signaling pathway is acknowledged as one of the main triggers of the obesity-induced inflammatory response. The aim of the present review is to describe the role that is played by the TLR4 signaling pathway in the inflammatory response and its modulation by saturated and omega-3 polyunsaturated fatty acids. Studies indicate that saturated fatty acids can induce inflammation by activating the TLR4 signaling pathway. Conversely, omega-3 polyunsaturated fatty acids, such as eicosapentaenoic acid and docosahexaenoic acid, exert anti-inflammatory actions through the attenuation of the activation of the TLR4 signaling pathway by either lipopolysaccharides or saturated fatty acids.

Keywords: inflammation; toll-like receptor 4; obesity; fatty acids

1. Obesity

Obesity is a multifactorial and polygenic condition that has become a very concerning public health issue that is affecting both developed and developing countries [1–3]. Overweight individuals (defined as body mass index (BMI) ≥ 25 kg/m^2) account for approximately 30% of the global population, i.e., 2.1 billion people, of whom more than 600,000 are classified as obese (defined as BMI ≥ 30 kg/m^2) [4]. The analysis conducted by the Global Burden of Disease Study 2013 showed that the overweight prevalence increased to 27.5% of adults and 47.1% of children in the past three decades [5]. The prevalence of obesity is currently higher in developed countries; nevertheless, approximately two-thirds of the obese population lives in developing countries [6]. Based on the current scenario, it is estimated that up to 50% of the global population will be classified as overweight or obese by 2030 [7]. Approximately 35% of adult individuals and 17% of children and adolescents (2 to 19 years old) are considered to be obese (defined by values above the 95th percentile of the BMI curve of these age groups) in the United States. It is estimated that approximately 300,000 people die due to obesity in the United States (U.S.) every year, which is the second highest cause of preventable death [8].

Cardiovascular diseases, type 2 diabetes (DM2), non-alcoholic fatty liver disease, and cancer stand out among the main health issues that are responsible for morbidity related to the obesity [9]. Obesity treatment and the treatment of its associated complications in developing countries has led to significant cost increases in healthcare. Costs that are linked to DM2, in particular, stand out, since 20–30% of overweight people present with a DM2 diagnosis, while 85% of diabetic patients are overweight or obese [10]. Calle et al. [11] conducted a prospective study of more than one million men and women and found that the lowest mortality rates, for all causes, in both men and women, occur in individuals with BMIs that are between 23.5 and 24.9 and 22.00 and 23.4 kg/m^2, respectively. Another study including 900,000 adult individuals found that BMIs that were above 25 kg/m^2 were associated with a 30% increase in general mortality rate per each 5 kg/m^2 increase [12].

Obesity results from the interactions of different factors, including genetic, metabolic, behavioral, and environmental ones. Accordingly, the dramatic increase in obesity prevalence rates suggests that behavioral and environmental components are the main factors that are responsible for obesity, with an emphasis on eating habits and exercise. With regard to eating, modern societies converge to an eating pattern called the Western diet, which is characterized by the intake of foods with high energy densities. Such densities derive from the high contents of fat and carbohydrate, especially sugars, that are found in these food types, a fact that contributes to obesity development [13,14].

The profile of fatty acids that are present in a diet may also be relevant to obesity. It is worth highlighting that, according to anthropological and epidemiological studies, humans from the Paleolithic Era—40,000 years ago—consumed a ratio of omega-6 (ω-6) to omega-3 (ω-3) polyunsaturated fatty acids of approximately 1, mainly due to a high intake of marine and vegetable sources of ω-3 polyunsaturated fatty acids (PUFAs). However, there was a significant increase in the intake of lipids, *trans* fatty acids, and ω-6 PUFAs after the Industrial Revolution, as well as a small increase in the intake of ω-3 fatty acids; meanwhile, intakes of vitamins C and E decreased. Such changes are particularly relevant if one takes into account the participation of these nutrients in the inflammatory response, which is linked to the physiopathology of different non-transmissible chronic diseases, such as obesity, DM2, cardiovascular diseases, hypertension, and cancer [15–17].

2. Inflammation, Adipose Tissue and Obesity

Inflammation is a central component of innate immunity, and microorganism destruction is the prime function of the inflammatory response, which is a process that involves the participation of effector cells in contact with pathogens that are living in the infected tissue. Microbial components, such as lipopolysaccharides (LPS) that are found in the cell wall of Gram negative bacteria, can trigger an inflammatory response through their interactions with cell-surface receptors found, for instance, in cells from the immune system, such as macrophages and neutrophils. Inflammation in response to microorganisms involves the increased synthesis and secretion of a number of mediators, including chemokines and cytokines. The latter include tumor necrosis factor (TNF)-α and interleukin (IL)-1, which act on endothelial cells and leukocytes to promote the recruitment and activation of leukocytes in the inflammatory area [18,19].

Inflammation can be classified as acute or chronic. Acute inflammation presents via three principal components: (i) changes in the vascular caliber, which result in increased blood flow in the inflammatory focus; (ii) structural changes in the microcirculation, which favor the exit of plasma proteins and leukocytes from the blood to the tissue; and, (iii) adhesion and transmigration of leukocytes from the microcirculation to the tissue, as well as their further activation, which allows the elimination of harmful agents. As soon as the infection is eliminated, or at least controlled, mechanisms are activated that act to limit any type of aggression against the host and to initiate the tissue repair process. Such a process aims to reduce the inflammation and it is termed resolution. Resolution is now known to be an active process involving the activation of negative feedback mechanisms, such as anti-inflammatory cytokine secretion, a reduction in receptor expression, activation of regulatory cells, and the production of pro-resolving lipid mediators [20–22].

Histamine, bradykinin, neuropeptides, prostaglandins, thromboxanes, leukotrienes, and platelet-activating factor stand out among the non-cytokine/chemokine mediators that are involved in the inflammatory response. The generation of eicosanoids initially occurs due to activation of phospholipase A2, which hydrolyzes membrane phospholipids to yield a free fatty acid. Arachidonic acid, an ω-6 PUFA, is predominant among the fatty acids released by phospholipase A2. The released fatty acids are used as a substrate by the cyclooxygenase enzymes (COX), which catalyze the synthesis of prostaglandins and thromboxanes, as well as by lipoxygenase (LOX) enzymes, which catalyzes the synthesis of leukotrienes. Such mediators are responsible for many aspects of the inflammatory response, such as vasodilation (prostaglandin E_2) and leukocyte migration (leukotriene B_4) [23–25].

Chronic inflammation involves the progressive changes in inflammatory cells as well as in tissue destruction and repair due to the on-going inflammatory process. Accordingly, inflammation can become pathologic because of the loss of tolerance or regulatory processes. As a result, there is an increase the plasma concentrations of many inflammatory biomarkers and in the number of activated inflammatory cells in the bloodstream as well as in the primary lesion area. Such changes can be easily observed, for instance, in patients with frank chronic conditions, like rheumatoid arthritis and inflammatory bowel diseases [26,27].

Chronic inflammation can also be present at lower intensities than has been seen in the classic inflammatory diseases. Evidence that obesity results in inflammation started emerging in the 1990s. This inflammation is directly involved in the etiology of cardiovascular diseases, DM2, and certain cancer types [28]. Hotamisligil et al. [29] found that genetically obese rodents, such as db/db and ob/ob mice and fa/fa rats, had increased expression of the TNF-α gene in white adipose tissue. They identified that the neutralization of TNF by anti-TNF-α antibodies mitigated the resistance of these animals to insulin action, establishing a link between inflammation, insulin resistance, and hyperglycemia. Macrophages from the stromal vascular fraction of adipose tissue appear to be the main cell type that is responsible for TNF-α and IL-6 release from the adipose tissue. The increased concentration of cytokines in this tissue is mostly derived from the infiltration of M1 macrophages, which are activated in the classical way and are characterized by the high expression of pro-inflammatory cytokines, like TNF-α, IL-1β and IL-6 [30–32] (Figure 1). It should be noted that macrophages correspond to about 40% of total white adipose tissue cells in obese mice and humans, as compared to only 18% in lean controls [33]. In the white adipose tissue, the expression of monocyte chemoattractant protein (MCP)-1 correlates positively with adiposity, and it is also higher in visceral adipose tissue when compared to subcutaneous adipose tissue [34,35]. The receptor for MCP-1, C-C chemokine receptor type 2 (CCR2), is expressed on monocytes present in peripheral blood and on adipose tissue macrophages. This implies that obesity favors the process of migration of blood monocytes into the visceral adipose tissue of obese individuals, which then differentiate into macrophages. This process is regulated by colony stimulating factors, such as macrophage-specific growth factor, called colony stimulating factor 1 (CSF-1) or macrophage colony-stimulating factor (M-CSF) [36].

In mammals, there are two types of adipose tissue: white and brown adipose tissue (BAT). BAT is specialized in the production of heat (thermogenesis) and, therefore, actively participates in the regulation of body temperature. BAT deposits are found in fetuses and newborns. In adult humans, there is a small volume of BAT in the cervical supra-clavicular, supra-adrenal, and para-spinal regions [37,38]. Brown and white adipocytes appear to have different physiology and opposing functions [39] Beiging/browning of white adipose tissue promotes energy expenditure by triggering thermogenesis, which suppresses diet-induced weight gain, as well as enhancing the efficiency of BAT activity [40]. In this context, individuals with low amounts of BAT would be prone to the development of obesity. Studies in animals lacking BAT or uncoupling protein 1 (UCP1) have clearly demonstrated the involvement of BAT thermogenesis in the protection against diet-induced obesity (DIO) [41]. Decreasing BAT activity or the removal of BAT in mice provokes increased glycemia and plasma triglyceride concentration and promotes insulin resistance [42]. Also, in humans, BAT activity was found to be inversely related to BMI and fat mass [43]. Furthermore, visceral adipose tissue inflammation may also be linked to the lower BAT volume, since TNF-α has been shown to induce brown adipocyte apoptosis and to hamper BAT differentiation [44].

Obesity is a relevant causal factor in the etiology of insulin-action resistance. Thus, obese patients present with reduced insulin action in the skeletal muscle due to lower phosphorylation of the tyrosine residues of the insulin receptor substrate (IRS)-1 and the reduced phosphatidylinositol-4,5-bisphosphate 3-kinase (PI3K) activity in this tissue. Such an outcome can cause a further reduction in insulin-induced glucose transport into the muscle tissue [45].

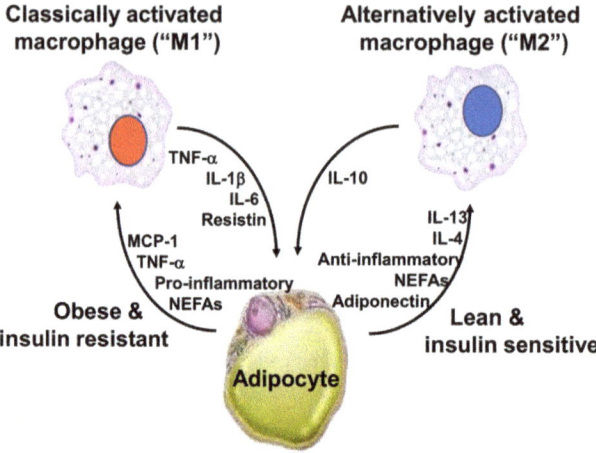

Figure 1. Interaction between M1 and M2 macrophages and adipocytes. Abbreviations: IL, interleukin; MCP, monocyte chemotactic protein; NEFAs, non-esterified fatty acids; TNF, tumor necrosis factor.

An increased inflammatory response is an important factor in the etiology of insulin-action resistance in obese patients. Such a response triggers the activation of protein kinases related to Toll signaling pathways and TNF-α receptors, such as the inhibitor of kappa B kinase (IKK) and c-jun N-terminal kinase (JNK)-1, which are capable of phosphorylating IRS-1 at the serine 307 residue. This reduces IRS-1 interaction with the insulin receptor beta subunit, and, consequently, causes decreased insulin signal transduction [46,47]. JNK knockout mice show lower adiposity, enhanced sensitivity to insulin and an increased capacity for insulin receptor signaling even when they are fed a lipid-rich feed. These findings suggest that activation through JNK is an important mechanism linked to insulin resistance in obese patients [48].

Among the inflammatory biomarkers that are related to obesity, IL-6 favors insulin-action resistance in obese individuals due to the induction of the cytokine signaling suppressor protein 3 (SOCS3), which physically associates itself with tyrosine phosphorylated proteins, such as the insulin receptor. In addition, SOCS3 decreases the phosphorylation of IRS-1 tyrosine, which weakens the IRS-1 coupling to the insulin receptor and the subsequent association between IRS-1 and phosphatidylinositol-3 kinase (PI3K). These findings suggest that SOCS3 is a relevant inhibitor of the insulin signaling pathway, as well as allowing a better understanding of the IL-6 effect on the insulin-action resistance that is induced by obesity [49].

Understanding that the immune system and different metabolic pathways are closely related to each other, as well as that they are functionally dependent, is essential for studies that are focused on obesity and on its possible metabolic repercussions. Thus, signaling pathways that are responsive to nutrient intake and the presence of pathogens are evolutionarily conserved and greatly integrated [50]. The excessive intake of obesity-associated nutrients can be detected by innate recognition receptors, and this results in the activation of pro-inflammatory signaling pathways as well as in stress responses in many parts of the body. This causes low-intensity chronic inflammation, defined by Hotamisligil et al. [30] as metabolic inflammation or as meta-inflammation, which is different from the classic inflammatory response. Moreover, the genesis of this inflammation is closely related to lifestyle and mainly to the quality of diet and exercise [51].

Meta-inflammation development is associated with a wide and integrated network of intracellular signal pathways, among which inhibitor of nuclear factor kappa-B kinase subunit beta (IKK-β) and c-Jun N-terminal kinase 1 (JNK-1) stand out. These proteins induce the synthesis of inflammatory mediators in different cell types. IKK-β and JNK-1 activation results in activating the transcription factors nuclear factor kappa B (NF-κB) and the activating protein (AP)-1, which translocate to the cell nucleus and activate the transcription of many genes encoding the proteins that are involved in inflammation, including TNF-α and COX-2. This process allows for the continuity of the inflammatory reaction, which is associated with conditions, such as atherogenesis and insulin-action resistance [52,53].

This systemic inflammatory response mainly originates from adipose tissue, which produces a wide variety of pro-inflammatory cytokines and chemokines, called adipokines [23]. However, currently, it is known that there are other tissues involved in meta-inflammation, such as the liver [54], pancreas [55], hypothalamus [56,57], and skeletal muscle [58]. It seems likely that the chronic low-grade inflammation that develops in adipose tissue with obesity is "transferred" to these other tissues through the appearance of active inflammatory mediators in the bloodstream.

In the context of inflammation and obesity, the role of gut microbiota in the development of metabolic disease should be noted. Studies have shown that certain bacteria populations produce enzymes that increase the efficiency of nutrient digestion, leading to an improved nutrient supply to the host, therefore, contributing to increased energy storage in the adipose tissue. The resulting increase in body adiposity can trigger the development of insulin resistance. There is also evidence that the gut microbiome can modulate that genes that are involved in energy storage and expenditure [59–62].

In 2004, Backhed et al. [61] reported that conventionally reared mice had a 42% increase in body fat and a 47% increases in periepididymal adipose tissue when compared to germ-free mice. Furthermore, transfer of the microbiota from the bowel of the conventional mouse to the gut of the germ-free mouse resulted in a 57% increase in body fat in two weeks, although feed consumption decreased. This result highlights the important role that the intestinal microbiota plays in energy homeostasis and its potential involvement in the etiology of obesity. Germ-free mice are resistant to diet-induced adiposity, which is associated with increased activity of AMP-activated protein kinase (AMPK) in liver and muscle and increased expression of adipose factor that is induced by fasting (Fiaf) in the small intestine [62]. On the other hand, the inoculation of the microbiota of conventional mice fed with this diet into germ-free animals results in an increase in adiposity [59].

It should also be noted that the dysbiosis that is associated with consuming a high-fat diet has been shown to increase intestinal permeability, which results in a greater translocation of LPS from the intestinal lumen to the blood circulation. This metabolic endotoxemia is associated with increased body fat, glucose intolerance, and increased expression of proinflammatory mediators and macrophage infiltration in white adipose tissue [60].

3. Toll-Like Receptor 4 and Inflammatory Response

The innate immune systems of mammals—which encompasses cells such as neutrophils and macrophages—use different strategies to recognize microorganisms. One of these strategies is based on recognizing general aspects of molecules associated with pathogens (pathogen-associated molecular patterns, or PAMPs) that result from microbial metabolism that is conserved throughout the evolution of the species. These molecules are widely distributed among pathogens; for instance, the LPS molecule is common in all Gram-negative bacteria, although it is not produced by the host [63–65].

Innate immune system receptors that are capable of recognizing PAMPs are called pattern recognition receptors, and these induce the expression of pro-inflammatory cytokines—for example, TNF-α and IL-1β—as well as activating the host's antimicrobial defense mechanisms, such as the synthesis of reactive oxygen and nitrogen species, including hydrogen peroxide and nitric oxide (NO), respectively [66,67]. PAMP recognition can induce cluster of differentiation 80 (CD80) and cluster of differentiation 86 (CD86) costimulatory molecules on the surface of cells, presenting antigens, as well as inducing small antigenic peptides that are linked to major histocompatibility complex (MHC) class II molecules in cell membranes that present antigens to CD4$^+$ T lymphocytes so activating adaptive immune responses [68].

The innate immune system recognizes PAMPs through toll-like receptors (TLRs) that are a family of transmembrane proteins that are responsible for playing an essential role in the innate immune system [69]. The main function of the TLR protein lies in controlling inflammatory and immunological responses. TLRs can recognize a whole variety of microbial PAMPs. Eleven different TLRs have been identified in humans and thirteen among all mammals [70]. TLRs belong to the IL-1 receptor (IL-1R) superfamily, which have a significant homology in their cytoplasmic regions, such as in the Toll/IL-1R (TIR) domain. The TIR domain is needed for the interaction and recruiting of many adaptive molecules that are involved in the activation of signaling pathways [67].

TLRs are expressed in different cell compartments and are recognized by many PAMPs deriving from viruses, pathogenic bacteria, fungi, and protozoa. TLR1, TLR2, TLR4, TLR5, TLR6, and TLR11 are expressed in the cellular membrane, whereas TLR3, TLR7, TLR8 and TLR9 are expressed in intracellular compartments, such as the endosome and the endoplasmic reticulum. Based on the amino acid sequence and on the genomic structure, TLRs can be divided into five subfamilies: TLR2, TLR3, TLR4, TLR5, and TLR9. The subfamily TLR2 comprises TLR1, TLR2, TLR6, and TLR10, whereas the subfamily TLR9 encompasses TLR7, TLR8, and TLR9 [71–73].

TLR4 was the first TLR reported in humans; it is expressed in innate immune cells, including monocytes, macrophages, and dendritic cells, as well as in other cell types, like adipocytes, enterocytes, and muscle cells. As indicated above, LPS is the primary agonist for TLR4 [74]. LPS is an integral structural component that is found in the external membrane of Gram-negative bacteria as well as representing one of the most powerful microbial inflammation indicators. It is a complex glycolipid composed of one hydrophilic polysaccharide and one hydrophobic domain called lipid A [75]. There is some evidence that saturated fatty acids can also bind to TLR4 and activate TLR4-mediated signaling pathways [76,77]. Also, there are other endogens ligands for TLR4, like heat shock protein (Hsp) 60, Hsp 70, type III repeat extra domain A of fibronectin, oligosaccharides of hyaluronic acid, polysaccharide fragments of heparan sulfate, and fibrinogen [78]. In the context of obesity, the increase in the plasma fibrinogen levels, which represents a positive acute phase protein, acts as a factor that is involved in the activation of the TLR4 pathway, and, consequently, in the amplification of the inflammatory response [79].

The interaction between LPS and TLR4 induces the synthesis of pro-inflammatory cytokines, such as TNF-α, IL-1β, IL-6, IL-8, and IL-12, which, in turn, work as endogenous inflammatory mediators by interacting with receptors found in different target cells. In addition to cytokines, macrophages release a whole variety of biological mediators in response to LPS, including platelet activation factor, prostaglandins, enzymes, and reactive oxygen and nitrogen species, such as superoxide anion and nitric oxide (NO). The synthesis of these pro-inflammatory mediators by monocytes and macrophages is designed to inhibit the growth and the dissemination of pathogens and to eliminate them either directly or through induction of adaptive immune responses [63,80].

LPS initially binds to the LPS-binding protein (LBP), which is found in the blood or in extracellular spaces. This protein promotes LPS binding to the CD14 molecule, which, in turn, is moored to the lipid bilayer by means of a glycophosphatidylinositol group that is found in most cells, except for endothelial ones. CD14 can also exist as a soluble protein, and, in this case, can lead LPS to the cell surface. The CD14 molecule is not found in transmembrane and intracellular domains; thus, it cannot trigger signal transduction processes on its own. When LPS binds to CD14, LBP dissociates itself and the LPS-CD14 complex physically associates with TLR4. Such a receptor needs an additional molecule, the so-called extracellular accessory protein (MD2), which binds to the TLR4 extracellular complex in order to recognize LPS [71].

Following ligand binding, TLRs dimerize and undergo conformational changes that are required for the subsequent recruitment of cytosolic TIR domain-containing adaptor molecules, including the cytoplasmic adapter protein MyD88. The association between TLR4 and MyD88 gathers proteins from the IL-1 receptor associated kinase (IRAK) family. Two members (IRAK4 and IRAK1) are phosphorylated in sequence, and this disrupts them from the receptor complex and promotes their association with TNF receptor associated factor 6 (TRAF6). TRAF6 then activates mitogen activated protein kinase (MAPK) proteins. These kinases can activate the AP-1 transcription factor [81].

The transcription factor NF-κB, which is found in a dimeric form in the cytoplasm of non-stimulated cells, is inactive when it is associated with κB inhibitors (IκB) (Figure 2). The family of IκB proteins includes IκBα, IκBβ, IκBε, and Bcl-3, as well as the carboxy-terminal regions of NF-κB1 (p105) and NF-κB2 (p100). The IκB proteins bind to different NF-κB dimers, although they have different affinities and specificities; therefore, besides the different NF-κB dimers that are found in a specific cell type, there are a large number of combinations of the IκB and the NF-κB dimers [82,83].

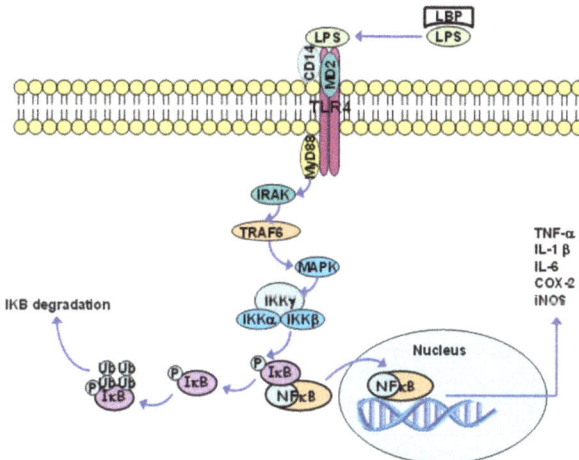

Figure 2. Toll-like receptor 4 (TLR4) induced signaling activates the transcription factor NFκB. LBP: LPS-binding protein; LPS: lipopolysaccharides; IRAK: IL-1 receptor associated kinase; TRAF6: TNF receptor associated factor 6; MAPK: mitogen activated protein kinase; IKK: inhibitor of nuclear factor kappa-B kinase; iNOs: inducible nitric oxide synthase.

Via MAPK, TRAF6 activates the IκB kinase complex (IKK), which is composed of two catalytic subunits (IKKα and IKKβ) and one regulatory subunit (IKKγ), and has the capacity to induce IκB phosphorylation. This phosphorylation results in IκB dissociation from the NF-κB complex and its subsequent polyubiquitination, which, in turn, leads to IκB degradation (mediated by the 26S proteasome) [73,81]. This process allows for the NF-κB dimer to translocate into the nucleus and to activate the transcription of many κB-dependent genes, such as the genes of pro-inflammatory cytokines, including TNF-α, IL-1β, IL-6, COX-2, and inducible nitric oxide synthase (iNOS) (Figure 2). NF-κB also stimulates the synthesis of IκB. Accordingly, the newly synthesized IκB binds to NF-κB and suppresses its activity, providing a feedback inhibition mechanism [74,81]. There are five members of the family of NF-κB transcription factors in mammals: NF-κB1 (p105/p50), NF-κB2 (p100/p52), RelA (p65), RelB, and c-Rel, which can dimerize to form homodimers and heterodimers that, in turn, are associated with specific transcriptional responses to different stimuli. NF-κB1and NF-κB2 do not contain transcriptional activation domains and their homodimers work as repressors. On the other hand, Rel-A, Rel-B, and c-Rel drive the transcriptional activation domain, and, except for Rel-B, are capable of forming homodimers and heterodimers along with other members of this family of proteins. Consequently, the balance between different NF-κB homodimers and heterodimers regulates the transcriptional activity level. It is worth highlighting that these proteins are expressed in a specific cell and tissue pattern, which leads to an additional level of regulation. NF-κB1 (p50) and RelA, for example, are broadly expressed, and, therefore, the p50/RelA heterodimer is the most common NF-κB-binding activity inducer [82,83].

Human monocytes express TLR1, TLR2, TLR4, TLR5, TLR6, TLR8, and TLR9; but TLR2 and TLR4 are the receptors that are most commonly expressed in these cells. The expression of TLR2 and TLR4 in the plasma membrane of monocytes has been confirmed by flow cytometry; TLR2 and TLR4-binding (by peptidoglycan and LPS, respectively) generates pro-inflammatory cytokine secretion in these cells. Moreover, TLR2 and TLR4 activation recruits monocytes and forms foam cells in murine models of atherosclerosis [30,84].

Studies that were conducted in vitro with cell cultures showed the negative effects of pro-inflammatory cytokines deriving from TLR4 signal pathway activation on glucose uptake and on the metabolism of fatty acids [33,85,86]. TLR4 gene deletion in mice has a protective effect against adipose tissue inflammation and against the resistance to insulin action that is induced by the intake of a high fat diet, a fact that points towards the causal role played by TLR4 in metabolic changes driven by over-eating and obesity [87,88].

Humans with type I diabetes exhibit a greater expression of TLR2 and TLR4 in the cellular membrane in monocytes, as well as greater MyD88 protein content and IRAK phosphorylation in monocytes in the peripheral blood than in control groups [89]. Individuals with DM2 show increased cellular membrane levels of TLR2 and TLR4 in blood monocytes, as well as a higher concentration of IL-1β, IL-6, IL-8, and TNF-α in serum than in controls [90]. Similarly, TLR2, TLR4, and MyD88 are more highly expressed in blood mononuclear cells and in the abdominal subcutaneous white adipose tissue in obese and diabetic individuals than in patients with normal weight [63,80]. Also, overweight and obese people showed increased expression of TLR2 and TLR4 on peripheral blood mononuclear cells and in adipose tissue in comparison with lean people; the expression levels of TLR2 and TLR4 increased significantly with increasing body mass index [91].

Furthermore, insulin-action resistance in obese individuals can increase the expression of TLR4, which depends on the designated PU.1 transcription factor, which, in turn, regulates the gene expression that is related to the activation and the differentiation of myeloid cells, including the TLR2, TLR4, and TLR9 receptors [92,93]. Insulin has a suppressive effect on the expression of TLR4 and on the activity of the PU.1 transcription factor; however, the suppressive effect of the hormone would be expected to be reduced due to the insulin-action resistance related to obesity. Such a reduction would increase the expression of TLR4 in peripheral blood monocytes [94]. In view of this, it seems that the increase of the inflammatory response favors the occurrence of resistance to the action of the insulin, through the activation of the IKK-β and JNK kinases that reduce the activation of IRS-1 in the insulin signaling pathway. Conversely, the presence of insulin resistance favors the expression of TLR4, suggesting that insulin resistance promotes inflammation.

As described earlier, the TLR4 pathway increases the expression of pro-inflammatory cytokines, such as TNF-α, IL-1, and IL-6, by activating the transcription factors NF-κB and AP-1. These cytokines, in turn, increase the hepatic synthesis of CRP, which is the classic positive acute phase reactant and the most studied and accepted inflammatory biomarker. CRP is often used in clinical practice due to its high stability (mean half-life of 19 hours) and its rapid production in response to inflammatory stimuli [95,96]. It is important to note that other inflammatory biomarkers, such as IL-6, TNF-α, the intercellular adhesion molecule (ICAM)-1, P-selectin, E-selectin, the monocyte chemotactic protein

(MCP)-1, fibrinogen, and soluble CD40, have been characterized as predictors of cardiovascular disease, regardless of other cardiovascular risk factors [19,26].

Dietary lipids can cause changes in the expression patterns of TLRs [97]. Ingestion of a high calorie (910 kcal), high lipid (51 g), and high carbohydrate (88 g) meal by normal weight individuals caused significant changes in TLR in the post-prandial period, with TLR2 and TLR4 increasing in blood mononuclear cells. This reinforces the potential importance of postprandial inflammation for obesity, DM2, and cardiovascular disease physiopathology [98,99]. A high-fat meal also leads to increased NF-κB activation in the post-prandial period, as well as increased leucocyte activation, as assessed by the surface expression of CD11a, CD11b, and CD62L [100], and metabolic endotoxemia (i.e., increased plasma LPS levels) [101].

4. Fatty Acids, Toll-Like Receptors and Inflammation

4.1. Saturated Fatty Acids

Saturated fatty acids, particularly lauric acid and palmitic acid, are capable of stimulating an inflammatory response through the TLR4 signaling pathway [102]. Lee et al. [103] published the first study that demonstrated the effect of different fatty acids on the TLR4 signaling pathway. In this study, it was verified that lauric, palmitic, and stearic acids could induce COX-2 expression through an NFκB-dependent mechanism in a macrophage cell line. Among the saturated fatty acids that were tested, lauric acid (C12:0) had the greatest activation capacity through TLR4. Different from saturated fatty acids, monounsaturated and polyunsaturated acids did not lead to TLR4 signal activation. Moreover, cell pretreatment in vitro for three hours with different polyunsaturated fatty acids, particularly the ω-3 fatty acid docosahexaeanoic acid (DHA: 22: 6 ω-3), or oleic acid (ω-9) significantly reduced the subsequent pro-inflammatory effect induced by lauric acid [103].

Saturated fatty acids represent an essential component of bacterial endotoxins. The lipid A portion of LPS has six saturated fatty acids coupled to this structure through ester or amide bonds. The carbon chain length of these fatty acids in lipid A varies from 12 to 16 carbons. Interestingly, the replacement of these saturated fatty acids by monounsaturated or polyunsaturated fatty acids stops the pro-inflammatory activity of the LPS [104].

Saturated fatty acids can also induce an inflammatory response through the activation of TLR2, which forms heterodimers in the plasma membrane, along with TLR1 or TLR6. Diacylated and triacylated lipoproteins, peptidoglycans, and lipoteichoic acid are among this receptor's agonists [76,105,106]. Lee et al. [107] reported that lauric acid induced activation through NF-κB when TLR2 was cotransfected with TLR1 or TLR6; however, this did not occur when TLR1, 2, 3, 5, 6, or 9 were individually transfected. On the other hand, the omega-3 polyunsaturated fatty DHA suppresses activation through the NF-κB signaling pathway, whether this is induced by LPS or by lauric acid [108]. Furthermore, the inhibition of TLR2 expression enhances the sensitivity to insulin action in the skeletal muscle and in the white adipose tissue of mice that were fed on a high fat diet as well as inhibiting the expression of this receptor. This process results in the partial reversal of palmitic acid-induced insulin resistance [23,109].

Erridge and Samani [110] suggested that saturated fatty acids would not directly stimulate TRL2 and TLR4, but that this effect could result from the contamination of the bovine serum albumin that was used to solubilize the saturated fatty acids in the studies conducted in vitro. However, Huang et al. [76] demonstrated that saturated fatty acids activate the inflammatory response in vitro through TLR2 and TLR4. Lauric acid—which was not solubilized in bovine serum albumin—induced the activation of the NF-κB signaling pathway through TLR2—which was dimerized with TLR1 or TLR6—and TLR4. In addition, there are current propositions addressing TLR4 activation by saturated fatty acids that depend on fetuin A, which is produced in the liver and works through endogenous TLR4-binding [77].

Palmitate acid that is bound to TLR4 activates the kinase proteins JNK and IKK-β, and increases the expression and secretion of pro-inflammatory cytokines [86]. Palmitic acid also impairs insulin signaling pathways by inducing IRS-1 phosphorylation at serine residue position 307 [111]. This process reduces its interactions with the insulin receptor, and, consequently, diminishes the insulin-induced signal transduction. Moreover, saturated fatty acids induce insulin-action resistance due to the antagonistic action of the peroxisome proliferator-activated receptor-gamma coactivator (PGC)-1 alpha. Such a process induces the expression of mitochondrial genes that are involved with oxidative phosphorylation and with glucose capture, which is mediated by insulin [112,113].

4.2. Polyunsaturated Fatty Acids

Polyunsaturated fatty acids consist of two families (ω-3 and ω-6) that are characterized by the double bond locations defined by the first double bond in relation to the methyl terminal group in the fatty acid molecule. α-Linolenic and linoleic acids are examples of polyunsaturated fatty acids belonging to the ω-3 and ω-6 families, respectively. These two fatty acids are not synthesized in humans, and the lack of ω-3 and ω-6 intake causes signaling and symptom deficits, indicating that such nutrients are essential to humans; therefore, they must be consumed through the diet [24,25,114,115]. However, studies have shown that the ratio of ω-6 to ω-3 fatty acids in the diet has implications for health since increased ratios are associated with an increased risk of chronic disease incidence and progression [116,117].

α-Linolenic acid is the precursor of the ω-3 polyunsaturated fatty acids with a longer chain and a high degree of unsaturation, such as eicosapentaenoic acid (EPA: 20: 5 ω-3) and DHA, which are found in seafood, especially fatty fish, and in fish oil supplements. It is important to note that the α-linolenic concentration in the blood, cells, and tissues is significantly lower than that of the EPA and DHA. This suggests that the primary biological function of α-linolenic is as a substrate in EPA and DHA synthesis [118]. However, evidence shows that α-linolenic conversion into EPA and DHA in humans is relatively low: conversion into EPA is estimated to only be around 8–12%, and conversion into DHA is lower than 1% [119,120].

The beneficial effects resulting from an increased intake of ω-3 fatty acids were originally associated with the suppression of thrombosis. However, epidemiologic evidence suggests that the intake of ω-3 fatty acids reduces the morbidity and mortality rates due to cardiovascular diseases, as well as reducing systemic blood pressure, triacylglycerol concentrations, and the risk of endothelial dysfunction [27,121–126]. The capacity to lower triacylglycerol concentrations, which is related to diminished hepatic VLDL secretion, stands out among the aforementioned possible metabolic effects resulting from the intake of ω-3 fatty acids. This effect is partially dependent on mechanisms that are related to nuclear receptors, particularly the peroxisome proliferator activated receptor (PPAR)-α [127].

An increased intake of ω-3 fatty acids results in the corresponding accumulation of these fatty acids in cell membranes and circulating lipids. They replace ω-6 fatty acids (such as linoleic and arachidonic acids) in blood lipids and in cell membranes, and also modulate/activate different signaling pathways [128].

The ω-3 and ω-6 polyunsaturated fatty acids generate relevant modulations in the inflammatory response because they are precursors to different series of eicosanoids, which have different effects on the intensity of the inflammatory response. Accordingly, ω-6 arachidonic acid generates even-series eicosanoids, such as prostaglandin E_2 and leukotriene B_4. These eicosanoids induce pro-inflammatory effects, such as increased vascular permeability, vasodilation, fever, and chemotaxis. It is important to note that prostaglandin E_2 also has anti-inflammatory effects, such as reduced IL-1 and TNF-α production. EPA is the precursor for odd-series eicosanoids, such as prostaglandin E_3, thromboxane A_3 and leukotriene B_5, which induce lower-intensity inflammatory responses. Leukotriene B_5, for example, is 10 to 100 times less potent as a chemotactic agent in neutrophils than leukotriene B_4 [23,27,129]. EPA also competes with arachidonic acid for COX-2 and 5-LOX; therefore, EPA reduces the synthesis of even-series eicosanoids [130]. In addition, higher EPA and DHA concentrations in the plasma membrane favor the production of mediators, such as resolvins, maresins, and protectins, which are involved in the resolution of inflammation and healing [21,25,131].

The ingestion of alpha-linolenic acid can also modulate the inflammatory response in humans. For example, Caughey et al. [132] observed a significant reduction of TNF-α, IL-1β, TXB$_2$, and PGE$_2$ production by LPS-stimulated mononuclear cell cultures that were obtained from healthy subjects who consumed approximately 14 g/day alpha-linolenic acid for four weeks as compared to baseline and to a control group. The effect of α-linolenic acid may have been mediated through its conversion to EPA.

With regard to the molecular effects of EPA and DHA on inflammatory-response modulation, studies have shown that these fatty acids inhibit the expression of inflammatory genes, such as COX-2, iNOS, and IL-1 in macrophages [103,108]. In contrast to the stimulating effect of saturated fatty acids on TLR2 and TLR4 activation, EPA and DHA are capable of mitigating the activation of the NF-κB transcription factor pathway that is induced by various agonists [103,133,134]. Thus, DHA reduces NF-κB pathway activation and the expression of cytokines and COX-2 induced by TLR agonists, such as lipopeptides (TLR2) and LPS (TLR4) in macrophages [89]. In addition, there is reduced gene expression of COX-2 that is induced by LPS in monocytes from the peripheral blood of individuals who use fish oil supplements [103,108]. The synthesis of the cytokines IL-1, IL-2, and TNF-α was also mitigated after stimulation with LPS in vitro by mononuclear cells from the peripheral blood from individuals that were supplemented with 18 g of fish oil per day for six weeks [135].

In addition, EPA and DHA present another mechanism to modulate the inflammatory response by binding to G-protein coupled receptor 120 (GPR120), which is also known as free fatty acid receptor 4 (FFA4). GPR120 activation induced by EPA or DHA leads to β-arrestin 2 recruitment to the plasma membrane, where this protein binds to GPR120. Subsequently, the GPR120/β-arrestin 2 complex is internalized into the cytoplasmic compartment, where this complex binds to the TAK1-binding protein (TAB1). This process impairs the association between TAB1 and the kinase activated by the growth factor beta (TAK1), and, consequently, results in reduced TAK1 activation and in reduced activity of the IKK-β/NF-κB and JNK/AP-1 signaling pathways. Accordingly, the TAB1/TAK1 binding is a convergence point of stimuli that are induced by the TLR4 signaling pathway and of the TNF receptor (TNFR). The mitigation of TAK-1 activation by DHA leads to the reduced expression of genes with pro-inflammatory actions, such as TNF-α and IL-6 [136,137].

Other mechanisms that are related to the EPA and DHA effects concern their capacities to bind to peroxisome proliferator activated receptors (PPARs), including the isoforms PPAR-alpha, PPAR-gamma, and PPAR-beta/delta. PPARs are a group of nuclear receptors that are coded for by different genes. PPAR isoforms form heterodimers with the retinoid X receptor (RXR) and bind to peroxisome proliferator response elements (PPRE) in the region that is responsible for promoting the target genes that are involved in lipid metabolism and in the inflammatory response; subsequently, they modulate the expression of these genes [138]. PPAR-alpha and PPAR-gamma activations reduce the expression of genes that code for proteins presenting pro-inflammatory actions through inhibition of NF-κB activation. It is worth emphasizing that EPA and DHA directly interact with PPARs, and, therefore, modulate the expression of genes that are involved in lipid metabolism and the inflammatory response [139]. Furthermore, the anti-inflammatory effects of EPA and DHA on this signaling pathway can occur due to diminished nicotinamide adenine dinucleotide phosphate (NADPH) oxidase activity, which leads to lower TLR4 recruitment for lipid rafts and TLR4 dimerization [102]. Moreover, the lower NADPH oxidase activity also decreases the production of reactive oxygen species, which, in turn, are necessary to activate the TLR4 signaling pathway. Another possible mechanism of action of the ω-3 fatty acids concerns the capacity of incorporating DHA into the plasma membrane, which can lead to reduced TLR4 translocation for lipid rafts formation. This decreases TLR4 pathway activation, and, consequently, decreases NF-κB activation [102,140,141].

Figure 3 shows the main molecular mechanisms related to the effects of saturated and omega-3 fatty acids on the TLR4 pathway.

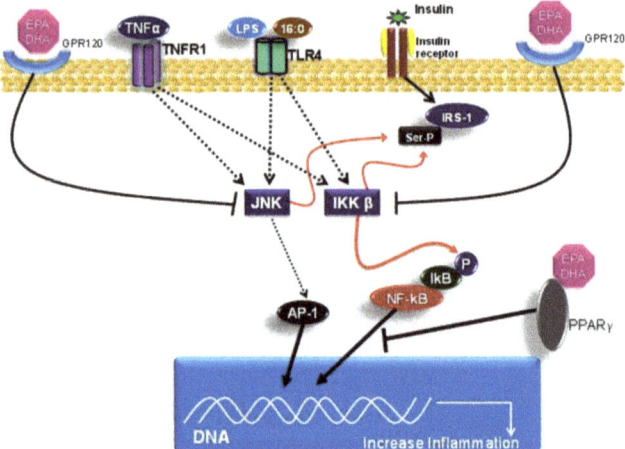

Figure 3. Molecular mechanism of the effects of saturated (16:0) and omega-3 polyunsaturated fatty acids (EPA, DHA) on the TLR4 and NFkB pathways. The arrows → indicate activation and the arrows ⊣ indicate inhibition. Abbreviations: TNFα, Tumor necrosis factor; TNFR1, Tumor necrosis factor receptor 1; LPS, Lipopolysaccharides; 16:0, palmitic acid; TLR4, Toll-like receptor 4; GPR120, G-protein coupled receptor 120; EPA, eicosapentaenoic acid; DHA, Docosahexaenoic acid; IRS-1, Insulin receptor substrate 1; Ser-P, phosphorylated *serine* residues; PPARγ, Peroxisome proliferator-activated receptor gamma; JNK, c-Jun N-terminal kinases; IKK β, inhibitor of nuclear factor kappa-B kinase subunit beta; IkB, NFKB Inhibitor; P, phosphate; AP-1, Activator protein 1.

5. Conclusions

The inflammatory process that occurs in obese people differs from the classical inflammatory response in certain respects. This inflammatory process manifests itself systemically and is characterized by a chronic low-intensity reaction. In this context, the TLR4 signaling pathway has been recognized as one of the main triggers in increasing the obesity-induced inflammatory response. This pathway responds to the increased exposure to saturated fatty acids and to LPS. Both of these are relevant in the context of obesity, with saturated fatty acids arising from within the adipose tissue triglyceride stores and the LPS arising from increased intestinal permeability perhaps due to an altered gut microbiota. Adipose tissue driven inflammation increases insulin resistance, both locally and systemically, so contributing to the co-morbidities of obesity, like DM2. Studies indicate that omega-3 fatty acids, namely EPA and DHA, have an anti-inflammatory effect, which involves attenuating the activation of the TLR4 signaling pathway. This has relevant implications for reducing meta-inflammation, and, consequently, resistance to insulin action and the risk of DM2 and cardiovascular disease in obese individuals. The omega-3 fatty acids can oppose the action of both classic TLR agonists (e.g., LPS) and saturated fatty acids in this regard.

Acknowledgments: The authors would like to thank The São Paulo Research Foundation and the Brazilian National Council for Scientific and Technological Development (CNPq) for the financial support.

Author Contributions: Literature searching and initial manuscript preparation were performed by M.M.R. The manuscript was revised and finalized by P.C.C. and M.M.R.

Conflicts of Interest: The authors declare that they have no conflict of interest.

References

1. Flegal, K.M.; Carroll, M.D.; Kit, B.K.; Ogden, C.L. Prevalence of obesity and trends in the distribution of body mass index among US adults, 1999–2010. *JAMA* **2012**, *307*, 491–497. [CrossRef] [PubMed]

2. Kopelman, P.G. Obesity as a medical problem. *Nature* **2000**, *404*, 635–643. [CrossRef] [PubMed]
3. Yach, D.; Stuckler, D.; Brownell, K.D. Epidemiologic and economic consequences of the global epidemics of obesity and diabetes. *Nat. Med.* **2006**, *12*, 62–66. [CrossRef] [PubMed]
4. WHO—World Health Organization. World Health Organization Obesity and overweight Fact Sheet (2016). Available online: http://www.who.int/mediacentre/factsheets/fs311/en/ (accessed on 30 January 2018).
5. Ng, M.; Fleming, T.; Robinson, M.; Thomson, B.; Graetz, N.; Margono, C.; Mullany, E.C.; Biryukov, S.; Abbafati, C.; Abera, S.F.; et al. Global, regional, and national prevalence of overweight and obesity in children and adults during 1980–2013: A systematic analysis for the Global Burden of Disease Study 2013. *Lancet* **2014**, *384*, 766–781. [CrossRef]
6. Alexandratos, N.; Bruinsma, J. *World Agriculture Towards 2030/2050: The 2012 Revision*; FAO: Rome, Italy, 2012.
7. United Nations News Centre, 2015. United Nations News Centre. Available online: http://www.un.org/sustainabledevelopment/blog/2015/07/un-projects-world-population-to-reach-8-5-billion-by-2030-driven-by-growth-in-developing-countries/ (accessed on 17 January 2018).
8. Ogden, C.L.; Carroll, M.D.; Curtin, L.R.; Lamb, M.M.; Flegal, K.M. Prevalence of high body mass index in US children and adolescents, 2007–2008. *JAMA* **2010**, *303*, 242–249. [CrossRef] [PubMed]
9. Mokdad, A.H.; Ford, E.S.; Bowman, B.A.; Dietz, W.H.; Vinicor, F.; Bales, V.S.; Marks, J.S. Prevalence of obesity, diabetes, and obesity-related health risk factors, 2001. *JAMA* **2003**, *289*, 76–79. [CrossRef] [PubMed]
10. Daousi, C.; Casson, I.F.; Gill, G.V.; MacFarlane, I.A.; Wilding, J.P.; Pinkney, J.H. Prevalence of obesity in type 2 diabetes in secondary care: Association with cardiovascular risk factors. *Postgrad. Med. J.* **2006**, *82*, 280–284. [CrossRef] [PubMed]
11. Calle, E.E.; Thun, M.J.; Petrelli, J.M.; Rodriguez, C.; Heath, C.W., Jr. Body-mass index and mortality in a prospective cohort of U.S. adults. *N. Engl. J. Med.* **1999**, *341*, 1097–1105. [CrossRef] [PubMed]
12. Prospective Studies Collaboration; Whitlock, G.; Lewington, S.; Sherliker, P.; Clarke, R.; Emberson, J.; Halsey, J.; Qizilbash, N.; Collins, R.; Peto, R. Body-mass index and cause-specific mortality in 900 000 adults: Collaborative analyses of 57 prospective studies. *Lancet* **2009**, *373*, 1083–1096. [CrossRef] [PubMed]
13. Amuna, P.; Zotor, F.B. Epidemiological and nutrition transition in developing countries: Impact on human health and development. *Proc. Nutr. Soc.* **2008**, *67*, 82–90. [CrossRef] [PubMed]
14. Vandevijvere, S.; Chow, C.C.; Hall, K.D.; Umali, E.; Swinburn, B.A. Increased food energy supply as a major driver of the obesity epidemic: A global analysis. *Bull. World Health Organ.* **2015**, *93*, 446–456. [CrossRef] [PubMed]
15. Roberts, C.K.; Barnard, R.J. Effects of exercise and diet on chronic disease. *J. Appl. Physiol. (1985)* **2005**, *98*, 3–30. [CrossRef] [PubMed]
16. Simopoulos, A.P.; DiNicolantonio, J.J. The importance of a balanced ω-6 to ω-3 ratio in the prevention and management of obesity. *Open Heart* **2016**, *3*, e000385. [CrossRef] [PubMed]
17. Galli, C.; Calder, P.C. Effects of fat and fatty acid intake on inflammatory and immune responses: A critical review. *Ann. Nutr. Metab.* **2009**, *55*, 123–139. [CrossRef] [PubMed]
18. Calder, P.C. Polyunsaturated fatty acids and inflammatory processes: New twists in an old tale. *Biochimie* **2009**, *91*, 791–795. [CrossRef] [PubMed]
19. Calder, P.C.; Ahluwalia, N.; Albers, R.; Bosco, N.; Bourdet-Sicard, R.; Haller, D.; Holgate, S.T.; Jönsson, L.S.; Latulippe, M.E.; Marcos, A.; et al. A consideration of biomarkers to be used for evaluation of inflammation in human nutritional studies. *Br. J. Nutr.* **2013**, *109*, 1–34. [CrossRef] [PubMed]
20. Molfino, A.; Amabile, M.I.; Monti, M.; Muscaritoli, M. Omega-3 Polyunsaturated Fatty Acids in Critical Illness: Anti-Inflammatory, Proresolving, or Both? *Oxid. Med. Cell. Longev.* **2017**, *2017*, 5987082. [CrossRef] [PubMed]
21. Serhan, C.N.; Chiang, N.; Dalli, J. New pro-resolving *n*-3 mediators bridge resolution of infectious inflammation to tissue regeneration. *Mol. Asp. Med.* **2017**. [CrossRef] [PubMed]
22. Calder, P.C. Omega-3 fatty acids and inflammatory processes. *Nutrients* **2010**, *2*, 355–374. [CrossRef] [PubMed]
23. Calder, P.C.; Ahluwalia, N.; Brouns, F.; Buetler, T.; Clement, K.; Cunningham, K.; Esposito, K.; Jönsson, L.S.; Kolb, H.; Lansink, M.; et al. Dietary factors and low-grade inflammation in relation to overweight and obesity. *Br. J. Nutr.* **2011**, *106*, 5–78. [CrossRef] [PubMed]
24. Calder, P.C. The role of marine omega-3 (*n*-3) fatty acids in inflammatory processes, atherosclerosis and plaque stability. *Mol. Nutr. Food Res.* **2012**, *56*, 1073–1080. [CrossRef] [PubMed]

25. Calder, P.C. Marine omega-3 fatty acids and inflammatory processes: Effects, mechanisms and clinical relevance. *Biochim. Biophys. Acta* **2015**, *1851*, 469–484. [CrossRef] [PubMed]
26. Calder, P.C. Fatty acids and inflammation: The cutting edge between food and pharma. *Eur. J. Pharmacol.* **2011**, *668*, 50–58. [CrossRef] [PubMed]
27. Calder, P.C.; Yaqoob, P. Marine omega-3 fatty acids and coronary heart disease. *Curr. Opin. Cardiol.* **2012**, *27*, 412–419. [CrossRef] [PubMed]
28. Emilsson, V.; Thorleifsson, G.; Zhang, B.; Leonardson, A.S.; Zink, F.; Zhu, J.; Carlson, S.; Helgason, A.; Walters, G.B.; Gunnarsdottir, S.; et al. Genetics of gene expression and its effect on disease. *Nature* **2008**, *452*, 423–428. [CrossRef] [PubMed]
29. Hotamisligil, G.S.; Shargill, N.S.; Spiegelman, B.M. Adipose expression of tumor necrosis factor-alpha: Direct role in obesity-linked insulin resistance. *Science* **1993**, *259*, 87–91. [CrossRef] [PubMed]
30. Hotamisligil, G.S. Inflammation and metabolic disorders. *Nature* **2006**, *444*, 860–867. [CrossRef] [PubMed]
31. Wellen, K.E.; Hotamisligil, G.S. Inflammation, stress, and diabetes. *J. Clin. Investig.* **2005**, *115*, 1111–1119. [CrossRef] [PubMed]
32. Zeyda, M.; Stulnig, T.M. Adipose tissue macrophages. *Immunol. Lett.* **2007**, *112*, 61–67. [CrossRef] [PubMed]
33. Lumeng, C.N.; Bodzin, J.L.; Saltiel, A.R. Obesity induces a phenotypic switch in adipose tissue macrophage polarization. *J. Clin. Investig.* **2007**, *117*, 175–184. [CrossRef] [PubMed]
34. Cancello, R.; Clement, K. Is obesity an inflammatory illness? Role of low-grade inflammation and macrophage infiltration in human white adipose tissue. *BJOG* **2006**, *113*, 1141–1147. [CrossRef] [PubMed]
35. Cave, M.C.; Hurt, R.T.; Frazier, T.H.; Matheson, P.J.; Garrison, R.N.; McClain, C.J.; McClave, S.A. Obesity, inflammation, and the potential application of pharmaconutrition. *Nutr. Clin. Pract.* **2008**, *23*, 16–34. [CrossRef] [PubMed]
36. Ferrante, A.W. Obesity-induced inflammation: A metabolic dialogue in the language of inflammation. *J. Intern. Med.* **2007**, *262*, 408–414. [CrossRef] [PubMed]
37. Cannon, B.; Nedergaard, J. Brown adipose tissue: Function and physiological significance. *Physiol. Rev.* **2004**, *84*, 277–359. [CrossRef] [PubMed]
38. Nedergaard, J.; Bengtsson, T.; Cannon, B. Unexpected evidence for active brown adipose tissue in adult humans. *Am. J. Physiol. Endocrinol. Metab.* **2007**, *293*, E444–E452. [CrossRef] [PubMed]
39. Cinti, S. The adipose organ. *Prostaglandins Leukot. Essent. Fatty Acids* **2005**, *73*, 9–15. [CrossRef] [PubMed]
40. Cao, L.; Choi, E.Y.; Liu, X.; Martin, A.; Wang, C.; Xu, X.; During, M.J. White to brown fat phenotypic switch induced by genetic and environmental activation of a hypothalamic-adipocyte axis. *Cell Metab.* **2011**, *14*, 324–338. [CrossRef] [PubMed]
41. Lowell, B.B.; Susulic, V.; Hamann, A.; Lawitts, J.A.; Himms-Hagen, J.; Boyer, B.B.; Kozak, L.P.; Flier, J.S. Development of obesity in transgenic mice after genetic ablation of brown adipose tissue. *Nature* **1993**, *366*, 740–742. [CrossRef] [PubMed]
42. Connolly, E.; Morrisey, R.D.; Carnie, J.A. The effect of interscapular brown adipose tissue removal on body-weight and cold response in the mouse. *Br. J. Nutr.* **1982**, *47*, 653–658. [CrossRef] [PubMed]
43. van Marken Lichtenbelt, W.D.; Vanhommerig, J.W.; Smulders, N.M.; Drossaerts, J.M.; Kemerink, G.J.; Bouvy, N.D.; Schrauwen, P.; Teule, G.J. Cold-activated brown adipose tissue in healthy men. *N. Engl. J. Med.* **2009**, *360*, 1500–1508. [CrossRef] [PubMed]
44. Nisoli, E.; Briscini, L.; Giordano, A.; Tonello, C.; Wiesbrock, S.M.; Uysal, K.T.; Cinti, S.; Carruba, M.O.; Hotamisligil, G.S. Tumor necrosis factor alpha mediates apoptosis of brown adipocytes and defective brown adipocyte function in obesity. *Proc. Natl. Acad. Sci. USA* **2000**, *97*, 8033–8038. [CrossRef] [PubMed]
45. Samuel, V.T.; Shulman, G.I. Mechanisms for insulin resistance: Common threads and missing links. *Cell* **2012**, *148*, 852–871. [CrossRef] [PubMed]
46. Guo, S. Insulin signaling, resistance, and the metabolic syndrome: Insights from mouse models into disease mechanisms. *J. Endocrinol.* **2014**, *220*, 1–23. [CrossRef] [PubMed]
47. Hotamisligil, G.S.; Davis, R.J. Cell Signaling and Stress Responses. *Cold Spring Harb. Perspect. Biol.* **2016**, *8*. [CrossRef] [PubMed]
48. Han, M.S.; Jung, D.Y.; Morel, C.; Lakhani, S.A.; Kim, J.K.; Flavell, R.A.; Davis, R.J. JNK expression by macrophages promotes obesity-induced insulin resistance and inflammation. *Science* **2013**, *339*, 218–222. [CrossRef] [PubMed]

49. Tilg, H.; Moschen, A.R. Insulin resistance, inflammation, and non-alcoholic fatty liver disease. *Trends Endocrinol. Metab.* **2008**, *19*, 371–379. [CrossRef] [PubMed]
50. Kirwan, A.M.; Lenighan, Y.M.; O'Reilly, M.E.; McGillicuddy, F.C.; Roche, H.M. Nutritional modulation of metabolic inflammation. *Biochem. Soc. Trans.* **2017**, *45*, 979–985. [CrossRef] [PubMed]
51. Egger, G.; Dixon, J. Obesity and chronic disease: Always offender or often just accomplice? *Br. J. Nutr.* **2009**, *102*, 1238–1242. [CrossRef] [PubMed]
52. Ertunc, M.E.; Hotamisligil, G.S. Lipid signaling and lipotoxicity in metaflammation: Indications for metabolic disease pathogenesis and treatment. *J. Lipid Res.* **2016**, *57*, 2099–2114. [CrossRef] [PubMed]
53. Hotamisligil, G.S. Inflammation, metaflammation and immunometabolic disorders. *Nature* **2017**, *542*, 177–185. [CrossRef] [PubMed]
54. Cai, D.; Yuan, M.; Frantz, D.F.; Melendez, P.A.; Hansen, L.; Lee, J.; Shoelson, S.E. Local and systemic insulin resistance resulting from hepatic activation of IKK-beta and NF-kappaB. *Nat. Med.* **2005**, *11*, 183–190. [CrossRef] [PubMed]
55. Ehses, J.A.; Perren, A.; Eppler, E.; Ribaux, P.; Pospisilik, J.A.; Maor-Cahn, R.; Gueripel, X.; Ellingsgaard, H.; Schneider, M.K.; Biollaz, G.; et al. Increased number of islet-associated macrophages in type 2 diabetes. *Diabetes* **2007**, *56*, 2356–2370. [CrossRef] [PubMed]
56. De Souza, C.T.; Araujo, E.P.; Bordin, S.; Ashimine, R.; Zollner, R.L.; Boschero, A.C.; Saad, M.J.; Velloso, L.A. Consumption of a fat-rich diet activates a proinflammatory response and induces insulin resistance in the hypothalamus. *Endocrinology* **2005**, *146*, 4192–4199. [CrossRef] [PubMed]
57. Milanski, M.; Arruda, A.P.; Coope, A.; Ignacio-Souza, L.M.; Nunez, C.E.; Roman, E.A.; Romanatto, T.; Pascoal, L.B.; Caricilli, A.M.; Torsoni, M.A.; et al. Inhibition of hypothalamic inflammation reverses diet-induced insulin resistance in the liver. *Diabetes* **2012**, *61*, 1455–1462. [CrossRef] [PubMed]
58. Varma, V.; Yao-Borengasser, A.; Rasouli, N.; Nolen, G.T.; Phanavanh, B.; Starks, T.; Gurley, C.; Simpson, P.; McGehee, R.E., Jr.; Kern, P.A.; et al. Muscle inflammatory response and insulin resistance: Synergistic interaction between macrophages and fatty acids leads to impaired insulin action. *Am. J. Physiol. Endocrinol. Metab.* **2009**, *296*, 1300–1310. [CrossRef] [PubMed]
59. Turnbaugh, P.J.; Bäckhed, F.; Fulton, L.; Gordon, J.I. Diet-induced obesity is linked to marked but reversible alterations in the mouse distal gut microbiome. *Cell Host Microbe* **2008**, *3*, 213–223. [CrossRef] [PubMed]
60. Cani, P.D.; Bibiloni, R.; Knauf, C.; Neyrinck, A.M.; Delzenne, N.M.; Burcelin, R. Changes in gut microbiota control metabolic endotoxemia-induced inflammation in high-fat diet-induced obesity and diabetes in mice. *Diabetes* **2008**, *57*, 1470–1481. [CrossRef] [PubMed]
61. Backhed, F.; Ding, H.; Wang, T.; Hooper, L.V.; Koh, G.Y.; Nagy, A.; Semenkovich, C.F.; Gordon, J.I. The gut microbiota as an environmental factor that regulates fat storage. *Proc. Natl. Acad. Sci. USA* **2004**, *101*, 15718–15723. [CrossRef] [PubMed]
62. Bäckhed, F.; Manchester, J.K.; Semenkovich, C.F.; Gordon, J.I. Mechanisms underlying the resistance to diet-induced obesity in germ-free mice. *Proc. Natl. Acad. Sci. USA* **2007**, *104*, 979–984. [CrossRef] [PubMed]
63. Basith, S.; Manavalan, B.; Lee, G.; Kim, S.G.; Choi, S. Toll-like receptor modulators: A patent review (2006–2010). *Expert Opin. Ther. Pat.* **2011**, *21*, 927–944. [CrossRef] [PubMed]
64. Pandey, S.; Kawai, T.; Akira, S. Microbial sensing by Toll-like receptors and intracellular nucleic acid sensors. *Cold Spring Harb. Perspect. Biol.* **2014**, *7*, a016246. [CrossRef] [PubMed]
65. Satoh, T.; Akira, S. Toll-Like Receptor Signaling and Its Inducible Proteins. *Microbiol. Spectr.* **2016**, *4*. [CrossRef]
66. Beutler, B.A. TLRs and innate immunity. *Blood* **2009**, *113*, 1399–1407. [CrossRef] [PubMed]
67. Moresco, E.M.; LaVine, D.; Beutler, B. Toll-like receptors. *Curr. Biol.* **2011**, *21*, 488–493. [CrossRef] [PubMed]
68. Lin, Q.; Li, M.; Fang, D.; Fang, J.; Su, S.B. The essential roles of Toll-like receptor signaling pathways in sterile inflammatory diseases. *Int. Immunopharmacol.* **2011**, *11*, 1422–1432. [CrossRef] [PubMed]
69. Carvalho, F.A.; Aitken, J.D.; Vijay-Kumar, M.; Gewirtz, A.T. Toll-like receptor-gut microbiota interactions: Perturb at your own risk! *Annu. Rev. Physiol.* **2012**, *74*, 177–198. [CrossRef] [PubMed]
70. Trudler, D.; Farfara, D.; Frenkel, D. Toll-like receptors expression and signaling in glia cells in neuro-amyloidogenic diseases: Towards future therapeutic application. *Mediators Inflamm.* **2010**, *2010*. [CrossRef] [PubMed]
71. Connolly, D.J.; O'Neill, L.A. New developments in Toll-like receptor targeted therapeutics. *Curr. Opin. Pharmacol.* **2012**, *12*, 510–518. [CrossRef] [PubMed]

72. Triantafilou, M.; Triantafilou, K. The dynamics of LPS recognition: Complex orchestration of multiple receptors. *J. Endotoxin Res.* **2005**, *11*, 5–11. [CrossRef] [PubMed]
73. Beutler, B. Innate immunity: An overview. *Mol. Immunol.* **2004**, *40*, 845–859. [CrossRef] [PubMed]
74. Dobrovolskaia, M.A.; Vogel, S.N. Toll receptors, CD14, and macrophage activation and deactivation by LPS. *Microbes Infect.* **2002**, *4*, 903–914. [CrossRef]
75. Triantafilou, M.; Triantafilou, K. Lipopolysaccharide recognition: CD14, TLRs and the LPS-activation cluster. *Trends Immunol.* **2002**, *23*, 301–304. [CrossRef]
76. Huang, S.; Rutkowsky, J.M.; Snodgrass, R.G.; Ono-Moore, K.D.; Schneider, D.A.; Newman, J.W.; Adams, S.H.; Hwang, D.H. Saturated fatty acids activate TLR-mediated proinflammatory signaling pathways. *J. Lipid Res.* **2012**, *53*, 2002–2013. [CrossRef] [PubMed]
77. Pal, D.; Dasgupta, S.; Kundu, R.; Maitra, S.; Das, G.; Mukhopadhyay, S.; Ray, S.; Majumdar, S.S.; Bhattacharya, S. Fetuin-A acts as an endogenous ligand of TLR4 to promote lipid-induced insulin resistance. *Nat. Med.* **2012**, *18*, 1279–1285. [CrossRef] [PubMed]
78. Gay, N.J.; Gangloff, M. Structure and function of Toll receptors and their ligands. *Annu. Rev. Biochem.* **2007**, *76*, 141–165. [CrossRef] [PubMed]
79. Al-ofi, E.; Coffelt, S.B.; Anumba, D.O. Fibrinogen, an endogenous ligand of Toll-like receptor 4, activates monocytes in pre-eclamptic patients. *J. Reprod. Immunol.* **2014**, *103*, 23–28. [CrossRef] [PubMed]
80. Könner, A.C.; Brüning, J.C. Toll-like receptors: Linking inflammation to metabolism. *Trends Endocrinol. Metab.* **2011**, *22*, 16–23. [CrossRef] [PubMed]
81. Kawai, T.; Akira, S. Pathogen recognition with Toll-like receptors. *Curr. Opin. Immunol.* **2005**, *17*, 338–344. [CrossRef] [PubMed]
82. Caamaño, J.; Hunter, C.A. NF-kappaB family of transcription factors: Central regulators of innate and adaptive immune functions. *Clin. Microbiol. Rev.* **2002**, *15*, 414–429. [CrossRef] [PubMed]
83. Li, Q.; Verma, I.M. NF-kappaB regulation in the immune system. *Nat. Rev. Immunol.* **2002**, *2*, 725–734. [CrossRef] [PubMed]
84. Cole, J.E.; Georgiou, E.; Monaco, C. The expression and functions of toll-like receptors in atherosclerosis. *Mediat. Inflamm.* **2010**, *2010*, 393946. [CrossRef] [PubMed]
85. Jager, J.; Grémeaux, T.; Cormont, M.; Le Marchand-Brustel, Y.; Tanti, J.F. Interleukin-1beta-induced insulin resistance in adipocytes through down-regulation of insulin receptor substrate-1 expression. *Endocrinology* **2007**, *148*, 241–251. [CrossRef] [PubMed]
86. Kim, F.; Pham, M.; Luttrell, I.; Bannerman, D.D.; Tupper, J.; Thaler, J.; Hawn, T.R.; Raines, E.W.; Schwartz, M.W. Toll-like receptor-4 mediates vascular inflammation and insulin resistance in diet-induced obesity. *Circ. Res.* **2007**, *100*, 1589–1596. [CrossRef] [PubMed]
87. Saberi, M.; Woods, N.B.; de Luca, C.; Schenk, S.; Lu, J.C.; Bandyopadhyay, G.; Verma, I.M.; Olefsky, J.M. Hematopoietic cell-specific deletion of toll-like receptor 4 ameliorates hepatic and adipose tissue insulin resistance in high-fat-fed mice. *Cell Metab.* **2009**, *10*, 419–429. [CrossRef] [PubMed]
88. Shi, H.; Kokoeva, M.V.; Inouye, K.; Tzameli, I.; Yin, H.; Flier, J.S. TLR4 links innate immunity and fatty acid-induced insulin resistance. *J. Clin. Investig.* **2006**, *116*, 3015–3025. [CrossRef] [PubMed]
89. Devaraj, S.; Dasu, M.R.; Rockwood, J.; Winter, W.; Griffen, S.C.; Jialal, I. Increased toll-like receptor (TLR) 2 and TLR4 expression in monocytes from patients with type 1 diabetes: Further evidence of a proinflammatory state. *J. Clin. Endocrinol. Metab.* **2008**, *93*, 578–583. [CrossRef] [PubMed]
90. Ahmad, R.; Al-Mass, A.; Atizado, V.; Al-Hubail, A.; Al-Ghimlas, F.; Al-Arouj, M.; Bennakhi, A.; Dermime, S.; Behbehani, K. Elevated expression of the toll like receptors 2 and 4 in obese individuals: Its significance for obesity-induced inflammation. *J. Inflamm. (Lond).* **2012**, *9*, 48. [CrossRef] [PubMed]
91. Dasu, M.R.; Devaraj, S.; Park, S.; Jialal, I. Increased toll-like receptor (TLR) activation and TLR ligands in recently diagnosed type 2 diabetic subjects. *Diabetes Care* **2010**, *33*, 861–868. [CrossRef] [PubMed]
92. Haehnel, V.; Schwarzfischer, L.; Fenton, M.J.; Rehli, M. Transcriptional regulation of the human toll-like receptor 2 gene in monocytes and macrophages. *J. Immunol.* **2002**, *168*, 5629–5637. [CrossRef] [PubMed]
93. Rehli, M.; Poltorak, A.; Schwarzfischer, L.; Krause, S.W.; Andreesen, R.; Beutler, B. PU.1 and interferon consensus sequence-binding protein regulate the myeloid expression of the human Toll-like receptor 4 gene. *J. Biol. Chem.* **2000**, *275*, 9773–9781. [CrossRef] [PubMed]

94. Ghanim, H.; Mohanty, P.; Deopurkar, R.; Sia, C.L.; Korzeniewski, K.; Abuaysheh, S.; Chaudhuri, A.; Dandona, P. Acute modulation of toll-like receptors by insulin. *Diabetes Care* **2008**, *31*, 1827–1831. [CrossRef] [PubMed]
95. Wang, C. Obesity, inflammation, and lung injury (OILI): The good. *Mediat. Inflamm.* **2014**, *2014*, 978463. [CrossRef] [PubMed]
96. Wu, Y.; Potempa, L.A.; El Kebir, D.; Filep, J.G. C-reactive protein and inflammation: Conformational changes affect function. *Biol. Chem.* **2015**, *396*, 1181–1197. [CrossRef] [PubMed]
97. Aljada, A.; Mohanty, P.; Ghanim, H.; Abdo, T.; Tripathy, D.; Chaudhuri, A.; Dandona, P. Increase in intranuclear nuclear factor kappaB and decrease in inhibitor kappaB in mononuclear cells after a mixed meal: Evidence for a proinflammatory effect. *Am. J. Clin. Nutr.* **2004**, *79*, 682–690. [CrossRef] [PubMed]
98. Ghanim, H.; Abuaysheh, S.; Sia, C.L.; Korzeniewski, K.; Chaudhuri, A.; Fernandez-Real, J.M.; Dandona, P. Increase in plasma endotoxin concentrations and the expression of Toll-like receptors and suppressor of cytokine signaling-3 in mononuclear cells after a high-fat, high-carbohydrate meal: Implications for insulin resistance. *Diabetes Care* **2009**, *32*, 2281–2287. [CrossRef] [PubMed]
99. Burdge, G.C.; Calder, P.C. Plasma cytokine response during the postprandial period: A potential causal process in vascular disease? *Br. J. Nutr.* **2005**, *93*, 3–9. [CrossRef] [PubMed]
100. Van Oostrom, A.J.; Rabelink, T.J.; Verseyden, C.; Sijmonsma, T.P.; Plokker, H.W.; De Jaegere, P.P.; Cabezas, M.C. Activation of leukocytes by postprandial lipemia in healthy volunteers. *Atherosclerosis* **2004**, *177*, 175–182. [CrossRef] [PubMed]
101. Erridge, C.; Attina, T.; Spickett, C.M.; Webb, D.J. A high-fat meal induces low-grade endotoxemia: Evidence of a novel mechanism of postprandial inflammation. *Am. J. Clin. Nutr.* **2007**, *86*, 1286–1292. [CrossRef] [PubMed]
102. Hwang, D.H.; Kim, J.A.; Lee, J.Y. Mechanisms for the activation of Toll-like receptor 2/4 by saturated fatty acids and inhibition by docosahexaenoic acid. *Eur. J. Pharmacol.* **2016**, *785*, 24–35. [CrossRef] [PubMed]
103. Lee, J.Y.; Sohn, K.H.; Rhee, S.H.; Hwang, D. Saturated fatty acids, but not unsaturated fatty acids, induce the expression of cyclooxygenase-2 mediated through Toll-like receptor 4. *J. Biol. Chem.* **2001**, *276*, 16683–16689. [CrossRef] [PubMed]
104. Hoshino, K.; Takeuchi, O.; Kawai, T.; Sanjo, H.; Ogawa, T.; Takeda, Y.; Takeda, K.; Akira, S. Cutting edge: Toll-like receptor 4 (TLR4)-deficient mice are hyporesponsive to lipopolysaccharide: Evidence for TLR4 as the Lps gene product. *J. Immunol.* **1999**, *162*, 3749–3752. [PubMed]
105. Mylona, E.E.; Mouktaroudi, M.; Crisan, T.O.; Makri, S.; Pistiki, A.; Georgitsi, M.; Savva, A.; Netea, M.G.; van der Meer, J.W.; Giamarellos-Bourboulis, E.J.; et al. Enhanced interleukin-1β production of PBMCs from patients with gout after stimulation with Toll-like receptor-2 ligands and urate crystals. *Arthritis Res. Ther.* **2012**, *14*, 158. [CrossRef] [PubMed]
106. Snodgrass, R.G.; Huang, S.; Choi, I.W.; Rutledge, J.C.; Hwang, D.H. Inflammasome-mediated secretion of IL-1β in human monocytes through TLR2 activation; modulation by dietary fatty acids. *J. Immunol.* **2013**, *191*, 4337–4347. [CrossRef] [PubMed]
107. Lee, J.Y.; Zhao, L.; Youn, H.S.; Weatherill, A.R.; Tapping, R.; Feng, L.; Lee, W.H.; Fitzgerald, K.A.; Hwang, D.H. Saturated fatty acid activates but polyunsaturated fatty acid inhibits Toll-like receptor 2 dimerized with Toll-like receptor 6 or 1. *J. Biol. Chem.* **2004**, *279*, 16971–16979. [CrossRef] [PubMed]
108. Lee, J.Y.; Plakidas, A.; Lee, W.H.; Heikkinen, A.; Chanmugam, P.; Bray, G.; Hwang, D.H. Differential modulation of Toll-like receptors by fatty acids: Preferential inhibition by n-3 polyunsaturated fatty acids. *J. Lipid Res.* **2003**, *44*, 479–486. [CrossRef] [PubMed]
109. Caricilli, A.M.; Nascimento, P.H.; Pauli, J.R.; Tsukumo, D.M.; Velloso, L.A.; Carvalheira, J.B.; Saad, M.J. Inhibition of toll-like receptor 2 expression improves insulin sensitivity and signaling in muscle and white adipose tissue of mice fed a high-fat diet. *J. Endocrinol.* **2008**, *199*, 399–406. [CrossRef] [PubMed]
110. Erridge, C.; Samani, N.J. Saturated fatty acids do not directly stimulate Toll-like receptor signaling. *Arterioscler. Thromb. Vasc. Biol.* **2009**, *29*, 1944–1949. [CrossRef] [PubMed]
111. Capurso, C.; Capurso, A. From excess adiposity to insulin resistance: The role of free fatty acids. *Vascul. Pharmacol.* **2012**, *57*, 91–97. [CrossRef] [PubMed]

112. Holland, W.L.; Bikman, B.T.; Wang, L.P.; Yuguang, G.; Sargent, K.M.; Bulchand, S.; Knotts, T.A.; Shui, G.; Clegg, D.J.; Wenk, M.R.; et al. Lipid-induced insulin resistance mediated by the proinflammatory receptor TLR4 requires saturated fatty acid-induced ceramide biosynthesis in mice. *J. Clin. Investig.* **2011**, *121*, 1858–1870. [CrossRef] [PubMed]
113. Patel, P.S.; Buras, E.D.; Balasubramanyam, A. The role of the immune system in obesity and insulin resistance. *J. Obes.* **2013**, *2013*, 616193. [CrossRef] [PubMed]
114. Calder, P.C. *n*-3 Fatty acids and cardiovascular disease: Evidence explained and mechanisms explored. *Clin. Sci. (Lond).* **2004**, *107*, 1–11. [CrossRef] [PubMed]
115. Calder, P.C.; Yaqoob, P. Understanding omega-3 polyunsaturated fatty acids. *Postgrad. Med.* **2009**, *121*, 148–157. [CrossRef] [PubMed]
116. Burghardt, P.R.; Kemmerer, E.S.; Buck, B.J.; Osetek, A.J.; Yan, C.; Koch, L.G.; Britton, S.L.; Evans, S.J. Dietary *n*-3:*n*-6 fatty acid ratios differentially influence hormonal signature in a rodent model of metabolic syndrome relative to healthy controls. *Nutr. Metab. (Lond).* **2010**, *7*, 53. [CrossRef] [PubMed]
117. Wan, J.B.; Huang, L.L.; Rong, R.; Tan, R.; Wang, J.; Kang, J.X. Endogenously decreasing tissue *n*-6/*n*-3 fatty acid ratio reduces atherosclerotic lesions in apolipoprotein E-deficient mice by inhibiting systemic and vascular inflammation. *Arterioscler. Thromb. Vasc. Biol.* **2010**, *30*, 2487–2494. [CrossRef] [PubMed]
118. Baker, E.J.; Miles, E.A.; Burdge, G.C.; Yaqoob, P.; Calder, P.C. Metabolism and functional effects of plant-derived omega-3 fatty acids in humans. *Prog. Lipid Res.* **2016**, *64*, 30–56. [CrossRef] [PubMed]
119. Burdge, G.C.; Wootton, S.A. Conversion of alpha-linolenic acid to eicosapentaenoic, docosapentaenoic and docosahexaenoic acids in young women. *Br. J. Nutr.* **2002**, *88*, 411–420. [CrossRef] [PubMed]
120. Goyens, P.L.; Spilker, M.E.; Zock, P.L.; Katan, M.B.; Mensink, R.P. Conversion of alpha-linolenic acid in humans is influenced by the absolute amounts of alpha-linolenic acid and linoleic acid in the diet and not by their ratio. *Am. J. Clin. Nutr.* **2006**, *84*, 44–53. [CrossRef] [PubMed]
121. Calder, P.C. The relationship between the fatty acid composition of immune cells and their function. *Prostaglandins Leukot. Essent. Fatty Acids* **2008**, *79*, 101–108. [CrossRef] [PubMed]
122. Casula, M.; Soranna, D.; Catapano, A.L.; Corrao, G. Long-term effect of high dose omega-3 fatty acid supplementation for secondary prevention of cardiovascular outcomes: A meta-analysis of randomized, placebo controlled trials [corrected]. *Atheroscler. Suppl.* **2013**, *14*, 243–251. [CrossRef]
123. Chowdhury, R.; Warnakula, S.; Kunutsor, S.; Crowe, F.; Ward, H.A.; Johnson, L.; Franco, O.H.; Butterworth, A.S.; Forouhi, N.G.; Thompson, S.G.; et al. Association of dietary, circulating, and supplement fatty acids with coronary risk: A systematic review and meta-analysis. *Ann. Intern. Med.* **2014**, *160*, 398–406. [CrossRef] [PubMed]
124. Marik, P.E.; Varon, J. Omega-3 dietary supplements and the risk of cardiovascular events: A systematic review. *Clin. Cardiol.* **2009**, *32*, 365–372. [CrossRef] [PubMed]
125. Studer, M.; Briel, M.; Leimenstoll, B.; Glass, T.R.; Bucher, H.C. Effect of different antilipidemic agents and diets on mortality: A systematic review. *Arch. Intern. Med.* **2005**, *165*, 725–730. [CrossRef] [PubMed]
126. Yokoyama, M.; Origasa, H.; Matsuzaki, M.; Matsuzawa, Y.; Saito, Y.; Ishikawa, Y.; Oikawa, S.; Sasaki, J.; Hishida, H.; Itakura, H.; et al. Effects of eicosapentaenoic acid on major coronary events in hypercholesterolaemic patients (JELIS): A randomised open-label, blinded endpoint analysis. *Lancet* **2007**, *369*, 1090–1098. [CrossRef]
127. Buettner, R.; Parhofer, K.G.; Woenckhaus, M.; Wrede, C.E.; Kunz-Schughart, L.A.; Schölmerich, J.; Bollheimer, L.C. Defining high-fat-diet rat models: Metabolic and molecular effects of different fat types. *J. Mol. Endocrinol.* **2006**, *36*, 485–501. [CrossRef] [PubMed]
128. Hartweg, J.; Farmer, A.J.; Holman, R.R.; Neil, A. Potential impact of omega-3 treatment on cardiovascular disease in type 2 diabetes. *Curr. Opin. Lipidol.* **2009**, *20*, 30–38. [CrossRef] [PubMed]
129. Yu, K.; Bayona, W.; Kallen, C.B.; Harding, H.P.; Ravera, C.P.; McMahon, G.; Brown, M.; Lazar, M.A. Differential activation of peroxisome proliferator-activated receptors by eicosanoids. *J. Biol. Chem.* **1995**, *270*, 23975–23983. [CrossRef] [PubMed]
130. Kalupahana, N.S.; Claycombe, K.; Newman, S.J.; Stewart, T.; Siriwardhana, N.; Matthan, N.; Lichtenstein, A.H.; Moustaid-Moussa, N. Eicosapentaenoic acid prevents and reverses insulin resistance in high-fat diet-induced obese mice via modulation of adipose tissue inflammation. *J. Nutr.* **2010**, *140*, 1915–1922. [CrossRef] [PubMed]

131. Caughey, G.E.; Mantzioris, E.; Gibson, R.A.; Cleland, L.G.; James, M.J. The effect on human tumor necrosis factor alpha and interleukin 1 beta production of diets enriched in *n*-3 fatty acids from vegetable oil or fish oil. *Am. J. Clin. Nutr.* **1996**, *63*, 116–122. [CrossRef] [PubMed]
132. Chiang, N.; Serhan, C.N. Structural elucidation and physiologic functions of specialized pro-resolving mediators and their receptors. *Mol. Asp. Med.* **2017**, *58*, 114–129. [CrossRef] [PubMed]
133. Sampath, H.; Ntambi, J.M. Polyunsaturated fatty acid regulation of gene expression. *Nutr. Rev.* **2004**, *62*, 333–339. [CrossRef] [PubMed]
134. Stryjecki, C.; Mutch, D.M. Fatty acid-gene interactions, adipokines and obesity. *Eur. J. Clin. Nutr.* **2011**, *65*, 285–297. [CrossRef] [PubMed]
135. Endres, S.; Meydani, S.N.; Ghorbani, R.; Schindler, R.; Dinarello, C.A. Dietary supplementation with *n*-3 fatty acids suppresses interleukin-2 production and mononuclear cell proliferation. *J. Leukoc. Biol.* **1993**, *54*, 599–603. [CrossRef] [PubMed]
136. Oh, D.Y.; Talukdar, S.; Bae, E.J.; Imamura, T.; Morinaga, H.; Fan, W.; Li, P.; Lu, W.J.; Watkins, S.M.; Olefsky, J.M. GPR120 is an omega-3 fatty acid receptor mediating potent anti-inflammatory and insulin-sensitizing effects. *Cell* **2010**, *142*, 687–698. [CrossRef] [PubMed]
137. Oh, D.Y.; Olefsky, J.M. Omega 3 fatty acids and GPR120. *Cell Metab.* **2012**, *15*, 564–565. [CrossRef] [PubMed]
138. Li, A.C.; Glass, C.K. PPAR- and LXR-dependent pathways controlling lipid metabolism and the development of atherosclerosis. *J. Lipid Res.* **2004**, *45*, 2161–2173. [CrossRef] [PubMed]
139. Martínez-Fernández, L.; Laiglesia, L.M.; Huerta, A.E.; Martínez, J.A.; Moreno-Aliaga, M.J. Omega-3 fatty acids and adipose tissue function in obesity and metabolic syndrome. *Prostaglandins Other Lipid Mediat.* **2015**, *121*, 24–41. [CrossRef] [PubMed]
140. Meital, L.T.; Sandow, S.L.; Calder, P.C.; Russell, F.D. Abdominal aortic aneurysm and omega-3 polyunsaturated fatty acids: Mechanisms, animal models, and potential treatment. *Prostaglandins Leukot. Essent. Fatty Acids* **2017**, *118*, 1–9. [CrossRef] [PubMed]
141. Puglisi, M.J.; Hasty, A.H.; Saraswathi, V. The role of adipose tissue in mediating the beneficial effects of dietary fish oil. *J. Nutr. Biochem.* **2011**, *22*, 101–108. [CrossRef] [PubMed]

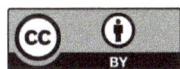

© 2018 by the authors. Licensee MDPI, Basel, Switzerland. This article is an open access article distributed under the terms and conditions of the Creative Commons Attribution (CC BY) license (http://creativecommons.org/licenses/by/4.0/).

MDPI
St. Alban-Anlage 66
4052 Basel
Switzerland
Tel. +41 61 683 77 34
Fax +41 61 302 89 18
www.mdpi.com

Nutrients Editorial Office
E-mail: nutrients@mdpi.com
www.mdpi.com/journal/nutrients

www.ingramcontent.com/pod-product-compliance
Lightning Source LLC
LaVergne TN
LVHW071938080526
838202LV00064B/6628